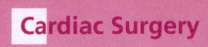

Cardiac Surgery

The material contained in this book is endorsed by AORN as a useful component in the ongoing education process of perioperative nurses.

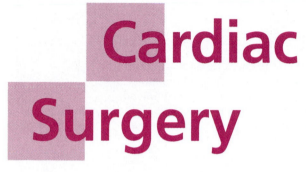

Cardiac Surgery

Patricia C. Seifert, RN, MSN, CRNFA, CNOR

Operating Room Coordinator, Cardiac Surgery
The Arlington Hospital
Arlington, Virginia

with **503** *illustrations*

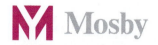 Mosby

St. Louis Baltimore Berlin Boston Carlsbad Chicago London Madrid
Naples New York Philadelphia Sydney Tokyo Toronto

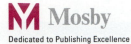

Editor: Michael S. Ledbetter
Senior Developmental Editor: Teri Merchant
Project Manager: Gayle May Morris
Production Editors: Judith Bange and Donna L. Walls
Series Designer: Jeanne Wolfgeher
Design Manager: Susan Lane
Manufacturing Supervisor: Betty Richmond

A NOTE TO THE READER:

The author and publisher have made every attempt to check dosages and nursing content for accuracy. Because the science of pharmacology is continually advancing, our knowledge base continues to expand. Therefore we recommend that the reader always check product information for changes in dosage or administration before administering any medication. This is particularly important with new or rarely used drugs.

Printed in the United States of America
Composition by Graphic World, Inc.
Printing/binding by Von Hoffmann Press, Inc.
Color separation by Color Associates, Inc.

Mosby–Year Book, Inc.
11830 Westline Industrial Drive
St. Louis, Missouri 63146

Library of Congress Cataloging in Publication Data

Seifert, Patricia C.
    Cardiac surgery / Patricia C. Seifert.
      p.   cm.—(Mosby's Perioperative nursing series)
    Includes bibliographical references and index.
    ISBN 0-8016-6542-6
    1. Heart—Surgery—Nursing. 2. Heart—Surgery. 3. Operating room nursing. I. Title. II. Series.
    [DNLM: 1. Heart Surgery—nursing. 2. Operating Room Nursing. WY 162 S459c 1994]
    RD598.S386 1994
    617.4'12059—dc20
    DNLM/DLC
    for Library of Congress   93-42494
                                          CIP

94 95 96 97 98 / 9 8 7 6 5 4 3 2 1

For Grace, Kathleen, and Francesca

Consultants

David C. Cleveland, MD
Pediatric Cardiovascular Surgeon,
Children's Medical Center of Dallas,
Dallas, Texas

Nancy B. Davis, RN, BSN, NP, CRNFA, CNOR
Nurse Practitioner, RNFA,
Cardiovascular and Chest Surgical Associates,
Boise, Idaho

JoAnn Desilets, RN
Cardiac Surgery Operating Room Head Nurse,
Children's Hospital of Philadelphia,
Philadelphia, Pennsylvania

Diane L. Fecteau-Wautel, RN, MSA
Assistant Director of Nursing, GOR/PACU/SDCC,
The Johns Hopkins Hospital,
Baltimore, Maryland

John R. Garrett, MD, FACS
Chief, Cardiac Surgery, and Chairman, Department of
Surgery,
The Arlington Hospital,
Arlington, Virginia

Cathie E. Guzzetta, RN, PhD, FAAN
Director, Holistic Nursing Consultants,
Dallas, Texas
Editor-in-Chief, *Capsules and Comments in Critical Care
Nursing*

Elizabeth Edwinia Ion, RN, CNOR
Cardiovascular Nurse Specialist,
QI Coordinator, Dunn/Main OR/PACU,
The Methodist Hospital,
Houston, Texas

Gail Kaempf, RN, MSN, CNOR
Perioperative Clinical Nurse Specialist,
Presbyterian Medical Center of Philadelphia,
Philadelphia, Pennsylvania

Edward A. Lefrak, MD
Chief, Cardiac Surgery Section;
Director, Heart and Lung Transplant Program,
The Virginia Heart Center at Fairfax Hospital,
Falls Church, Virginia;
Assistant Clinical Professor of Surgery,
Georgetown University School of Medicine,
Washington, DC

Jill O. Montgomery, RN, CNOR
Senior Staff Nurse II,
The Cardiac Surgical Nursing Team,
The Children's Hospital,
Boston, Massachusetts

John O'Connell, BS, CCP
Cardiovascular Perfusionist,
The Arlington Hospital,
Arlington, Virginia

Jane C. Rothrock, DNSc, RN, CNOR
Professor and Program Coordinator, Perioperative
Nursing,
Delaware County Community College,
Media, Pennsylvania

Ann P. Weiland, MSN, MBA, ANP-C
Assistant Vice President,
Washington Hospital Center,
Washington, DC

William M. Yorde, BS, CCP
Cardiovascular Perfusionist,
The Arlington Hospital,
Arlington, Virginia

Preface

Cardiac surgery places the patient in a uniquely vulnerable situation, and the perioperative nurse plays a vital role as patient advocate within the continuum of care. Among the numerous texts written by nurses, physicians, and perfusionists addressing the needs of patients undergoing cardiac surgery, none has been devoted to perioperative nursing care. *Cardiac Surgery* is intended to close a gap in the cardiac literature.

The purpose of this book is twofold: (1) to identify the needs of adult patients during surgery and (2) to demonstrate the perioperative nursing considerations and interventions that form the basis for professional practice in the cardiac operating room. Although adult congenital lesions (and infant patent ductus arteriosus) are included, pediatric cardiac surgery is not discussed in detail; the special needs of this patient population warrant a book devoted solely to the subject. Medical/surgical nursing care, critical care, and rehabilitation have been thoroughly discussed elsewhere and thus are only briefly mentioned in this book.

Part One of *Cardiac Surgery* addresses the foundations of cardiac surgical nursing, including a historical perspective (Chapter 1); attributes of perioperative cardiac nurses and the cardiac team (Chapters 2 and 3); surgical anatomy and physiology (Chapter 4); environment, instrumentation, and equipment, including structural standards (Chapter 5); and elements of the nursing process, including process and outcome standards (Chapters 6 through 10).

Part Two describes surgical interventions that focus on generic procedures (Chapter 11); surgery for coronary artery disease (Chapter 12), valvular heart disease (Chapters 13 through 15), and thoracic aortic aneurysms and dissections (Chapter 16); ventricular assist devices for the failing heart (Chapter 17); transplantation of the heart and lungs (Chapter 18); surgery for conduction disturbances (Chapter 19), adult congenital heart disease (Chapter 20), and trauma and emergencies (Chapter 21); and miscellaneous procedures (Chapter 22).

The procedures discussed include those commonly done for frequently encountered disorders, as well as those performed for rarer disorders. No single method of repair is universally suited to a particular problem, and each operation will be influenced by the training and experience of team members. However, there are basic principles that can be applied to many situations. The appropriate operation depends on the lesion, anatomic features, patient factors, and available resources. Moreover, surgical procedures are constantly evolving. When the underlying rationale for familiar techniques is understood, the nurse should be able to modify current practices and adapt to new ones in light of this rationale.

Some of the special features of *Cardiac Surgery* are:
- Comments and reminiscences about the history of cardiac surgery from perioperative nurses who participated in the formation of cardiac surgery programs
- Competency statements for perioperative nurses based on AORN's Standards and Recommended Practices and the American Nurses Association and American Heart Association's Council on Cardiovascular Nursing Standards of Cardiovascular Nursing Practice
- Characteristics of cardiac perioperative nurses based on the Benner/Dreyfus model for progressing from novice to expert
- A cardiac surgery course outline and pretests and posttests for nurses learning the perioperative cardiac role
- Anatomic drawings illustrating a surgical perspective
- Nursing standards of care for cardiac procedures
- Step-by-step procedures with rationales and possible alternative maneuvers
- RN first assistant considerations related to cardiac surgery
- "Pearls" by nurses and surgeons who are experts in their fields, and by others, that provide special insights into the subject under discussion

In performing the perioperative role, the nurse focuses on issues related to patient safety, protection from hazards, comfort, prevention of infection, emotional support, and educational needs regarding the surgery and its impact on the patient's functional status postoperatively. Although these issues have global significance, within the context of surgery they take on a distinctive character requiring special interventions. Alterations in myocardial oxygen supply and demand, temperature, and blood flow to major organs are only a few of the stressors affecting patients during surgery. Perioperative nurses must understand the underlying pathoanatomy, monitor hemodynamic status, anticipate patient needs, and intervene appropriately and quickly. Responding effectively requires knowledge, skill, compassion, and clinical judgment.

Of special concern to all cardiac team members are the temporal constraints imposed by the need for induced cardiac arrest. "Time is muscle," and the difference between reversible and irreversible ischemic myocardial injury is difficult to determine with precision. That cardiac surgery is considered "stressful" is due in large part to the tyranny of the clock. This consideration places great importance on mental and manual skill, efficiency, and, above all, teamwork.

The public and professional esteem enjoyed by cardiac surgeons has been greatly influenced by their manual skill, as well as their mental acumen. Such skill and acumen are equally important in the perioperative nurse. The patient's safety and welfare depend both on the nurse's critical thinking skills and on the safe and appropriate use of the myriad instruments, equipment, prosthetics, and other items within the cardiac technologic armamentarium.

The concept of the "team" is essential to a cardiac service. The team is the primary unit and one that exemplifies the principle that the whole is greater than the sum of its parts. Nurses and surgeons alike consistently emphasize the necessity of teamwork. Team members may have special roles and responsibilities, but these are interdependent and necessitate flexibility and an appreciation of one another's duties and functions if successful outcomes are to be achieved. The strong bonds that often develop among team members are evidence of the mutual support and respect that characterize the group.

Although, out of necessity, proportionately more time is devoted to the physiologic needs of patients who are anesthetized, meeting psychosocial needs is also a critical component of the perioperative nurse's role. Comfort measures and anxiety-reducing interventions preoperatively are integral components of perioperative nursing practice. They reflect not only a compassionate attitude, but also a means of reducing endogenous catecholamine release and myocardial oxygen consumption. Communicating with the family of a critically ill patient requires the ability to provide a realistic appraisal of the situation without taking away all sense of hope for a successful outcome. When patients die in the operating room, it is the perioperative nurse who routinely prepares the body and is there to support the family and loved ones when they make their final farewells.

Cardiac surgery has a profound physiologic and emotional impact on the patient, the family, and friends. Probably no other organ carries with it such deep psychologic and spiritual significance. As it was centuries ago, the heart is still believed to be the seat of the soul and the wellspring of emotion. An awareness of what the patient experiences during surgery and the appropriate nursing care that is provided in collaboration with surgeons, anesthesiologists, perfusionists, and other members of the surgical team enhances continuity of care and facilitates recovery, recuperation, and rehabilitation. *Cardiac Surgery* has been written as a testament to the outstanding contributions of perioperative nurses and to the art and science that are reflected in their practice.

Acknowledgments

The decision to write *Cardiac Surgery* on my own was based on the desire to achieve consistency throughout the book and to reflect certain beliefs about the demands of cardiac disease, surgery, and the clinicians who participate in surgical procedures. It has been my good fortune throughout my professional life to have a diverse and flexible job description that allowed me to engage in a variety of practice roles: staff nurse, RN first assistant, educator, clinical coordinator, and administrator. These experiences have given me valuable insights into the needs of patients and families, as well as professional associates. They also inspired me to write about the special needs of surgical patients and the vital role played by perioperative cardiac surgical nurses. I am especially indebted to my present and former colleagues at The Arlington Hospital, the Fairfax Hospital, and the Washington Hospital Center.

However, this book could not have been written without the help of many persons. Few have the knowledge and experience to treat as complex a subject as cardiac surgery completely without relying on those with expertise in the field; I am no exception. I am most grateful to the consultants listed in the front of this book who have reviewed the manuscript and offered valuable suggestions and comments.

I would like to thank my nursing colleagues for their unstinting support and encouragement in the development of this book. Their compassion and competence have made them exemplary role models: Nancy Abou-Awdi, Ursula Anderson, Sonia Astle, Gwyn Baumgarten, Alice Cannon, Nancy Davis, Jodee Desilets, Diane Fecteau, Dr. Cathie Guzzetta, Chris Esperson, Peggy Hartin, Kim Hill, Nancy Holloway, Dena Houchin, Edwinia Ion, Gail Kaempf, Cecil King, Linda Lewis-Sims, Brad Manuel, Dr. Rosemary McCarthy, Jill Montgomery, Cheryl Nygren, Pat Palmer, Dottie Platt, Leanna Revell, Pat Rogers, Dr. Jean Reeder, Dr. Jane Rothrock, Bridget Schall, Anne Weiland, Chizuko Williams, and the nursing colleagues with whom I have had the privilege of working.

I am deeply grateful to the surgeons for whom I have been a first assistant. Their patience and their faith in me during thousands of operations have provided me with learning opportunities afforded to few.

They have demonstrated the art and the science of surgery elegantly and skillfully: Drs. David C. Cleveland, John R. Garrett, Cleland Landolt, Edward A. Lefrak, Quentin Macmanus, and Alan M. Speir. I also wish to express my great appreciation to the many surgeons, anesthesiologists, cardiologists, and other physicians who responded to my requests and who generously shared with me their knowledge and experiences: in particular, Drs. W. Gerald Austen, Richard Bjierke, Peter Conrad, Denton A. Cooley, Paul Corso, Willard Daggett, Richard DeWall, Paul A. Ebert, Rene Favaloro, O.H. Frazier, Ted Friehling, Jorge Garcia, Nevin M. Katz, C. Walton Lillehei, Robert S. Litwak, Luis Mispretta, Albert Pacifico, William S. Pierce, John D. Randolph, Bruce A. Reitz, William C. Roberts, Emil Roushdy, Sandy Schaps, Mohammed Shakoor, John A. Walhausen, and Scott Walsh.

The assistance of perfusionists has been invaluable, and I am especially thankful to Aaron Hill, Bob Groom, John O'Connell, and William Yorde.

The contributions of artists Peter Stone, M. La-Waun Hance, SA, Dan Beisel, and Edna Hill, and photographers Howard Kaye, Kip Seymour, and Doug Yarnold, CRNA, have been vital to the book.

To Leo Rosenbaum, a special thank you.

No book can be written without the assistance of librarians. I am indebted to Cecelia Durkin, Donna Giampa, Susan Osborn, Sue Polucci, Nell E. Powell, Alice Sheridan, and Norma Stavetski.

Supporters within the business community have provided valuable information and generously shared resources: Steve Aichele, Barry Hopper, Bertie Janney, William Merz, Alan Mock, William Pilling, Dick Reid, and Charles Riall.

I am most grateful to the individuals at Mosby who worked on this project. Their attention to detail and guidance in no small way helped to make this book a reality; thank you, Nancy Coon, Beverly Copland, Suzie Epstein, Michael Ledbetter, Teri Merchant, Judi Bange, Donna Walls, Gayle Morris, and Susan Lane.

Finally, to my husband and children, thank you for your patience and love.

Patricia C. Seifert

Contents

PART TWO

Surgical Interventions

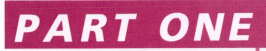

PART ONE

Foundations of Cardiac Surgical Nursing

1

History of Cardiac Surgery

I may have made the progress reported sound easy, effortless, and unobstructed. That most certainly was not the case. There were innumerable failures, disappointments, frustrations, and obstacles—nature's as well as man's. The only solution was a mixture of persistence and stubbornness.

C. Walton Lillehei, MD, 1986 (p. 21)

Many of the innovations came from surgeons themselves and their helpers.

Harris B. Shumacker, MD, 1992 (p. 366)

Probably no other achievement focused the public's attention on the world of cardiac surgery as did the first human heart transplant performed by Christiaan Barnard (1967) on December 3, 1967, in Cape Town, South Africa (Fig. 1-1). Not only was this hailed as a technologic miracle, it also had a profound emotional impact, because the object of attention was no less than what was considered the seat of the soul.

For centuries curiosity about the structure and function of the heart had been tempered by injunctions against touching it and by reverence for it as the principal and most noble organ of the body (Shumacker, 1992). Although William Harvey studied the hearts of animals, his deduction that dual pumps—the right and left heart—propelled the blood to the body in a continuous cycle through the interconnecting pulmonary and systemic circulations was the result of human experiments on the valves of veins and not on the heart itself (Comroe, 1983).

As late as 1896 surgeons were hesitant to perform cardiac procedures and risk the wrath or ridicule of their peers. Theodor Billroth, the noted abdominal surgeon, is reported to have said in 1880 that "a surgeon who would attempt the suture of a heart should lose the respect of his colleagues because the operation is not compatible with a surgeon's responsibility" (Nissen, 1963). And as if that were not enough to chill the enthusiasm of surgeons, Sir Stephen Paget predicted in that same year that "surgery of the heart has probably reached the limits set by Nature to all surgery; no new method, and no new discovery can overcome the natural difficulties that attend a wound of the heart" (Paget, 1896, p. 121).

These statements were not without some foundation, given the obstacles to open chest surgery during that era—infection, hemorrhage, and the difficulty of avoiding the lethal cardiopulmonary consequences of pneumothorax (Brieger, 1991). Ironically, the beginning of heart surgery is often considered to have been in 1896, when a German, Ludwig Rehn, successfully sutured a stab wound to the right ventricle of a young man. In doing this, Rehn demonstrated that touching the heart would not necessarily cause a lethal dysrhythmia and that the myocardium could hold sutures (Rashkind, 1982). The first cardiac surgical procedure in the United States occurred in 1902 and was also the closure of a stab wound.

In a world rarely free from fighting and war, it is not surprising that early attempts at cardiac repair often focused on battle injuries. One of the most famous wartime accomplishments was Dwight Harkin's World War II series of 134 operations to remove retained missiles from the heart and great vessels: there were no deaths, and all patients were discharged from the chest surgery hospital (Johnson, 1970).

These and other achievements—from Rehn's 1986 myocardial suture repair to Barnard's 1967 cardiac transplantation to Denton Cooley's 1969 and William DeVries' 1982 (DeVries, 1988) implantation of a total artificial heart—are singular examples of the progress made in cardiac surgery, which, as Lillehei (1986) has noted, sounds "easy, effortless, and unobstructed" (p. 21). Such was not the case, however, as these pioneers would surely agree. The history of cardiac surgery is the result of many investigations that paved the way for momentous achievements. It is meticulous research and serendipitous discoveries. It is numerous trials and errors by physicians and technicians in experimental laboratories and imaginative solutions to seemingly insurmountable problems by surgeons,

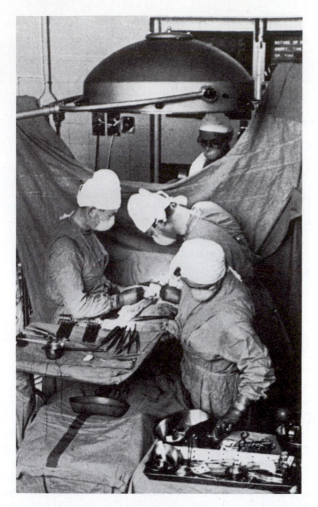

Fig. 1-1 Dr. Christiaan N. Barnard performing the world's first heart transplant in Capetown, South Africa, on Dec. 3, 1967. (Courtesy Berchtold Corp.)

nurses, and others involved in surgery. Whether they were elucidating anatomy and physiology, enhancing diagnostic capabilities, developing surgical techniques, creating prosthetic replacements, or designing instruments and sutures, many persons were responsible for transforming ideas into clinical reality. Often, brilliant insights had to await the development of the appropriate technology that would allow their implementation.

EARLY CRUCIAL DEVELOPMENTS

A number of developments laid the groundwork for cardiac surgery as we know it today. From the electrocardiogram to vascular clamps that would not traumatize blood vessels, numerous inventions and discoveries paved the way for the successful treatment of congenital and acquired heart disease (Comroe and Dripps, 1977; Table 1-1).

Electrocardiography, Chest Radiographs, and Selective Coronary Arteriography

The invention of the stethoscope by Laennec in 1819 brought medicine into the age of physical examination. Physicians could begin to understand *what* was happening, but the *why* and *how* of cardiac disease required new methods of detection.

Electrocardiography

Investigations in the 1850s uncovered the electrical current that accompanied cardiac contraction. By the 1870s scientists were familiar with the electrical activity of the heart. Measurement of these electrical currents was first achieved by recording the activity on the exposed hearts of experimental animals. In 1887 Augustus Waller made a surface recording, which he called an "electrogram" or "cardiogram" (Johnson, 1970, p. 17). It was not until Willem Einthoven's work in the late 1890s, however, that normal and abnormal waveforms and deflections of the electrocardiogram were described. Studies of the cardiac dysrhythmias were greatly expanded by Sir Thomas Lewis in a 1912 monograph entitled *Clinical Disorders of the Heart Beat*, and by 1920 the electrocardiogram was an established component of the cardiac examination.

Chest radiographs

The diagnosis and treatment of heart disease was greatly simplified by Wilhelm Roentgen's discovery of x-rays in 1895. Within a short time x-ray films were used to evaluate cardiomegaly, aneurysms, pericardial and pleural fluid, and pulmonary edema (Johnson, 1970).

Selective coronary arteriography

Radiographic opacification of the vascular system allowed diagnosticians to analyze a problem affecting the systemic circulation and plan appropriate treatment. Probably the most significant advancement affecting the treatment of heart disease was F. Mason Sones' 1958 development of selective coronary arteriography. As with many discoveries, this one was quite unexpected, but Sones and his colleagues were quick to recognize the tremendous potential of this technique. Not only did it improve the diagnosis of coronary artery disease and other cardiac pathologic conditions, but most important, according to Effler (1970), "it defined the needs of the individual patient" (p. xi). Thus clinicians could tailor surgical therapy (e.g., number and location of bypass grafts) and individualize patient teaching needs (e.g., life-style/risk factor modification and/or genetic counseling).

Cardiac Resuscitation and Thoracic Anesthesia

Cardiac resuscitation

Cardiac arrests during the administration of chloroform or ether for general anesthesia had been documented from the mid-1800s, but the cause of these

Table 1-1 ■ *Clinical advances in cardiovascular surgery: surgical instruments, supplies, and prostheses*

Date	Scientist	Event (and citation)
1902-1912	Carrel	Used arteries, veins, metal tubes, rubber tubes, and gold-plated aluminum tubes as vascular grafts in animals; developed atraumatic needles and clamps, petrolatum-coated sutures (*Lyon Med* 98:859, 1902; *Surg Gynecol Obstet* 2:266, 1906; with Guthrie: *Bull J Hopkins Hosp* 18:18, 1907; *J Exp Med* 16:17, 1912; *Surg Gynecol Obstet* 15:245, 1912)
1910	Stewart	Devised clamp to permit blood flow to continue through one channel of a large artery while remainder was closed and available for surgical procedures (partial occlusion clamp); rediscovered in 1946 by Potts (*JAMA* 55:647, 1910)
1946	Potts, Smith, and Gibson	Used Stewart clamp (see above) for anastomosis of aorta to pulmonary artery (*JAMA* 132:627, 1946)
1947	Hufnagel	Used rigid tubes of methyl methacrylate for permanent intubation of thoracic aorta (*Arch Surg* 54:382, 1947)
1948	Potts	Designed clamp to permit surgical division of ductus arteriosus (*Q Bull Northwestern U Med School* 22:321, 1948)
1949	Donovan and Zimmerman	Used polyethylene as an artificial surface to replace arteries (*Blood* 4:1310, 1949; *Ann Surg* 130:1024, 1949)
1949	LaVeen and Barberio	Studied tissue reaction to plastics used in vascular surgery (Ann Surg 129:74, 1949)
1950	Dubost and others	Used preserved human aortas to replace narrowed arteries; first blood vessel bank (*Semin Hop Paris* 26:4497, 1950)
1951	Grindlay and Waugh	Used Ivalon plastic sponge as framework (*Arch Surg* 63:288, 1950)
1951	Hufnagel	Inserted plastic (methyl methacrylate) valve in descending aorta of dogs (*Bull Georgetown U Med Center* 4:128, 1951)
1952-1954	Vorhees, Jaretzki, and Blakemore; Blakemore and Voorhees	Used Vinyan "N" cloth in dogs to bridge arterial gap; fashioned first synthetic artery from a woven material (fibroblasts grew over cloth to form "new" intima); used clinically; used woven material to replace metal or plastic (*Ann Surg* 135:332, 1952; 140:324, 1954)
1955	Deterling and Bhonslay	Made first objective evaluation of nylon and 15 other fabrics being used or proposed as prosthetic materials (*Surgery* 38:71, 1955)
1955	Hufnagel	Introduced flexible, seamless vascular prosthesis to replace an arterial bifurcation (*Surgery* 37:165, 1955)
1955	Edwards and Tapp	Used crimped accordian nylon tubing to provide flexibility without kinking (crimped graft) (*Surgery* 38:61, 1955)
1955-1960	Ethicon, Inc.	Developed miniaturization of sutures; used monofilaments in small diameters (*The Ethicon contribution to cardiac, vascular, and pulmonary surgery during the last 25 years*, Somerville, N.J., 1972, Ethicon)
1956	Wesolowski and Sauvage	Studied mesh versus solid materials for prostheses (*Ann Surg* 143:65, 1956)
1956	Murray	Used homografts for mitral and aortic valves (*Angiology* 7:466, 1956)
1960s	Various instrument companies	Manufactured microforceps, clamps, scissors, and apparatus for tying knots for microsurgery
1960	Harken and others	Devised prosthesis for replacing regurgitant aortic valve (*J Thorac Cardiovasc Surg* 40:744, 1960)
1960	Starr and Edwards	Devised caged ball-valve to replace stenotic mitral valve (*Ann Surg* 154:726, 1961)
1962	Usher and others	Used polypropylene monofilament suture to close wounds (*JAMA* 179:780, 1962)
1962	Ross	Developed homograft replacement of aortic valve (*Lancet* 2:487, 1962)
1963	Gott, Whiffen, and Dutton	Used heparin bonding on colloidal graphite surfaces (*Science* 142:1297, 1963)
1964	Barratt-Boyes	Used homografts of aortic valves to replace stenotic or regurgitant valves (*Thorax* 19:131, 1964)
1965	Simmons and others	Used Teflon terry cloth to encourage growth of neointima (*Surg Forum* 16:128, 1965)
1965	Binet and others	Used preserved aortic valves from pig to replace human valves (*Acad Sci Paris* 261:5733, 1965)
1966	Liotta and others	Used Dacron prostheses (woven, knitted, velour, flocked) to encourage growth of a "new" intima (*Cardiovasc Res Center Bull* 4:69, 1966)
1968	Carpentier and others	Performed mitral valve replacement with frame-mounted aortic heterograft (*J Thorac Cardiovasc Surg* 56:388, 1968)
1969	Carpentier and others	Denatured proteins in porcine valves by treating with glutaraldehyde to prevent antigenic reactions (*J Thorac Cardiovasc Surg* 58:467, 1969)
1970	Björk	Created Björk-Shiley valve, a tilting disk mitral valve prosthesis (*J Thorac Cardiovasc Surg* 60:355, 1970)
1970	Gonzalez-Lavin and others	Used autologous pulmonary valve to replace diseased aortic valve (*Circulation* 42:781, 1970)

Modified from Comroe JH, Dripps RD: *The top ten clinical advances in cardiovascular-pulmonary medicine and surgery between 1945 and 1975: how they came about.* Final report, Bethesda, Md, Jan 31, 1977, National Heart and Lung Institute. An article describing this information was also published by the authors entitled: Scientific basis for the support of biomedical science, *Science* 192:105, 1976.

arrests was not determined until 1911, when ventricular fibrillation (which was already familiar to scientists) was implicated. Early attempts at resuscitation were largely unsuccessful until Morris Schiff described a method of open cardiac massage. The first successful attempt at cardiac massage was made in the early 1900s by a surgeon who performed an emergency thoracotomy to gain access to the heart. The intracardiac injection of epinephrine was first attempted a few years later, and drug treatment for cardiac arrest with epinephrine and calcium chloride eventually gained popularity. It seems strange that closed cardiac massage should be introduced years after open chest resuscitation, but the closed method (with artificial respiration) was not known until 1960, when it was introduced by William Kouwenhoven, James Jude, and Guy Knickerbocker (1960).

Defibrillation

Research on induced ventricular defibrillation with alternating current, as well as termination of the dysrhythmia with a larger amount of the same type of current, was published in 1900. This work was largely ignored until the 1930s, when Kouwenhoven, Donald Hooker, O.R. Langworthy, and colleagues from Johns Hopkins Hospital in Baltimore started experiments on ventricular fibrillation in open and closed chests of animals. Although there was little initial success in electrically terminating the dysrhythmia, they did learn about the damaging effects of hypoxia on cardioversion. Work by Carl Wiggers in the 1930s showed that combining cardiac massage (to perfuse the heart) with electrical shock resulted in the revival of fibrillating animal hearts. Claude Beck first applied these findings to the clinical arena, but it was not until 1947 that he succeeded in performing the first successful operative defibrillation in a human (Johnson, 1970). The direct-current defibrillator used today was introduced a few years later. Direct current was much less traumatic and more efficient than alternating current (Harkin, 1989). Theo Raber (1992), a nurse working at Hahnemann Hospital in Philadelphia in the 1950s, recalls the frequent shocks received by surgeons using defibrillators that were plugged into ordinary wall (alternating-current) outlets.

Thoracic anesthesia

Before thoracic anesthesia became available, operations on the chest wall were limited by the constraints imposed by an open thorax and the body's need for a constant supply of oxygenated blood. At the time chest surgery consisted mainly of incision and drainage for empyema or pleural effusion. The problem of opening the pleura and exposing the lungs to atmospheric pressure, which would cause the lungs to collapse, was solved in two ways in the early 1900s. Ferdinand Sauerbruch designed a complex subatmospheric pressure chamber in which the thorax could be opened without the lungs collapsing and causing asphyxia. The apparatus enclosed all of the patient's body except the head; the surgeon would

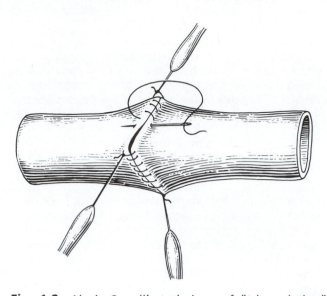

Fig. 1-2 Alexis Carrell's technique of "triangulation" (see text). (Modified from Comroe JH: Who was Alexis who? Cardiovascular diseases, *Bull Tex Heart Inst* 6[3]:251, 1979; based on Carrell A: La technique operatoire des anastomoses vasculaires et la transplantation des visceres, *Lyon Med* 98:859, 1902.)

operate by placing his hands in gloves that allowed entry into the chamber without loss of negative pressure. The introduction of closed, positive-pressure endotracheal anesthesia in the early 1900s provided a preferable alternative to the cumbersome and impractical Sauerbruch apparatus and eventually became the accepted standard for thoracic surgery anesthesia (Frost, 1985). The impact of these two types of anesthetic management is evident in the 1921 *Textbook of Surgical Nursing*, written by Ralph Colp and by Manela Wylie Keller, former chief operating room nurse at St. Luke's Hospital in New York. In describing operations for pulmonary lobectomy, the authors refer to both negative-pressure chambers and positive-pressure endotracheal inflation of the lungs, adding in an understated manner that the latter "is successful, and does not require as much time or preparation as the negative-pressure variety of operations" (p. 129).

Blood Vessel Surgery

Developments in vascular surgery had a major impact on cardiac surgery. Early attempts to anastomose blood vessels had failed mainly because of thrombosis and infection. In the early 1900s Alexis Carrel, often in collaboration with Charles Guthrie, devised techniques of end-to-end anastomoses that resulted in a smooth intraluminal lining that did not contain excess tissue that could become the focus for clot formation. The suture method (Fig. 1-2), still used today, consisted of triangulating the rounded openings of blood vessels by inserting three equidistant retraction sutures close to the open end of the vessel. By gently retracting the stay sutures, a triangle was formed, allowing Carrel to sew along straight lines rather than in a circle. He would sew one side of the triangle, then the second side, and then complete the third side of the anastomosis. Another improvement was to include all three layers of the vessel wall in the anastomosis. Carrel's success is often attributed to his dexterity, gentle handling of tissue, and strict asepsis in an era before antibiotics were available. He also designed special instruments and sutures, which he coated with petrolatum to facilitate their sliding through blood vessels. One of his few innovations that has not been widely adopted was his preference for black surgical attire to reduce the glare from operating lights and enhance visibility (Comroe, 1979).

Improved surgical management of thoracic aortic aneurysms was greatly influenced by the work of Houston surgeons Michael DeBakey and Denton Cooley in the mid-1950s (Brieger, 1991). Their techniques have been widely adopted, and the prosthetic grafts that they designed have become a standard component of the cardiac surgical inventory.

Blood, Blood Transfusions, and Heparin

Blood typing and transfusions

Blood transfusions had been attempted for centuries with little success because of transfusion reactions and blood clotting. Although by the end of the nineteenth century scientists had learned about the mechanism of such reactions and had begun to use citrate experimentally to prevent clotting, blood tranfusions were still dangerous and rarely performed. Delays in finding a solution to the problem were partly due to the introduction in 1875 of intravenous saline infusion to treat hemorrhage. Progress was made when George Crile, using Carrel's vascular anastomotic techniques, connected donor arteries to recipient veins. The resulting smooth inner lining of the conjoined blood vessels prevented clotting, but the method was time consuming and impractical. Also, the problem of transfusion reaction remained. It was Karl Landsteiner who first discovered, in 1900, three of the four blood groups (which he called A, B, and C); the fourth blood group, O, was discovered in 1902 by Alfred von Decastello and Adriano Strurli. The discovery of blood groups was largely unappreciated by all except a few until 1911, when cross-agglutination testing prior to blood infusions demonstrated significant reductions in transfusion reactions (Johnson, 1970).

Blood preservation was first developed around World War I, and the first blood bank was created in 1937 at Cook County Hospital in Chicago. During World War II whole-blood transfusions to treat shock gained widespread use, and methods were devised to prolong the storage life of blood.

Heparin and protamine

Both blood banking and the discovery of heparin by Jay McLean in 1915 were crucial to the development of cardiac surgery. Early use of McLean's discovery provided a means of anticoagulating postoperative patients, whose recovery was often complicated by thromboembolism. Later use of this knowledge enabled cardiopulmonary bypass circuits to remain free of blood clots. The discovery in 1937 by Erwin Chargoff and Kenneth Olson that protamine sulfate neutralized the effects of heparin was another milestone that allowed animal experimentation on the heart and enabled the development of John Gibbon's heart-lung machine.

Cardiopulmonary Bypass

Early investigations

Although thoracic anesthesia gave investigators surgical access to the lungs, it could do little more than provide clear visualization of the surface of the beating heart. Stopping the heart with cessation of blood flow to the coronary and systemic circulations created a risk for ventricular fibrillation and anoxia of the brain and other organs. In the absence of a method to perfuse the body without having to rely on cardiac contraction, surgeons were limited to "closed" procedures that could be performed without stopping or opening the heart. Surgery for acquired diseases was mainly limited to closed mitral commissurotomy for mitral stenosis, pericardiectomy for constrictive pericarditis, and drainage of pericardial effusion. Procedures for intracardiac congenital lesions (such as tetralogy of Fallot) were generally limited to extracardiac palliative operations. Only those congenital defects outside the heart, such as patent ductus arteriosus and coarctation of the aorta, could be repaired directly.

Techniques to repair atrial septal defects were developed that reduced the possibility of air embolus during surgery, but these were "blind" procedures that were technically difficult. The poor results associated with these and other procedures to repair intracardiac defects made investigators continue to look for a method of performing "open" procedures. Surgeons needed a quiet, dry operating field (Johnson, 1970).

Two techniques had the potential to make this a reality. One was occlusion of venous return, introduced into clinical practice in the late 1940s; the vena cavae were clamped, and the repair was performed. This method could be used for pulmonary valve stenosis and other right-sided lesions wherein air embolus was less of a danger than it was on the left side of the heart. However, the danger of anoxia still limited safe operating time. The other technique was the institution of total-body hypothermia, which had been shown to reduce myocardial oxygen demand and thereby prolong the "safe" anoxic period. Studies by W.G. Bigelow and his associates in Toronto around the same time had demonstrated the feasibility of this technique. Interest became widespread, and researchers attempted to develop methods to avert the ventricular fibrillation and air embolism that plagued the method (Litwak, 1970).

A workable technique was finally devised by the early 1950s. Patients were anesthetized, intubated, and immersed in an ice-water bath. When the desired temperature was reached, the patients were removed from the ice-water bath and placed on the operating table where the surgery was performed. Although the introduction of cardiopulmonary bypass a few years later superceded the use of hypothermia as the principal method of performing open heart surgery, the concept of reducing myocardial (and systemic organ) oxygen consumption by using hypothermia eventually became an important addition to bypass technology for protecting the myocardium (as well as the brain and other organs) during surgery.

Extracorporeal circulation

Research by physiologists and others had shown that the idea of extracorporeal circulation was feasible. (Alexis Carrel and Charles Lindbergh had collaborated in the 1930s on an early heart-lung apparatus.) The "azygos (low) flow principle" had shown that when the vena cavae were occluded, enough blood returned to the heart via the azygous vein (which empties into the superior vena cava) to provide a sufficient (albeit greatly reduced) cardiac output to sustain life. The significance of this was appreciated by those wondering whether reduced bypass flows would produce irreversible injury. A number of investigators were interested in devising a mechanical means of removing carbon dioxide and adding oxygen to the blood. Different methods of gas exchange had been tried, but none seemed to be workable in humans until John Gibbon (1954) introduced his heart-lung machine in Philadelphia on May 6, 1953, to close an atrial septal defect in an 18-year-old woman. Venous blood drained into the pump from the superior vena cava and was returned, freshly oxygenated, to the body through the femoral artery. Gibbon and his wife, Maly, had worked for nearly two decades on the project; what seems simple today was exceedingly difficult then. According to Shumacker (1992), who has described one of the last talks Gibbon gave before his death, Gibbon received almost no encouragement from his colleagues; heparin had recently become available, but not its antagonist, protamine; there was no plastic, so the system was mainly rubber and glass; circuit components were purchased from secondhand shops!

It seems incredible today, but few surgeons initially understood or accepted the significance of this achievement, perhaps partly because Gibbon's original paper was published in a regional journal (rather than one with a national circulation) and because few surgeons had the knowledge or resources to use the device (Dobell, 1990; Shumacker, 1992). The popularity of the machine increased in a few years, however, when John Kirklin and his colleagues at the Mayo Clinic in Rochester, Minnesota, built a similar machine, which they used in a series of successful operations. Richard DeWall, with the encouragement of C. Walton Lillehei of the University of Minnesota, simplified the device by creating a bubble oxygenator that was nontoxic, inexpensive, and disposable. This

modification enabled many surgeons to use extracorporeal techniques (Litwak, 1970). Obstacles persisted, however, one of the greatest being the need for large amounts of blood to "prime" the pump. Denton Cooley (1989) had described having to draw blood from seven or eight donors on the morning of surgery in the 1950s. Cooley himself made an important contribution when he started to prime the pump with intravenous solutions rather than blood. This was not only safer and more efficient, but it also enabled him to operate on Jehovah's Witnesses. Membrane oxygenators, which produce less adverse physiologic alterations than the bubble method, were introduced in the late 1950s and early 1960s. Continuous-flow, roller-type pump heads, widely used today for blood propulsion, were popularized by Michael DeBakey, who at the time was at Tulane University (but later went to the Methodist Hospital in Houston) (Shumacker, 1992).

Cross-circulation

One cannot discuss the subject of extracorporeal circulation without mentioning the cross-circulation studies of Lillehei and others at the University of Minnesota. The idea of using a human donor as a biologic oxygenator was conceived in the early 1950s. In April 1954, the first successful operation using this technique was performed on a 1-year-old boy with his father as the donor. The first total correction of tetralogy of Fallot was accomplished with this technique. Although the heart-lung machine became the standard for extracorporeal circulation, Lillehei's group, using the cross-circulation technique, showed what could be achieved with a dry, quiet operative field. They made remarkable advancements in the surgical correction of a number of congenital defects and malformations that previously had been considered "uncorrectable."

Surgical Instruments, Supplies, and Prostheses

Instruments

Many surgical techniques could not be perfected until appropriate instruments and supplies became available that would allow the surgeon to perform new, more complex procedures. Early failures were often partly due to clamps that slipped or tore delicate tissue. Because atraumatic jaws did not exist before the 1940s, surgeons in that era used rubber boots ("rubbershods") over the jaws of clamps to reduce their crushing effects. These difficulties led to many working relationships between instrument makers, and surgeons and nurses looking for a particular clamp or retractor.

Willis Potts enabled patent ductus ligations to be performed with less risk of massive hemorrhage with a clamp he designed in 1944 that could grasp the tissue firmly. Potts also introduced the partial-occlusion clamp for shunt palliation of congenital defects such as tetralogy of Fallot. The clamp isolates the portion of the blood vessel to be repaired or anastomosed, while allowing blood flow through the unclamped portion of the vessel.

Many nurses were also involved in these endeavors. Instruments were frequently borrowed from other specialty services; the Himmelstein retractor, used by some as a sternal retractor, was originally designed for neurosurgery. Theo Raber (1992) from Hahnemann Hospital recalls "inventing" many instruments in collaboration with surgeons and instrument manufacturers. Alice Cannon (1992) (Fig. 1-3), a nurse working with Albert Starr at the University of Oregon Hospital in Portland, developed, in collaboration with two of the surgical residents, a pediatric retractor, as well as arterial catheters and the use of orthopedic stockinette as sternal wound towels for cardiac surgery. Gwyn Baumgarten (1992) (Fig. 1-4) was a nurse at St. Luke's Hospital working with Denton Cooley, when she designed numerous instruments, including the aorta clamp that bears her name (Fig. 1-5) and a wire twister needle holder, first made by Hoenig Instruments, and presently manufactured by the V. Mueller Company and the Pilling Company. These and many other nurses were frequently called on to design and develop clamps, retractors, and other instruments that would enhance the operative procedure. Master craftsmen such as William Merz from the V. Mueller Company and William Pilling from the Pilling Company, along with numerous engineers working in hospitals, made important contributions. The number of cardiovascular instruments that bear the surname of Cooley, Potts, DeBakey, or Baumgarten—to name a few—also attest to the mutually rewarding efforts between clinicians and manufacturers.

Suture

Early sutures consisted mainly of catgut and silk. These materials and the free needles that were used often traumatized blood vessels and fostered thrombosis at the anastomotic site. Operating room nurses were also called on to consult with suture companies to devise less traumatic needles and suture material (Raber, 1992). With the introduction of monofilaments (such as polypropylene) and multifilaments of braided Dacron, as well as swedged-on needles (that reduced the size mismatch between suture and needle), vascular anastomoses could be performed that were not only less traumatic, but also stronger, less irritating to surrounding tissue, less likely to become infected, and longer lasting.

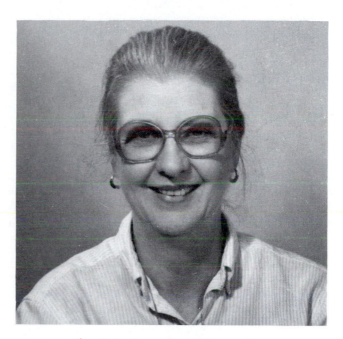

Fig. 1-4 Gwyn Baumgarten, RN.

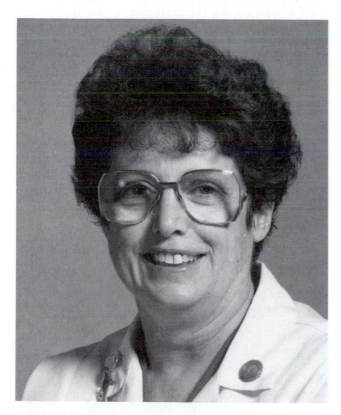

Fig. 1-3 Alice Cannon, RN.

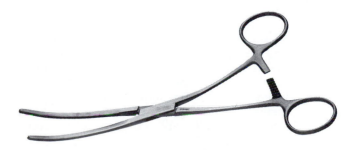

Fig. 1-5 Cooley-Baumgarten aorta clamp. (Courtesy Baxter Health Care Corp., V. Mueller Div., Chicago, Ill.)

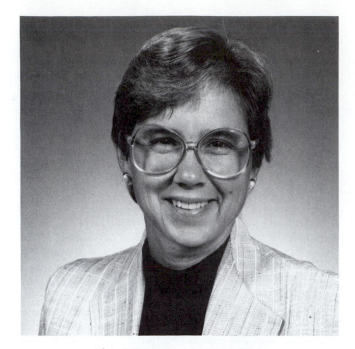

Box 1-1   *Four periods in the development of heart surgery*

Period 1 (1956 to 1962)
Homologous blood bypass pump prime
Reusable equipment
Surgery for congenital heart disease

Period 2 (1963 to 1969)
Nonblood pump prime
Disposable equipment
Surgery for acquired valvular heart disease

Period 3 (1970 to 1979)
Moderate hypothermia for myocardial protection
Surgery for coronary atherosclerotic heart disease
Cardiac transplantation and mechanical circulatory assistance

Period 4 (1980 to Present)
Cardioplegia
Impact of interventional cardiology (PTCA, balloon valvuloplasty)
Refinement of surgical techniques
Surgery for atrial and ventricular dysrhythmias

Modified from Cooley DA: Recollections of early development and later trends in cardiac surgery, *J Thorac Cardiovasc Surg* 98 (5, pt 2):817, 1989.

Fig. 1-6   Nancy Davis, RN, NP.

In a 1951 article entitled "Surgery of the Heart and Great Vessels," Lisbeth Brandt, head nurse of the operating room at The Presbyterian Hospital in Chicago, described existing cardiac procedures and outlined the supplies and instruments required. The only types of suture listed were silk and catgut.

Supplies and equipment

Interestingly, most of the items listed by Brandt (1951) are still familiar to contemporary perioperative nurses; what is remarkable is what is omitted by Brandt: synthetic sutures, sternal retractors (rib spreaders are included), pacemaker wires, disposable drapes, prosthetic implants, cautery, and a defibrillator. Pacemaker wires in the early 1950s and 1960s consisted of bare wire attached to the heart and pulled through the chest wall. Raber (1992) has described insulating these early leads with polyethylene tubing so that patients (or staff) would not be inadvertently shocked. In addition to these items, the creation of plastics and synthetic fibers, as well as improvements in existing materials, broadened the array of surgical supplies and led to refinements that made surgery more efficient and effective. Reusable equipment and supplies, common during the early period of heart surgery, were eventually replaced by disposable items (Cooley, 1989; Box 1-1).

Nancy Davis (1992) (Fig. 1-6), a nurse practitioner who worked with Albert Starr at St. Vincent's Hospital in Portland, Oregon, in the mid 1960s and later started a cardiac surgery service in Boise, Idaho, recalls the numerous, complex supplies needed for operative procedures. To make the process more efficient, especially as it related to turnover time, the nurses designed special packs for various types of supplies: bypass tubing packs, drape packs, sponge and gown packs, and suture packs. This change streamlined the process for preparing the operating room, and it has become a concept that has been widely implemented in cardiac operating rooms (see Chapter 5).

Prosthetic implants

The development of vascular substitutes was important for the fields of both vascular and cardiac surgery. Early tube grafts to replace portions of diseased aortas and peripheral blood vessels were made from Vinyon "N", a fine, porous nylon derivative. These grafts were introduced by Arthur Voorhees, Alfred Jaretzki, and Arthur Blakemore in a 1952 report. Although aortic homografts had been used for bridging arterial defects, their supply was scarce and their insertion technically challenging. Voorhees' contribution was significant because he was one of the first to find an arterial substitute that would act like a native vessel and not cause thrombosis or anastomotic breakdown (Voorhees, 1988).

Nylon, Orlon, and Ivalon (a styrofoam-like material) proved disappointing because prolonged exposure to body fluids caused them to lose tensile strength and to degenerate; Dacron and polyester (Teflon) were more successful and are now the most widely used synthetic materials for vascular conduits (Cooley, 1986). Patch grafts to repair intracardiac defects were also made from Dacron and Teflon, but many early procedures used Ivalon to patch atrial and ventricular septal defects.

Further refinements included crimping to avoid kinking of the graft, different porosities to either allow rapid tissue ingrowth or to prevent interstitial hemorrhage (depending on the degree of heparinization), and improved sterilization techniques (Cooley, 1986). Cooley and DeBakey both made many contributions to the development of these prosthetic materials, and tube and patch grafts of woven, knitted, and velour material are now widely used for arterial repair.

Nurses contributed to these developments in a number of ways. Baumgarten (1992), who recalls late nights in the hospital kitchen slicing graft material to make arterial conduits, instituted a system of tracking the names and serial numbers of prosthetic implants in the 1960s—a standard practice today.

In 1976 Edwinia James Ion (Fig. 1-7) designed and received a patent for a set of graduated graft sizers made of stainless steel. Before this time grafts were delivered to the operating room unsterilized. The surgeon would have to compare the diseased vessel with the available grafts, and then the appropriate graft would be sterilized; this delay prolonged cross-clamp time and led to the practice of an array of grafts in various sizes being sterilized first and placed on the field; as a result, many blood-soiled, but unused, grafts were wasted or had to be soaked in peroxide and resterilized for future use (Cardiovascular nurse, 1976; Ion, 1992). Use of the sizers enhanced patient safety by reducing cross-clamp time, eliminating the guess work in the selection of grafts, and reducing the risk of infection posed by resterilized grafts; also, they saved money.

Cardiac valve prostheses. Because the introduction of the heart-lung machine in the 1950s enabled surgeons to expose the inside of the heart, interest in a substitute heart valve grew. Reparative procedures were insufficient for valves that were too calcified or immobile. Early substitutes to replace individual cusps were made of pericardium, Teflon, and Dacron. Even artificial chordae tendineae from silk suture were devised. Most of these attempts failed because of thrombosis, dehiscence, or loss of leaflet mobility (Lefrak and Starr, 1979).

Hufnagel implanted a ball-valve in the descending thoracic aorta of a patient with aortic insufficiency (see Chapter 14), but it only partly corrected the physiologic problem. A substitute was needed that could be implanted in the native position (e.g., the aortic root or the mitral annulus). Dwight Harkin solved the problem for aortic valve disease by implanting a ball-cage valve (see Chapter 14) in the subcoronary position in 1960. Around the same time, Albert Starr implanted a mitral ball-cage valve (see Chapter 13). Over the next few years, Starr's aortic and mitral (Starr-Edwards) prostheses were implanted throughout the United States and abroad.

Davis (1992) (see Fig. 1-6), working with Cannon (see Fig. 1-3) and Starr, remembers the excitement as

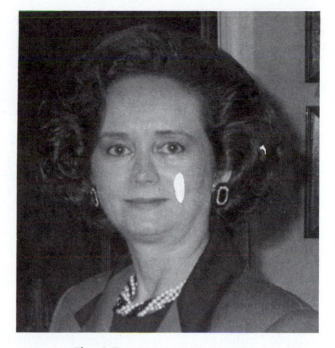

Fig. 1-7 Edwinia James Ion, RN.

visitors from all over the world came to Portland to observe the new valve procedure and learn about the use of these prostheses.

The work of Starr, Harkin, and other researchers confirmed that valvular problems, rather than intrinsic myocardial disease, were the cause of disability and that valve replacement instead of drugs alone could improve morbidity and mortality (Lefrak and Starr, 1979). This idea provided incentive to Donald Ross and Brian Barratt-Boyes to use aortic homografts in the mid 1960s to replace stenotic or regurgitant valves. Within a few years Carpentier and his colleagues in Paris introduced the porcine valve and made valve replacement a reality for patients who could not undergo the chronic anticoagulation required with mechanical valves (see Table 1-1).

SURGICAL PROCEDURES
Congenital Heart Disease

Patent ductus arteriosus

Before Robert Gross and John Hubbard of Boston performed the first successful suture ligation of a patent ductus in 1938, many physicians were knowledgeable about the effects of this persistent connection between the aorta and the pulmonary artery after birth. The function of the ductus was understood in the first century AD; the "machine-like" murmur had been described in 1898; and a ligating procedure had been suggested in 1907. According to Rashkind (1982), one of the factors that enabled Gross to attempt the procedure was the collaborative relationship that had been established with pediatricians and cardiologists; this was to help others perform daring surgical procedures in the future. Also contributing to the success of these procedures were the ductus clamps that had been designed by Potts (see earlier discussion).

Coarctation of the aorta

Like the patent ductus, coarctation of the aorta was known to physicians, but its consequences were unappreciated until Maude Abbott classified these disorders in her *Atlas of Congenital Heart Disease* in 1936. Both Gross and Alfred Blalock at Johns Hopkins had considered operations that would either bypass the narrowed segment of the descending aorta or resect it and reconnect the cut ends. Resection was a problem because no one had cross-clamped (totally occluded) an aorta for fear of causing vascular injury or lower-extremity paralysis. Clarence Crafoord of Stockholm discovered that the aorta could be clamped temporarily without the development of these complications and in 1944 used the technique to resect the coarctation and reanastomose the aorta with Carrel's suture techniques (Johnson, 1970; Shumacker, 1992). Crafoord's techniques also had a tremendous impact on vascular surgery for aortic and other blood vessel diseases.

Tetralogy of Fallot

In 1888 Étienne-Louis Arthur Fallot described the cardinal manifestations of the "blue malady": stenosis of the pulmonary artery, ventricular septal defect, right ventricular hypertrophy, and dextroposition of the aorta. The idea for a surgical intervention came from Helen Taussig, a physician at Johns Hopkins Hospital. Realizing that the degree of cyanosis was inversely proportional to the amount of pulmonary blood flow, she thought that if there were a way to connect a systemic artery and the pulmonary artery to increase blood flow to the lungs, the severity of the disorder could be reduced. She proposed her idea of creating a systemic artery–pulmonary artery anastomosis to Blalock. With the assistance of Vivian Thomas, Blalock's laboratory technician, Blalock performed the first shunt procedure in 1944. With modification of the procedure—anastomosing the innominate artery, and later the subclavian artery, to the pulmonary artery—results improved, and the Blalock-Taussig palliative shunt became firmly established. Potts' side-to-side descending aortic–left pulmonary artery anastomosis (with the partial occlusion clamp he designed) and other procedures followed (Johnson, 1970; Shumacker, 1992).

Credit to Blalock and Taussig for devising the procedure did not appear right away in nursing texts. It was described, but not named, by Stafford and Diller in 1947 as a "brilliant recent advance [that] has been made in extending the benefits of surgery to 'blue babies' " (p. 167); it was again described, but not attributed to Blalock and Taussig, in West, Keller, and Harmon's 1950 text.

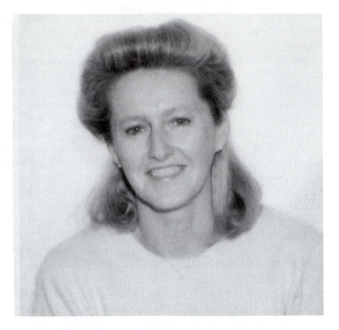

Fig. 1-8 Jill Gorman Montgomery, RN.

Atrial septal defects

Various operations to repair atrial septal defects were attempted, but the risk of air traveling to the left side and embolizing to the systemic circulation hampered these efforts. One of the most intriguing procedures, developed in the early 1950s by Robert Gross in Boston, was described in the 1962 book, *Cardiovascular Surgical Nursing*, by Mary E. Fordham. A "well," a funnel-shaped receptacle, was sewn to a right atriotomy, and blood was allowed to fill the container. Surgeons could insert their fingers through the blood-filled well and attempt to repair the defect using this "underwater" technique. The method was complicated, and the results were difficult for other surgeons to duplicate. The use of caval occlusion and hypothermia finally allowed John Lewis and Richard Varco from the University of Minnesota to repair the defect under direct vision in 1952 (Johnson, 1970).

Palliation for other defects

Excessive pulmonary blood flow, as well as restricted pulmonary flow, could be a problem, and the artificial creation of pulmonary stenosis by banding the artery was introduced in 1952. Creation of an atrial septal defect to increase mixed pulmonary-systemic blood flow in babies with transposition of the great arteries was introduced in 1950.

Correction of defects became possible with the introduction of cardiopulmonary bypass and with Lillehei's cross-circulation techniques. Often bypass was used in conjunction with surface cooling. Jill Gorman Montgomery (1992) (Fig. 1-8), a nurse working with Robert Gross and Aldo Castenada, has described surface cooling techniques used in Boston during the early 1970s. Infants were placed in a large green plastic bag—with endotracheal tube and intravascular lines in place—and immersed in a bathtub of ice slush. When the infants were cooled to the desired temperature (or when they fibrillated), they were taken out of the bag and placed on the operating table. The chest was opened, cardiopulmonary bypass was instituted, and the operation was performed. Postoperative neurologic sequelae were rare, even 20 years later.

Improved operative results permitted the development of corrective procedures for ventricular septal defects (VSDs), tetralogy of Fallot, transposition of the great arteries (TGA), and many other intracardiac disorders. In her 1962 book Fordham describes the palliative procedures (shunts) that had been developed and lists corrective operations for VSD, TGA, tetralogy of Fallot, partial and total anomalous pulmonary venous return, and partial and complete atrioventricular canal (Fordham had been head nurse of the intensive care unit for cardiovascular patients at St. Mary's Hospital in Rochester, Minnesota; supervisor at the Chest Hospital in London, England; and supervisor of the Brooklyn Chest Hospital in Cape Town, South Africa).

VALVULAR HEART SURGERY
Early Procedures

The surgical treatment of valvular heart disease was first directed toward the problems created by rheumatic valvulitis, which produced mitral stenosis.

Mitral valve surgery

Early attempts to treat mitral valve stenosis were encouraged by Rehn's successful suturing of a heart wound. A number of researchers had considered the possibility of relieving the obstruction to blood flow caused by mitral stenosis by excising portions of the deformed valve. Surgeons began to use finger dilatation, valvotomy, or partial valvectomy on aortic, pulmonary, and mitral valves. Elliott Cutler, Claude Beck, and Samuel Levine built a device called a cardiovalvulotome, which was inserted through the left ventricle to excise a portion of a stenotic mitral valve. In 1923 they used the device on an 11-year-old girl with severe mitral stenosis. She survived the operation but succumbed 4½ years later from progression of her disease. Other instruments were developed, and expectations were high that surgical correction of mitral stenosis had finally become a reality (Johnson, 1970).

In 1929 Cutler and Beck published their summary of the results of 12 operations for chronic valvular heart disease performed between 1913 and 1928. The dismal results (only three patients were alive after 1 week, and most died within a few hours after surgery) caused a furor, and attempts to relieve mitral stenosis were halted during the next 15 years (Shumacker, 1992).

The modern era of mitral valve surgery was initiated by Charles Bailey in the 1940s. While at the Hahnemann Medical School in Philadelphia, Bailey realized that a left atrial approach to the mitral valve would avoid damage to the left ventricle. Ventricular dysfunction was of concern because patients were almost always severely debilitated, and defibrillation, safe thoracic anesthesia, blood transfusion, antidysrhythmic drugs, and other advancements taken for granted today were unavailable or in the early stages of development.

After working on dogs to refine techniques for enlarging the mitral valve orifice without creating severe mitral regurgitation, Bailey performed his first procedure in 1945 on a 37-year-old man. The operation was a failure, in large part because of the lack of vascular clamps that would not tear friable cardiac tissue (Johnson, 1970). The next three patients also died, but his fifth patient, a 24-year-old woman, survived. The procedure, called a commissurotomy, was significant because it involved splitting the valve commissures, rather than removing a portion of the leaflet or digitally enlarging the valve orifice, which often led to severe regurgitation. Around the same time, similar successful attempts by Dwight Harken in Boston and Lord Brock in London confirmed the feasibility of surgery for mitral stenosis, and closed mitral commissurotomy became an established procedure (Lefrak and Starr, 1979).

Aortic valve surgery

Surgical correction for aortic stenosis was first attempted in humans by Theodore Tuffier, a French surgeon, in 1912. When he opened the chest of a young man and palpated the aorta, it felt soft rather than firmly calcified as expected, and Tuffier decided to invaginate the aortic wall into the aortic valve to dilate it. (Alexis Carrel was present at the operation.) After he had done this, Tuffier noticed an appreciable reduction in the intensity of the vibratory "thrill" that is caused by blood squirting through a stenotic valve and hitting the wall of the aorta. The patient survived and recovered. However, it was not until the 1950s that Charles Bailey, spurred on by the death of a colleague with aortic stenosis, performed the first successful aortic valve commissurotomy (Johnson, 1970; Shumacker, 1992).

Correction of aortic insufficiency was attempted by Charles Hufnagel at the Georgetown University Hospital in Washington, D.C. Although his prosthesis (see earlier discussion and Chapter 14) provided only partial relief, it did set the stage for Harkin's and Starr's accomplishments. The development of prostheses that could perform the function of their natural counterparts enabled clinicians to treat severe valvular heart disease. Improvement in the surgical outcome for aortic valve disease is shown in Table 1-2.

Coronary artery disease

Angina pectoris and its symptoms were named and described by Herberden in 1768, and coronary thrombosis was diagnosed 100 years later.

Table 1-2 ■ *Aortic valve replacement: elective procedure—first operation*

Characteristics	Mid 1960s	Early 1990s
Average patient age	50-55 yr	65-70 yr
Length of operation	6-7 hr	3-4 hr
Hospital mortality	10%-15%	2%-3%
Postoperative hospital stay	14 days	7 days
Thromboembolic rate (mechanical valves)	4%-5%/pt-yr	1%-2%/pt-yr

From Austen WG: Presidential address: Surgery is a great career, *Am Coll Surg Bull* 77(12):6, 1992. Based on data from:
1. Herr RH and others: A review of 6 years' experience with the ball-valve prosthesis, *Ann Thorac Surg* 6:199, 1968.
2. Cooley DA and others: Total cardiac valve replacement using SCDK-Cutter prosthesis: experience with 250 consecutive patients, *Ann Surg* 164:428, 1966.
3. Effler DB, Favaloro R, Groves LK: Heart valve replacement: clinical experience, *Ann Thorac Surg* 1:4-24, 1965.
4. Akins CW and others: Late results with Carpentier-Edwards procine bioprosthesis, *Circulation* 82(suppl IV):IV65, 1990.
5. Akins CW: Mechanical cardiac valvular prostheses, *Ann Thorac Surg* 52:161, 1991.
6. End results in cardiac surgery, Massachusetts General Hospital, Boston, unpublished data.

Indirect methods. Cervical and upper dorsal sympathectomy was an early attempt to alleviate anginal pain. This method of pain relief for angina pectoris was described in 1947 by surgeon Edward S. Stafford and nurse Doris Diller in *A Textbook of Surgery for Nurses:* the sensory nerve fibers were interrupted by alcohol injection of the upper thoracic sympathetic ganglia. The book also refers to "surgical methods to improve the circulation of the heart following coronary occlusion [that] are now under trial. . . . Perhaps the future will bring success" (p. 168).

Another indirect method was to excise the thyroid gland to lower the body's metabolic requirements. Sympathectomy and alcohol injection for pain relief and thyroidectomy for decreasing metabolic activity (and myocardial oxygen demand) were listed as surgical options by surgeon Walter Modell in his 1952 *Handbook of Cardiology for Nurses,* but the author noted that these attempts had not been very successful. The author also included the Beck procedure but noted that it had been unsuccessful for the problem of "deficient coronary circulation" (p. 210).

Direct myocardial revascularization for atherosclerotic coronary artery disease had to await the development of extracorporeal techniques and selective coronary arteriography. Since the 1930s Claude Beck had been aware of the vascular interconnections between the coronary arteries and extracardiac portions at the base of the heart, and within adhesions between the heart and the pericardium. He theorized that grafting adjacent tissues to the myocardium would provide a new blood supply to the heart (Beck, 1935). Beck would roughen the surface of the heart with a

burr or bone rasp to remove the visceral pericardium and then graft parietal pericardium, pericardial fat, or pectoral muscle directly onto the exposed myocardium.

A similar technique was tried in the 1930s by Laurence O'Shaughnessy in England. He pulled omentum up through the diaphragm and sutured it to the myocardial surface ("cardio-omentopexy"). O'Shaughnessy and others stimulated the formation of adhesions with powdered bone, talc, and other abrasive substances. Results of these operations were generally poor, but the work was a stimulus to others to find more direct methods to increase the coronary blood supply.

A brief allusion to the Beck procedure is made by surgeon John West, nurse Manelva Keller (who had coauthored the 1921 text with Colp), and nurse Elizabeth Harmon in their 1950 book, *Nursing Care of the Surgical Patient:*

> Attempts have been made to establish a collateral blood supply in such cases [e.g., narrowing or occlusion of a coronary artery] by placing muscle or other well vascularized tissues in contact with the heart, but the results have not been very satisfactory. The *chief surgical interest in the disease* is related to the danger of carrying out operative procedures upon patients with damaged coronary arteries. The increased risk in such cases is considerable but by no means prohibitive (pp. 191-192).

Although the authors could not envision a bright future for the surgical repair of hearts afflicted with coronary artery disease, they did reflect a growing awareness of the increased morbidity and mortality resulting from preexisting ischemic heart disease in patients undergoing surgery on other body systems.

Arthur Vineberg from McGill University in Montreal devised a different approach to coronary artery disease. He speculated that tunneling the internal mammary artery (IMA) into the myocardium would stimulate the development of new blood vessels between the artery and the myocardium. He first performed the operation clinically in 1950, and by 1964 he reported impressive results. Others attempted similar procedures using a variety of arterial sources such as the IMA and the gastroepiploic artery; surgeons even experimented with autogenous vein grafts attached to the aorta at one end and implanted into a myocardial tunnel at the other end. Beck interposed a segment of autogenous systemic artery between the descending thoracic aorta and the coronary sinus to increase myocardial blood flow retrogradely. Although these indirect procedures were never reliable, they did increase the knowledge and skill of surgeons. Information about coronary sinus retrograde perfusion, flow characteristics of arterial grafts (IMA and the gastroepiploic), intraoperative rhythm disturbances, anatomic variations, and other findings eventually enhanced methods of direct revascularization and myocardial protection (Shumacker, 1992).

Although Fordham's 1962 book has an extensive section on surgical repair of congenital heart disease, the section on acquired disorders is limited to valvular heart disease and aortic aneurysms; there is no discussion of coronary artery disease. In the 1969 publication by Maryann Powers and Frances Storlie (both nurses in Portland, Oregon) entitled *The Cardiac Surgical Patient*, three "revascularization procedures for coronary artery disease" (p. 74) are included: (1) the Vinebery procedure (using IMA and gastroepiploic pedicle grafts), as well as "more direct attack[s] on coronary occlusion" (p. 76); (2) coronary endarterectomy; and (3) incision and patch enlargement of an obstructed coronary artery. Direct anastomoses are not mentioned.

Direct methods. Direct revascularization techniques came under investigation in the 1950s. Once again, Carrel's studies in the early 1900s provided a foundation for future techniques. He had performed aortocoronary bypass grafting in dogs with carotid artery grafts attached proximally to the descending aorta and distally to the left coronary artery. Other early attempts were aimed at replacing diseased portions of a coronary artery with venous or arterial grafts. Some tried embolectomy or Carrel's carotid-coronary anastomoses. Direct IMA—coronary artery anastomoses were performed in dogs by a number of Russian and American investigators, but they had to contend with sewing on a beating heart, which hindered the transference of the techniques to humans. Investigators sought a way to achieve cardiac standstill so that they could work on a quiet field. This was made possible with the introduction of cardiopulmonary bypass.

As early as 1958, William Longmire and John Cannon from the University of California at Los Angeles described an IMA—coronary bypass. Shumacker (1992) has attributed the first successful aortocoronary bypass with autogenous saphenous vein to Michael DeBakey of The Methodist Hospital (Houston) in 1964; Austen (1992) has attributed this feat to Edward Garrett (a colleague of DeBakey's). Publication of Garrett and DeBakey's results did not occur until 1973 (Garrett, Dennis, and DeBakey, 1973). Others—George Green, Rene Favaloro, Dudley Johnson—followed quickly, and with the heart-lung machine and the creation of microsurgical instruments, saphenous vein bypass grafting spread rapidly. Favaloro's report (1968) of his operation in 1967 at the Cleveland Clinic is often considered the beginning of the coronary bypass era (Austen, 1992). Direct anastomoses with the IMA were slower to take hold, but their use became widespread when their long-term patency was demonstrated (Loop and others, 1986).

Transplantation

Carrel and Guthrie had performed cardiac transplantation in animals early in the twentieth century. Solid organ transplantation in humans started with kidney transplants in 1954, but problems with rejection limited the procedure to identical twins, who were least likely to reject each other's organs. With the introduction of azathioprine (Imuran) and steroid immunosuppression in 1962, survival rates improved in patients receiving organs from donors who were not

identical twins, and interest in heart transplantation began to grow. Tissue-typing and studies on the histocompatibility of antigens were shown to affect outcomes positively, but finding and matching donors to recipients remained difficult. During a presentation Norman Shumway from Stanford University recalled his early experiences with transplantation in dogs (starting in 1958) and the uncertainty of immune responses. Shumway stated, "At the outset we thought the dog would be wise enough not to reject something as important to his survival as an orthotopically transplanted heart, [but] the usual laws of immunology . . . prevailed" (Shumway, 1992).

Because of rejection problems, efforts were increased to develop more nonspecific immunosuppressive agents (Austen, 1992). The discovery of antilymphocyte serum in the 1960s resulted in a third immunosuppressive agent that, when added to the other two drugs, enabled surgeons to attempt other organ transplants. Barnard (1967) performed his historic human transplantation in 1967, and there was tremendous interest in the procedure.

One of the first nursing texts to include transplantation of the human heart, entitled *Cardiovascular Nursing: Rationale for Theory and Nursing Approach*, was published in 1970 and written by Jeanette Kernicki, Barbara Bullock, and Joan Matthews (all nurses at The Methodist Hospital in Houston). The authors provided a detailed description with drawings of the transplant operation that no doubt was helpful to operating room nurses familiarizing themselves with the steps of the procedure. Kernicki, Bullock, and Matthews were also among the first to discuss the legal ramifications of "brain death," ethical questions surrounding the procedure, and the emotional stress felt by families and the nurses and physicians caring for the recipient and the donor. The operative setup and preparation was also described in 1972 by Virginia Higgins (a nurse at Barnes Hospital in St. Louis) in her chapter on cardiothoracic operations in the fifth edition of *Alexander's Care of the Patient in Surgery* (Higgins, 1972).

But problems of rejection quickly reduced the global fervor for cardiac transplantation. Shumway, Richard Lower (who later continued his transplant investigations at the Medical College of Virginia in Richmond), and colleagues from Stanford continued to study the problem and improved the 1-year survival rate from 22% in 1968 to almost 70% in 1978 (Jamieson, Stinson, and Shumway, 1979). They were among the few during this period, however, who continued to study transplantation techniques.

By 1975 and the publication of Ouida King's *Care of the Cardiac Surgical Patient* (King had been a critical care nurse at the Texas Heart Institute), the poor results of transplantation were reflected in the one-paragraph discussion of the subject. Tissue rejection and limited donor availability were cited, and mention was made of the search for a mechanical heart as an alternative cardiac pump. This trend was echoed in Rita Chow's 1976 book, *Cardiosurgical Nursing Care*, which also briefly referred to heart transplantation and the possibility of total mechanical heart replacement for end-stage heart disease.

The introduction of cyclosporine and monoclonal antibody immunosuppression in the late 1970s had a significant impact on survival rates, and transplantation moved from experimental status to clinical reality. In 1981 Bruce Reitz and his colleagues at Stanford University Hospital performed the first successful long-term heart-lung transplant (Reitz, Pennock, and Shumway, 1981). Cooley had performed a heart-lung transplant in the late 1960s on a young child, but rejection developed not long afterward, according to Ion (1992), who was the scrub nurse during the procedure. Joel Cooper and his associates in Toronto achieved the first successful long-term lung transplant in 1983 (Toronto Lung Transplant Group, 1988).

The excitement of these early transplant procedures is still vivid for Baumgarten and Ion, who worked with Cooley in Houston. According to Ion, one of the operating rooms was converted into a "sterile" room for recuperating transplant patients (Baumgarten, 1992; Ion, 1992).

Peggy Hartin, (Fig. 1-9), who was at Stanford during the early transplant era also remembers the excitement. In 1968 at AORN's Boston Congress, Hartin, along with Ludmilla Davis, Operating Room Director of Stanford University Hospital, participated in a panel on "The Role of the Nurse in Heart Transplant." Nationwide press coverage, including coverage in *Life* and *Time* magazines, was given to this conference, largely because of the enthusiasm surrounding the recent heart transplantation that had been performed by Shumway at Stanford (Driscoll, 1990).

Hartin had come to Stanford University Hospital in 1959 and had joined the cardiac team in 1964. One of her most memorable experiences concerning that cardiac transplant procedure (the first at Stanford and the third in the world) was keeping away from the operating room and the intensive care unit the newspaper reporters who had resorted to climbing the walls of the hospital and dressing as central service attendants. In contrast, when Shumway and Reitz performed the first heart-lung transplant, the news media and curiosity seekers were conspicuously absent (Hartin, 1992).

DEVELOPMENT OF CARDIAC SURGICAL NURSING: THE PERIOPERATIVE ROLE
Early Operating Room Nursing

The history of perioperative cardiac nursing is as brief as the specialty of cardiac surgery itself. Its origins can be found in the development of surgery that "specializes in the treatment of physical disorders through mechanical measures" (West, Keller, and Harmon, 1950, p. 5).

The era of modern surgery—and consequently perioperative nursing—began with the introduction

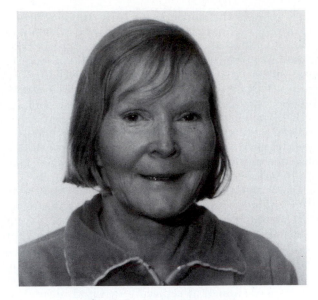

Fig. 1-9   Peggy Hartin, RN.

of anesthesia and antisepsis, and the subsequent development of surgical techniques that were made possible by these advancements. Operative procedures had been performed for centuries prior to the mid-1900s, but usually as a last resort, because pain, hemorrhage, and infection exacted a high toll. Early surgery was limited to excision of superficial lesions, amputation, and drainage of infected fluid. Operative procedures on the heart were rare, and like Rehn's suture closure of a myocardial laceration, were performed in emergent situations. Surgical gloves, hats, and masks were unknown.

Change came with Louis Pasteur's discovery of bacteria as the causative agent in infection and Joseph Lister's application of this knowledge to the treatment of wounds (West, Keller, and Harmon, 1950). The introduction of antisepsis "made it absolutely necessary that nurses should be of such an intellectual calibre and development as would permit them to be trained in the prevention of infection through absolute cleanliness" (Metzger, 1976; Walsh, 1929, p. 125).

Operating room nursing education began in 1876 at the Massachusetts General Hospital in Boston, when student nurses participated in an extensive operating room rotation. Operating room nursing as a specialty, and the concept of an operative "team" consisting of surgeons, nurses, and assistants, originated at Johns Hopkins Hospital in Baltimore (Lee, 1976). During this initial period nurses accompanied patients from their units to the operating room to assist surgeons with the technical tasks of surgery. After the operation, these same nurses followed the patient back to the surgical ward and provided care until the patient was discharged. A few nurses might be permanently assigned to the surgical suite to supervise the visiting nurses and manage the operational details of the suite (Kneedler, 1987).

Early Textbooks

Surgical textbooks before the mid-twentieth century reflected this continuum and discussed the patient's entire surgical experience from admission to post-operative recuperation and discharge. Intraoperative duties were described in detail, from organizing the operating room to sterilization procedures (steam sterilizers), antisepsis and asepsis, instrument passing, and dressing of wounds. These early texts even addressed preparation and management of surgery in the home, including "improvised operative positions" (Colp and Keller, 1921, table of contents). In addition to the content addressing surgical nursing, Colp and Weller's (1921) table of contents listed common operations on the following body systems: alimentary, glandular, nervous, osseous, reproductive, respiratory, skin and appendages, and urinary. Omission of the cardiovascular system reflected the relative lack of knowledge about surgery on the heart and blood vessels. This omission was gradually rectified as scientists learned more about the cardiovascular system and surgical techniques were devised to treat a growing number of congenital and acquired disorders.

Surgical nursing textbooks published in 1947 by Stafford and Diller and in 1950 by West, Keller, and Harmon continued to reflect the relative lack of cardiac surgical experience. Although these books did include chapters on surgery for heart disease, the sections were brief and amounted to three and four pages, respectively. However, by this time diseases and malformations of the heart were being widely investigated, and the clinical application to surgery—spurred on by the introduction of extracorporeal circulation—soon became evident. This in turn fostered the development of the specialty of cardiovascular nursing.

Development of Cardiovascular Nursing

With the progress made in understanding cardiovascular disorders came the need to meet the educational needs of nurses caring for this patient population. By the end of the 1940s, cardiovascular disease had become a national concern, stimulating the creation of The American Heart Association (AHA). In January of 1950 the "First National Conference on Cardiovascular Diseases" was held by the AHA in Washington, D.C. The purpose of the meeting was to summarize existing knowledge, find ways to use that knowledge more effectively, and define areas where research was most needed to answer basic questions (AHA, 1950). In keeping with the goals of the conference, the planners stressed the preparation of nurses to participate effectively in prevention, "assistance to the physician in diagnosis and treatment" (p. 247), nursing care, administration, rehabilitation, and research. "Each one of these areas of service involves special relationships and specialized knowledge" (p. 247), and a listing of essential abilities emphasized specialization and teamwork. Among these were:

. . . carrying out technical and social procedures for prevention, cure, or rehabilitation, and managing the nurse's role in the teamwork process for the care of the family and patient, and for program planning in the cardiovascular field. (p. 248)

The abilities required to care for cardiovascular patients promoted by the AHA were applicable to the operating room nurse, but formal educational programs for nurses were starting to delete the operating room component from their curricula. This trend was reflected in general surgical nursing textbooks. Whereas Keller's earlier text (Colp and Keller, 1921) had included an extensive section on the operating room nurse's duties, her 1950 text (West, Keller, and Harmon, 1950) reflected this change. In their preface to the fifth edition, the authors wrote, "The section on the operating room has been omitted since it was felt that such a highly specialized field of nursing could be more effectively presented in a separate text." The 1943 publication of Edythe Louise Alexander's *Operating Room Technique* (known in later editions as *Alexander's Care of the Patient in Surgery*) provided a reference text devoted to the operative care of surgical patients. Neither the first (1943) nor the second (1949) edition of Alexander's book included cardiac procedures ("heart" was not listed in the index of either edition). Chapters in these editions entitled "Chest Operations" discussed breast surgery and a few thoracotomy procedures. In the first edition Carrel's anastomotic techniques (with credit to Carrel) appeared in the chapter on "Vascular Operations" under the section discussing open embolectomy procedures (p. 377). Extracardiac repairs for patent ductus arteriosus and coarctation of the aorta appeared in the second edition, as did pericardiectomy.

The third (1958) edition of Alexander's book was the first to include a chapter on "Cardiovascular Operations," but it did not refer to extracorporeal circulation or the heart-lung machine. The focus was mainly on surgery for congenital heart disease, which did not require cardiopulmonary bypass.

Publication of the fourth edition (1967), which was coauthored with Wanda Burley, Dorothy Ellison, and Rosalind Vallari, greatly expanded the number and complexity of cardiovascular operations and included extracorporeal technology. In addition to the congenital malformations, acquired diseases and their treatment were described. However, revascularization of the coronary arteries was limited to descriptions of the Beck procedure, endarterectomy, and myocardial implantation of the IMA. The section on valvular heart disease included an extensive array of valve prostheses that were being used at the time.

Formation of AORN

Meeting the special educational needs of perioperative nurses and transmitting the knowledge required to provide operative care was a major motivating force in the development of The Association of Operating

Room Nurses (AORN), which held its first national Congress in 1954. In one effort to accomplish the goal of providing continuing education for operating room nurses, AORN's Audiovisual Committee, in collaboration with the Davis and Geck Company, premiered its first film in 1959 at the sixth annual AORN Congress in Houston (Driscoll, 1990). Entitled *Cardiac Surgery and the OR Nurse,* it featured Denton Cooley; Marie Ellison, Operating Room Supervisor at St. Luke's Episcopal–Texas Children's Hospitals in Houston; and Mary Schwendeman, editor of *OR Supervisor.* The film depicted the operating room nurse's role as a member of the cardiac surgery team and emphasized operating room nursing involvement before and during surgery (Nineteen years of AORN films, 1978). The *AORN Journal* and other perioperative nursing journals continue to publish articles pertinent to the cardiac nurse, and AORN has formed a Specialty Assembly to meet the needs of cardiovascular perioperative nurses.

Cardiovascular Nursing Literature

Other than the educational opportunities provided by AORN, book chapters, and published articles, there were few resources devoted exclusively to the special needs of perioperative cardiac nurses. There were, however, a number of excellent nursing texts and papers devoted to the preoperative and postoperative care of these patients. Most had no perioperative component, but these books were valuable resources in expanding the knowledge base of operating room nurses interested in cardiac surgery.

Fordham's 1962 text, *Cardiovascular Surgical Nursing,* reflecting the impact of Gibbon's heart-lung machine, is probably one of the earliest dealing with this subject. Fordham related the advancements of the heart-lung machine, the use of hypothermia, and the development of "adequate" cardiovascular prostheses to the evolution of a "more specialized and intensive type of [nursing] care . . . Modern cardiovascular care can be provided only by the highly skilled and trained nursing attendant" (p. v).

Articles started to appear in journals. Edwinia Ion (see Fig. 1-7), under her maiden name of Edwinia E. James, contributed to furthering cardiovascular knowledge by writing "The Nursing Care of the Open Heart Patient" in the *Nursing Clinics of North America* in 1967 as a result of her experiences as a private-duty cardiovascular nurse.

The demand for knowledge, skill, physical strength, and emotional stability were stressed by Powers and Storlie (1969) as necessary qualities for cardiac intensive care nurses. It was also becoming increasingly evident that there was a shift from "training" nurses to perform duties, to "educating" them to solve problems. Powers and Storlie emphasized the importance of questioning: *why* is a drug used, *what* is the mechanism of a particular dysrhythmia, *how* does a surgical procedure affect the heart? Such questions were not viewed as encroaching on the "tradi-

tional province of the physician" (p. 111), but as a means of making effective observations that, when correlated with basic knowledge, enabled the nurse to form (in the authors' words) a "nursing diagnosis" (p. 110).

This philosophy was reiterated in the 1970 publication of *Cardiovascular Nursing* by Kernicki, Bullock, and Matthews, which emphasized the "rationale for therapy and nursing approach"—the book's subtitle. In the book's preface, the authors noted a change from the primary role of executing physician's orders to a more collaborative role in the care of patients. This role required active participation rather than passive observation.

Mary Jo Aspinall's 1973 book, *Nursing the Open-Heart Surgery Patient,* also focused attention on the nurse's need for theoretical knowledge and the ability to use it in making clinical decisions. According to Aspinall, "[The nurse] must understand the operation of the machines . . . , recognize critical physiological changes, make interpretive judgments, and take necessary action" (preface).

Ouida M. King wrote in the preface of *Care of the Cardiac Surgical Patient,* which was also published in 1973, that her book was "designed to present a discussion of the principles involved in cardiac disease, thereby providing a background on which skill in caring for the cardiac surgical patient may be developed" (p. ix).

The need for skilled and informed nurses was echoed by their surgeon colleagues. Albert Starr and Denton Cooley each wrote a foreword in Powers and Storlie's book and in King's book, respectively, attesting to the importance of the cardiovascular nurse's professional role. In their surgical text, *Coronary Artery Surgery,* John Ochsner and Noel Mills (1978) highlighted the role of the cardiovascular nurse specialist and referenced research from the nursing literature (Elsberry, 1972) in their chapter on patient education for coronary artery bypass surgery.

Perioperative Cardiac Nurse

Although the role of the perioperative nurse appeared in few cardiovascular-specific nursing texts of the period, there were exceptions. One was Chow's 1976 book, *Cardiosurgical Nursing Care,* which included a short paragraph on preoperative visits by operating room nurses. Chow wrote:

> It is encouraging that some operating room nurses visit patients who are scheduled for major surgical procedures. This practice helps to alleviate the patient's anxieties, and helps the nurse to make observations about the mental and physical status of the patient and to anticipate his needs in personalized care. (p. 319)

Chizuko Williams (Fig. 1-10), former operating room supervisor at Deborah Heart and Lung Center in Brown Mills, New Jersey, recognized the importance of the preoperative visit early in her 25-year tenure at the center. Her staff visited "each surgical

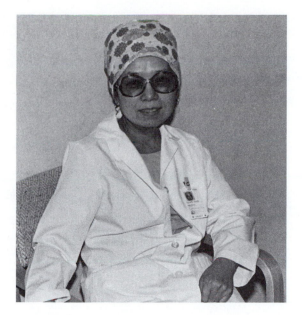

Fig. 1-10 Chizuko Williams, RN.

patient preoperatively to perform a nursing assessment and [develop] a nursing care plan. This enabled them to provide highly individualized care to their patients intraoperatively" (Williams, 1992). Her philosophy was described in an article in 1985 (Williams, Czapinski, and Graf, 1985) and in an accompanying interview (Conversation with the author, 1985).

Awareness of the profound physiologic effects of cardiac surgery, as well as the emotional effects of fear and anxiety, prompted other nurses (including those represented in this chapter) participating in the development of cardiac surgery programs to promote patient and family interactions. This trend was reflected in the perioperative nursing literature, which stressed the need to incorporate a psychosocial component in preoperative patient assessments.

In addition to relying on available nursing and surgical literature to expand their knowledge, periop-

erative cardiac nurses worked closely with the surgeon to increase their skill and experience within the surgical setting. These interactions with surgeons, perfusionists (not mentioned in this chapter, but deserving much credit), and other members of the cardiac team were important in achieving successful patient outcomes. Surgeons were among the first to support the development of a professional perioperative nursing role that would foster a calm, competent, and efficient operative environment. Shumacker (1992) reflected the need for knowledge, as well as skill, when he wrote that "especially trained nurses, assistants, and technicians superseded willing but untutored ones" (p. 366).

Perioperative cardiac nurses were highlighted in a book describing the history of the Texas Heart Institute (THI) (THI Foundation, 1989), one of the most well known cardiac centers in the world. Susan J. Kadow, at the time an assistant nurse manager of cardiovascular surgery at THI, was one of the many nurses depicted and quoted in the book. Her emphasis on the importance of close working relationships with the surgeon and the ability to anticipate needs, represents some of the critical attributes of perioperative cardiac nurses.

These attributes are among those considered most important for team members (Box 1-2). These qualities and the importance of consistency in the performance of operations were factors that led to expanded perioperative nursing roles. The RN First Assistant (RNFA) is one such role that has been widely adopted by perioperative cardiac nurses. The efforts of Nancy Davis (see Fig. 1-6) have been crucial to the development of the role and its widespread acceptance throughout the United States. The establishment of a college-level educational program for the RNFA by Jane Rothrock (1993) has enabled numerous perioperative nurses to engage in first-assisting duties that are based on a sound theoretical foundation, as well as extensive clinical practice. RNFA Christine Espersen (1993) describes the range of responsibilities of the RNFA during the preoperative, intraoperative, and postoperative periods and illustrates the positive impact that the RNFA has on patient care.

Box 1-2 *Important attributes of the perioperative cardiac nurse**

Theo Raber, RN   Hahemann Hospital, Philadelphia, Pa.   1954-1967

Ready to meet challenges
Levelheaded and cool in emergency situations
Can work closely with a team
A hard worker

Chizuko Williams, RN   Deborah Heart and Lung Hospital, Brown Mills, N.J.   1958-1990

Fosters working relationships between professional and nonprofessional staff to provide the highest quality operating room care
Visits each surgical patient preoperatively to perform a nursing assessment and nursing care plan
Continuously learns about new procedures and equipment
Dedicated and hard-working

Continued.

Box 1-2 *Important attributes of the perioperative cardiac nurse**—cont'd

Peggy Hartin, RN   Stanford University Hospital, Stanford, Calif.   1959-present

Enjoys the challenge of each case and anticipates the surgeon when procedures change
Has a long attention span and can stand for long periods of time
A supportive team player

Alice Cannon, RN   Oregon Health Sciences University, Portland, Ore.   1962-1984
Willamette Falls Hospital, Oregon City, Ore.   1984-1986
Portland VA Medical Center, Portland, Ore.   1986-present

Has absolute honesty and integrity
Willing to work hard and study on own time
Has the drive and determination—on own time—to attend rounds and conferences so that patients can expect and
receive excellent care by excellent, dedicated perioperative nurses.

Gwyn Baumgarten, RN   St. Luke's, Texas Children's Hospitals, Texas Heart Institute   1963-1974
Presently with Medtronic, Inc., Houston Tex.

A team player
"Thick-skinned," but compassionate toward others
Able to remain calm
Able to think under great pressure
Loyal
Dedicated

Edwinia Ion, RN   Jackson Memorial Hospital, Miami, Fla.   1963-1965
Independent Cardiovascular Nurse, Miami, Fla.   1965-1967
Texas Children's Hospital, St. Luke's Hospital, Houston, Tex.   1967-1969
The Methodist Hospital, Houston, Tex.   1969-present

Able to use knowledge and expertise to make sound judgments
A partner to the surgeon in developing a plan to coordinate care
Has a sense of humor, tolerance, humility, and a kind heart
The link between patient and family

Nancy Davis, RN NP   St. Vincent's Hospital, Portland, Ore.   1964-1968
St. Luke's Hospital, Boise, Idaho   1968-1974
RNFA, private practice   1974-present

Curious
A high achiever
Wants to do a good job consistently
Anticipates and plans ahead
Wants to understand what is happening; thrives on the challenge of learning and the joy of "meaningful work"

Jill Montgomery, RN   Boston Children's Hospital, Boston, Mass.   1971-present

Able to communicate with many different people—verbally and nonverbally
Approachable by patients, parents, other staff, ancillary help, and others
Able to "punt"
Flexibility and intelligence
Committed to the process of learning
Possesses honesty and integrity
Prepared for anything, anytime

*Certification (CNOR, CRNFA), degrees of nurses not listed.

CONCLUSION

The history of cardiac surgery and the role of the perioperative nurse have been largely associated with technical achievements. But these achievements, important as they are, do not reflect the essence of what cardiac surgery is, or what cardiac surgery team members do. A truer representation can be found in the personal characteristics of its participants: Davis' "curiosity," Montgomery's "flexibility," Baumgarten's "compassion" (Table 1-3), and Lillehei's "persistence." These qualities have enabled surgeons and nurses to perform the technical feats for which they are justifiably esteemed. Such qualities have motivated persons to go beyond what was expected and to extend their responsibilities above what was considered allowable. These are the significant achievements that represent cardiac surgery. Perioperative cardiac nurses need to be aware of their heritage so that they can appreciate how important their contributions have been and how necessary it is for them to continue to contribute to the welfare of patients with cardiac disease.

REFERENCES

Abbott M: *Atlas of congenital heart disease*, New York, 1936, American Heart Association.

Alexander EL: *Operating room technique*, ed 1, St Louis, 1943, Mosby.

Alexander EL: *Operating room technique*, ed 2, St Louis, 1949, Mosby.

Alexander EL: *The care of the patient in surgery including techniques*, ed 3, St Louis, 1958, Mosby.

Alexander EL and others: *Care of the patient in surgery including techniques*, ed 4, St Louis, 1967, Mosby.

American Heart Associaton: *Proceedings of the first national conference on cardiovascular diseases*, New York, 1950, AHA.

Aspinall MJ: *Nursing the open-heart surgery patient*, New York, 1973, McGraw-Hill.

Austin WG: Presidential address: surgery is a great career, *Am Coll Surg Bull* 77(12):6, 1992.

Barnard CN: A human cardiac transplant: an interim report of a successful operation performed at Groote Schuur Hospital, Cape Town, *S Afr Medi J* 41:1271, 1967.

Baumgarten G: Personal communication, 1992.

Beck CS: The development of a new blood supply to the heart by operation, *Ann Surg* 102:801, 1935.

Brandt L: Surgery of the heart and great vessels, *OR Supervisor*, Dec 1951.

Brieger GH: The development of surgery. In Sabiston DC, editor: *Textbook of surgery*, ed 14, Philadelphia, 1991, WB Saunders.

Cannon A: Personal communication, 1992.

Cardiovascular nurse designs graft sizers, *Methodist J*, April 9, 1976.

Chow RK: *Cardiosurgical nursing care: understandings, concepts, and principles for practice*, New York, 1976, Springer.

Colp R, Keller MW: *Textbook of surgical nursing*, New York, 1921, Macmillan.

Comroe JH: Who was Alexis who? Cardiovascular diseases, *Bull Tex Heart Inst* 6(3):251, 1979.

Comroe JH: Doctor, you have six minutes, *Science*, p 64, Jan/Feb 1983.

Comroe JH, Dripps RD: *The top ten clinical advances in cardiovascular-pulmonary medicine and surgery between 1945 and 1975: how they came about*. Final report, Bethesda, Md, Jan 31, 1977, National Heart and Lung Institute.

Conversation with the author (Chizuko Williams, R.N.), *Cardiothorac Nurse* 3(1):5, 1985.

Cooley DA: *Surgical treatment of thoracic aneurysms*, Philadelphia, 1986, WB Saunders.

Cooley DA: Recollections of early development and later trends in cardiac surgery, *J Thorac Cardiovasc Surg* 98:817, 1989.

Cooley DA and others: Organ transplantation for advanced cardiopulmonary disease, *Ann Thorac Surg* 8:300, 1969.

Cutler E, Beck C: The present status of the surgical procedures in chronic valvular disease of the heart, *Arch Surg* 18:403, 1929.

Davis N: Personal communication, 1992.

DeVries WC: The permanent artificial heart: four case reports, *JAMA* 259:849, 1988.

Dobell ARC: Surgery in the era of technology, *Am Coll Surg Bull* 75(4):8, 1990.

Driscoll J: *Preserving the legacy: AORN 1949-1989*, Denver, 1990, Association of Operating Room Nurses.

Effler DB: Introduction. In Favaloro RG: *Surgical treatment of coronary arteriosclerosis*, Baltimore, 1970, Williams & Wilkins.

Elsberry JL: Psychological responses to open heart surgery, *Nurs Res* 21:220, 1972.

Espersen CC: The RN First Assistant in cardiac surgery. In Rothrock JC: *The RN first assistant: an expanded perioperative nursing role*, ed 2, Philadelphia, 1993, JB Lippincott.

Favaloro R: Saphenous vein autograft replacement of severe segmental coronary artery occlusion, *Ann Thorac Surg* 5:334, 1968.

Fordham ME: *Cardiovascular surgical nursing*, New York, 1962, Macmillan.

Frost EAM: *Essays on the history of anesthesia*, Georgetown, Conn, 1985, McMahon.

Garrett EH, Dennis EW, DeBakey ME: Aortocoronary bypass with saphenous vein grafts: seven-year follow-up, *JAMA* 223:792, 1973.

Gibbon J: Application of a mechanical heart and lung apparatus to cardiac surgery, *Minn Med* 37:171, 1954.

Harkin DE: The emergence of cardiac surgery, *J Thorac Cardiovasc Surg* 98(5, pt 2):805, 1989.

Hartin P: Personal communication, 1992.

Higgins V: Cardiothoracic operations. In Ballinger WF, Treybal JC, Vose AB: *Alexander's care of the patient in surgery*, ed 5, St Louis, 1972, Mosby.

Ion E: Personal communication, 1992.

James EE: The nursing care of the open heart patient, *Nurs Clin North Am* 2(3):543, 1967.

Jamieson SW, Stinson EB, Shumway NE: Cardiac transplantation in 150 patients at Stanford University, *Br Med J* 1(6156):93, 1979.

Johnson SL: *The history of cardiac surgery: 1896-1955*, Baltimore, 1970, Johns Hopkins University Press.

Kernicki J, Bullock BL, Matthews J: *Cardiovascular nursing: rationale for therapy and nursing approach*, New York, 1970, GP Putnam's Sons.

King OM: *Care of the cardiac surgical patient*, St Louis, 1975, Mosby.

Kneedler JA: Origins of operating room nursing. In Kneedler JA, Dodge GH: *Perioperative patient care: the nursing perspective*, ed 2, Boston, 1987, Blackwell Scientific Publications.

Kouwenhoven WB, Jude JR, Knickerbocker GG: Closed-chest cardiac massage, *JAMA* 173:1064, 1960.

Lee RM: Early operating room nursing, *AORN J* 24(1):124, 1976.

Lefrak EA, Starr A: *Cardiac valve prostheses*, New York, 1979, Appleton-Century-Crofts.

Lillehei CW: Discussion of Lillehei CW and others: The first open-heart repairs of ventricular septal defects, atrioventricular communis, and tetralogy of Fallot using extracorporeal circulation by cross-circulation: a 30-year follow-up, *Ann Thorac Surg* 41(1):4, 1986 (p 21).

Litwak RS: The growth of cardiac surgery: historical notes, *Cardiac Surg (Cardiovasc Clin)* 1(2):6, 1970.

Loop FD and others: Influence of the internal mammary artery graft on 10-year survival and other cardiac events, *N Engl J Med* 314:1, 1986.

Metzger RS: The beginnings of OR nursing education, *AORN J* 24(1):73, 1976.

Modell W: *Handbook of cardiology for nurses*, New York, 1952, Springer.

Montgomery JG: Personal communication, 1992.

Nineteen years of AORN films, *AORN J* 27(3):511, 1978.

Nissen R: *Billroth and cardiac surgery*, Lancet 2:25, 1963.

Ochsner JL, Mills NL: *Coronary artery surgery*, Philadelphia: 1978, Lea & Febiger.

Paget S: *Surgery of the chest*, London: 1896, John Wright.

Powers M, Storlie F: *The cardiac surgical patient*, London, 1969, Macmillan.

Raber T: Personal communication, 1992.

Rashkind WJ: Historical aspects of surgery for congenital heart disease, *J Thorac Cardiovasc Surg* 84:619, 1982.

Reitz BA, Pennock JL, Shumway NE: Simplified operative method of heart and lung transplantation, *J Surg Res* 31:1, 1981.

Rothrock JC: *The RN first assistant: an expanded perioperative nursing role*, ed 2, Philadelphia, 1993, JB Lippincott.

Shumacker HB: *The evolution of cardiac surgery*, Bloomington, 1992, Indiana University Press.

Shumway NE: *Transplantation of the heart and heart-lung*. Paper presented at Cardiac Surgery: 1993 "State of the Art," The Academy of Medicine of New Jersey, Division of Cardiothoracic Surgery, School of Cardiovascular Perfusion, Department of Nursing Education and Quality Assurance, Cooper Hospital/University Medical Center, St Thomas, Virgin Islands, Nov 14, 1992.

Stafford ES, Diller D: *A textbook of surgery for nurses*, Philadelphia, 1947, WB Saunders.

Texas Heart Institute Foundation: *Twenty-five years of excellence: a history of the Texas Heart Institute*, Houston, 1989, THI Foundation.

Toronto Lung Transplant Group: Experience with single lung transplantation for pulmonary fibrosis, *JAMA* 259:2558, 1988.

Voorhees AB: The origin of the permeable arterial prosthesis: a personal recollection, *Surg Rounds*, p 79, Feb 1988.

Voorhees AB, Jaretzki A, Blakemore AH: The use of tubes constructed from Vinyon "N" cloth in bridging arterial defects, *Ann Surg* 135(3):332, 1952.

Walsh JJ: *History of nursing*, New York, 1929, PJ Kennedy.

West JP, Keller MW, Harmon E: *Nursing care of the surgical patient*, New York, 1950, Macmillan.

Williams C: Personal communication, 1992.

Williams C, Czapinski N, Graf D: Perioperative nursing: implications for open-heart surgery, *Cardiothorac Nurs* 3(1):1, 1985.

2

The Cardiac Nurse

Perioperative patient care is a complex and comprehensive physiologic and psychologic undertaking; it is at times precise and scientific, and at times fluid, intuitive, and subjective.

Jane C. Rothrock, RN, 1990 (p. xii)

Nursing roles have been influenced by collaborative practice models and the multidisciplinary integration of resources. This is especially evident in the cardiac operating room, where patient outcomes are dependent on shared decision making and responsibility for judging the appropriateness of interventions. This emphasis on clinical nursing judgment implies that nurses demonstrate the knowledge and skills required to function as partners in collaborative efforts.

Cardiac surgery represents a unique meshing of cognitive, psychomotor, and affective skills. In this setting the nurse must have knowledge of an extensive array of cardiovascular disorders and their treatment, be able to manipulate complex equipment, and interact effectively with patients and families coping with illnesses that have a profound physiologic and emotional impact on their lives (Fig. 2-1). These skills are acquired gradually through the performance of the traditional roles of circulator and scrub nurse and form the basis for expanded clinical nursing practice represented by the RN first assistant (RNFA).

DEVELOPMENT OF CLINICAL SKILL

Clinical skill develops as one learns to integrate theoretical knowledge and experience in the perioperative arena. Nurses specializing in cardiac surgery progress from a beginner's level to an advanced level of practice as they apply these "head and hand" skills to patient situations. Benner (1984) identified five stages of proficiency to describe this progression: novice, advanced beginner, competent, proficient, and expert (Box 2-1). The model has been applied to numerous clinical settings, including the operating room (Byrne, 1986).

These designations are situational. A perioperative nurse, proficient in general surgery, would enter a cardiac surgery service as a novice or advanced beginner because the patient population, the operative

procedures, and the cardiac team would be unfamiliar. The nurse with past open heart surgery experience in another institution would be likely to adapt more quickly to the new setting but would still function as a beginner. Specific attributes of the environment and the team would need to be learned. Among these would be the structure of the unit, location of supplies, surgeon preferences, and personalities of individual team members.

The RNFA novice would have demonstrated proficiency as a scrub nurse and circulator (Association of Operating Room Nurses [AORN], 1990), but as a beginning cardiac RNFA, the novice would need to develop new skills specific to the practice of cardiac first assisting.

Other characteristics of developing proficiency include (1) a shift from relying on abstract principles to using past concrete experiences, (2) viewing the sit-

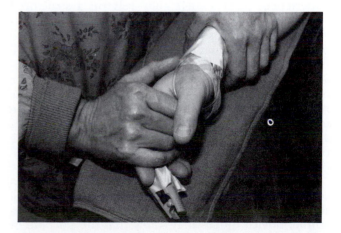

Fig. 2-1   The patient is wearing a pulse oximeter finger cot. Perioperative cardiac nursing combines high tech with high touch. (Photograph by Howard Kaye.)

Box 2-1   *Five stages of proficiency*

Novice: The nurse has no experience with cardiac surgery and bases performance on rules and instructions from the preceptor. The novice is unable to place patient situations into context.

Advanced beginner: The nurse has had limited experience with cardiac surgery and is able to identify critical activities but is unable to discern subtle cues or to prioritize actions.

Competent nurse: The nurse has sufficient experience to formulate an efficient and organized plan of care but still lacks flexibility and speed in unusual situations.

Proficient nurse: The nurse is capable of placing actions in context and sees situations holistically rather than as a series of steps. The proficient nurse works interdependently with other members of the cardiac team.

Expert: The nurse has a wealth of experience and responds automatically to familiar situations rather than depending on analysis and rules. Performance is fluid and flexible. The expert works interdependently with professionals within and outside the cardiac operating room.

Modified from Benner P: *From novice to expert,* Menlo Park, Calif, 1984, Addison-Wesley.

---

uation more as a whole rather than as a compilation of bits, and (3) moving from detached observation to involved performance (Benner, 1982, 1984). Typical comments made by cardiac perioperative nurses at various skill levels are highlighted throughout this chapter.

NOVICE

Novices orienting to cardiac surgery have had no previous open heart surgery experience on which to base their performance. Because of the complexity of patients' problems, most beginning cardiac nurses come to a cardiac service with some perioperative nursing experience. At this stage they rely on a structured educational process that focuses on checklists and textbook rules, such as instrument and supply lists, or patient vital signs and blood values. Novices may have minimal theoretical knowledge of cardiac disease, diagnostic studies, or surgical techniques; the course outline in Box 2-2 lists knowledge basic to cardiac nursing. A pretest/posttest (see Appendix A) can be used to identify specific learning needs. Often novices are not aware of their knowledge or skills, because they are too unfamiliar with the situation to ask questions.

A preceptor can help the novice to begin the process of transforming abstract knowledge into clinical skill by applying theory to patient situations. For example, novice nurses may know that the purpose of coronary artery bypass surgery is to improve blood

flow to the myocardium, but they may not know how this is achieved with bypass grafts. In planning preoperative teaching for the patient, the novice will need to understand the goal of the planned surgery, how that goal is to be met, and what the patient's responses may be to the intervention.

Psychomotor skills are enhanced by frequent hands-on practice and return demonstration with instruments and equipment such as vascular clamps, bypass lines, sternal saws, defibrillators, and autotransfusion systems. Over time the nurse develops habits that enhance the efficient use of these devices.

Psychosocial skills can be developed by role playing and interacting with patients under the guidance of the preceptor. The preceptor can adapt the novice's previous experience and level of understanding to the situation, making it a learning experience for both patient and nurse.

Often the best preceptors for novices and advanced beginners are those at the competent and proficient level because they can relate better than experts to the structured learning needs of beginners (Urden, 1989). They are able to assimilate the novice into the unit culture by interpreting new experiences in light of what the novice knows and what the novice needs to learn. The preceptor provides a balanced perspective and helps the novice to make the transition from detached observer to involved performer.

The following are typical comments of a novice circulating nurse:

"I couldn't believe how many machines and how much equipment there was in the room."

"There were a lot of people, but they didn't seem to get in each other's way. They made it look easy."

"I was afraid the patient would have a cardiac arrest and I'd be all alone."

The novice observes the situation but does not feel capable of becoming an active participant. Thoughts are disjointed and do not reflect a focus on achieving a goal. The novice's anxiety level is increased by a lack of practice in using the equipment and supplies common to cardiac surgery and by the fear of being expected to do something for which he or she has had no preparation. The novice is not yet aware that patient care requires both individual actions and mutually shared responsibilities. Commonly, there is a feeling of sensory overload that can be overwhelming without the guidance and support of the preceptor and other members of the team.

ADVANCED BEGINNER

The advanced beginner still follows preset rules but is starting to perceive patterns, set priorities, and anticipate needs based on patient cues during routine procedures. Both the novice and the advanced beginner learn basic skills by focusing on tasks. The competencies outlined in Appendix B have been developed to reflect the basic knowledge and skills required

---

Box 2-2 *Cardiac surgery course outline*

Unit 1
Introduction to the cardiac service
Anatomy and physiology
Perioperative nursing roles
Competency skill checklist
Standards of clinical practice
Standards of professional performance
Supplies and equipment
Prostheses
　Grafts
　Valves and homografts
　Obturators
Room setup
Basic instrumentation
Table setup

Unit II
Cardiovascular disease/pathophysiology
　Congenital
　　Normal fetal circulation
　　Circulation after birth
　　Increased pulmonary blood flow
　　Decreased pulmonary blood flow
　　Malformations
　Acquired
　　Coronary artery disease
　　Valvular heart disease
　　Thoracic aneurysms
　　Pacemakers and conduction disturbances
　　Emergencies
　　Miscellaneous
Diagnostic studies
　Noninvasive (electrocardiogram, echocardiogram, nuclear studies, computed tomography, magnetic resonance imaging, etc.)
　Invasive (cardiac catheterization)

Interventional cardiology
　Percutaneous transluminal coronary angioplasty (PTCA)
　Stents, atherectomy devices
　Occlusive devices for congenital defects
Laboratory tests
Blood bank
Cardiovascular drugs
Infection control
Perioperative care
Cardiac anesthesia
Hemodynamic monitoring
Generic cardiac procedure
Extracorporeal circulation
Myocardial protection

Unit III
History of cardiac surgery
Procedures for congenital heart disease
　Special patient/family needs
　Special equipment and supplies
　Special instrumentation
Procedures for acquired heart disease
　Special patient/family needs
　Special equipment and supplies
　Special instrumentation
Emergency procedures
　Trauma
　Postoperative hemorrhage
Pacemakers, internal cardioverter defibrillators (ICDs)
Patient teaching
Discharge planning and rehabilitation
The Mended Hearts (support group)
Research
Ethical issues

---

of the perioperative cardiac nurse. These competencies reflect AORN's *Standards and Recommended Practices* (1993), and the American Nurses' Association and American Heart Association (AHA) Council on Cardiovascular Nursing's *Standards of Cardiovascular Nursing Practice* (1981).

The nurse at the advanced beginner level may be able to perform the skills but is not able to make associations between them. For instance, the proficient or expert nurse continuously assesses the hemodynamic status of the patient by comparing the information displayed on the monitor with the directly observable beating heart. (The expert may not even be conscious of doing this unless questioned). Correlating subtle, progressive alterations in pressures (decreasing systemic pressure, increasing pulmonary pressure) to a distended, sluggish heart alerts the expert to anticipate the use of supportive measures, such as inotropic drugs, cardiopulmonary bypass, intraaortic balloon counterpulsation, or other interventions to rest the heart and conserve its energy resources. The

expert prepares for these procedures before being specifically requested to do so by the surgeon. The advanced beginner may be aware of these clinical signs but is unable to recognize their significance or identify available options and interventions appropriate to the clinical situation.

Preceptors help beginning nurses to identify recurring aspects of situations. The advanced beginner starts to differentiate between what is normal and what is abnormal, and between what is significant and what is not, but is still learning to judge the relative importance of these different aspects.

A circulating nurse at this level remarks:

"It was hard to remember when to turn the warming blanket off and when to turn it back on, when to pour the cold solutions and when to give warm saline."

"I tried to stay with the patient on induction, but I had to leave him to count or open more supplies."

"I tried to do all the things I had to do, but I was always behind."

In this case the advanced beginner knows that the principles of temperature control and patient safety are important but cannot integrate them efficiently.

Another difficulty encountered by the advanced beginner is the formulation of a procedural timetable for completing tasks sequentially and in order of priority. A scrub nurse at this level typically remarks:

"When the chest is being closed, I have to keep up with the sternal wires, do the counts, prepare the dressings, get the chest tubes hooked up, clean up my back table, unlock the clamps. . . . I feel I have to get everything done at the same time."

"My preceptor tries to help me prioritize and do the most important things first, but I have a hard time trying to determine what's important. And there isn't enough time to figure it out, anyway!"

The scrub nurse is attempting to complete these tasks without identifying what has to be done first and what can wait. While it may be obvious to the proficient nurse that the sternal wires need to go in before the dressing is applied, or that cleaning up the table can be done after the case is completed, that kind of "common sense" is the result of participating in enough cases to be able to view the situation as a whole and not as a set of separate and unrelated activities.

It is not uncommon for the advanced beginner to forget certain basic activities or go through a transient dip in the learning curve. The scrub nurse may omit a step during the cannulation procedure (e.g., tying the cannula to the tourniquet); the circulator may neglect to apply the dispersive pad; the RNFA may forget when to use the cardiotomy suction in preference to the discard suction. One reason for this regression is that the nurse at this stage is trying to focus on both the particular and the general. He or she is trying to remember numerous details while at the same time attempting to plan ahead, perceive the situation on a more global scale, and group individual activities into sets (e.g., performing cannulation, opening or closing the chest, inserting temporary pacing wires). Such "lapses" are disconcerting to the nurse, and it is helpful to review basic steps with an emphasis on why actions are performed. When previously learned "rules" are explained in the context of situations experienced, nurses arrive at a deeper and more meaningful understanding of their performance.

COMPETENT NURSE

The competent nurse is able to place aspects of the situation into perspective and formulate a deliberate plan that is efficient and organized. Tasks are incorporated into the plan and are no longer the center of attention. Although lacking in speed and flexibility, the nurse has sufficient knowledge and skill to organize care, as illustrated by this nurse's comments:

"We were getting a patient from the cath lab for emergency surgery. We asked the cath lab tech if blood had been ordered and what lines were in place; then we called the front desk to have them page the perfusionist and the anesthesia staff. We opened the packs while the scrub nurse scrubbed her hands. She came in from the scrub sink just as the patient entered the room. I helped the patient onto the bed and tried to calm him while anesthesia inserted pressure lines and prepared to intubate; the other circulator counted with the scrub nurse. Once he was asleep, we grounded him, and while I tucked his arms and shaved and prepped his chest, the other circulator inserted the urinary catheter and washed his legs. The scrub nurse had finished her setup when the surgeon arrived. We were able to start the case right away."

Emergency cases are not atypical, and a nurse who has been with a cardiac service for 2 or 3 years will have encountered a number of such cases. These experiences allow nurses to develop a perspective, to put actions into terms of goals. In a situation such as that described, the goal is to minimize the patient's myocardial damage and improve blood flow to the heart. This is commonly achieved by putting the patient on bypass and revascularizing the myocardium as expeditiously as possible. Nursing interventions of the circulator are aimed at facilitating this process by focusing on activities pertinent to the goal, such as comfort, safety, and anxiety-reducing measures, as well as monitoring and patient preparation procedures. The scrub nurse focuses on preparing instruments and supplies for the incision, cardiopulmonary bypass, and coronary anastomoses. Activities not directly related to the goal (dressings, chest tubes, pacing wires) can be deferred. The nurse is capable of judging what is and is not critical for preparation of an emergency case.

At this level nurses benefit from simulations and decision-making exercises (see Appendix C). Various imagined scenarios enable the nurse to detect the problem and define it, collect and analyze information, select options, identify available resources, develop plans, and evaluate the relative effectiveness of these plans. By placing the problem within a context (e.g., a particular surgeon's preferences, unit-specific characteristics, team members' designated responsibilities), nurses can avoid actions not pertinent. They can focus on plans that are congruent with the structure of the unit and the performance of team members.

These simulations can be practiced with a proficient or expert mentor, or they can be done alone. The value of these exercises is that the nurse can think through a problem without the attendant stress of real-life situations and reduce the margin for error by narrowing the selection to only the most appropriate options.

Such "what if?" exercises are helpful not only to the competent nurse, but also to the novice and advanced beginner, who are often being precepted by the nurse at the competent level. Deliberate, conscious planning enables the competent nurse to verbalize step-by-step the rationale for actions to the novice and to put those actions into context. Compared with the expert, the competent nurse still relies on a linear analysis of performance that can be broken down into discrete bits. She or he is not yet capable of seeing the situation as a seamless whole.

PROFICIENT NURSE

Proficient nurses have learned from experience what to expect in a given situation and how to make modifications in response to changes in the patient's status. They know what the usual course of events is and plan appropriately without obvious effort. They are not deterred by unusual circumstances or untoward events. Unlike the competent nurse, the proficient nurse has advanced beyond a checklist mentality and has an overall picture of the situation. This holistic view is a hallmark of the proficient nurse.

The proficient nurse considers fewer options in deciding how to proceed, even in complex situations. In the case of a patient with a dissecting thoracic aortic aneurysm, the proficient nurse will want to determine the location of the aneurysm, because many nursing actions will be dictated by this. For instance, if the patient has a descending thoracic aneurysm, the nurse knows that the patient will be placed laterally and will require thoracotomy instruments and equipment to accomplish a lateral thoracotomy position.

Perfusion of the kidneys and other organs distal to the aneurysm may require extracorporeal techniques while the aorta is cross-clamped. The nurse does not dwell on gathering instruments and supplies for a median sternotomy and induced cardiac arrest, because in this situation the aneurysm is approached from the left lateral thoracotomy incision and the heart does not need to be stopped.

Conversely, the nurse awaiting a patient with an ascending aortic aneurysm knows that the position will be supine, that sternotomy instruments will be used, and that cardiopulmonary bypass will be used to perfuse the body's organs while the heart is arrested. The size and the location of the aneurysm will dictate cannulation techniques, which in turn will affect skin preparation, surgical exposure, and instrumentation. If the aneurysm has dilated the aortic annulus to the point of valvular incompetence (as evidenced during cardiac catheterization by dye regurgitating into the left ventricle), aortic valve replacement may be indicated, necessitating valve instruments. If the aortic root and ascending aorta must be resected, obliterating the entrance to the coronary arteries, aortocoronary continuity must be reestablished by either coronary ostial reimplantation or bypass grafts (if coronary artery disease is documented). This situation would necessitate coronary bypass instruments and exposure of the saphenous vein if bypass grafts are required.

The description of these activities is linear, but the thought processes of the nurse do not proceed in such a step-by-step manner. The proficient nurse will focus on the salient features (ascending/descending) and consider the multiple options available almost simultaneously. In considering the important aspects of a case, proficient nurses will talk to each other in a way that may not be easily understood by less-experienced clinicians. In discussing plans for a dissecting ascending aortic aneurysm with the scrub nurse and circulator, the RNFA might make the following comments:

"The dissection originates in the lateral aspect of the ascending aorta, close to the root. The ventricle was opacified, so we'll probably replace the valve. The coronaries were clean, so grafts are unlikely; we'll reimplant the ostia. Plan on cannulating the groin before we open the chest."

The RNFA is stating that because of the location and extent of the aneurysm, the ascending aorta and the aortic valve will be replaced. Because there is a danger of lacerating this aneurysm during sternotomy and because placing a cannula in the aneurysmal aorta would risk rupture, the surgeon will first cannulate the femoral artery to initiate cardiopulmonary bypass. To reestablish blood flow to the coronary arteries (necessitated by excision of the aortic root, which contains the entrance to the coronary system), the entrance of the coronary arteries will be anastomosed to the prosthetic graft. Coronary bypass grafts are not indicated, because the patient has no evidence of significant coronary artery disease.

The circulator comments:

"I'll pull the graft valve prostheses as well as individual valves and grafts. I'll order the FFP so it's ready when we need to preclot. The sizers have been opened. I'll prep the groin for cannulation. After we've gotten started, I'll talk to the family and let them know what's going on. I saw them in the cath lab, and they were understandably upset."

The circulating nurse knows that the patient will probably require a prosthesis (and appropriate sizers) that combines a woven graft and a manufactured valve. The circulator will also have separate grafts and valves available in the event that these are indicated. Because the patient will be systemically heparinized, the grafts will be preclotted with fresh frozen plasma (or some other method) in order to reduce interstitial hemorrhage. The nurse is familiar with such cases and knows to cleanse the groin for exposure of the femoral artery for cannulation. Patients with ascending aneurysms frequently present emergently, so family members' anxiety levels tend to be high during this high-risk procedure. The nurse is aware of this and can talk to the family once the procedure is underway.

Comments of the proficient scrub nurse may include:

"The femoral lines are ready. It's a big aneurysm, so we may need another sucker."

The scrub nurse is referring both to the cannulation technique that will be required and to the potential for severe hemorrhage. The request for "another sucker" refers to setting up an additional cardiotomy suction line that can be used to return shed blood to the pump quickly if there is excessive bleeding.

All three nurses are anticipating what can be expected and what modifications may be required. At this stage nurses demonstrate the following characteristics: basing performance on experience, viewing the situation as a dynamic whole, and becoming actively involved. With extensive knowledge and experience, proficient nurses are flexible enough to develop contingencies when surgical procedures do not proceed as planned, whereas novices may not be able to understand why and how such modifications were chosen. Only when nurses have attained a competent level of skill can they grasp the holistic nature of the proficient nurse's or expert's performance. Case studies enable nurses to decipher the decision-making process in selecting interventions to meet specific patient needs, and they test their ability to compare the expected with what actually occurs. In addition, they identify the most important aspects of the situation and focus on them.

EXPERT

Experts have attained a level of skill that is difficult to describe because of the many contextual nuances associated with their clinical interventions. They respond automatically to situations and rarely analyze their decisions. Only when they have had little or no previous experience with a situation will experts need to reduce a situation to its component parts. Through repeated practice, experts have acquired habits that are ingrained in their performance.

The grace and rhythm of many experts and their seeming ability to read minds are the result not only of extensive experience with patient situations, but also of working closely with their team members. Excellence in the health care setting is often the result of collaborative relationships, as well as individual efforts. This is especially evident in the cardiac service, where mutual trust and respect, based on clinical competence, are themselves factors that promote positive patient outcomes.

RNFAs who have worked with a surgeon make few unnecessary motions and facilitate the performance of highly exacting surgical techniques such as anastomosis and cannulation. The expert scrub nurse displays a graceful familiarity with the stages of a procedure and is unlikely to be directed by the surgeon in any but those situations where the surgeon has not yet decided how to proceed. The expert circulator is known by the controlled calmness created in the operating room and the efficient progression of the surgery.

Unlike less-skilled nurses, experts and proficient nurses approach a situation with the self-assurance that comes from knowing what is happening and what can (or cannot) be done about it.

"I was in the cafeteria just after finishing a mitral valve replacement. I heard the STAT overhead page calling the surgeon to the unit. I knew something must have happened, and I ran to the ICU. The patient had suddenly put out a liter of blood. I opened the emergency chest set on the overbed table and put on a gown and gloves. Another nurse from the OR had heard the page and came in; she sprayed the chest, and I draped while the surgeon gowned. We opened the chest and saw a tear in the ventricle near the location of the valve prosthesis. We tried to patch it, but it kept tearing. The patient was too unstable to transport to the OR, so we put her on bypass to perfuse her organs and decompress the heart. She kept bleeding, so we discussed replacing the valve prosthesis in the ICU and came to a quick decision to do it there. We had no choice. We arrested her, got some instruments from the OR, and replaced the prosthesis right there in the ICU. Six months later she walked out of the hospital."

In viewing this situation, the novice might be appalled at the perceived lack of attention to the "basics," but in fact the basic consideration was to fix the ventricular tear and stop the bleeding so that the patient could survive. Deliberating over appropriate sterile technique or the optimal surgical environment would have hindered the eventual successful outcome for this patient. What is significant in this instance is the shared responsibility and the collaborative plan that was implemented for the patient. Had there not been both competence and good working relationships, the outcome might not have been as positive.

This anticipation of problems and the selection of appropriate interventions characterize the expert. But outlining or explaining the mental progression from problem identification to implementation of clinical strategies is difficult for experts to do. Much of their practice is based on well-formed habits and intimate knowledge of co-workers' problem-solving processes, as well as extensive clinical experience. For this reason, the use of case studies relating to actual events are recommended teaching/learning strategies for experts. Experts can describe their experiences to proficient nurses, who in turn can interpret the expert's performance in a way that is understandable to nurses with less contextual experience. The expert can identify clinical situations where his or her actions made a difference. The proficient or competent nurse can reduce those actions into quantifiable sets of activities that can be more easily comprehended by the novice or advanced beginner.

CONCLUSION

The development of expertise in perioperative cardiac surgery nursing is quantitative and qualitative. It is knowing and using the knowledge to provide care. It is understanding the needs of the patient, as well as the requirements of the surgical procedure and fellow team members. It is a continuing process that depends not only on self-reliance but also on the support and encouragement of those who know the environment. The next chapter discusses the cardiac team and the importance of that fellowship.

APPENDIX A
Pretest/Posttest

Use the following terms to answer questions 1 through 14.

Epinephrine	Tricuspid valve
Left ventricular aneurysm	Lesser saphenous vein
Supine	Dopamine
Superior vena cava	Pulmonary valve
Lateral	Inferior vena cava
Right atrium	Aorta
Left atrium	Aortic valve
Mediastinum	Right ventricle
Cephalic vein	Ventricular septal
Mitral valve	defect
Air	Left ventricle
Lungs	Right ventricle
Blood	Calcium chloride
Internal mammary artery	Mitral regurgitation
Dobutamine	Greater saphenous vein
Mechanical valve	Pulmonary veins
prosthesis	Biologic valve
	prosthesis

1. Describe the movement of blood through the heart and lungs from the inferior and superior vena cava to the ascending aorta.

2. Which valves are in the right side of the heart?

3. Which valves are in the left side of the heart?

4. Which valve(s) is (are) most likely to become diseased in the adult?

5. What type of valve prosthesis generally requires postoperative chronic anticoagulation?

6. Complications of myocardial infarction include the following (list three):

7. The patient position for coronary bypass surgery is _____ .

8. Which *vein* is most likely to be used as a graft/conduit in coronary artery bypass grafting?

9. Which coronary bypass graft/conduit displays the greatest long-term patency?

10. The patient position for an ascending aortic thoracic aneurysm is _____ .

11. The patient position for a descending aortic thoracic aneurysm is _____ .

12. During typical cardiopulmonary bypass, blood is diverted from the _____ and _____ , oxygenated, and pumped into the _____ .

13. The *main* reason for inserting chest tubes into the cardiac surgical patient is to remove _____ from the _____ .

14. Which drug(s) is (are) most likely to be given via the intracardiac route?

15. The most *common* setting (in watt seconds) for internal defibrillation in the adult is (circle the best answer):
a. 10 b. 30 c. 60 d. 250 e. 400
16. Complications of cardiac surgery include perioperative myocardial infarction, stroke, hemorrhage, and death.
a. True b. False
17. Immediately postoperatively, patients will appear pale and feel warm and clammy.
a. True b. False

Answer key

1. Right atrium → tricuspid valve → right ventricle → pulmonary valve → pulmonary artery → lungs → pulmonary veins → left atrium → mitral valve → left ventricle → aortic valve
2. Mitral, aortic
3. Tricuspid, pulmonary
4. Mitral, aortic
5. Mechanical valve prosthesis
6. Left ventricular aneurysm, ventricular septal defect, mitral regurgitation
7. Supine
8. Greater saphenous vein
9. Internal mammary artery
10. Supine
11. Lateral
12. Inferior vena cava and superior vena cava, aorta
13. Blood, mediastinum
14. Epinephrine
15. a
16. a
17. b

APPENDIX B
Competency Statements in Perioperative Cardiac Nursing

Assessment

1. Competency to assess the physical health status and physiologic response of the patient
    1.1. Assesses physical cardiovascular risk factors
        Age
        Obesity
        Hypertension
        Smoking
        Alcohol intake
        Drug abuse (e.g., cocaine)
        Hypercholesterolemia
        Diabetes
    1.2. Identifies current medical diagnosis and therapy
    1.3. Identifies other congenital and acquired conditions
    1.4. Assesses previous health state
        Past medical history (angina, MI, CHF, vascular disease, syncope, TIA, stroke)
        Hospitalizations
        Surgery (sternotomy, thoracotomy, vein stripping, transurethral resection)
        Injuries
        Chronic illnesses (lupus, arthritis, multiple sclerosis, (myasthenia gravis, pulmonary disease, thyroid disorders)
        Infectious diseases (rheumatic fever, endocarditis)
    1.5. Identifies presence of prostheses/implants
        Pacemaker, internal defibrillator
        Prosthetic heart valve
        Joint prostheses (hip, knee)
    1.6. Assesses medication history
        Antiplatelets
        Aspirin
        Dipyridamole
        Anticoagulants
        Nitrates
        ACE inhibitors
        Digitalis
        Diuretics
        Antidysrhythmics
        Beta blockers
        Calcium channel blockers
        Inotropes
        Antihypertensives
        Immunosuppressants
        Steroids, antiinflammatories
    1.7. Notes diagnostic studies
        Electrocardiogram
        Exercise stress test
        Echocardiogram
        Cardiac catheterization
        Nuclear studies
        Arteriograms
        Pulmonary function studies
        Roentgenograms
    1.8. Reports deviation of laboratory studies
        Complete blood count
        Blood glucose
        Coagulation profile (prothrombin time, partial thromboplastin time, platelets)
        Urinalysis
        BUN, creatinine
        Liver function studies
        Serum enzymes
        Serum lipid levels
        Serum electrolytes
        Arterial blood gases
        Reports blood type (units available, cold antibodies, donor-directed units)
    1.9. Verifies allergies (medications, chemical, food, contact)
    1.10. Assesses cardiovascular status
        Blood pressure(s) (legs and arms, bilaterally)
        Pulse (legs and arms, bilaterally)
        Dysrhythmias
        Presence of monitoring lines
        Edema
        Pain in the chest, arms, shoulders, back, neck, jaw, stomach
        Murmurs
        Fatigue
        Claudication
        Bruits
        Cyanosis
    1.11. Assesses respiratory status
        Respiratory rate
        Intercostal retractions, bulging
        Use of accessory respiratory muscles
        Breath sounds
        Chest tubes
        Shortness of breath, dyspnea, cough
        Prolonged expiration
        Increased anterior/posterior diameter
    1.12. Assesses skin condition
        Previous incisions
        Rashes, bruises
        Skin turgor
        Diaphoresis
        Petechiae
        Temperature
        Skin color
        Nail beds
        Clubbing
        Invasive lines
    1.13. Assesses urinary/renal status
        History of benign prostatic hypertrophy, prostate surgery
        Intake and output
        Serum creatinine and BUN
    1.14. Assesses neuropsychiatric status
        Syncope, dizziness
        Level of consciousness
        Confusion, restlessness
        Numbness, tingling
        Anger
        Anxiety, fear
        Tension, depression
    1.15. Notes weight and height

Modified from AORN: Competency statements in perioperative nursing; standards of perioperative nursing: clinical practice/professional. In AORN: *standards and recommended practices for perioperative nursing,* Denver, 1993, AORN.

1.16. Notes sensory impairments (hearing, vision, tactile)
1.17. Assesses nutritional status
    Weight
    NPO status
1.18. Determines mobility of body parts
    Presence of indwelling catheters
    History and physical
    Medication
1.19. Communicates/documents physical health status

2. Competency to assess the psychosocial health status and psychophysiologic response of the patient
    2.1. Assesses psychosocial cardiovascular risk factors
        Family history
        Stressful life events
        Sedentary living
    2.2. Assesses personal and social factors
        Meals, caffeine intake
        Sleep patterns
        Occupation, activities, hobbies
        Economic status, insurance
        Living arrangements
        Geographic location
        Cultural/spiritual beliefs
        Education
        Basic language
    2.3. Identifies coping mechanisms
        Denial, withdrawal, anger
        Information seeking
    2.4. Identifies support systems
        Family, significant others
        Nurse liaison (preoperative, intraoperative, and postoperative)
        Support groups (The Mended Hearts)
        Counseling/pastoral services
    2.5. Assist significant others with postmortem care
        Prepare body for viewing
        Provide private viewing area
        Respect refusal to see deceased
        Allow mothers/fathers to hold babies/children
        Accompany to chapel or other suitable area
        Refer to appropriate personnel for support/assistance
    2.6. Assesses ability to comply with prescribed therapy
    2.7. Elicits perception of surgery
    2.8. Elicits expectation of care and verifies consent
    2.9. Determines knowledge level of patient
        Diagnosis
        Therapy, surgery
        Postoperative care
        Rehabilitation
    2.10. Communicates/documents psychosocial health status

3. Competency to analyze and interpret health status data in determining nursing diagnoses
    3.1. Analyzes and interprets assessment data
        Selects pertinent data
        Sets priorities for data based on acuity
        Emergent
        Semiemergent
        No acute distress

3.2. Identifies nursing diagnoses/patient problems consistent
    With clinical manifestations
    With human responses to cardiovascular problems
3.3. Validates diagnoses with patient, significant others, and cardiac team members, when possible
3.4. Supports nursing diagnoses with scientific knowledge
    Nursing
    Medical
    Physical sciences
    Social sciences
3.5. Communicates/documents nursing diagnoses to health care team in a manner that facilitates the determination of outcomes and plan of care

Planning
4. Competency to identify expected outcomes unique to the patient
    4.1. Develops outcome statements based on nursing diagnoses and related to needs of cardiac surgery patients in collaboration with patient, significant others, and cardiac team members, when possible
    4.2. Identifies outcomes that are consistent with patient's cardiovascular history and therapeutic interventions
    4.3. Formulates outcomes that are measurable
    4.4. Develops outcomes that provide direction for continuity of care
    4.5. Sets priorities for outcome achievement based on
        Clinical signs
        Laboratory data
        Patient preference, physical capabilities, and behavior patterns
        Human and material resources available to patient
    4.6. Directs interventions to correct, alter, or maintain the nursing diagnoses
    4.7. Communicates and documents outcomes to appropriate persons in retrievable form
5. Competency to develop a plan of care that prescribes nursing actions to achieve patient outcomes
    5.1. Coordinates planned activities with patient, significant others, and cardiac team members
    5.2. Identifies nursing actions in a logical sequence specific to type of surgery
        Coronary bypass grafting
        Valve surgery
        Thoracic aneurysms
        Congenital defects
        Conduction disturbances
        Trauma/emergencies
        Other cardiac conditions
    5.3. Identifies nursing actions to achieve patient outcomes
    5.4. Identifies patient teaching needs to achieve expected outcomes
    5.5. Maintains availability of appropriate sterile equipment, instruments, and supplies
    5.6. Maintains equipment in functional order
    5.7. Coordinates scheduling of elective and emergency cases

5.8. Notifies control desk and team members of possible cases/unstable patients
5.9. Organizes instruments, equipment, and supplies to facilitate rapid and efficient room preparation
5.10. Controls environment to meet patient needs
  Temperature/humidity
  Traffic patterns
  Noise level
5.11. Prepares for potential emergencies
  Certified in CPR
  Follows assigned call schedule
  Maintains backup instruments, supplies, equipment
5.12. Assigns activities to personnel based on
  Qualifications
  Demonstrated competency
  Patient needs
  Availability of personnel
5.13. Communicates/documents patient's plan of care to appropriate personnel in retrievable form

Implementation

6. Competency to implement nursing actions in transferring the patient to the OR according to the prescribed plan
  6.1. Confirms identity of patient
  6.2. Selects personnel for transport depending on need
    Sufficient number
    Patient acuity
  6.3. Determines appropriate and safe method according to need
    Nitroglycerin available
    Transport personnel CPR certified
    Use of monitoring devices as indicated
  6.4. Provides for emotional needs during transfer
    Allows significant others to accompany patient to entrance of cardiac suite
    Used comfort measures and touch
    Greets patient by name and introduces self
  6.5. Communicates/documents patient's transfer
7. Competency to participate in patient and family teaching
  7.1. Identifies teaching/learning needs of cardiac surgical patient and family related to
    Expected sequence of events
    Surgical procedure
    Immediate postoperative events
    Prevention of complications
    Discharge planning
  7.2. Assesses readiness to learn
    Anxiety level
    Acuity level
    Level of consciousness
  7.3. Provides instructions based on identified needs, readiness to learn, and desires of patient and significant others
  7.4. Determines teaching effectiveness
  7.5. Respects patient's use of therapeutic coping strategies
  7.6. Communicates/documents patient/family teaching to provide for continuity of care
8. Competency to create and maintain a sterile field
  8.1. Maintains sterility of bypass lines
  8.2. Confines and contains instruments used in groin

8.3. Maintains sterility while supplying sterile items for procedure
  Heart valves
  Grafts
  Donor organs
  Solutions and supplies
  Other items as needed
8.4. Uses aseptic technique to preclot grafts
8.5. Changes gown and gloves after contamination from
  Team member's back
  Groin procedures
  OR bed elevated or lowered
8.6. Maintains sterility of setup until patient exits OR
8.7. Follows procedure for culturing tissue or solutions per institutional protocol
8.8. Follows procedure for rinsing glutaraldehyde-preserved tissue or valve prostheses per institutional protocol
8.9. Keeps instruments clean of blood and particulate matter during procedure
8.10. Communicates/documents maintenance of sterile field

9. Competency to provide equipment and supplies based on patient needs
  9.1. Ensures equipment is functioning properly before use
    Defibrillator, cords, and paddles
    Fibrillator
    Sternal saw and power source
    Overhead lights
    Headlight and light source
    Autotransfusion system
    Discard suction system
    Electrosurgical equipment
    External pacemaker generator
    OR bed
    Hypothermia/hyperthermia unit
    Refrigerator (for cold solutions)
    Cooling unit (for iced solutions)
    Blood refrigerator
    Blanket warmer
    Positioning equipment
    Other items as requested
  9.2. Operates and maintains equipment (above) according to manufacturer's instructions
  9.3. Selects instruments appropriate to procedure and size of patient in organized and timely manner
    Basic sternotomy
    Coronary artery bypass
    Valve surgery
    Thoracic aneurysm
    Congenital defects
    Conduction disturbances
    Trauma/emergencies
  9.4. Ensures instruments are functioning properly before use
    Vascular clamps
    Retractors
    Forceps
    Scissors and needle holders
  9.5. Anticipates the need for equipment and supplies
    Suture
    Prostheses and sizers
    Patch material (synthetic and biologic)

Medications

Special items per protocol

9.6. Documents lot and serial numbers of all prosthetic implants

9.7. Completes implant documentation forms for patient identification

9.8. Uses supplies judiciously and cost-effectively

As indicated from discussion with surgeon

According to surgeon preference

According to surgical technique

9.9. Ensures emergency equipment and supplies are available at all times

Items checked daily

Replacements/backups available

Replacements ordered promptly

9.10. Follows policy for reporting unsafe medical devices

9.11. Communicates/documents provision of equipment and supplies

10. Competency to account for sponges, "sharps," instruments, and other items as indicated per protocol

10.1. Accounts for sponges, "sharps," instruments

10.2. Accounts for specialty items per protocol

Bulldog clamps

Hypodermic needles

Umbilical tapes

Vessel loops

Rubbershods

Cannulas

Stopcocks

Prosthetic sizers/handles

Other items per policy and procedure

10.3. Communicates/documents results of counts according to institutional protocol

11. Competency to administer drugs and solutions as prescribed

11.1. Identifies drugs and solutions used

Heparin solution

Heparin bolus

Protamine

Papaverine

Calcium chloride

Epinephrine

Antibiotic solution

Cardioplegia solution

Topical cold solutions (normal saline, lactated Ringer's)

Topical hemostatic agents

Antidysrhythmic medications

11.2. Provides medications and solutions at proper temperature per protocol

Cold during induced arrest

Warm before or after induced arrest/when danger of producing fibrillation with cold solutions

11.3. Avoids ice chips in slush or liquid cold topical solutions

11.4. Communicates/documents administration of drugs and solutions

12. Competency to monitor the patient physiologically during surgery

12.1. Monitors physiologic status of patient

Skin color

Temperature (skin, esophageal, rectal, urinary, septal, within bypass lines)

Systemic blood pressure

Mean arterial pressure

Pulmonary artery systolic/diastolic/mean pressures

Pulmonary artery wedge pressure

Central venous pressure

Intracardiac pressure (left atrial, coronary sinus)

Oxygen saturation of arterial hemoglobin

Cardiac output, cardiac index

Electrocardiogram

12.2. Identifies lethal dysrhythmias

Ventricular fibrillation

Ventricular tachycardia

Asystole

12.3. Calculates intake and output

Blood loss, blood salvaged/reinfused

Urinary output

Pericardial effusion

Irrigating solutions

12.4. Assists/monitors behavioral changes preoperatively and during induction of anesthesia

Restlessness

Anxiety

Tenseness

12.5. Initiates nursing actions based on interpretation of physiologic changes

Anxiety-reduction measures

Comfort measures

CPR

Defibrillation

Notification of surgeon, anesthesiologist, perfusionist, and other team members as indicated

12.6. Operates monitoring equipment according to manufacturers' instructions

12.7. Communicates/documents physiologic responses

13. Competency to monitor and control the environment

13.1. Regulates room temperature as indicated

Cool during cardiopulmonary bypass

Warmer before and after bypass (as indicated)

13.2. Communicates with engineering department as necessary to maintain room temperature/humidity

13.3. Regulates hypothermia/hyperthermia unit as indicated

13.4. Implements OR sanitation policies

13.5. Confines and contains contaminated items (e.g., those used in the groin, lung biopsies)

13.6. Properly disposes of waste materials

"Sharps"

Bloody or body fluid–soiled items

Infected material

13.7. Maintains traffic patterns that

Avoid contamination

Provide sufficient space for operative preparation

Facilitate smooth transport of patient to and from OR

13.8. Avoids pressure on body parts from heavy instruments or leaning on patient

13.9. Follows policy for observers in OR (or in a special viewing area): number, purpose, etc.

13.10. Communicates/documents environmental controls

14. Competency to implement nursing actions in transferring the patient to the SICU according to the prescribed plan.
    14.1. Reports patient status to SICU prior to patient's leaving OR; includes
        Patient's name
        Procedure (bypass grafts, valves, grafts, etc)
        Difficulties associated with operative procedure (poor-quality saphenous vein, small aortic root, etc.)
        Weight, height
        Allergies
        Location of central and peripheral lines
        Intraoperative problems
            Excessive blood loss
            Dysrhythmias
            Blood pressure
            Difficulty cardioverting/defibrillating
            Bypass problems
        Blood/blood products (given and available)
        Urinary output
        Medications: used and required, dosage, route
            Nitroprusside
            Dopamine
            Dobutamine
            Nitroglycerin
            Lidocaine
            Additional medications
        Tubes, drains, catheters
        Temporary pacing leads
            Atrial
            Ventricular
        Most recent electrolyte levels
            Potassium
            Sodium
        Patient problems/concerns
        Notification of family members of patient's status
        Pertinent past medical history
        Pertinent past psychosocial history
    14.2. Selects personnel for transport based on patient acuity and staff needs
    14.3. Transports remaining blood/blood products to SICU (or blood bank) as indicated by hospital policy
    14.4. Ensures patient safety, privacy, and dignity during transport
    14.5. Verifies SICU bed is ready for transport
        Properly made
        Warming blanket applied
        X-ray cassette applied (if requested)
        Sufficient oxygen in portable tank
        Transport monitor
        Defibrillator
    14.6. Covers patient with warm blankets
    14.7. Accompanies patient to SICU with anesthesia and surgical staff (per protocol)
    14.8. Communicates physiologic and psychosocial data relevant to discharge planning to SICU staff and documents in perioperative records
    14.9. Assesses patient's physiologic stability prior to departing for SICU
15. Competency to respect the patient's rights
    15.1. Demonstrates consideration of patient's rights
        American Nurses' Association: *Code for Nurses*
        American Hospital Association: *A Patient's Bill of Rights*
    15.2. Provides privacy through confidentiality and physical protection
    15.3. Identifies cultural and spiritual beliefs
        Attitudes toward blood transfusions
        Heart as "seat of the soul"
        Family support
        Expressions of fear/anxiety
        Desire for religious counseling
    15.4. Communicates/documents respect for patient's rights

Evaluation

16. Competency to perform nursing actions that demonstrate professional accountability
    16.1. Completes an orientation based on individualized learning needs
    16.2. Remains current with newer trends in
        Cardiovascular technology
        Nursing/medical research
        Patient care practices
    16.3. Demonstrates flexibility and adaptability to changes in patient's status
    16.4. Demonstrates tact and understanding when dealing with the public, patients, and staff
    16.5. Communicates appropriate information to team members and representatives of other departments
    16.6. Seeks new learning opportunities for personal and professional development
    16.7. Promotes nursing research and incorporates research findings in practice
    16.8. Bases judgments and decisions on knowledge, skill, and experience
    16.9. Fosters professional growth of team members, peers, colleagues, and others
    16.10. Practices within ethical and legal guidelines
    16.11. Participates in self-evaluation and peer review
    16.12. Seeks and provides constructive feedback
    16.13. Demonstrates accountability for maintaining competency as a cardiac team member
    16.14. Seeks assistance when needed
    16.15. Fosters collaborative working relationships in delivery of patient care
    16.16. Considers factors related to efficient and effective use of human and material resources
    16.17. Communicates/documents nursing accountability
17. Competency to evaluate patient outcomes
    17.1. Develops criteria for outcome measurement
    17.2. Measures outcome achievement in collaboration with patient, significant others, and cardiac team members, when possible
    17.3. Evaluates patient responses to nursing interventions
    17.4. Communicates/documents degree of goal achievement as appropriate to promote continuity of care
18. Competency to measure effectiveness of nursing care
    18.1. Establishes criteria to measure quality of nursing care through a systematic quality assessment/improvement process

18.2. Evaluates practice in context of standards of clinical practice and professional performance, and relevant statutes and regulations, including but not limited to

AORN: *Standards and Recommended Practices for Perioperative Nursing*

American Nurses' Association and American Heart Association Council on Cardiovascular Nursing: *Standards of Cardiovascular Nursing Practice*

JCAHO standards

Other standards relevant to care of patients undergoing cardiac surgery

18.3. Assesses patient postoperatively

18.4. Evaluates effectiveness of nursing actions in relation to desired patient outcomes

18.5. Communicates/documents results of nursing care

19. Competency to reassess continuously all components of patient care based on new data

19.1. Reassesses physiologic and psychosocial health status

19.2. Revises nursing diagnoses based on changes in health status

19.3. Reestablishes outcomes based on changes in signs and symptoms/laboratory data/patient preferences

19.4. Revises plan of care to reflect changes in priorities

19.5. Implements revised plan of care

19.6. Reevaluates patient outcomes and outcome criteria

19.7. Communicates/documents process of reassessment

Abbreviations

ACE (inhibitor) Angiotensin-converting enzyme
AORN Association of Operating Room Nurses
BUN Blood urea nitrogen
CHF Congestive heart failure
CPR Cardiopulmonary resuscitation
JCAHO Joint Commission on Accreditation of Healthcare Organizations
MI Myocardial infarction
NPO Nothing by mouth
OR Operating room
SICU Surgical intensive care unit
TIA Transient ischemic attack

APPENDIX C
"What If?" Simulations and Decision-Making Exercises

SITUATION 1 The surgeon is about to split the sternum, and the saw will not work.

QUESTIONS TO ASK:

Was the saw power source connected?

Was the saw put together correctly?

Is there a procedure for testing the saw before use?

Is there a sterile backup saw available?

What other resources are available in the operating room?

SITUATION 2 The patient, recently transported to the surgical intensive care unit (SICU), has just arrested.

QUESTIONS TO ASK:

What are the responsibilities of the cardiac OR staff?

What supplies and instruments are available in the SICU?

How would you best set up for an emergency sternotomy?

What supplies and instruments need to be brought from the OR?

How are nursing roles and responsibilities differentiated?

What information needs to be communicated to the OR? To the blood bank?

SITUATION 3 You are preparing for a repair of an atrial septal defect. You notice that the anesthesiologist is getting ready to insert a pulmonary artery catheter.

QUESTIONS TO ASK:

Where will the surgical site be located in the heart?

Why might a pulmonary artery catheter not be inserted in a patient with a right-sided lesion?

What technical difficulties would be associated with the presence of the catheter?

Why might a pulmonary artery catheter be indicated?

Could the placement of the catheter be adjusted?

Could the catheter be inserted postoperatively?

SITUATION 4 You are visiting a patient preoperatively, and the family starts to ask you questions about the surgery (including how long it will last; if the surgeon is competent).

QUESTIONS TO ASK:

What is it that the patient and family want to know?

Are you qualified (legally and professionally) to answer their questions?

What should you do if you are unable to answer their questions? Whom would you contact?

What can you do to reduce their level of anxiety?

SITUATION 5 While you are assisting the surgeon in incising the pericardium near the innominate vein, there is sudden, copious bleeding.

QUESTIONS TO ASK:

What do you do first?

What aspects of the situation are pertinent?

Does it make a difference who the surgeon is?

Are there surgeon's preferences that would dictate your response? Are there universally accepted responses that you could rely on?

Could you have done anything differently to lessen the possibility of cutting a blood vessel?

REFERENCES

American Nurses' Association and American Heart Association Council on Cardiovascular Nursing: *Standards of cardiovascular nursing practice,* Kansas City, Mo, 1981, ANA.

Association of Operating Room Nurses: *Core curriculum for the RN first assistant,* Denver, 1990, AORN.

Association of Operating Room Nurses: *Standards and recommended practices for perioperative nursing,* Denver, 1993, AORN.

Benner P: From novice to expert, *Am J Nurs* 82(3):402, 1982.

Benner P: *From novice to expert,* Menlo Park, Calif, 1984, Addison-Wesley.

Bryne B: Skill acquisition: students in the OR, *AORN J* 43(6):1312, 1986.

Rothrock JC: *Perioperative nursing care planning,* St Louis, 1990, Mosby.

Urden LD: Knowledge development in clinical practice, *J Contin Educ Nurs* 20(1):18, 1989.

3

The Cardiac Team

Success in cardiac surgery depends on a team effort.

Denton A. Cooley, MD, 1984, (p. 1)

Cardiac surgery typifies the team concept as does no other surgical specialty. Complex technologic resources, distinctive patient problems, and, frequently, sudden and life-threatening physiologic alterations require that individual efforts be integrated efficiently and effectively into a unified plan of action.

DEVELOPMENT OF THE TEAM

A team is more than a collection of people. It is a cohesive group of individuals whose personal and professional goals are congruent with the overall goal of the service (Sullivan and Decker, 1985): to achieve optimal patient outcomes by providing knowledgeable and skilled care in a safe and therapeutic environment to patients with cardiovascular disease. Among individual team members, goals may include meeting the challenges presented by these patients, being rewarded for performance, and receiving recognition for contributions to patient care.

The qualities that are sought in prospective team members reflect the values of the service and the organization (Box 3-1). The ability to function within the group depends not only on knowledge and skill, but also on qualities such as flexibility, dedication, a sense of humor, and the ability to reset or modify priorities.

Integrating individual and team goals is achieved through a process that fosters camaraderie among group members. It is influenced by frequent interaction, interesting work, effective communication, a history of success, high performance standards, team members' knowledge and experience, and support and encouragement from group leaders (Uliss, 1991).

As a result of the ego strength derived from clinical competence, team members are often highly motivated and possess strong characters. Such personal qualities lend themselves to environments where independent thinking is encouraged. A structured environment is suitable during the formative stages of a cardiac program, but decentralized units provide a more appropriate forum for the problem solving and decision making required in an established cardiac surgical service. Communication must be open and information shared freely if team members are to be able to make appropriate decisions and resolve problems individually and collectively.

TEAM MEMBERS

The core of a cardiac service consists of nurses, surgeons, surgical assistants, anesthesiologists, anes-

---

Box 3-1 Comments about the members of a cardiac team

Dena Houchin, RN
Texas Heart Institute
Houston, Texas

Whether interviewing nurses, prospective residents, or clerical staff, we favor those with a positive attitude, an appreciation for quality, and a respect for loyalty. We search for those who want to be part of an upbeat, progressive program. The tempo is fast and demanding, and a solid work ethic is essential. If these performance traits are present, clinical knowledge and skills can be imparted successfully.

We look for chemistry that enables colleagues to maximize their skills, making the outcome greater than the aggregate. Among our nurses, one is a workhorse who makes the best juggler look boring! Another offers "TLC" in a warm, reassuring manner second to none. A third has that snappy repartee that keeps everyone grinning with anticipation. Each one joined our service with good, though not exceptional, cardiovascular knowledge. Within their first year, each became invaluable to the service. As you might expect, turnover among these positions is rare.

thetists, and perfusionists. (Nursing roles are discussed in more detail in Chapter 2.) Assistive personnel such as surgical technicians, as well as support staff such as aides and orderlies, perform many vital functions and should also be considered cardiac team members.

The surgical staff is represented by the attending cardiac surgeon, who has received extensive training in cardiac procedures. Cardiac training programs often have a uniquely characteristic philosophy and methodology that is transmitted to the surgeon-in-training. Familiarity with that training offers useful insights into preferences for instruments and supplies, perceptions about roles and functions of team members, and procedural considerations, such as cannulation for bypass and anastomotic techniques. Discussing aspects of the service with the surgeon, as well as contacting a colleague from the surgeon's "alma mater," can be very helpful to nurses who are establishing a new service or preparing for the arrival of an additional member of the surgical staff.

Depending on the nature of the institution, another surgeon may perform first-assisting duties. Fellows, residents, and medical students are often involved in university training programs. In some hospitals surgical (physicians') assistants and/or RN first assistants (RNFAs), employed by the surgeon or the hospital, or self-employed, provide assistance during, before, and after the procedure.

Anesthesiologists and certified registered nurse anesthetists provide relief from pain, monitor patient functions, and create safe operative conditions for the patient. Cardiovascular anesthesiologists have specialized knowledge of the circulatory dynamics of the patient with cardiac disease. They may serve as teachers for anesthesia students.

Perfusionists are technologists who are specially trained in the use of extracorporeal circulation. They run the cardiopulmonary bypass machine (the "pump"), which oxygenates returning venous blood and pumps it back into the arterial system. They may have additional responsibilities related to the intraaortic balloon pump and other ventricular support devices.

Where available, cardiopulmonary technologists assist the perfusionist and the anesthesiologist by performing intraoperative laboratory analyses of blood gas levels, electrolyte levels, bleeding times, and heparin concentration levels. They may also aid with hemodynamic monitoring by preparing systems for intravascular venous and arterial pressure measurements.

Within the immediate surgical environment, supportive staff may have tasks delegated to them by anesthesia or nursing personnel for the preparation, maintenance, and cleaning of equipment, instruments, and supplies. Surgical technicians perform scrub role duties. Environmental service employees help with the rapid room turnovers required for emergency cases and perform terminal, as well as routine, cleaning duties.

Because many cardiac services operate under a separate budget, supply coordinators enhance inventory control by keeping track of the numerous items used during surgery. When such a position is unavailable, responsibility for these items is often divided among nursing team members.

The cardiac team can also be thought of on a more global scale. In addition to the surgical team members are the staff of the nursing units caring for patients before and after surgery, cardiologists and other referring physicians, and members of other departments, such as the pathology laboratory, the blood bank, the cardiac catheterization and electrophysiology laboratories, the noninvasive diagnostic laboratories, the pharmacy, and the respiratory therapy, radiology, and cardiac rehabilitation departments.

Cardiac surgery places demands on practically every department within a hospital. Political sensitivity and group process skills facilitate productive interdepartmental and interdisciplinary relationships.

STRESS AND STRESS REDUCTION WITHIN THE CARDIAC TEAM

A cardiac service is stressful, and for many this provides an opportunity to excel. (It is not difficult to understand why some describe the cardiac team as "type A's working on type A's"—alluding to the compulsive and competitive qualities ascribed by Friedman [1969] to coronary-prone personalities.)

There are times, however, when challenges may become burdens. Cardiac procedures routinely last longer than 3 hours and may be especially prolonged in complex cases. It should not be surprising that disharmony appears occasionally.

Considerable literature is devoted to the causes of stress and its effects in the workplace. Stress factors pertaining to cardiac surgery in particular are related to the work environment, equipment and material resources, patient factors, and staff dynamics.

Work Environment

Weinger and Englund (1990), who studied anesthesia performance, described a number of stressful factors affecting surgical team members that are applicable to a cardiac service. Among the most stressful were noise level, temperature and humidity, ambient lighting, and the arrangement of equipment and furniture.

Noise levels tend to be prolonged and loud, given the combined sounds of the bypass machine, electrosurgical units, physiologic monitors, light sources, suction equipment, autotransfusion systems, and sternal saws. In settings with similar noise levels, short-term memory losses and distractions during critical periods were noted (Weinger and Englund, 1990). The effect of background music is variable. Music with a quick tempo and strong percussion may increase tension, whereas slower tempos and more melodic rhythms may enhance performance and reduce anxiety (Kaempf and Amodei, 1989; Moss, 1985).

Adjustments to ambient temperature levels are common. It is not unusual to have thermostats set at 55° F (12° C) for most adult and pediatric procedures to conserve patient energy resources. During rewarming of the patient, room temperatures may be increased. Radiant heaters are sometimes used to provide additional heat. Extremes in temperature can produce an increase in errors, according to Weinger and Englund (1990). When indicated, room temperatures can be adjusted up or down to achieve a more comfortable level. Low humidity can also be a problem, leading to dehydration when access to fluids is limited.

Illumination of the surgical field requiring up to 20,000 lux can produce uncomfortable glare (Weinger and Englund, 1990). Excess lighting (e.g., continued illumination of the leg after the saphenous vein has been excised) may cause discomfort.

The arrangement of equipment and furniture may present a problem, especially in a small operating room (OR). The array of machines is staggering when one considers the routine and specialized equipment required, such as the defibrillator, the intraaortic balloon pump, and supply carts for anesthesia, perfusion, and nursing needs. On occasion, additional equipment is needed for electrophysiology studies or transesophageal echocardiography. (And if there is an incorrect count, room must be made for the portable x-ray machine!) Moreover, storage space is often inadequate, necessitating creativity in the arrangement of supplies. Throughout the procedure the circulating nurse is responsible for using and repositioning many of these items; this can be a source of frustration in a confined work area and may increase the risk of infection.

Storage problems may be improved with the use of exchange carts, which obviate the need for maintaining the entire inventory in the cardiac suite. Custom packs (see Chapter 5) save shelf space and reduce the need for excess inventory; they also save time that would be needed for opening numerous individual supplies (especially beneficial during emergencies), and they reduce the number of lost charges by consolidating multiple items.

Although one may have little control over many of these factors (and adapt remarkably well), there are methods to reduce stress that combine relaxation techniques, regular physical exercise, and sound nutritional habits (Moss, 1985). A physical technique to alleviate tension is alternative tensing and relaxing of muscles; autogenic relaxation is a mental exercise that enables the nurse to imagine pleasant feelings or situations. Rhythmic breathing can also have a calming effect.

Equipment and Material Resources

Nonfunctioning equipment, lost or unavailable instruments and supplies, and dirty equipment have been identified as major stressors in the OR (Moss, 1989). Nurses have recounted anxiety-producing sit-

uations such as a sternal saw or a defibrillator that would not operate (and with no replacement available). As the array of cardiovascular products increases, nurses are faced with the prospect of maintaining an increasing inventory of equipment and supplies.

Thorough cleaning and careful checking of instruments before surgery, along with a regular maintenance program for equipment, will avoid many problems, but unexpected events may still occur. There should be at least two basic sternotomy sets that will enable the surgeon to open the chest and place the patient on cardiopulmonary bypass. Individually wrapped sterile instruments can provide immediate replacements. Backup equipment should be available for critical items such as bypass machines, defibrillators, saws, and electrosurgical units. Even new programs with small caseloads cannot afford to rely on a single sternal saw or defibrillator. Backup units should be available on the unit. The same-model defibrillator may be available on another nursing unit; receiving prior permission from that unit's department head will help facilitate borrowing the machine if the need arises. A list of similar-model defibrillators throughout the hospital can be helpful, but the perioperative nurse must confirm that the defibrillator is compatible with the internal paddles used in the OR. Internal paddles will not function in a dissimilar defibrillator.

Borrowing critical items such as a valve or graft prosthesis may be necessary when the supply of a particular-size prosthesis has been depleted unexpectedly. Establishing a collaborative network with nurses in other institutions can form the basis for a mutually beneficial system of borrowing (and loaning) needed items for emergencies. Perfusionists also may be able to rely on colleagues in other institutions, or on manufacturers, to provide immediate repair or replacement of critical devices.

System flaws related to equipment may jeopardize patient outcomes. Not infrequently, patients present emergently. Patients requiring immediate surgical intervention, whether because of a failed percutaneous transluminal coronary angioplasty (PTCA), acute dissecting aneurysm, or postoperative hemorrhage, need a cardiac team that can be ready within minutes. The stress of such urgency can be unnecessarily aggravated by delays in notification, nonfunctioning beepers, inadequate room preparation, and missing instruments or supplies. Problems in alerting team members for emergency procedures should be resolved expeditiously by the cardiac manager and the department head responsible for notification of on-call personnel.

Adequate room preparation (with no missing supplies or instruments) is a team responsibility and an individual obligation. Because emergencies are not uncommon, it is helpful at the conclusion of scheduled procedures to have the room cleaned and fully stocked with sterile items that are ready to be opened. After a long and strenuous day, when staff have been working beyond their scheduled shift time, it is understandable that they would want to leave. However, when called for an emergency, the staff will appreciate having the OR clean and ready for another case with suction setup and sterile instruments, supplies, and other items available. The patient should not have to wait unnecessarily for a room to be cleaned and prepared.

Patient Factors

Patient factors may be among the most stressful: patients die. Ranging in age from a few hours to 90 years old, cardiac surgery patients are at greater risk for complications because of the underlying severity of most heart conditions requiring surgery. The nurse and other team members often must deal with feelings of powerlessness or loss, and it is normal to reflect on one's performance and its effect, if any, on the final outcome.

Moral conflicts may add to the personal suffering felt by nurses in association with caring for dying patients and their families when one must balance obligations to others with obligations to one's self. Clarifying these obligations with a counselor or an ethics consultant and turning to a compassionate listener or other support systems may assist the nurse in dealing with these situations (Rushton, 1992).

Other patient-related factors include the potential for transmission of blood-borne diseases, such as hepatitis and the human immunodeficiency virus (HIV). Strict adherence to universal precautions and the standards set by the Occupational Safety and Health Administration (OSHA, 1991) and the Association of Operating Room Nurses (1992) helps to minimize the risk to both patients and health care workers. Additional methods to reduce exposure to patients and health care workers continue to be investigated. Fernsebner (Schlepp, 1989) and Pate (1990) have offered suggestions to decrease occupational exposure: greater use of disposable scalpels and electrosurgical units for incising and dissecting tissue, disposable containers for sharp items in all ORs, impervious gowns, better gloves, modifications in the design of surgical instruments, and more self-defensive surgical techniques.

Many of these patient-related issues may produce ethical dilemmas concerning patient rights and staff rights, just and equitable distribution of technologic resources and organs for transplantation, end-of-life considerations, noncompliance with "do not resuscitate" orders, informed consent, and interventions that benefit or potentially harm the patient. These issues are becoming more complex with the enactment of state and federal laws that often apply to cardiac surgery patients. Among these are The Patient Self-Determination Act of 1990 and the Uniform Anatomical Gift Act (Commissioners on Uniform State Laws, 1987; Sadler, Sadler, and Stason, 1968). The former was enacted to ensure that patients are informed of their right to consent or refuse treatment and to make their wishes known through advance directives. These are instructions concerning what course of treatment they would desire should they become incompetent or should their condition become terminal. The most common forms of advance directives are the Living Will and the Durable Power of Attorney for Health Care (McKenzie, 1989). AORN's (1993) explication of nursing's code of ethics can provide guidance to perioperative nurses.

The Uniform Anatomical Gift Act, revised in 1987, enables the next of kin of expired patients to consider organ, tissue, and eye donation. State and federal laws require that family members be offered the option of making such a donation. The act also makes anatomic gifts by the donor before death irrevocable; consent of the family is not required after the death of the donor (Hawke, Kraft, and Smith, 1990).

Staff Dynamics

Mariano (1989) has described problems associated with interdisciplinary collaboration. Teams composed of highly diverse, skilled professionals may be hindered in accomplishing their functions by four factors: goal conflicts, role conflicts, problems with decision making, and problems with interpersonal communication.

Goals

Although the main goal of a cardiac team is to provide quality care to patients, individual and group goals contribute to this. Among these goals are task and maintenance goals, short- and long-term goals, and client, professional, and organizational goals. Conflict can arise when goals are not clearly specified or when team members' perceptions of the goals and their achievement are incongruent. Often these differences are related to dissimilar philosophic, religious, or professional values.

Clear identification of goals, assessment of individuals perceptions about desired goals, consensus regarding which goals are most important, and unity on actions to be taken are some of the things that can foster a less divisive environment (Mariano, 1989).

Roles

Disagreement about role performance can exist between nurses, physicians, and other team members, as well as among nurses themselves (Chaska, 1990). In the cardiac arena this may be compounded by the presence of physician assistants (PAs) and perfusionists—all highly trained professionals. Often there is an overlapping of roles. For example, first-assisting duties may be performed by other surgeons, by PAs, or by RNFAs. The scrub role may be fulfilled by a surgical technician or a registered nurse (RN). Differing expectations of persons performing within the same role can produce ambiguity, frustration, and distrust. This may be aggravated by inequalities in reward systems (monetary or nonmonetary), recognition of performance, little opportunity for career growth, and varying degrees of autonomy, responsibility, and accountability.

Methods to reduce role conflicts focus on clarifying role perceptions and expectations, identifying members' professional competencies, exploring overlapping responsibilities, and possibly renegotiating role assignments (Mariano, 1989). Position descriptions and competency-based evaluations can help reduce role ambiguity and provide objectivity. Persons responsible for assigning their respective staffs, such as nurses or PAs, should jointly discuss staffing needs on a case-by-case basis or through a mutually agreed-on schedule. Flexibility and cooperation promote collaborative working relationships that enhance professional harmony and improve team function (Seifert, 1993).

Emergencies are often good examples of flexibility: PAs, perfusionists, or anesthesia personnel can assist the circulating nurse or the RNFA in preparing the patient for surgery or in elevating the legs of a patient requiring vein harvest for a coronary artery bypass procedure. Nurses can assist in procuring medications or assisting with endotracheal intubation.

It is evident from research on collaborative practice models that a solid knowledge base in one's discipline and an appreciation of the knowledge and skills required in others' disciplines offer a strong foundation for effective interdisciplinary working relationships. In a cardiac service, as in other specialized services, there is a large overlapping knowledge base from which all members can draw. The depth and scope of that knowledge may vary, and its application to practice may distinguish one discipline from another, but the concepts are mutually understood. Consider the concept of balancing myocardial oxygen supply and demand and how implementing that goal is interpreted by different disciplines. Anesthesia staff engage in the pharmacologic manipulation of intravascular pressures and resistances; perfusionists prepare and infuse cardioplegia solutions that preserve and protect myocardial function; nurses employ anxiety-reducing measures that diminish endogenous catecholamine release; surgeons use techniques that minimize cross-clamp time. These interventions all aim at optimizing the balance between oxygen supply and demand.

Decision making

Achieving successful outcomes is hampered if problems are not clearly identified or if team members' roles in the decision-making process are poorly defined. Consensus is achieved, not by unanimity, but by providing an opportunity for all members to participate, based on sufficient and relevant data, discussion of alternatives, commitment to action, and mutual respect for all members' contributions (Mariano, 1989).

Such a process may not be appropriate during an emergency situation; but neither can the resolution of emergencies be entirely satisfactory if consensus building has not already been established as a team value. A patient with a life-threatening problem is more likely to have a successful outcome when team members are sure of their roles, individual strengths are promoted, their knowledge base is secure, and appropriate interventions are implemented.

The cultural norms of the group will promote or hinder joint problem solving. In teams where nursing managers and staff freely discuss problems and possible solutions, a favorable climate is likely to exist. Nurses in such an atmosphere are more comfortable discussing treatment alternatives with physician colleagues. One's understanding of the rationales for treatment can be enhanced by attending cardiac catheterization conferences, surgical grand rounds, or critical care meetings. Insight into why a surgeon makes a certain patient care decision is invaluable in preparing for an operative procedure. One is better able to anticipate the needs of both the surgeon and the patient if one is aware of the options a surgeon is likely to consider. What are the individual surgeon's indications for selecting a particular valve prosthesis? For returning a patient to the OR for mediastinal exploration? For inserting a ventricular assist device? By better understanding the surgeon's decision-making process, the nurse becomes more capable of anticipating the most likely options and preparing for them. Similarly, nurses can plan and jointly implement care with anesthesia personnel based on a knowledge of preferred vasoactive medications, the sequence of inserting central pressure lines and endotracheal tubes, and the transportation of patients to postoperative care units.

Surgeons, anesthesiologists, and other team members can be made aware of issues of importance to nurses and be made aware of the need to coordinate and integrate the elements of the service. For example, nurses who include a psychosocial assessment of the patient often obtain information crucial to the successful outcome of the procedure. They may discover that for a particular patient, the optimal placement of a pacemaker generator is the abdomen rather than the chest wall, or that geographic location may preclude insertion of a valve prosthesis requiring follow-up laboratory testing for anticoagulation-related bleeding times. This process also enables patients to participate in the decision-making process affecting their care.

Communication

Communication between the clinical staff fosters continuity of patient care. It is also the vehicle for reassessing and redefining how the team functions. It is necessary for the reappraisal process that includes improving knowledge and skill, engaging in frank self-evaluation, and offering constructive and issue-oriented criticism. Team members communicate by speaking and listening, negotiating, and expressing opinions and feelings without recrimination (Mariano, 1989).

Forums for communication may be formal or informal. Committees may be organized to discuss problems on a regular basis. Informal meetings between two or more people can be held as the need arises. Interpersonal problems are best handled by those involved. Managers should intervene only when a resolution cannot be found and the ongoing antagonisms affect team function and patient care. Managers should not attempt to force mutual admiration, but they do have a duty to ensure fair treatment of staff, to communicate acceptable levels of performance by team members, to offer unit orientations and continuing education, and to provide the resources necessary for the nurse to practice effectively and efficiently.

CONCLUSION

Cardiac surgery is a team process that reflects a comprehensive approach to patient care. Problems affecting performance can be resolved through communication and strategies that foster participation by all members of the team.

REFERENCES

Association of Operating Room Nurses: ANA code for nurses with interpretive statements—explications for perioperative nursing, AORN J 58(2):369, 1993.

Association of Operating Room Nurses: Revised statement on the patient and health care workers with human immunodeficiency virus (HIV) and other blood borne diseases, AORN J 55(1):52, 1992.

Chaska NL: *The nursing profession: turning points*, St Louis, 1990, Mosby.

Commissioners on Uniform State Laws: *Uniform Anatomical Gift Act of 1987*. National Conference of Commissioners on Uniform State Laws, Newport Beach, Calif, July 1987.

Cooley DA: *Techniques in cardiac surgery*, ed 2, Philadelphia, 1984, WB Saunders.

Friedman M: *Pathogenesis of coronary artery disease*, New York, 1969, McGraw-Hill.

Hawke D, Kraft J, Smith SL: Tissue and organ donation and recovery. In Smith SL: *AACN tissue and organ transplantation: implications for professional nursing practice*, St Louis, 1990, Mosby.

Kaempf G, Amodei ME: The effect of music on anxiety, AORN J 50(1):112, 1989.

Mariano C: The case for interdisciplinary collaboration, Nurs Outlook 37(6):285, 1989.

McKenzie CL: The ethics of advance directives: what every nurse needs to know, Va Nurse 57(1):18, 1989.

Moss VA: Stress and the OR nurse, Surg Rounds, p 108, Sept 1985.

Moss VA: Burnout: symptoms, causes, prevention, AORN J 50(5):1071, 1989.

OSHA (Occupational Safety and Health Administration, Department of Labor): Final rule: occupational exposure to bloodborne pathogens, 19 CFR Part 1910.1030, Federal Register, pp 64004-64182, Dec 6, 1991.

Pate JW: Risks of blood exposure to the cardiac surgical team, Ann Thorac Surg 50:248, 1990.

Patient Self-Determination Act; Omnibus Budget Reconciliation Act of 1990, Title IV, Section 4602, Congressional Record, 136, H12456-H12457, Oct 26, 1990.

Rushton CH: Care-giver suffering in critical care nursing, Heart Lung 21(3):303, 1992.

Sadler AM, Sadler BL, Stason EB: The uniform anatomical gift act: a model for reform, JAMA 206:2501, 1968.

Schlepp S: AORN participates in hearing on blood borne diseases, AORN J 50(6):1264, 1989 (legislation column).

Seifert PC: Collaborative practice and the R.N. first assistant. In Rothrock JC: The *R.N. first assistant: an expanded perioperative nursing role*, ed 2, Philadelphia, 1993, JB Lippincott.

Sullivan EJ, Decker PJ: *Effective management in nursing*, Menlo Park, Calif, 1985, Addison-Wesley.

Uliss D: What leadership style best suits critical care nurses? Nurs Manage 22(6):56D, 1991.

Weinger MB, Englund CE: Ergonomic and human factors affecting anesthetic vigilance and monitoring performance in the operating room environment, Anesthesiology 73:995, 1990.

4

Anatomy and Physiology

. . . The motion of the heart is as follows: first of all, the auricle contracts, and . . . throws the blood . . . into the ventricle, which, being filled, the heart raises itself straightway, makes all its fibres tense, contracts the ventricles, and performs a beat, by which beat it immediately sends the blood supplied to it by the auricles into the arteries . . .

William Harvey, 1628*

LOCATION OF THE HEART

The heart and the origins of the great vessels are commonly approached through a median sternotomy incision (Fig. 4-1). The sternum consists of three parts: the bony **manubrium** and **sternal body** attaching at the second costal cartilage (angle of Louis), and the cartilaginous **xiphoid process** (Fig. 4-2). The superior edge of the sternum is known as the **suprasternal notch.** Coursing behind and parallel to the lateral border of the sternum are the right and left **internal mammary** (thoracic) **arteries,** which can be used as conduits during coronary revascularization procedures.

Pericardium

When the sternum is divided, it exposes the **pericardial sac,** which is situated within the middle portion of the mediastinal compartment of the thorax. The pericardium is fused inferiorly to the central tendon of the diaphragm, partially overlapped laterally by the lungs in their pleural sacs, and protected anteriorly by the sternum and the costal cartilages of the third, fourth, and fifth ribs. Behind the pericardium are the esophagus, posterior mediastinum, descending aorta, and vertebral column.

The pericardium consists of serous and fibrous layers (Fig. 4-3). The **visceral pericardium** is a serous layer that is closely adherent to the outer surface of the heart. It extends superiorly onto the great vessels, where it is reflected forward to form the **parietal peri-**

cardium, which fuses to the fibrous pericardial wall. The area between the visceral and parietal serous layers, the pericardial cavity, contains about 50 ml of clear, thin, lubricating fluid that enables the heart to move freely within the space (Hurst, 1988). Adhesions from prior surgery or inflammatory processes can produce thickening of the pericardium or obliteration of the cavity, which, in extreme cases, may constrict the ventricles and impair diastolic filling. When the pericardium is incised during surgery, care is taken to avoid the underlying structures, which include the innominate vein, ascending aorta, proximal pulmonary artery, and right ventricle.

Running vertically along the lateral pericardium are the right and left **phrenic nerves,** which innervate the diaphragm. Identifying these nerves is important for protecting the diaphragm during procedures in which the lateral pericardium is incised or excised.

SIZE AND POSITION OF THE HEART

The heart itself is about the size of a person's fist. Depending on the age, sex, height, nutritional status, and amount of epicardial fat, the weight of the heart is variable, but in the average man it is about 325 g, and in the average woman, it is about 275 g (Schlant, Siverman, and Roberts, 1990).

The cardiac wall is composed of three layers (see Fig. 4-3). The outermost layer is the **epicardium** (visceral pericardium); the **myocardium** is the functional muscular layer; and the innermost layer, the **endocardium,** covers the inside of the cardiac chambers and is continuous with the lining of the blood vessels.

Approximately two thirds of the heart is to the left of the midline. It is tilted forward and to the left with

---

On the Motion of the Heart and Blood. Cited in Clendening (1942, p. 161).

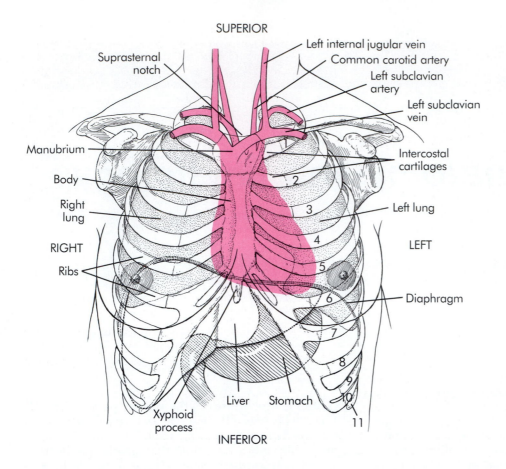

Fig. 4-1 Location of the heart. (Drawing by Peter Stone.)

Fig. 4-2 **Lateral view of the pericardium within the mediastinum.** (Drawing by Peter Stone.)

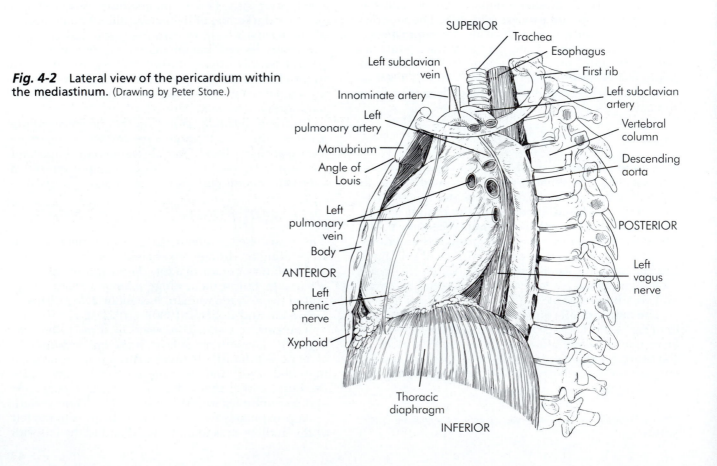

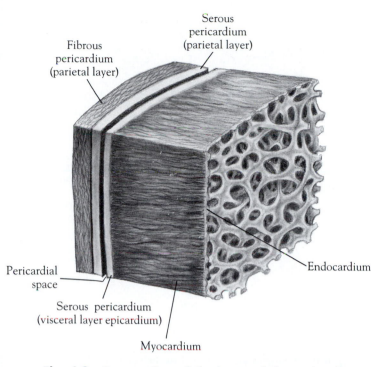

Fibrous
pericardium
(parietal layer)

Serous
pericardium
(parietal layer)

Endocardium

Pericardial
space

Serous pericardium
(visceral layer epicardium)

Myocardium

Fig. 4-3 Cross section of the layers of the pericardium and the heart (epicardium, myocardium, and endocardium). (From Thompson JM and others: *Mosby's clinical nursing,* ed 3, St Louis, 1993, Mosby.)

the **apex,** the lower tip of the left ventricle, anterior to the rest of the heart (Fig. 4-4). The apex is located in the fifth intercostal interspace, about 3½ inches from the left sternal border. From the front, one sees the right ventricle in the center with the aorta and the pulmonary artery above it; the superior vena cava, right atrium, and atrial appendage on the right; and a sliver of the left ventricle on the left with the tip of the left atrial appendage high on the left heart border. Thus the right ventricle lies anteriorly, and the greater portion of the left ventricle is situated posteriorly. When the cardiac silhouette is viewed on a chest x-ray film, the right cardiac border is formed by the right atrium, the inferior border is formed by the right ventricle, and the left border is almost entirely formed by the apex of the left ventricle (Fig. 4-5).

The **base,** or upper portion, of the heart is fixed by attachment of the right and left atria to the superior and inferior venae cavae, and the pulmonary veins, respectively (Fig. 4-6). The outflow portion of the right ventricle is attached superiorly to the pulmonary artery, and the outflow tract of the left ventricle is connected to the aorta. The apex is free, which enables the surgeon to elevate the heart for surgical exposure.

Fig. 4-4 Pericardium open to expose the heart and roots of the great vessels. (Drawing by Peter Stone.)

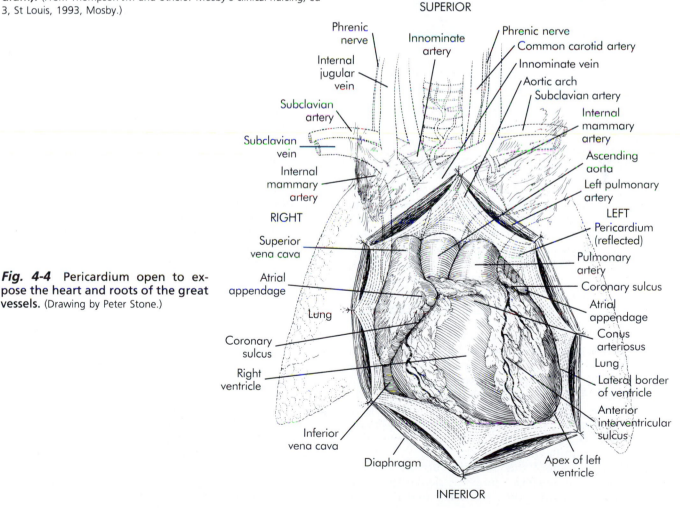

SUPERIOR

Phrenic nerve

Innominate artery

Phrenic nerve

Common carotid artery

Internal jugular vein

Innominate vein

Aortic arch

Subclavian artery

Subclavian artery

Subclavian vein

Internal mammary artery

Internal mammary artery

Ascending aorta

Left pulmonary artery

RIGHT

LEFT

Pericardium (reflected)

Superior vena cava

Pulmonary artery

Atrial appendage

Coronary sulcus

Lung

Atrial appendage

Coronary sulcus

Conus arteriosus

Right ventricle

Lung

Lateral border of ventricle

Anterior interventricular sulcus

Inferior vena cava

Diaphragm

Apex of left ventricle

INFERIOR

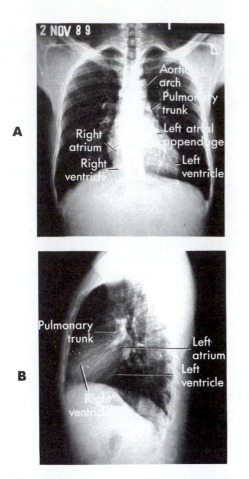

Fig. 4-5   Normal chest x-ray films. **A,** Anteroposterior. **B, Lateral.** (From Cannobio MM: *Cardiovascular disorders,* St Louis, 1990, Mosby.)

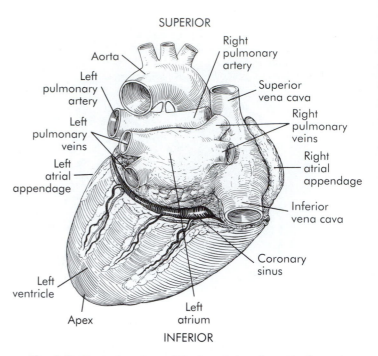

Fig. 4-6   Posterior view of the heart showing attachment of cardiac structures. (Drawing by Peter Stone.)

EXTERNAL FEATURES OF THE HEART

Externally the atria are separated from the ventricles by the **coronary sulcus,** also called the **atrioventricular groove.** The proximal portions of the right coronary artery and the left circumflex coronary artery can be found within this groove. The right and left ventricles are divided by the **interventricular sulcus,** which lies over the interventricular septum. It descends from the coronary sulcus toward the apex and is often obscured by epicardial fat in the adult.

Just to the left side of the anterior interventricular groove is the left anterior descending coronary artery, which courses down to the apex, where it curves around to the posterior interventricular groove on the diaphragmatic surface of the heart.

The posterior interventricular groove is the pathway for the posterior descending coronary artery, which is commonly the distal branch of the right coronary artery or, less commonly, the terminal portion of the left circumflex artery.

In the area where the posterior atrioventricular groove meets the posterior interventricular groove is the **crux.** It is at this point internally that the atrial

septum meets the ventricular septum. It is an important landmark for the surgeon performing coronary bypass grafting, because it is at this point that the posterior descending (interventricular) coronary artery turns to course downward toward the apex.

CARDIAC CHAMBERS
Right Atrium

Internally, the right atrium contains both a smooth surface and a rough area formed by the **pectinate muscles.** The two areas are separated by a muscular bundle called the **crista terminalis.** Externally this corresponds to the **sulcus terminalis,** which extends vertically from the superior vena cava to the inferior vena cava (Fig. 4-7).

The smoother posterior and medial (septal) walls contain the orifices of venous channels. The **superior vena cava (SVC)** enters the atrium superiorly, and the **inferior vena cava (IVC)** enters inferiorly. Both cavae receive systemic venous drainage. The IVC is guarded by the **eustachian valve;** occasionally this valve impedes cannulation of the IVC for cardiopulmonary bypass (Kirklin and Barratt-Boyes, 1993).

Medial to the IVC, coronary venous return drains through the coronary sinus, which is guarded by a flap of tissue called the **thebesian valve.** Cardioplegia solution for intraoperative myocardial protection (see Chapter 11) may be infused retrogradely through a cannula inserted directly (or indirectly via the right atrium) into the sinus. The thebesian valve may partially obstruct the entrance to the coronary sinus, making retrograde cannula insertion difficult.

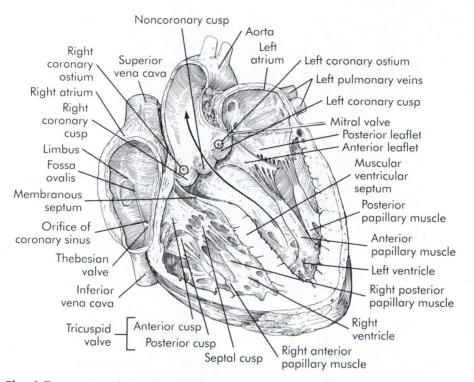

Fig. 4-7 Interior of the heart (pulmonary artery removed). (Drawing by Peter Stone.)

Also within the septal wall is the **atrioventricular (AV) node** of the conduction pathway. The node is located anterior and medial to the coronary sinus and above the septal leaflet of the tricuspid valve. Because the AV node is not grossly visible, extreme caution is used to avoid injury to the node and other conduction tissue during surgical manipulation of the atrial septum. The atrial septum additionally contains what was the fetal **ostium secundum** and the **foramen ovale,** surrounded anteriorly by a thickened ridge called the **limbus.**

Protruding anteromedially and overlapping the aortic root is the triangular **right atrial appendage.** For the surgeon, the appendage is a convenient entry point for venous cannulation and can be severed without functional impairment of the heart (Bharati, Lev, and Kirklin, 1983).

The lower portion of the right atrial wall is occupied by the tricuspid valve orifice. During ventricular systole the tricuspid valve is closed and the right atrium functions as a holding chamber for blood. During ventricular diastole blood from the right atrium flows through the opened valve into the right ventricle.

Right Ventricle

The right ventricle, normally the most anterior of the cardiac chambers, is located directly behind the sternum. It is a crescent-shaped chamber with a wall 4 to 5 mm thick. The inflow portion, originating at the tricuspid valve, contains numerous thick, muscular tissue bands, **trabeculae carneae.** From these arise two to four **papillary muscles** and multiple threadlike

chordae tendineae, which attach to the tricuspid valve. The outflow portion of the right ventricle, called the **infundibulum,** or **conus arteriosus,** is relatively smooth walled and exits at the **pulmonary valve** (Fig. 4-8).

A number of prominent muscular bands form the demarcation between the inflow and outflow portions: the **crista supraventricularis,** the **parietal band,** the **septal band,** and the **moderator band.** The right bundle branch of the conduction system travels through the moderator band toward the right ventricular endocardium. The moderator band, crossing from the lower ventricular septum to the anterior wall, joins the anterior papillary muscle projecting from the inner ventricular wall. Attached to this muscle are the anterior chordae tendineae, which anchor the tricuspid valve leaflets and prevent them from everting into the right atrium during ventricular systole.

Left Atrium

Desaturated blood flows from the right ventricle through the pulmonary valve orifice to the right and left branches of the **pulmonary artery** and into the lungs (see Fig. 4-7). From the lungs, oxygenated blood drains into the left atrium by way of the **pulmonary veins,** usually two on either side of the left atrium. Like the right atrium, the left atrium serves as a collecting chamber for blood during ventricular systole and as a conduit during ventricular diastole.

The left atrium is superior and posterior to the other cardiac chambers and, as a result, is not normally seen in the frontal chest x-ray film. If, as a conse-

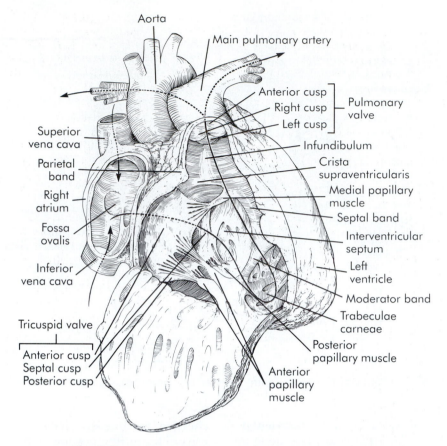

Fig. 4-8   **Right ventricle opened.** (Drawing by Peter Stone.)

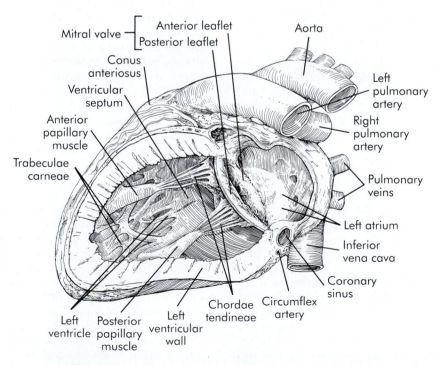

Fig. 4-9   **Left ventricle opened.** (Drawing by Peter Stone.)

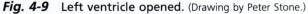

quence of the increased pressure or volume associated with severe mitral stenosis or regurgitation, it becomes massively dilated, the enlarged lateral borders of the left atrium will be evident on the roentgenogram.

The endocardial surface is smooth with the exception of the **left atrial appendage,** which is lined with pectinate muscles. This appendage, like the one on the right atrium, can be sacrificed with little consequence to myocardial function. In the left atrium the **fossa ovalis** (the remnant of the foramen ovale) is a central shallow area in the atrial septum.

Left Ventricle

The left ventricle receives blood from the left atrium via the orifice of the mitral valve, whose leaflets create a funnel-shaped inflow tract into the left ventricle (Fig. 4-9). The exit of the outflow tract, the aortic valve, is adjacent to the mitral valve. The aortic and mitral valves are separated by a fibrous band from which originates most of the anterior leaflet of the mitral valve and portions of the left and posterior (noncoronary) cusps of the aortic valve. This intimate relationship is important during procedures on the mitral or aortic valve.

The left ventricular chamber is conical and is surrounded by thick muscular walls between 8 and 15 mm thick, approximately three times the thickness of the right ventricular wall. The tip of the apex may be thin, measuring 2 mm or less. The left ventricle is posterior to and to the left of the right ventricle, and inferior to, anterior to, and to the left of the left atrium.

The ventricular **septum** forms the medial wall and normally bulges into the right ventricle. It is almost entirely muscular except for the superiorly located **membranous septum** just below the right and posterior (noncoronary) cusps of the aortic valve. On the left ventricular side the demarcation between the membranous septum and the **muscular septum** is called the **limbus marginalis.**

The membranous septum is both interventricular and atrioventricular. The former portion lies between the left ventricle and the right ventricle (behind the supraventricular crest). The latter, superior, part of the membranous septum lies between the left ventricle and the right atrium.

Trabeculae carneae are found in the left ventricle, but they are finer and more numerous than those of the right ventricle. Arising from the trabeculae are two papillary muscles which, with their attached chordae, anchor the mitral valve. These papillary muscles are stronger than those on the right and, with the chordae, help to maintain coaptation of the valve leaflets during ventricular systole. Because the papillary muscles receive their blood supply from the distal portion of the coronary arterial system, impaired blood flow due to coronary artery disease may produce ischemia with subsequent papillary muscle dysfunction.

CARDIAC VALVES

The four valves within the base of the heart are designed to maintain forward blood flow and prevent regurgitation into the originating chamber (Fig. 4-10).

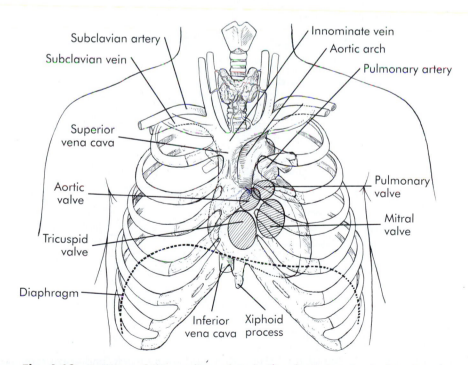

Fig. 4-10 Position of the cardiac valves in the chest. (Drawing by Peter Stone.)

Essentially this is a passive process that depends on changing pressure gradients. As blood accumulates behind the valve, the pressure increases to a point where it becomes greater than the pressure in front of the valve. The valve then opens to allow transvalvular flow. Increasing pressure beyond the valve forces the leaflets to close.

The atrioventricular **mitral valve** and the **tricuspid valve** are structurally and functionally similar to each other. The two semilunar valves, the **aortic valve** and the **pulmonary valve,** are also similar to each other and are located at the exits of their respective left and right ventricular outflow tracts.

A consistently uniform relationship exists between the four valves, with the aortic valve centrally wedged between the tricuspid and mitral valves (Fig. 4-11). The pulmonary valve is located anterior to, to the left

of, and superior to the aortic valve. The merger of the valve annuli forms the **central fibrous skeleton** of the heart. This fibrous body, also known as the **right fibrous trigone,** is pierced by the conduction **bundle of His.** A **left fibrous trigone** is formed by connective tissue coursing from the central fibrous body to the left, posteroinferiorly and anteriorly.

Mitral Valve

Situated at the entrance to the left ventricle, the mitral valve allows blood from the right atrium to enter the lower chamber. The area of the mitral valve orifice in adults is 4 to 6 cm² (Lake, 1985) and will permit insertion of the tips of two fingers (Thorek, 1983). The valve consists of two fibroelastic leaflets that originate from the annulus fibrosus encircling the left atrioven-

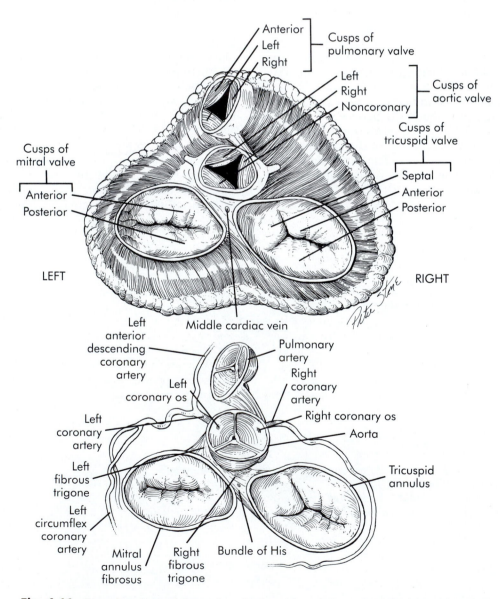

Fig. 4-11 Superior view of the valves (atria, pulmonary trunk, and aorta removed). (Drawing by Peter Stone.)

tricular orifice (see Fig. 4-9). The leaflets are pale yellow, thin glistening membranes whose atrial surface is relatively smooth. The ventricular surface is very irregular because of the attachment of the chordae tendineae.

The triangular **anterior leaflet,** also called the anteromedial, septal, or aortic leaflet, stretches across the ventricular cavity from the septum to the anterolateral wall of the left ventricle. The leaflet is continuous with the supporting tissues of the posterior aortic valve cusp lying above it and is visible during surgery on the aortic valve.

The quadrangular **posterior leaflet,** otherwise known as the posterolateral or mural leaflet, is longer and less mobile than the anterior leaflet. It encircles about two thirds of the valve circumference from the anterolateral to the posteromedial ventricular wall. Although differing in shape, both leaflets have similar surface areas, with the combined leaflet area being twice that of the mitral orifice. This provides a large area of approximation, or coaptation, during ventricular systole.

Mitral valve function during ventricular diastole and systole is regulated by the interaction of an intricate system consisting of not only the valve leaflets and their annular attachment, but also the chordae tendineae, the papillary muscles, and the ventricular wall (see Fig. 4-9). These components form the **mitral apparatus,** or **mitral complex,** and contribute to maintaining the normal geometry and mechanical function of the left ventricle (David, 1989).

At the end of ventricular systole, when the pressure of accumulated blood in the left atrium exceeds the pressure in the left ventricle, the mitral valve leaflets are forced open, allowing blood to enter the ventricular chamber. Near the end of ventricular filling, the atrium contracts, increasing ventricular volume by an additional 30%. Left ventricular systole then begins with the contraction of the papillary muscles. These muscles, as well as the chordae tendineae, which insert into the valve leaflets, prevent the leaflets from everting into the atrium. As intraventricular pressure rises, the free edges of the valve leaflets coapt along their atrial surfaces to form a tight closure. If chordae rupture as a result of infection or ischemia, severe valvular regurgitation with heart failure ensues. Dilatation of either the valve annulus or the left ventricle can also impair valve closure.

Tricuspid Valve

The orifice of the right atrioventricular valve is larger than that of the mitral valve and will permit entry of three fingertips in the adult—approximately 10 cm² (Thorek, 1988; see Fig. 4-8). The tricuspid valve has three leaflets, the **anterior, posterior,** and **medial** (septal) **leaflets,** which are unequal in size. The **anterior papillary muscle** and the **medial papillary muscle** are the two main attachments for the tricuspid valve; the medial (conal) papillary muscle may also be well developed. The proximity of the septal leaflet to the

His bundle of the conduction system warrants special consideration to avoid heart block during surgery on the tricuspid valve or the septal walls.

Although similar in form and function to the mitral valve, the leaflets and chordae of the tricuspid valve complex (see Fig. 4-8) are thinner and more translucent. The anterior leaflet stretches downward from the infundibulum to the inferolateral wall of the right ventricle. The posterior leaflet is usually the smallest, with its chordae originating from the posterior and anterior papillary muscles. The septal (medial) leaflet attaches to the membranous septum, as well as the muscular septum; it may obscure small ventricular septal defects.

Aortic Valve

Each of the semilunar valves is composed of three cusps, which open passively when the pressure behind them exceeds that in front of them. They are similar in form except that the aortic valve cusps are thicker than the pulmonary valve cusps. The normal adult aortic orifice area is 3 to 4 cm². The cusps are suspended from the annulus, a fibrous ring that encircles the proximal portion of the aorta, known as the **aortic root** (see Fig. 4-9). Within the root and behind each cusp the vessel wall forms pouchlike dilatations called the **sinuses of Valsalva** (Fig. 4-12). Because the openings, or ostia, of the right and left coronary arteries originate in two of the sinuses, the cusps are designated the **right, left,** and **noncoronary** (posterior) **cusps.** During ventricular systole, when blood pushes the cusps upward into the aorta, obstruction of the coronary ostia is prevented by the sinus of Valsalva dilatations. The right and noncoronary sinuses are proximal to the medial wall of the right atrium (see Fig. 4-7).

Pulmonary Valve

The pulmonary valve cusps are called **anterior, right,** and **left cusps** (see Fig. 4-8). The valve orifice area is usually about 4 cm². During ventricular diastole, when pulmonary artery pressure exceeds right ventricular pressure, the valve cusps fall passively backward and coapt to support the column of blood above. This closing mechanism is similar to that of the aortic valve. A discrete annulus is absent in the pulmonary valve.

CORONARY ARTERIES

Oxygen and nutrients are supplied to the myocardium by the **right** and **left coronary arteries** (Fig. 4-13; see also Fig. 4-12), originating in the aortic root. The **left main coronary artery** (whose ostium is slightly higher than the right coronary ostium), passes between the main pulmonary artery and the left atrial appendage before dividing into the **left anterior descending (LAD) coronary artery** and the **circumflex coronary artery.** Obtuse marginal branches of the circumflex artery supply blood to the left lateral wall of the heart.

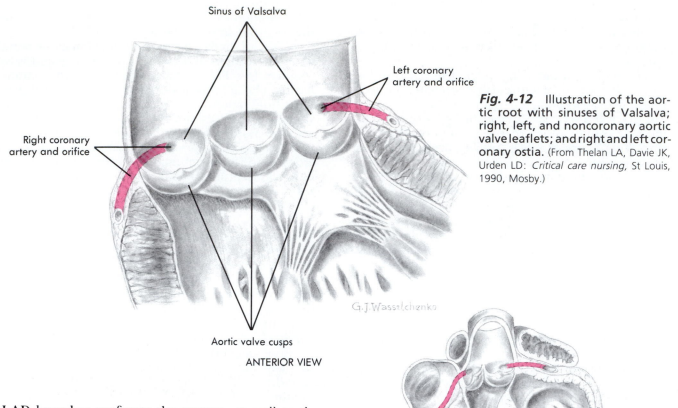

Sinus of Valsalva

Left coronary artery and orifice

Right coronary artery and orifice

Aortic valve cusps

ANTERIOR VIEW

G.J.Wassilchenko

Fig. 4-12 Illustration of the aortic root with sinuses of Valsalva; right, left, and noncoronary aortic valve leaflets; and right and left coronary ostia. (From Thelan LA, Davie JK, Urden LD: *Critical care nursing*, St Louis, 1990, Mosby.)

LAD branches perforate the septum, as well as the free walls of the left atrium and left ventricle, and supply portions of the conduction system and the anterior papillary muscle of the mitral valve. Other branches between the left coronary artery and the right coronary artery provide anastomotic connections to supply parts of the anterior right ventricular wall; in the presence of coronary atherosclerosis, these anastomoses are a source of collateral circulation.

The right coronary artery travels within the right atrioventricular groove before branching into the sinus node and acute marginal arteries to perfuse the right side of the heart. The **posterior descending coronary artery,** which supplies the posterior interventricular septum, is commonly the terminal branch of the right coronary artery. When this is the case, patients are said to have a "right dominant" system. When the posterior descending branch is a continuation of the (left) circumflex coronary artery, the patient is said to be "left dominant"; when both arteries supply the posterior septum, coronary distribution is said to be "balanced."

Dominance assumes significance in patients with ischemic heart disease affecting the dominant coronary distribution. Thus obstructive lesions of the left main coronary artery are especially critical in those patients with left dominant systems, because so much of the myocardium (particularly the anterior and posterior portions of the "workhorse" left ventricle) is dependent on flow from branches of the left coronary artery.

The LAD, circumflex, and right coronary arteries represent the three main vessels of the coronary artery

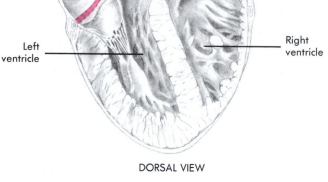

Left ventricle

Right ventricle

DORSAL VIEW

system. "Triple-vessel" coronary artery disease refers to the presence of obstructive lesions in all three of these arteries.

Variations in the branching pattern of the coronary arteries are common. Occasionally only one coronary artery originates from the aortic root, and anomalies of the coronary system are not uncommon in pediatric cardiac patients.

Coronary Blood Flow

In contrast to the other vascular beds of the body, myocardial blood flow is greater during diastole than it is during systole. The epicardial segment of the coronary arteries is perfused during systole, but the blood vessels within the myocardium are subject to compression by the left ventricular muscle during contraction (Fig. 4-14). This compression is especially evident in the subendocardium, where there is almost a

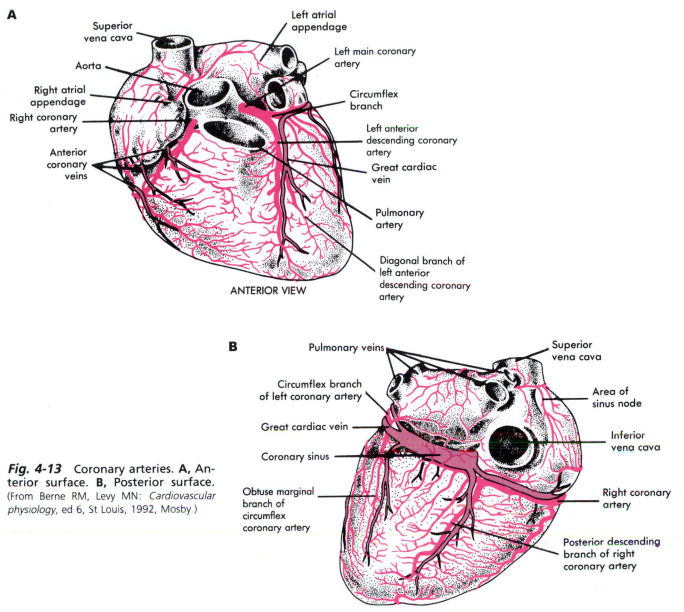

A

Superior
vena cava

Aorta

Right atrial
appendage

Right coronary
artery

Anterior
coronary
veins

Left atrial
appendage

Left main coronary
artery

Circumflex
branch

Left anterior
descending coronary
artery

Great cardiac
vein

Pulmonary
artery

Diagonal branch of
left anterior
descending coronary
artery

ANTERIOR VIEW

B

Pulmonary veins

Circumflex branch
of left coronary artery

Great cardiac vein

Coronary sinus

Obtuse marginal
branch of
circumflex
coronary artery

Superior
vena cava

Area of
sinus node

Inferior
vena cava

Right coronary
artery

Posterior descending
branch of right
coronary artery

POSTERIOR VIEW

Fig. 4-13 Coronary arteries. **A,** Anterior surface. **B,** Posterior surface. (From Berne RM, Levy MN: *Cardiovascular physiology*, ed 6, St Louis, 1992, Mosby.)

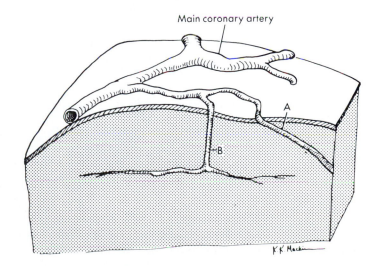

Main coronary artery

A

B

Fig. 4-14 Myocardial distribution of the coronary arteries. *A,* Epicardial arteries arise at acute angles from the main coronary vessels to supply the surface of the heart. *B,* Smaller vessels branch from the main vessels and epicardial arteries to penetrate deeper into the myocardium and endocardium. (From Quaal SJ: *Comprehensive intra-aortic balloon pumping*, St Louis, 1984, Mosby.)

total lack of flow during systole. When the heart relaxes in diastole, intramyocardial vessels fill with blood. In the presence of obstructive coronary artery disease, subendocardial perfusion suffers most. If there is concomitant heart failure, and if rising left ventricular diastolic pressures further compress the inner ventricular wall, blood flow is further jeopardized and can result in cellular death (Guyton, 1991).

Another factor affecting myocardial blood flow is the aortic pressure, which is generated by the heart itself. When diastolic pressure is low, coronary perfusion suffers. This is evident in patients with an aortic valve that does not completely close: regurgitating blood causes the aortic pressure to drop and the intraventricular pressure to increase, creating a double threat to the myocardium.

CARDIAC VEINS

Blood enters the cardiac venous system after the exchange of oxygen and other substances in the dense capillary network of the heart. The principal cardiac veins, the **greater** and **middle cardiac veins** and the **posterior left ventricular vein,** enter the right atrium via the coronary sinus.

The veins of the anterior right ventricular wall enter the right atrium independently of the coronary sinus. This is an important consideration when cardioplegia solution is infused retrogradely through the coronary sinus, because theoretically the right side of the heart would not be adequately permeated by the solution and therefore would not be sufficiently protected (Mohl and others, 1990). This hypothesis has been challenged, however, since there is an extensive network of venous collateral vessels that could allow a sufficient amount of cardioplegia to be delivered (Menasche, 1993).

Although the coronary sinus is the major venous drainage pathway, it is one of a number of drainage routes. Individual variability and a large network of venous interconnections provide routes (Mohl and others, 1990). A number of small venous channels **(thebesian veins)** within the atrial and ventricular septal walls open directly into the cardiac chambers, most often the right atrium.

Veins draining into the left side of the heart create a mixing of unoxygenated blood with freshly oxygenated blood from the lungs to produce a physiologic shunt. Deoxygenated bronchial blood also drains into the pulmonary veins. This is normal and explains why the expected oxygen saturation of blood leaving the left ventricle is slightly less than 100%. (Abnormal shunts occur when there is a defect producing communication between the right and left sides of the heart.)

CONDUCTION SYSTEM

Excitation, conduction, and contraction are characteristic of cardiac tissue (see Chapter 19). The ability to initiate a beat **(automaticity),** and generate it on a regular basis **(rhythmicity)** are properties of the excitation mechanism that begins on about the twenty-second day of gestation (DeHaan, 1990).

Once these electrical impulses are generated, they are conducted rapidly throughout the heart via specially differentiated muscle fibers. The initiation and propagation of electrical impulses precedes (and controls) the mechanical activity of contracting myocardial cells, enabling the heart to function as a pump.

The conduction system consists of the **sinoatrial (SA) node,** the **atrioventricular (AV) junction,** the **bundle of His,** the right and left **bundle branches,** and the **Purkinje fibers** (Fig. 4-15).

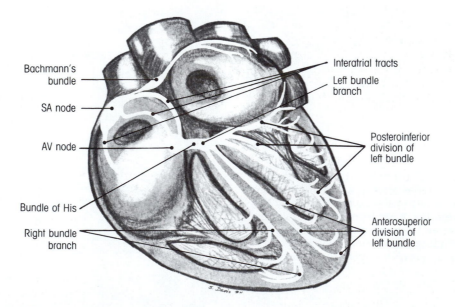

Fig. 4-15 Conduction system of the heart. (From Guzzetta CE, Dossey BM: *Cardiovascular nursing: holistic practice,* St Louis, 1992, Mosby.)

The SA node, known as the natural pacemaker of the heart, demonstrates self-excitation to the greatest degree. Although all conduction tissue possesses the property of automaticity, the SA node initiates impulses at a faster rate and ordinarily controls the rate of the heartbeat. It lies within the sulcus terminalis of the right atrial wall at the junction of the superior vena cava. There is little risk to the node during venous cannulation unless a clamp is placed too low on the appendage (Bharati, Lev, and Kirklin, 1983).

It is theorized that internodal pathways spread the electrical impulses between the SA node and the AV junction. Branches of these pathways conduct impulses to the left atrium. As the impulse spreads, the atria depolarize and contract (seen as the P wave on the electrocardiogram [ECG]).

Conduction slows momentarily when the impulse reaches the **AV node** within the AV junction, which is situated between the upper part of the coronary sinus and the septal (medial) leaflet of the tricuspid valve. This brief pause, reflected on the ECG by the PR interval (Fig. 4-16), allows sufficient time for atrial contraction (atrial "kick") to contribute to ventricular filling. AV nodal delay also protects the ventricle by limiting the transfer of abnormally excessive impulses associated with atrial fibrillation or atrial flutter. If every atrial fibrillation or atrial flutter impulse produced ventricular contraction, the increased workload and reduced cardiac output eventually would produce cardiac failure and cellular death (Feeney, 1992).

On emerging from the AV node, the impulse is conducted rapidly through the bundle of His penetrating the central fibrous body (right trigone). His bundle fibers travel down the right side of the interventricular septum for approximately 1 cm and then divide into the right and left bundle branches. The right bundle branch extends almost to the apex of the right ventricle, where it becomes a profuse terminal network of Purkinje fibers to supply the right ventricular endocardium. The thicker left bundle branch arises almost perpendicularly from the bundle of His and crosses the septum to enter the left ventricle. It then subdivides into anterior and posterior branches, or **fascicles,** terminating in Purkinje fibers throughout the ventricular subendocardium (Berne and Levy, 1992; Thelan, Davis, and Urden, 1990).

The impulse spreads uniformly throughout the Purkinje fibers and at a high rate of velocity throughout the ventricular cells; the ventricles depolarize and contract, forming the electrocardiographic QRS complex. Ventricular relaxation (the T wave) occurs with repolarization and a return to the resting electrical state. When one of the fascicles of the left bundle branch does not conduct impulses properly, it is referred to as a hemiblock. Conduction defects affecting the bundle branches are termed bundle-branch blocks.

It should be emphasized that the ECG does not provide direct information about the mechanical activity of the heart; it simply reflects the course of the cardiac impulse by recording variations in electrical

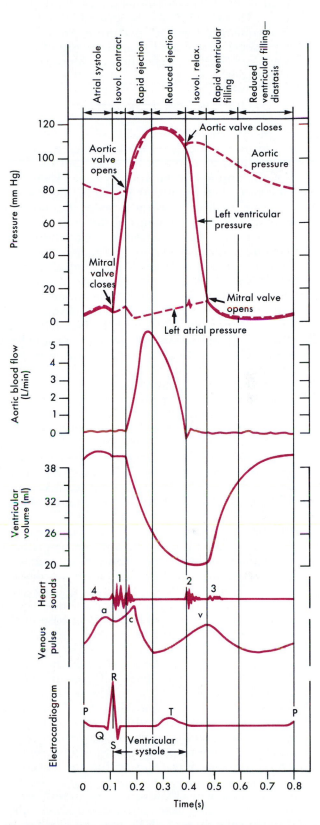

Fig. 4-16 Left atrial, aortic, and left ventricular pressure pulses correlated in time with aortic flow, ventricular volume, heart sounds, venous pulse, and the electrocardiogram for a complete cardiac cycle. (From Berne RM, Levy MN: *Cardiovascular physiology,* ed 6, St Louis, 1992, Mosby.)

potential from various locations on the body (Berne and Levy, 1992). The ECG also proves an indication of the adequacy of coronary perfusion. For example, in the presence of ischemia, changes in the ECG tracing, such as ST segment elevation or depression, are often apparent.

INNERVATION OF THE HEART

Although a denervated heart will continue to beat (as evidenced by the success of cardiac transplantation), it cannot adjust its rate efficiently without the influence of the **autonomic nervous system (ANS).** The ANS plays an important role in regulating the rate and vigor of each contraction to meet the moment-to-moment metabolic demands of the body.

Sensory nerves are found in the pericardium, ventricular walls, coronary vessels, and major blood vessels. These transmit impulses to the **central nervous system (CNS).** Autonomic motor fibers of the **sympathetic nervous system** stimulate increased contractility **(inotropy),** as well as heart rate **(chronotropy)** (Fig. 4-17). Stimulation of the right and left **vagus nerves** of the **parasympathetic nervous system** produces a slower (bradycardic) heart rate and prolonged conduction through the AV node. Ordinarily, parasympathetic tone predominates in healthy, resting persons. Blocking parasympathetic influences with atropine generally results in an increased heart rate, although reducing the effects of sympathetic influences (e.g., with propranolol) usually has only a slight effect on the heart rate. When both the sympathetic and parasympathetic divisions are blocked in a young, healthy adult, the heart reverts to an intrinsic heart rate of approximately 100 beats per minute (Berne and Levy, 1992).

The cardiac parasympathetic fibers originate in the **medulla oblongata** of the brain, and the sympathetic fibers originate in the thoracic and cervical segments of the **spinal cord.** Fibers from both divisions combine to create a complex network of nerves that travel to the heart. Sympathetic fibers are also found within the adventitia of the great vessels at the base of the heart (Berne and Levy, 1992).

Cardiac function is also regulated by receptors found in the walls of the aortic arch and the carotid sinus, which sense changes in blood pressure. Other receptors in various parts of the body respond to changes in the chemical composition of the blood (e.g., levels of oxygen, carbon dioxide, or hydrogen). These changes initiate impulses to the cardiovascular center of the brain, which responds by adjusting pressure, rate, flow, and/or contractility within the cardiovascular system (Thelan, 1990).

Another control mechanism is found in certain cells of the cardiac atria. These secrete a hormone, called **atrial natriuretic factor (ANF),** into the blood in response to increased atrial volumes. This produces a marked increase in urinary sodium and water excretion and acts as a potent vasodilator (Athanassopoulos and Cokkinos, 1991). The body can rid itself of excess

extracellular volume and enable the veins to restore intravascular blood volume (Thelan, 1990).

The higher centers of the brain also affect heart activity, as evidenced by the cardiovascular responses to intense emotions such as fear and anxiety. These responses are probably initiated by the hypothalamus and the limbic system (Guzzetta and Dossey, 1992).

EXCITATION-CONTRACTION OF THE CELL

Although extracardiac factors affect cardiac function, it is at the cellular level that excitation-contraction occurs. The conduction system typifies one kind of cardiac tissue. **Contractile units** make up the second

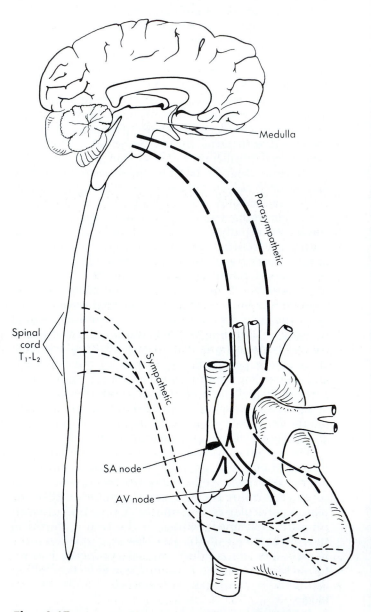

Fig. 4-17 Autonomic nervous system innervation of nodal tissue and myocardium by parasympathetic vagus nerve fibers and sympathetic fibers. (From Quaal SJ: *Comprehensive intra-aortic balloon pumping,* St Louis, 1984, Mosby.)

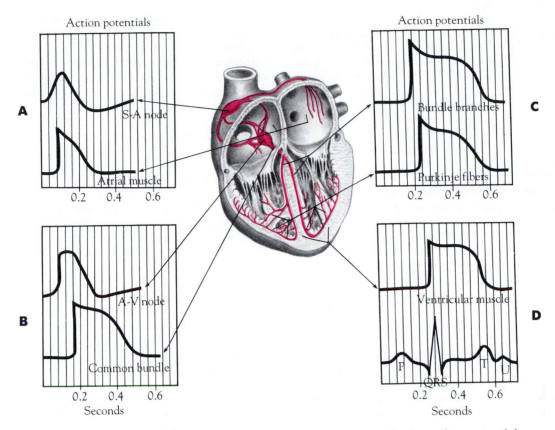

Fig. 4-18 Normal cardiac conduction pathways and transmembrane action potential of **A,** SA node; **B,** AV node; **C,** bundle branches; and **D,** ventricular muscle. (From Thompson JM and others: *Mosby's clinical nursing,* ed 3, St Louis, 1993, Mosby.)

major group of cells. These two types of cells are related in that conducted electrical impulses are converted into the mechanical work of myocardial contraction.

The composition of fluid inside and outside the cellular membrane of contractile cells differs with respect to the concentration of electrolytes, especially sodium (Na^+), potassium (K^+), and calcium (Ca^{++}). When dissolved in fluid, these electrolytes become ions, which are good conductors of electricity. Na^+ and Ca^{++} are more concentrated in the extracellular fluid, whereas K^+ is more highly concentrated inside the cell. (The energy required to achieve this is produced during the breakdown of adenosine triphosphate [ATP].) Although there is some passive movement of sodium and potassium across the cell wall when the cell is at rest, the cell membrane actively prevents the equalization of these ions by pumping sodium out of and potassium back into the cell via the sodium-potassium pump. Because of the imbalance in the concentration of specific ions, the inside of the cell is more negative than the outside, producing an electrical gradient. The cell depolarizes (producing cellular contraction) when it is stimulated by an impulse. The cell membrane becomes more permeable to both Na^+ and Ca^{++} ions entering the cell through selective channels, thereby producing an action potential (Fig. 4-18).

During the early phase of depolarization, sodium rushes in via the **"fast" sodium channel** and neutralizes some of the negative charges inside the cell. This allows even more sodium to enter until the fast sodium channels are inactivated, contraction ceases, and the cell becomes refractory to further excitation. Until the cell has repolarized, the heart is unable to contract again, thereby preventing sustained, tetanic myocardial contraction (Berne and Levy, 1992).

Following the opening of the fast sodium channels, the **"slow" sodium channels** then open and allow Ca^{++} (and some Na^+) to enter the cell after the initial fast entry of Na^+. Activation, inactivation, and recovery of the slow channels is slower than that of the fast channels. Calcium channel—blocking medications (for example, verapamil, nifedipine) reduce Ca^{++} inflow and thereby diminish cardiac contractility. Conversely, catecholamines increase the inward current of Ca^{++} and enhance contractility (Berne and Levy, 1992).

During this period of repolarization, potassium diffuses out of the cell, a process that culminates in the restoration of the resting membrane potential. The sodium/potassium pump restores Na^+ and K^+ to their appropriate concentration inside and outside the cell membrane, and the cycle is ready to start again.

CARDIAC CYCLE

Depolarization stimulates muscles to contract, producing the systolic phase of the cardiac cycle, whereas repolarization allows the myocardium to relax, producing the diastolic phase of the cardiac cycle. With each heartbeat, the ventricles propel blood through the vascular system. (See Fig. 4-16 for the relationship between the successive electrical and mechanical events during one cardiac cycle.) Approximately 70% of the ventricular volume flows directly into the ventricles from the atria. Atrial systole contributes another 30% to the total volume of blood in the ventricle at the end of ventricular diastole. Although atrial contraction is not essential in the normal heart, it contributes significantly to left ventricular filling in the presence of a narrowed (stenotic) mitral valve.

The onset of ventricular contraction (systole) is termed **isovolumic contraction.** During this brief period, ventricular volume is constant, but ventricular pressure rises and closes the mitral (and tricuspid) valve. When the pressure within the ventricle is sufficient to open the aortic and pulmonary valves, the **ejection phase** begins. Ejection of blood into the aorta (or pulmonary artery) is rapid at first and then is reduced. In the systemic circulation, aortic pressure declines as blood flow is transmitted to the vascular periphery. Left ventricular pressure also decreases, and a gradient develops, with the relatively higher aortic pressure closing the aortic valve. The ventricle does not completely empty during systole. Approximately 40% of the end-diastolic volume remains; the amount of blood ejected is called the **ejection fraction** and is commonly used to indicate ventricular function (Table 4-1).

Isovolumic relaxation is the period between closure of the semilunar valves and opening of the atrioventricular valves. Ventricular volume remains constant, but ventricular pressure drops dramatically (Berne and Levy, 1992).

Atrial pressure rises with the blood accumulated during the previous systolic period to open the AV valves and cause rapid filling of the relaxed ventricles. The **rapid filling phase** is followed by the period of **diastasis,** during which there is slow filling of the ventricles by venous return from the lungs and the periphery. An increase in ventricular volume and pressure initiates the repetition of the cycle.

CARDIAC OUTPUT

The cardiac output is the volume of blood pumped by the heart per minute. It is determined by multiplying the **stroke volume** (the amount of blood ejected with each contraction) by the **heart rate.** Thus the cardiac output of a subject who ejects 70 ml of blood 80 times a minute is 5600 ml, or 5.6 L/min. Because patients vary in size, the metabolic requirements for blood differ. The cardiac output can be corrected for differences in body size by dividing it by the body surface area to compute the **cardiac index.** (The stroke volume index can be computed by dividing the stroke volume by the body surface area.)

Normally the right and left ventricles eject equal amounts of blood per minute, but individual stroke outputs may vary. If the right ventricle momentarily pumps more blood than the left ventricle, the minute output will equalize because the increased right ventricular volume will increase left ventricular filling and thereby increase the left ventricular stroke volume (Schlant and Sonnenblick, 1990).

Determinants of Cardiac Output

Depending on the needs of the body, cardiac output is increased or decreased by four interrelated factors: heart rate, preload, afterload, and contractility.

Heart rate

Heart rate refers to the frequency of contraction, reflected by the pulse rate. Although the sinus node usually determines the heart rate, neural and humoral factors also play a role in determining the heart rate. A change in the heart rate will alter the following three factors.

Preload

Preload is the amount of blood in the ventricle before it contracts. It is also known as the **left ventricular end-diastolic volume (LVEDV).** Because it is technically easier to measure pressure than it is to measure volume, **left ventricular end-diastolic pressure (LVEDP)** is commonly used to measure preload (although it is not synonymous with LVEDV [Lake, 1985]). The greater the preload, within physiologic limits, the more the myocardial fibers stretch, and subsequently, the more forcefully the fibers shorten to produce an increase in stroke volume. The relationship between volume, stretch, and subsequent contraction is known as the **Frank-Starling law.**

Because the heart is composed of two pumps, it is necessary to distinguish between right and left ventricular preload. Venous return to the right atrium, measured with a central venous pressure (CVP) catheter, represents the right filling pressure, or preload. The preload of the left ventricle is inferred with a pulmonary artery catheter containing an inflatable balloon at its tip. The balloon can be inflated and wedged temporarily in a branch of the pulmonary artery. Because there are no valves between the pulmonary artery and the left atrium, this **pulmonary artery wedge pressure (PAWP),** measured when the mitral valve is open, reflects both left atrial pressure and LVEDP.

Preload is also dependent on the amount of circulating blood and its distribution throughout the body. Conditions that decrease blood volume (e.g., hemorrhage) decrease venous return and cardiac output. The distribution of blood can be affected by contracting external muscles, body position, and venous tone. Veins are capable of dilating and sequestering

Table 4-1 ■ *Concepts related to cardiac output*

	Normal values		
	Adult	Child	
Cardiac Output (CO) Amount of blood (in liters) ejected by left ventricle per minute; product of heart rate times stroke volume	4-8 L/min	Newborn: 1 yr: 5 yr: 10 yr:	0.8-1.0 L/min 1.3-1.5 L/min 2.5-3.0 L/min 3.8-4.0 L/min
Heart Rate Number of contractions (beats) per minute; chronotropy	70-100 bpm	Newborn: 1 yr: 5 yr: 10 yr:	145 bpm 115 bpm 95 bpm 75 bpm
Cardiac Index (CI) Cardiac output per square meter of body surface area; used to compare CO of different-sized persons	2.5-4.0 L/min/m2	Divide CO by body surface area	
Preload Volume of blood in ventricle at end of diastole Right-sided heart preload: measured by central venous pressure (CVP) Left-sided heart preload: measured by pulmonary artery wedge pressure (PAWP)	Mean 0-5 mm Hg Mean 4-12 mm Hg	Mean 0-4 mm Hg Mean 4-8 mm Hg	
Afterload Impedance to contraction; vascular resistance the heart must overcome to pump blood into circulation; wall tension during systole Right ventricular afterload is reflected by pulmonary vascular resistance (PVR) Left ventricular afterload is reflected by systemic vascular resistance (SVR)	2.0 Wood units* 20.0 Wood units	Infant: Child: Infant: Toddler: Child:	25-40 Wood units 0.5-4 Wood units 35-50 Wood units 25-35 Wood units 15-25 Wood units
Contractility Ability of ventricle to pump; inotropic state of the heart			
Stroke Volume Amount of blood ejected per heartbeat	60-130 ml/beat	Newborn: 1 yr: 5 yr: 10 yr:	5 ml/beat 13 ml/beat 31 ml/beat 50 ml/beat
Ejection Fraction Percentage of end-diastolic volume ejected into (systemic) circulation; indicator of left ventricular function	60%-70%		

Modified from Guzzetta CE, Dossey BM: *Cardiovascular nursing: holistic practice*, St Louis, 1992, Mosby; and Hazinski MF: *Nursing care of the critically ill child*, ed 2, St Louis, 1991, Mosby.
*Multiply Wood units by 80 to convert to dynes sec/cm^{-5}.

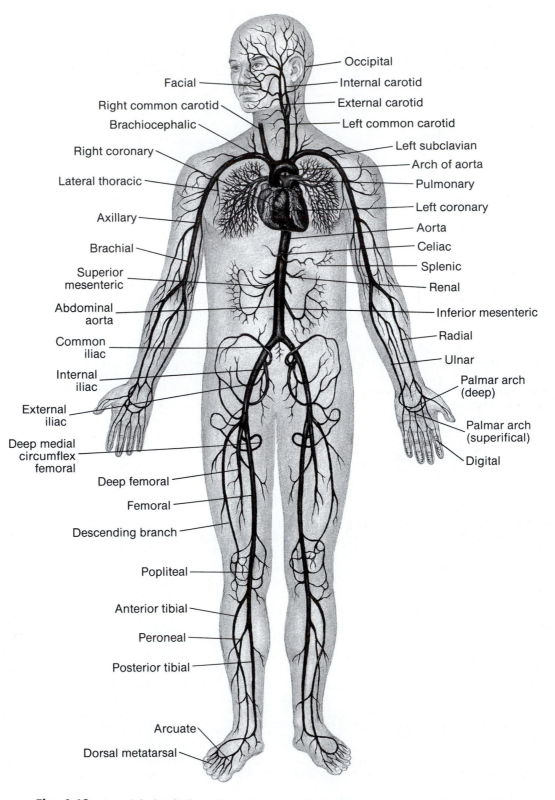

Fig. 4-19   **Arterial circulation.** (From Cannobio MM: *Cardiovascular disorders,* St Louis, 1990, Mosby.)

large amounts of blood in dependent portions of the body (Braunwald, 1992).

Finally, ventricular wall compliance plays a role in diastolic filling of the ventricle. When the heart is relaxed, rapid diastolic filling can be achieved. However a stiff or thickened ventricle, found in patients with left ventricular hypertrophy, coronary artery disease, or cardiac tamponade, is less compliant and impairs diastolic filling.

Afterload

Afterload is the ventricular wall tension created during ejection; it is the resistance the ventricles must overcome during contraction. Resistance is created by aortic distensibility, the systemic vascular bed, and blood volume and viscosity. Left ventricular or right ventricular outflow tract obstructions (such as aortic valve stenosis or pulmonary valve stenosis) also increase the workload of the heart. Calculation of the systemic vascular resistance is commonly performed to indicate afterload. Because of the great energy requirements of the left ventricle, pharmacologic manipulation of the afterload is frequently performed in the operating room and the critical care setting to decrease the workload of the ventricle.

When left ventricular function is impaired and the ventricle cannot eject adequately, blood backs up in the lungs. This raises pulmonary vascular pressure and hence pulmonary vascular resistance, which increases right ventricular afterload. In very young patients with congenital lesions producing increased blood flow to the lungs, pulmonary hypertension and elevated right ventricular afterload can produce heart failure in a short period of time.

Contractility

Contractility refers to the inotropic state of the ventricle, independent of changes in heart rate, preload, or afterload. Sympathetic stimulation or inotropic agents such as digitalis, calcium, and dobutamine hydrochloride increase contractility and cardiac output. When pharmacologic agents such as barbiturates, halothane, beta blockers, or calcium channel blockers are given or, when there is a loss of functioning ventricular muscle, as in myocardial infarction or left ventricular aneurysm, contractility is decreased.

Whether extrinsic or intrinsic, manipulation of the heart rate, preload, afterload, and contractility to achieve optimum cardiac output helps to ensure adequate perfusion of the tissues.

MYOCARDIAL OXYGEN CONSUMPTION

Closely related to the determinants of cardiac output is **myocardial oxygen consumption (MVo$_2$)**. Oxygen is required to do the work associated with contraction and relaxation. When the oxygen demand exceeds the supply, hypoxemia results. Mechanisms are instituted to return the myocardium to a balanced state by either reducing the oxygen demand or increasing the oxygen

supply. In patients with ischemic heart disease (where reduced blood flow produces a decrease in oxygen supply), beta-blocking drugs can reduce the demand, whereas surgical revascularization of the myocardium increases the supply. Without surgery, the ability to increase the oxygen supply is limited because of the obstructive lesions and the already high rate of myocardial oxygen extraction from the blood. In patients with left ventricular hypertrophy, the increased thickness of the myocardial wall (without a commensurate increase in the vascular network supplying the tissue) adversely affects the distribution of coronary blood flow to the subendocardium. When the supply of oxygen cannot be readily increased via coronary artery blood flow, balancing the supply/demand equation focuses on reducing the demand.

MVo$_2$ is primarily determined by the heart rate, wall tension, and contractility—all factors associated with cardiac output. Myocardial wall tension is affected by conditions that increase pressure (aortic stenosis) or volume (aortic regurgitation) loads on the heart. Both pharmacologic and psychologic interventions are warranted in decreasing myocardial oxygen demands.

CIRCULATORY SYSTEM

The heart pumps blood to the tissues to provide nourishment and to remove the waste products of metabolism. The transportation route for the distribution and exchange of these substances is formed by the circulatory system.

Systemic Circulation

The systemic circulation supplies all the tissues of the body except the lungs. Blood is ejected from the left ventricle into the aorta, from which arteries branch off to perfuse the head, upper extremities, abdominal organs, and lower extremities (Fig. 4-19). Arteries transport blood under high pressure and have strong muscular walls (Fig. 4-20).

Arteries subdivide into **arterioles,** whose function is to control the release of blood into the capillaries. Internal respiration occurs in the **capillaries,** where fluids, nutrients, electrolytes, oxygen, and other substances are exchanged through their single-layer walls for the end-products of cellular metabolism. Blood then collects in the **venules** and flows into progressively larger veins to return to the right atrium (Fig. 4-21). Flap valves within the veins help to maintain unidirectional blood flow. Contracting external muscles propel venous blood toward the heart.

Pulmonary Circulation

In the pulmonary circulation, blood is pumped from the right ventricle into the main pulmonary artery, which divides into the right and left pulmonary arteries. These further subdivide into the arterioles and capillaries of the lungs. External respiration occurs in

ARTERY   VEIN

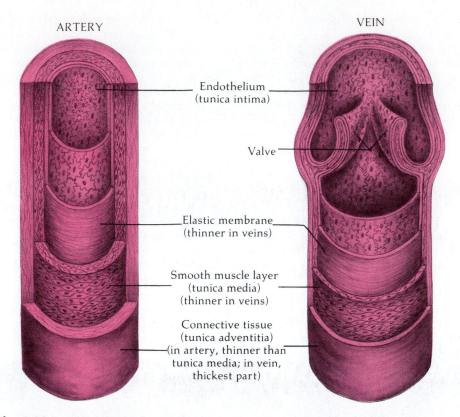

Endothelium
(tunica intima)

Valve

Elastic membrane
(thinner in veins)

Smooth muscle layer
(tunica media)
(thinner in veins)

Connective tissue
(tunica adventitia)
(in artery, thinner than
tunica media; in vein,
thickest part)

Fig. 4-20 Cross section of an artery and vein showing the three layers: tunica intima, tunica media, and tunica adventitia. Larger veins and arteries have their own blood supplies provided by tiny blood vessels (vasa vasorum) distributed throughout the vessel walls. (From Thompson JM and others: *Mosby's clinical nursing*, ed 3, St Louis, 1993, Mosby.)

the capillary beds, where carbon dioxide is exchanged for oxygen. Oxygenated blood from the lungs flows through the pulmonary veins into the left atrium. After birth, direct contact between blood from the right side of the heart and blood from the left side occurs only at the capillary level.

Fetal Circulation

In utero there is mixing of blood from both sides of the heart through the **foramen ovale,** which becomes the fossa ovalis (Fig. 4-22). In addition, there is a communication between the aorta and the pulmonary artery, called the **ductus arteriosus.** In fetal life deoxygenated blood is oxygenated in the placenta (rather than the lungs). The lungs are relatively nonfunctional; thus perfusion of this organ is not critical. At birth, however, the lungs assume responsibility for oxygenation. Expansion of the lungs with air decreases pulmonary vascular resistance and therefore resistance to flow from the right atrium and the right ventricle. Studies by Rudolph (1970) have shown that pulmonary vascular resistance decreases mainly in response to the elevated oxygen levels within the pulmonary vessels.

At the same time systemic vascular resistance and aortic pressure increase because the tremendous blood flow through the placenta ceases. This increased pressure is reflected in the left ventricle and the left atrium. Because blood flows from areas of higher pressure to areas of lower pressure, blood preferentially travels from the right side of the heart into the lower-pressure right ventricle and pulmonary bed rather than into the higher-pressure region of the left side of the heart. Increased left atrial pressure closes the flap that lies over the foramen ovale on the left atrial wall.

Cessation of flow through the ductus arteriosus is not related to pressure gradients, however. It is due to changes in the muscular wall of the ductus that cause it to constrict. Over the next few months, fibrous ingrowth occludes the lumen altogether; the remaining structure is called the **ligamentum arteriosum.** Occasionally a ductus remains patent, causing excessive pulmonary blood flow. The ductus can be ligated to close the communication; surgery can be performed in the neonatal intensive care unit or the operating room (see Chapter 20).

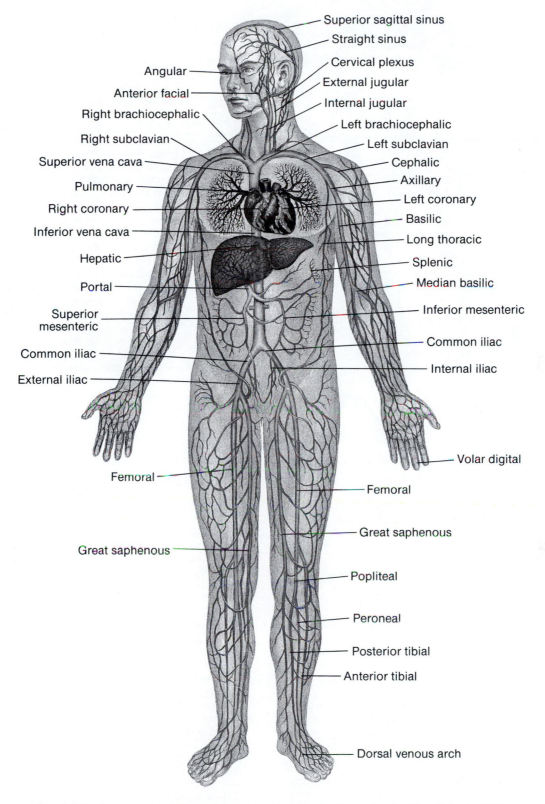

Fig. 4-21 **Venous circulation.** (From Cannobio MM: *Cardiovascular disorders,* St Louis, 1990, Mosby.)

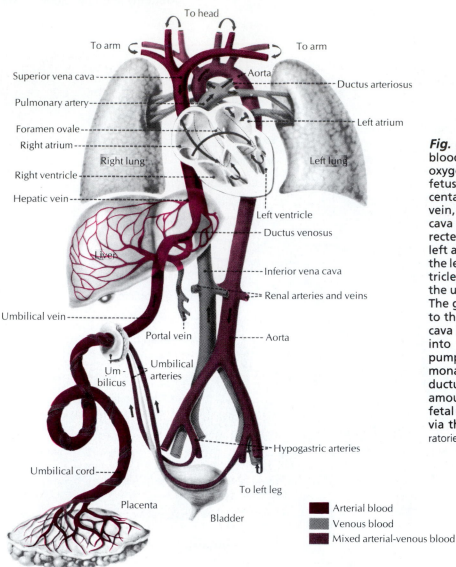

To head

To arm

To arm

Superior vena cava

Aorta

Ductus arteriosus

Pulmonary artery

Left atrium

Foramen ovale

Right atrium

Right lung

Left lung

Right ventricle

Hepatic vein

Left ventricle

Ductus venosus

Liver

Inferior vena cava

Renal arteries and veins

Umbilical vein

Portal vein

Aorta

Um-bilicus

Umbilical arteries

Hypogastric arteries

Umbilical cord

To left leg

Placenta

Bladder

■ Arterial blood

■ Venous blood

■ Mixed arterial-venous blood

Fig. 4-22 Fetal circulation. The mother's blood is circulated to the placenta, where oxygen and nutrients are exchanged for the fetus's metabolic products. From the placenta, blood flows through the umbilical vein, fetal ductus venosus, and inferior vena cava to the right atrium. This blood is directed through the foramen ovale into the left atrium, bypassing the fetal lungs. From the left atrium blood flows into the left ventricle, which pumps it into the aorta and the umbilical arteries, back to the placenta. The greater portion of the blood returning to the right atrium from the superior vena cava is directed through the tricuspid valve into the right ventricle. From here it is pumped into the pulmonary artery. Pulmonary blood flow is shunted through the ductus arteriosus into the aorta. A small amount of pulmonary blood flow enters the fetal lungs and returns to the left atrium via the pulmonary veins. (Courtesy Ross Laboratories, Columbus, Ohio.)

REFERENCES

Athanassopoulos G, Cokkinos DV: Atrial natriuretic factor, *Prog Cardiovasc Dis* 33(5):313, 1991.

Berne RM, Levy MN: *Cardiovascular physiology*, ed 6, St Louis, 1992, Mosby.

Bharati S, Lev M, Kirklin J: *Cardiac surgery and the conduction system*, New York, 1983, John Wiley & Sons.

Braunwald E: *Heart disease: a textbook of cardiovascular medicine*, ed 4, Philadelphia, 1992, WB Saunders.

Clendening L: *Sourcebook of medical history*, New York, 1942, Dover Publications.

David TE: Preservation of the posterior chordae tendineae in mitral valve replacement. In Grillo HC and others: *Current therapy in cardiothoracic surgery*, Toronto, 1989, BC Decker.

DeHaan RL: The embryonic origin of the heartbeat. In Hurst JW, editor: *The heart, arteries and veins*, ed 7, vols 1 and 2, New York, 1990, McGraw-Hill.

Feeney MK: Dysrhythmias. In Guzzetta CE, Dossey BM: *Cardiovascular nursing: holistic practice*, St Louis, 1992, Mosby.

Guyton AC: *Textbook of medical physiology*, ed 8, Philadelphia, 1991, WB Saunders.

Guzzetta CE, Dossey BM: The critical link between body and mind. In Guzzetta CE, Dossey BM: *Cardiovascular nursing: holistic practice*, St Louis, 1992, Mosby.

Hurst JW, editors: *Atlas of the heart*, New York, 1988, Gower.

Kirklin JW, Barratt-Boyes BG: *Cardiac surgery*, ed 2, New York, 1993, Churchill Livingstone.

Lake CL: *Cardiovascular anesthesia*, New York, 1985, Springer-Verlag.

Menasche P: Coronary sinus retroperfusion for myocardial protection: pragmatic observations and caveats based on a large experience. In Karp RB, Laks H, Wechsler AS, editors: *Advances in cardiac surgery*, vol 4, St Louis, 1993, Mosby.

Mohl W and others: Current status of coronary sinus interventions. In Karp RB, Laks H, Wechsler AS, editors: *Advances in cardiac surgery*, vol 2, St Louis, 1990, Mosby.

Rudolph AM: The changes in the circulation after birth, *Circulation* 41:343, 1970.

Schlant RC, Silverman ME, Roberts WC: Anatomy of the heart. In Hurst JW, editor: *The heart, arteries and veins*, ed 7, vols 1 and 2, New York, 1990, McGraw-Hill.

Schlant RC, Sonnenblick EH: Normal physiology of the cardiovascular system. In Hurst JW, editor: *The heart, arteries and veins*, ed 7, vols 1 and 2, New York, 1990, McGraw-Hill.

Thelan LA, Davis JK, Urden LD: *Textbook of critical care nursing*, St Louis, 1990, Mosby.

Thorek P: *Anatomy in surgery*, ed 3, New York, 1983, Springer-Verlag.

5

Environment, Instrumentation, and Equipment

Why should a cardiac surgical unit be organized or developed? Where should such units be organized? When should they be organized? With what resources should they be developed? Finally, how does one go about it and what does it take to make it go?

Arthur E. Baue, MD, Alexander S. Geha, MD, and Hugh O'Kane, MD, 1974 (p. 31)

Questions asked in 1974 about organizing a cardiac surgical unit remain pertinent today because of the intense demands that such a service places on a hospital's human, material, and fiscal resources. As medical costs escalate and reimbursement decreases, the appropriateness and expense of diagnosing and treating cardiovascular disease have come under intense scrutiny.

One consequence of this is the public's demand for greater accountability by health care professionals for their clinical performance and the results of their interventions. Professional organizations such as the American Nurses Association (ANA) and the Association of Operating Room Nurses (AORN) (1993) have developed standards to guide nurses in their practice. Standards specific to cardiovascular nursing practice have been published by the ANA and the American Heart Association (AHA) Council on Cardiovascular Nursing (ANA/AHA, 1981). Accrediting agencies such as the Joint Commission on Accreditation of Healthcare Organizations (JCAHO, 1993) and federal and state governments require specific evidence of acceptable standards of clinical practice and patient outcomes.

This emphasis on the process and outcome of care is reflected in standards that, respectively, guide the way care is provided and monitor the results that are achieved. In addition to **process** and **outcome standards, structural standards** exist that relate to the material aspects of the clinical arena. Interest in these guidelines has been exemplified by the enactment of The Safe Medical Devices Act of 1990 (Public Law 101-629), which demonstrates the public's concern about the development and use of technologic re-sources and makes users of these devices accountable for their actions.

Cardiac perioperative nurses use a wide array of machines and equipment, and they must ensure that they are operated not only in a safe manner, but also efficiently, effectively, and cost-consciously. AORN's Standards of Administrative Nursing Practice (AORN, 1993) reflect those structural standards that assist nurses in providing a safe operating room environment and in using available resources appropriately. This chapter discusses the material resources of a cardiac operating room, including the cardiac suite, equipment, instruments, supplies, and prosthetic implants. Suggested policies and procedures for a cardiac service are listed in Box 5-1.

THE CARDIAC SUITE

What the minimum requirements should be for performing cardiac procedures has come under debate on numerous occasions, but standards for the construction of a cardiac suite have remained fairly constant since the publication of guidelines by the Inter-Society Commission for Heart Disease Resources of the American College of Cardiology (ACC) and the AHA (ACC/AHA, 1991; Scannel and others, 1975). These guidelines (Box 5-2) reflect the intensive demand for adequate monitoring, electrical safety, protected power supplies, availability of hot and cold water, infection control mechanisms, and other resources that support an optimal cardiac surgical environment.

Diagnosis and treatment facilities should be closely linked both geographically and operationally to pro-

Box 5-1 *Policies and procedures related to cardiac surgery*

Policies and procedures specific to cardiac surgery are listed below. When policies and procedures are already available in the main operating room (such as those related to counts, electrosurgical safety, and positioning), they can be used by the cardiac service and need not be reformulated.

Autotransfusion system
Blood refrigerator
Hypothermia/hyperthermia unit
Preparation of iced saline/"slush"
Rinsing and preparation of glutaraldehyde-preserved valve prostheses
Preclotting of vascular grafts
Policy for compliance with The Safe Medical Devices Act of 1990
Borrowing and lending of cardiac supplies and equipment
Availability/maintenance of sterile cardiac instrument sets during steam shutdown
Use of emergency generators during power failure
Use of internal/external defibrillator
Posting of cardiac procedures: scheduled, emergent
Position descriptions for cardiac staff (circulating and scrub nurses, RN first assistants)
Orientation program to the cardiac service
Staffing of the cardiac suite(s)
Staffing coverage for percutaneous transluminal coronary angioplasties and atherectomies
Emergency sternotomy outside the cardiac operating room (e.g., intensive care unit, emergency room)
Use of cardiac personnel in noncardiac operating rooms
On-call policy for cardiac personnel
Notification of on-call personnel in emergency situations
Visitor policy for the cardiac operating room
Death procedure/procedure for family viewing of the deceased
Preoperative patient assessment
Patient/family teaching of the cardiac surgery patient
Postoperative report to the surgical intensive care unit
Postoperative patient assessment
Sterilization methods, recommendations for cardiac instruments/supplies/equipment
Policy for compliance with the Anatomical Gift Act
Policies related to organ transplantation/retrieval of donor organs
Cardiac quality improvement
Policy on Patient Self-Determination Act

mote the flow of information and continuity of care. Interdisciplinary cooperation and communication between the operating room (OR) and units such as the emergency department, the coronary care unit, the surgical and/or neonatal intensive care unit, the laboratory, and the cardiac catheterization and angiographic suites enhance patient outcomes.

Traffic patterns are of special concern within the operating room, as well as to and from other departments. Transport routes should be preplanned to avoid delays. For instance, the fastest routes from the cardiac catheterization laboratory and the surgical intensive care unit to the cardiac OR should be identified, because patients requiring emergency surgery often come from these areas. (Mock runs can be practiced to test the system.) If an elevator must be used, it should be called to the floor and held so that the patient can be moved into it without delay. It should be of sufficient size to accommodate the patient, the staff, and equipment such as monitors and ventricular support devices. In some hospitals freight elevators may provide the only adequately sized lifts.

Occasionally, cardiovascular procedures are performed outside the OR suite because patients are too critically ill to be transported. Such cases include emergency sternotomies for postoperative cardiac tamponade in the surgical intensive care unit, portable cardiopulmonary bypass for failed angioplasty patients in circulatory collapse (Regas, 1990) and patent ductus arteriosus ligations in the neonatal intensive care unit (Huddleston, 1991). In planning procedures to be performed outside the OR, perioperative nurses must consider (1) how sterility is to be maintained; (2) how to supply all necessary equipment, instruments, and other items; and (3) how to work within the confines of an unfamiliar environment (Box 5-3).

FURNITURE

Standard furnishings found in the cardiac OR include the OR bed and accessories, small and standard-size tables, kick buckets, ring stands, Mayo stands, linen and waste hampers, intravenous (IV) poles, suction, sitting and standing stools, patient monitors, and anesthesia machines. Additional tables and stands may be needed for extra basins, instrument containers, and drapes (Pierson, 1991). They may also be needed to provide surfaces for setting up a sterile field to insert intravascular lines by anesthesia personnel, or for rinsing biologic valve prostheses, thawing cryopreserved homografts, or arranging components of ventricular assist devices. Portable carts may be used to store suture, prosthetic implants, or other supplies.

The OR bed may be modified to enable it to be raised higher than usual for exposure of the internal mammary arteries (located on either side of the retrosternal borders). Surgery on neonates and infants may require a special, smaller bed with a hood to reflect and maintain body temperature (Firkins and Joy, 1989).

Cardiac ORs are typically dedicated to open heart procedures. Furniture is selected and arranged according to the preference and needs of the staff and often is consistent with an established plan. Some ORs use one or more Mayo stands and a back table; others may use an overbed table without a Mayo stand. The staff can determine what works best for them.

Whatever the plan, it can be diagrammed for environmental service employees to assist them in returning items to their proper location after cleaning. This diagram should include instructions about re-

---

Box 5-2 *Recommended resources for cardiac surgery*

Cardiac Operating Room

600 to 800 square feet

Large enough to accommodate 8 to 12 (or more) staff members

Large enough to maneuver without contamination of sterile areas

Storage space

Sufficient for cardiac instrument, supplies, and equipment

Easily accessible to cardiac staff

Pump Room

Adequate for storage of pump oxygenator(s) and assist devices

Located within surgical suite

Accessible from inside and outside suite

Plumbing

Installation of plumbing to provide hot, cold, and waste water for pump oxygenator

Suction

3 to 4 separate and independent sources of suction

1 dedicated suction source for anesthesia

Anesthesia Utility Pedestal

Ceiling-mounted units for gasses, oxygen, suction, electrical outlets, and/or

Floor-mounted multipurpose pedestals

Blood Gas Core Laboratory

Capable of performing analyses of blood gasses, pH, and electrolytes

Located adjacent to or near operating suite

Capable of providing blood gas results within 5 to 10 minutes during cardiopulmonary bypass

Infection Control

Installation of air-handling equipment capable of at least 25 operating room air changes per hour

Maintenance of temperature between 20° and 24° C (68° and 75° F), with capability of attaining 15.5° C (60° F)

Maintenance of humidity between 50% and 55%

Installation of high-efficiency particulate air filtering of incoming air (state codes may vary)

Unobstructed exhaust vents

Higher air pressure in operating room than outside operating room

Compliance with dress codes

Appropriate sterilization techniques

Electrical Hazard Control

Sufficient electrical outlets for equipment

90 to 120 amperes for peak load electrical current

Availability of alternative sources of power in case of power failure

Compliance with national electric codes

Electrical Interference and Shielding

Avoidance of monitoring signal distortion

Operating Room Illumination

Capability of lighting two operating fields simultaneously

200 to 250 foot candles for ambient light in operating room

2500 to 4000 foot candles for operative site

Instruments and Prostheses

Preventive maintenance and repair program

Appropriate storage and sterilization

Monitoring

Capability to monitor cardiorespiratory systems, blood gasses, pH, electrolytes, temperature, renal function, and coagulation abnormalities

Communication

Capability for direct audio communication with blood bank and operating room control desk

Data Handling

Capability to input and retrieve patient data

Pump Oxygenator

Availability of backup pump oxygenator

Preventive maintenance program

Record system for each pump oxygenator

Radiology

Capability of flexibility and maintenance of sterility of surgical field

Availability of a rapid processing unit in close proximity to operating room

Preventive Maintenance Program

Availability of policies and procedures for preventive maintenance of equipment and plant of operating room

Regular surveillance of medical devices for safety and efficacy

Availability of policies and procedures for emergency repairs and replacement of equipment

Data from ACC/AHA Task Force (1991); Department of Health, Education, and Welfare (1978); and Inter-Society Commission for Heart Disease Resources (1975, 1976).

---

connecting electrical cords that have been unplugged during cleaning. A diagram is also useful for OR personnel who are not familiar with the routine arrangement and must begin the initial room preparation for an emergency procedure. This may occur on the evening or night shifts when cardiac staff are not yet in-house. Orientation to the cardiac OR will enable those unfamiliar with the cardiac routine to help during emergencies. Of special importance is the location of supplies, instruments, medications, etc., and the identification of what items to open. Wasted supplies can be minimized if only those items that need to be opened are set around the room when the cardiac staff leaves for the day.

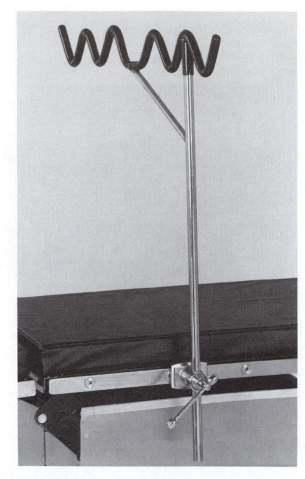

Fig. 5-1 "Picket fence" used to elevate one or both legs for circumferential skin preparation. Other models have two legs that attach to the OR bed. (Courtesy OSI, Orthopedic Systems, Inc., Hayward, Calif.)

EQUIPMENT
Positioning Equipment

The patient position for most cardiac procedures is supine, because that position affords the best exposure of the heart and great vessels. Positioning supplies and padding for hands and elbows can be kept near the OR bed. If the lower extremities do not need to be exposed, an anesthesia screen placed at the foot of the bed will keep heavy drapes off the feet. In obese patients padded sleds may be needed to keep the arms tucked next to the body. Armboards attached to the bed can provide extra width for very large patients. Very tall patients may require a footboard to extend the length of the bed.

An anesthesia screen or IV poles keep drapes off the face and provide access to the airway and intravascular lines. Some services use an overbed frame that is placed over the patient's head. These frames may have a shelf that, after being draped, can be used

by the surgeon and assistant to place instruments. Splints may be used to maintain the position of the wrist in which a radial arterial monitoring line has been inserted.

When saphenous leg vein must be excised for coronary bypass grafting, leg holders can be used to elevate the legs for circumferential skin preparation (Fig. 5-1). Elevating or flexing the legs may be contraindicated when a femoral artery sheath is in place, so the nurse should first confer with the surgeon about which skin preparation and positioning technique to use. Foam rubber leg supports that elevate and externally rotate the legs are available for intraoperative use to provide optimal exposure for harvesting saphenous leg veins (see Chapter 12).

Cardiovascular lesions such as those involving the descending thoracic aorta are best approached through a left lateral thoracotomy incision. Lateral positioning equipment and supplies include overarm boards (or Mayo stands), axillary rolls, and pillows to support the legs and feet. A vacuum pillow on the bed that hardens into the desired shape when suction is applied is useful for lateral positioning. A modified

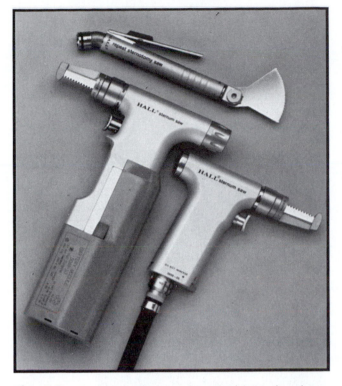

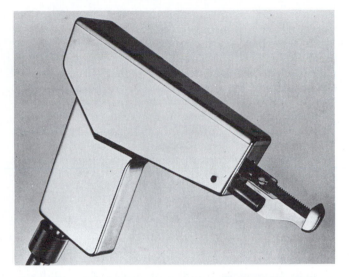

Fig. 5-3 Electric (reciprocating) sternal saw with a foot-control pedal. (Courtesy Sarns 3M Health Care, Ann Arbor, Mich.)

Fig. 5-2 *Clockwise, from right:* Air-driven, hand-controlled sternal saw powered by nitrogen from a portable tank; battery-powered (reciprocating) sternal saw (convenient for sternal splitting during distant procurement of donor hearts for transplantation); oscillating saw often used for repeat sternotomies. (Courtesy Zimmer, Hall Surgical Div., Carpinteria, Calif.)

lateral position can be achieved with a small roll, sandbag, or IV bag placed under the operative side, thereby slightly tilting the chest to provide the necessary exposure.

Headlight, Loupes

A fiberoptic headlight and light source offer supplemental lighting, which is usually necessary for illuminating deep chest cavities. In addition to the surgeon, the assistant may also require a headlight. Loupes with $2\frac{1}{2}\times$ to $3\frac{1}{2}\times$ magnification are commonly used and may be stored in the cardiac suite.

Sternal Saw

To expose the mediastinum, the sternum is divided from the xiphoid process to the sternal notch with a saw that is air driven (Fig. 5-2, *A*), battery powered (Fig. 5-2, *B*), or electrically powered (Fig. 5-3). The blade is inserted with the teeth facing up. Some surgeons prefer to saw from the sternal notch to the xiphoid process; in this case, the toothed edge of the blade is inserted downward. (In neonates and infants, heavy scissors can be used to transect the cartilaginous sternum.)

An oscillating saw with sagittal saw blades (Fig. 5-2, *C*) may be used for repeat sternotomies, where the presence of adhesions from a previous sternotomy increases the risk of injuring underlying structures adhering to the sternum. The action of the saw allows the bone to be divided from the anterior table of the sternum to the posterior table. Saw blades may be wide or narrow depending on surgeon preference. Some surgeons prefer to use the reciprocating saw (Fig. 5-3) for repeat sternotomies.

When a saw is unavailable, a Lebsche knife and mallet may be the only available means of splitting the sternum to expose the heart in acute settings such as an emergency room (see Chapter 21). Thoracotomy incisions are made with a knife.

Hypothermia/Hyperthermia Units

The ability to control the temperature of both the patient and the environment is critical to the success of cardiac surgery. External patient cooling and warming is achieved with mobile hypothermia/hyperthermia units. Some units have only a warming function. A disposable or nondisposable thermia blanket is placed under a sheet (or other padding) on the OR table and connected to hoses running to the unit. The desired temperature is selected, and water within the machine's reservoir is pumped through the hoses into the channels within the blanket. The unit must be kept filled with water to function properly. The unit should be turned on early so that it will be warm when the patient is positioned on it. (And the filling process will be completed more quickly if the unit is activated before the blanket is compressed by the patient's weight.) Recommended temperature settings are between 38° and 40° C (100.4° and 104° [Stellar, 1991]). In addition to monitoring water temperature, some machines also monitor the patient's temperature via a rectal probe that is inserted before the patient is draped.

Hypodermic needles, towel clips, or other sharp objects stuck into the blanket will cause the circulating water to leak out of the thermia pad and may pose an electrosurgical hazard. Thermal burns are a potential danger, although most hyperthermia units do not exceed the safe setting of 41° to 42° C. A more probable cause of injury from these units is pressure necrosis. Recommendations for preventing such injuries include placing additional padding between the patient and the blanket, confirming the proper position of the temperature probe, and maintaining electrical safety practices when electrosurgical instruments are used (Hyperthermia devices and skin injury, 1990).

Radiant Heaters

Radiant heaters may be employed as an additional heat source for maintaining body temperature. These are often used in pediatric procedures. Precautions are necessary to avoid burns or insensible water loss from prolonged use.

Saline Ice Units

Cold topical solutions enhance cooling of the myocardium during induced hypothermia. Various methods of cooling normal saline (or lactated Ringer's solution) are available, such as refrigerator or freezer storage of bags or bottles, or using dry ice or isopropyl alcohol as the cooling agent. The unit shown in Fig. 5-4 is self-contained and specifically designed for cardiovascular procedures.

Cold topical solutions are also available in dispenser bags (Fig. 5-5), making them especially useful for transplant organ preservation during the procurement period. The bags can be cooled, transported to the procurement site, and opened to expose a sterile wrapped solution container. The wrapping is removed, and the contents are poured or squeezed into a basin.

Defibrillator

Defibrillation by the external or internal application of a direct-current (DC) electrical shock to the myocardium is instituted when the heart fibrillates. It is the only reliable therapy for persistent ventricular tachycardia and ventricular fibrillation (Bojar, 1989). The amount of current selected will vary depending on the size of the patient and on whether internal or external defibrillation is being performed (Table 5-1). It should be noted that defibrillation will not convert a heart that is asystolic; the heart must be fibrillating. (A pacemaker would be needed for the heart to start beating.)

Defibrillators (Fig. 5-6) should be tested before use. The unit may not function if the power cord has been disconnected and there is insufficient battery power. The unit should be inspected routinely to ensure that it is connected to line power when it is not in use.

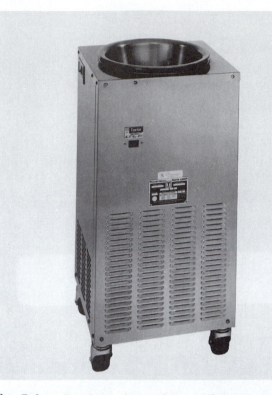

Fig. 5-4 Saline ice unit. Coolants such as isopropyl alcohol and water are placed in the basin, which is covered with a sterile drape and a basin filled with normal saline or lactated Ringer's solution. The solution is cooled to the desired temperature and consistency (liquid or soft slush) and poured over the heart to provide topical cooling of the myocardium. (Courtesy Taylor Co., Rockton, Ill.)

Both external and internal paddle tips come in an assortment of sizes (Fig. 5-7). Disposable defibrillator electrodes (Fig. 5-8, *E*) can be applied securely to the chest. Some manufacturers make pediatric adaptors that slip over the standard external paddles (Fig. 5-8, *B*). Internal paddles (Fig. 5-8, *D*) are screwed into handles attached to cords that are connected to the defibrillator (or the adapter [Fig. 5-8, *A*] that inserts into the defibrillator). Ethylene oxide is indicated for sterilizing handles and cords; internal paddle tips can be steam sterilized. However, to avoid the separation of tips, handles, and cords, it is recommended that a set of tips, handles, and cords be sterilized as a unit. External paddles sterilizable by ethylene oxide are available (Fig. 5-8, *C*). These can be used when the recently draped patient fibrillates and the sternum is not yet opened to allow placement of internal paddles.

For defibrillation, direct electrical current must traverse the myocardium. To achieve this, internal paddles are commonly placed laterally on the right atrium and the left ventricle. They do not need to be moistened with conductive paste, since the heart is already lubricated with blood and pericardial fluid. Personnel should stand away from the table to avoid being shocked. In the presence of pericardial effusions from prior sternotomy, sterile external paddles can be used.

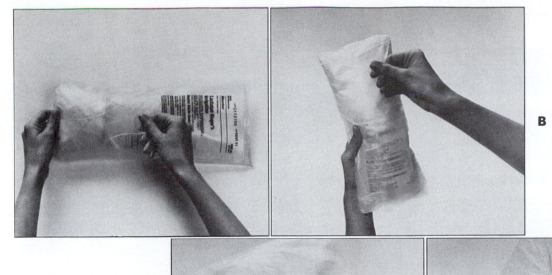

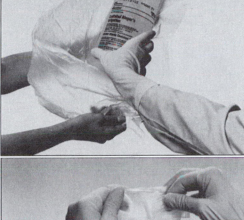

Fig. 5-5 Sterile dispensing system for cold topical solutions. **A,** The overwrap is removed to expose the dispensing bag. **B,** The ridged tab is grasped and pulled to expose the wrapped container. **C,** The point of the wrap is pulled forward and back to expose the sterile container. **D,** The sterile nurse removes the container from the wrap. **E,** The sterile nurse opens the container by pulling the tab directly across the bag. (Courtesy Baxter Healthcare Corp., IV Systems Div., Round Lake, Ill.)

Table 5-1 ■ *External/internal defibrillator settings for children and adults*

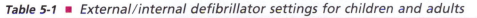

	Setting
	External Setting
Infants*	2 watt seconds/kg
Children*	2 watt seconds/kg
Older children	100-300 watt seconds
Adults	200-400 watt seconds
	Internal Setting
Neonates and children:	Lowest possible setting should be used, starting at 3 watt seconds for neonates and 5 watt seconds for children, and increasing the energy in slow increments; no definitive data are available for defibrillation energy requirements in neonate and child
Older children and adults†	10 to 20 watt seconds

*Data from the American Academy of Pediatrics Committee on Drugs: Emergency drug doses for infants and children, *Pediatrics* 81(3):462, 1988.
†Data from Kerber RE and others: Open chest defibrillation during cardiac surgery: energy and current requirements, *Am J Cardiol* 46:393, 1980.

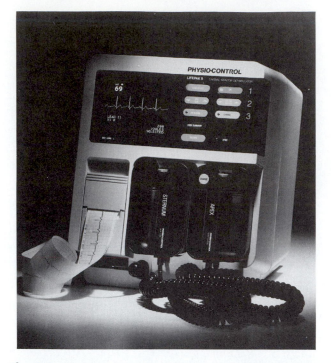

Fig. 5-6 Defibrillator. The unit provides internal and/or external defibrillation or cardioversion. (Courtesy Physio-Control Corp., Redmond, Wash.)

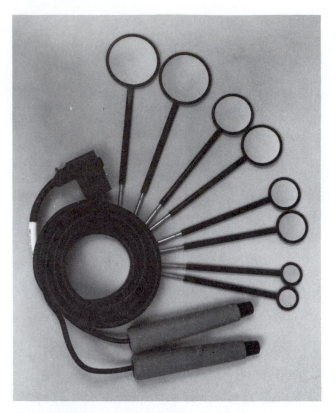

Fig. 5-7 Internal defibrillator paddle tips come in an array of sizes. Smaller tips are used for infants and children. A large tip placed under the patient's back and a standard adult tip placed directly on the heart provide external-internal defibrillation. Paddles will work only in defibrillator units for which they were designed. (Courtesy Hewlett-Packard Co., Medical Products Group, Andover, Mass.)

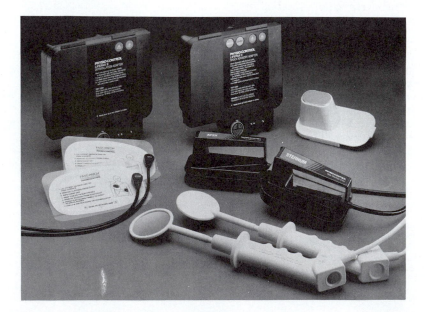

Fig. 5-8 Accessories for LifePak 9 defibrillator. *Clockwise, from top:* Defibrillator adapter cassette (required for internal paddles); pediatric clip-on external paddles, which slide over adult paddles; sterilizable external paddles (ethylene oxide is recommended for sterilization); internal defibrillator handles and tips with remote discharge control; disposable defibrillator/ECG electrodes for external defibrillation. (Courtesy Physio-Control Corp., Redmond, Wash.)

Another method is to perform anteroposterior defibrillation with a large, flat external paddle placed against the patient's back and an internal paddle placed on top of the heart (Fig. 5-7). Precautions should be taken to pad the handle of the external paddle so as not to cause pressure injury to the patient's back. If the patient fibrillates during dissection of the adhesions, anteroposterior defibrillation with internal-external paddles can be performed. Or, the pleura can be opened and the internal paddles placed on the pleural surface and pressed against the heart.

The defibrillator can also be used for cardioversion. The difference between defibrillation and cardioversion is that the former delivers an unsynchronized shock to the heart. A patient requiring cardioversion has a pulse (e.g., the ventricle is not fibrillating), and the shock is synchronized with the R wave of the QRS complex. In the OR the procedure is most commonly indicated to convert recent-onset atrial fibrillation to normal sinus rhythm. When cardioversion is to be performed, the patient is attached by electrocardiogram (ECG) cables to the defibrillator, which has been set to the "synchronous" mode. This is done to synchronize the delivery of electrical current to the R wave of the QRS complex (ventricular systole). If the shock is not synchronized to the R wave, it can produce ventricular fibrillation if it is discharged during the vulnerable period (the T wave of the ECG).

The unit is then charged and activated. Successful cardioversion depolarizes all excitable myocardium, interrupts abnormal electrical circuits, and establishes electrical homogeneity, which fosters normal sinus rhythm (Zipes, 1992). When no QRS complex exists (e.g., in ventricular fibrillation), the defibrillator will not discharge if it is in the synchronous mode, because there is no regular waveform that the machine can "read" and synchronize to. If the patient fibrillates, valuable time may be lost trying to change settings to "asynchronous"; therefore it is recommended that the defibrillator routinely be kept in the asynchronous mode unless cardioversion specifically is performed.

Fibrillator

Under controlled conditions, induced fibrillation is a useful technique in the control of hemorrhage, which can occur when the myocardium or a major artery is lacerated and cardiopulmonary bypass has been discontinued. The beating heart produces a systolic force and a pulse wave that can disrupt sutures as they are being inserted or tied. A cardiac fibrillator capable of delivering 25 to 50 V of alternating current (AC) produces a fine fibrillation, enabling the surgeon to repair the injury on a quiescent field (Fig. 5-9).

To perform this technique, the surgeon uses the temporary epicardial ventricular pacing lead wires that have been attached prior to termination of cardiopulmonary bypass. The distal ends of the leads are passed off the field and attached to the fibrillator. The fibrillator is activated, producing fine fibrillation. Once the repair is accomplished and the bleeding con-

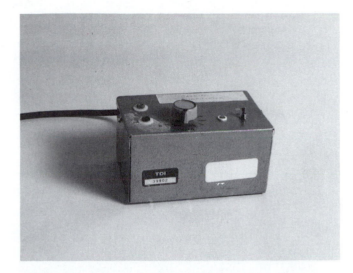

Fig. 5-9 Electrical fibrillator delivers direct current to produce fine fibrillation, allowing the surgeon to work on a relatively quiescent field. (Courtesy Edward A. Lefrak, MD.)

trolled, cardiac massage followed by defibrillation with DC countershock (with internal paddles) will cause cardiac action to resume. (The pacing leads may then be removed from the fibrillator and attached to an external pacemaker for pacing if indicated.)

Nurses must understand the different indications for fibrillation and defibrillation if serious accidents are to be avoided. Fibrillation is used to produce a relatively motionless field so that tissue being repaired is not torn; defibrillation is used to reverse fibrillation and initiate cardiac contractions. To reduce confusion between the fibrillator and the defibrillator, one author has suggested painting the fibrillator red and referring to it as the "red box" (Cooley, 1984).

Electrosurgical Unit

Electrosurgical units use high-frequency electrical current to cut tissue and cauterize bleeding vessels. The development of solid-state generators has significantly decreased the potential for burns and electrical shocks that were associated with spark-gap units (although not all cardiac surgeons have welcomed this modification).

Two electrosurgical units may be used when more than one surgical site is being exposed. This may occur during coronary artery bypass procedures where the saphenous vein is being excised simultaneously with opening of the chest and preparation for cannulation. When two units are in use, each unit must be connected to its own dispersive pad that has been applied to the patient. Commonly, dispersive pads are applied bilaterally to the patient's buttocks. When two units are in use, caution must be taken to ensure that changes in current settings are made only to the unit being used by the surgeon making the request and that the unused electrosurgical pencil is not discharged inadvertently by leaning on the control but-

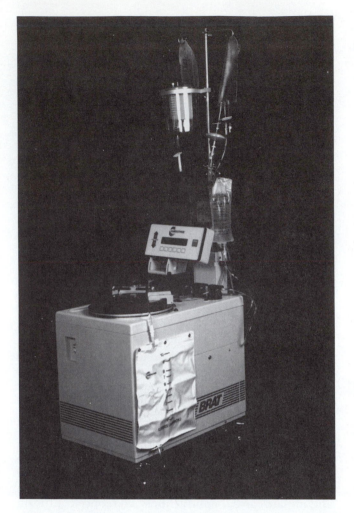

Fig. 5-10   Baylor Rapid Autologous Transfusion (BRAT) System. (Courtesy COBE Cardiovascular, Inc., Arvada, Colo.)

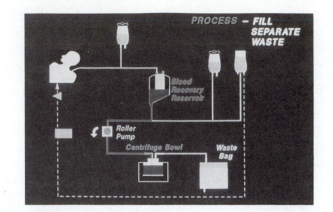

Fig. 5-11   Autotransfusion system. (Courtesy Haemonetics Corp., Braintree, Mass.)

ton. The amount of current needed will vary during the operation depending on the type of tissue being cauterized. Often the surgeon will request a lower setting when cauterizing close to vascular structures such as the aorta or internal mammary artery.

Precautions are warranted in patients with permanent pacemakers. Problems that have been encountered with the use of electrocautery include damage or alterations to pulse generator functions, electrical and thermal burns at the myocardial insertion site of the electrode, and ventricular fibrillation. Some authors have suggested the use of bipolar cautery to reduce the amount of electricity transmitted to surrounding tissue. When monopolar probes are used, precautions include placing the dispersive pads as far as possible from the pulse generator, using short bursts of electrocautery, monitoring pacer function frequently, and having ready access to a pulse-generator programmer (Levine and others, 1986). If possible, the type and manufacturer of the pacemaker should be identified in the event that reprogramming or other alterations have to be made.

Recent innovations have included argon-enhanced coagulation, which produces less charring and more controlled hemostasis. Proposed benefits of this technology include greater efficiency in controlling bleeding from small vessels and capillaries such as those in the internal mammary artery bed of the retrosternum.

Autotransfusion System

Autotransfusion systems (Fig. 5-10) that salvage, process, and return blood back to the patient have several advantages, including avoidance of incompatible bank blood, decreased risk of infection, and less danger of donor-related disease. Contraindications to the use of autologous blood transfusions include sepsis, severe coagulopathy, renal failure, bowel perforation, and cancer (Martin and others, 1989).

Blood is collected by suction, filtered, and anticoagulated with a heparin solution or citrated phosphate dextrose. A cell processor separates and packs the red blood cells, which have been washed to remove the anticoagulant and reinfused as indicated (Fig. 5-11). Precautions should be taken to avoid suctioning topical hemostatic agents such as thrombin, fibrin glue, or microfibrillar collagen compounds into the reservoir, since they can trigger clotting mechanisms (Girard, Morgan, and Orr, 1988). The aspiration of topical antibiotics should be avoided as well.

Another method of autotransfusion is used postoperatively to salvage mediastinal shed blood. Chest tube drainage is collected, filtered, and reinfused within a 1- or 2-hour period (Sympson, 1991). The collecting chamber (Fig. 5-12) may be a unit designed solely for chest tube drainage, or it may be the venous reservoir used during the bypass procedure and modified for autotransfusion. Collection systems should be labeled with the patient's name.

Pump Oxygenator

The pump oxygenator (Fig. 5-13), also called the heart-lung machine, bypass pump, or the "pump,"

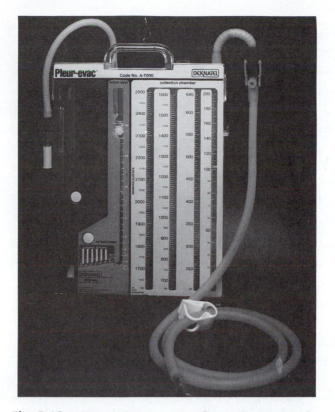

Fig. 5-12 Chest drainage system for mediastinal and/or pleural chest tubes. Chest tubes are connected to the tubing from the collecting chamber; gentle suction is applied. The unit can be modified to provide autotransfusion capability. (Courtesy Deknatel, Inc., Fall River, Mass.)

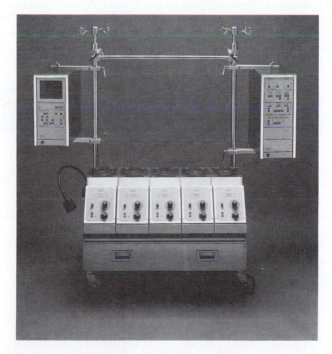

Fig. 5-13 Cardiopulmonary bypass pump. (Courtesy Sorin Biomedical, Irvine, Calif.)

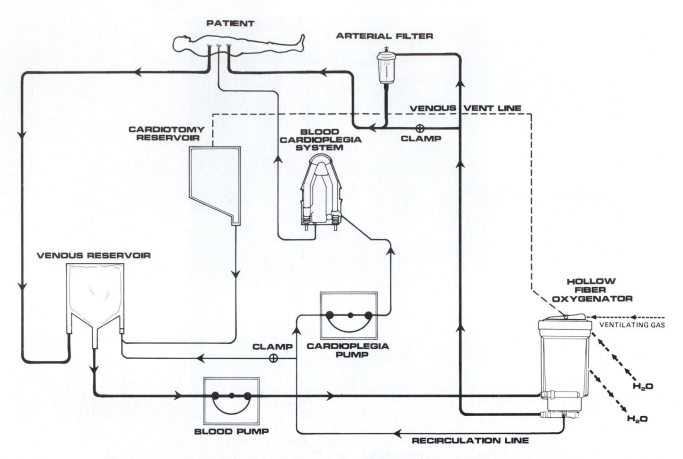

Fig. 5-14 Typical extracorporeal blood circuit used during cardiac surgery. Venous blood exits the patient and drains by gravity into a venous reservoir. The blood is then pumped into the oxygenator. The oxygenator's heat exchanger controls the temperature of the blood during surgery. The ventilating gas flowing into the oxygenator removes carbon dioxide and adds oxygen to the blood. The oxygenated blood then flows through the arterial filter and back to the patient. Oxygenated blood is also taken from the oxygenator and mixed with a cardioplegia solution before being pumped through the blood cardioplegia system heat exchanger, where it is cooled. The blood is then periodically infused into the coronary arteries antegradely and/or retrogradely to nourish the heart while it is arrested during the cardiac repair. (Courtesy Sorin Biomedical, Irvine, Calif.)

supports the patient's cardiorespiratory function during cardiac surgery. It does this by draining or siphoning venous blood, removing waste gases, oxygenating and filtering the blood, and pumping it back into the patient's arterial system (Fig. 5-14). The unit incorporates an oxygenator, a heat exchanger to warm or cool the blood, a device to propel the blood into the arterial system, and monitoring and safety devices.

Returning blood is diverted from the right atrium via one or two cannulas attached to tubing that leads to the pump. A single, two-stage cannula (Fig. 5-15) is used in many procedures where the right atrium is not opened. The cannula is inserted through the right atrium with the fenestrated distal end placed in the inferior vena cava to collect returning blood from the lower body. The portion of the cannula sitting in the right atrium also has openings, which collect blood from the superior vena cava and coronary sinus. The

cannula is attached to tubing that goes to the pump.

The inferior and superior venae cavae may be cannulated separately, with the cannulas "Y'd" to the venous return tubing. This is necessary when the right atrium is the surgical site and must remain free of excess blood.

Various kinds of cannulas are available depending on the size of the patient, the exposure required, and the flow rates needed. Because inflow with oxygenated blood is dependent on the amount of venous outflow, the surgeon optimizes returning blood flow by inserting as large a catheter as possible into the venous system. (Larger catheters also produce less-shear forces and are less traumatic to the formed elements in the blood.)

Arterial catheters (Fig. 5-16) to return oxygenated blood commonly are inserted into the ascending aorta. When entry into the thorax of a patient who has pre-

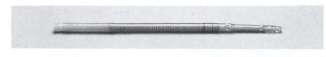

Fig. 5-15 Single two-stage cannula for venous drainage. The distal tip of the cannula is placed in the inferior vena cava; superior vena cava drainage exits through the proximal openings in the catheter. (Courtesy Bard Cardiopulmonary Div., Tewksbury, Mass.)

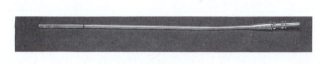

Fig. 5-16 Arterial cannula. The most common insertion site is the anterior ascending aorta. (Courtesy Bard Cardiopulmonary Div., Tewksbury, Mass.)

viously undergone a sternotomy poses a risk of injuring the heart or aorta, the surgeon may cannulate the femoral artery. Arterial cannulas (femoral or aortic) are secured to the drapes or the patient's skin to aid in preventing the accidental removal of the catheter. Both venous and arterial cannulas may be reinforced with wire to avoid kinking.

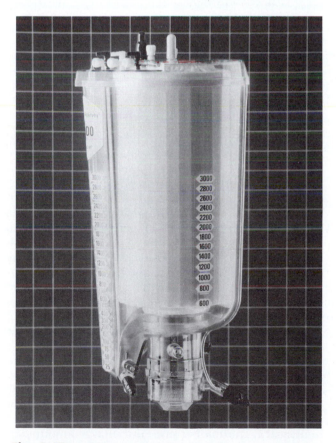

Fig. 5-17 Bubble oxygenator. (Courtesy Bard Cardiopulmonary Div., Tewksbury, Mass.)

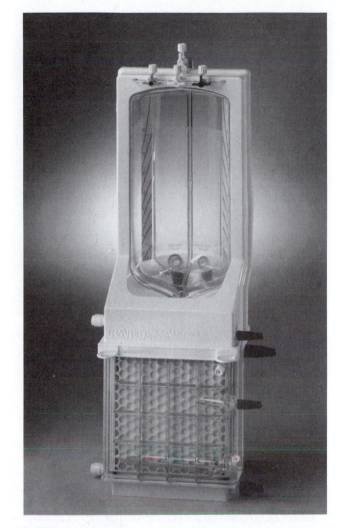

Fig. 5-18 Membrane oxygenator. (Courtesy Bard Cardiopulmonary Div., Tewksbury, Mass.)

Two methods of blood oxygenation have evolved to remove carbon dioxide and restore oxygen: the bubble method (Fig. 5-17) and the membrane method (Fig. 5-18). The bubble method works by pumping oxygen directly through a column of venous blood. This creates a foam of air bubbles, necessitating the use of a chemical surfactant to defoam the blood and filters to remove the bubbles. Membrane oxygenators use a gas-permeable membrane through which oxygen diffuses into, and carbon dioxide diffuses out of, the desaturated blood. Advocates of the membrane method stress that because of the absence of a direct blood-gas interface, there is a reduced risk of air emboli, as well as less trauma to the cellular components of the blood, resulting in improved renal function and less use of bank blood. Membrane technology also facilitates control of oxygen (PaO_2) and carbon dioxide ($PaCO_2$) levels in the blood during hypothermia (Kirklin and Kirklin, 1990). These are among the major reasons why membrane oxygenators are more commonly used.

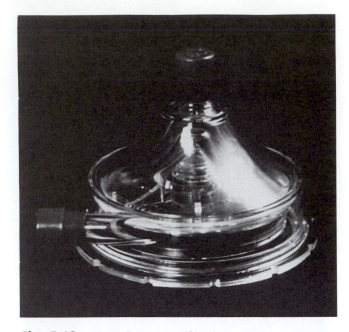

Fig. 5-19 Biomedicus centrifugal pump. (Courtesy Medtronic, Inc., Minneapolis, Minn.)

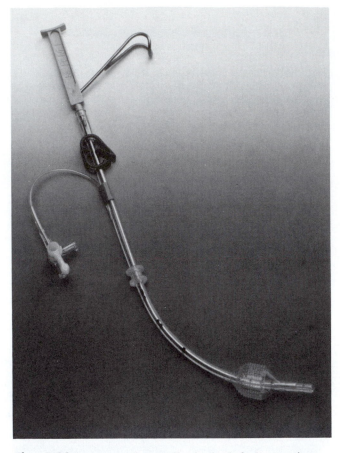

Fig. 5-20 Retrograde cardioplegia infusion catheter. The distal tip is inserted through an incision in the right atrial wall and into the orifice of the coronary sinus. (Courtesy Research Medical, Inc., Midvale, Utah.)

A heat exchanger may be incorporated into the oxygenator. This is used to alternatively cool and rewarm the blood within the bypass circuit. Hoses connected at one end to a water supply built into the operating room are attached to the heat exchanger at the other end. The temperature is controlled by the regulation of warm or cold water circulating around the tubing encasing the blood.

In most extracorporeal circuits the roller pump is used to propel oxygenated blood through polyvinylchloride (PVC) tubing. Blood inside the tubing is displaced by the compression of the rotating pump head. Although some damage occurs to the blood, relatively atraumatic blood flow can be achieved with careful calibration and judicious use. (Cellular trauma may be attributed more to prolonged pump runs and overuse or misuse of suctioning devices [Frazier and Colon, 1988]).

In many cases a centrifugal pump (Fig. 5-19) rather than a roller head is used for maintaining blood flow. Centrifugal pumps use kinetic energy that transfers high volumes of flow at low pressure. Rotating cones within the pump create centrifugal force, which provides the energy to drive the blood. Safety features such as the prevention of excessive pressures in the arterial line have resulted in widespread use of this pumping device (Kirklin and Barratt-Boyes, 1993).

Although blood normally flows in pulsatile waves with systolic and diastolic phases (seen on the arterial waveform), blood flow with roller heads or centrifugal pumps is nonpulsatile (no phasic waveform is seen). This is manifested by a "mean" arterial waveform on the oscilloscope during total cardiopulmonary bypass. Pulsatile bypass systems are available, but research findings have yet to establish a significant benefit with pulsatile versus nonpulsatile flow.

Additional components of the bypass system include blood filters and bubble traps, which are incorporated into the circuit to trap gaseous and particulate matter that could produce emboli. Cardioplegia infusion devices are added to the system as well. Catheters are available for antegrade (aortic root infusion) and retrograde (coronary sinus infusion) cardioplegia delivery (Fig. 5-20). Monitoring devices are used to measure blood gases, pH, temperature, and intravascular pressures. Suction lines return shed blood to the cardiotomy filter and then to the oxygenator for reinfusion. Other suction lines can be used to vent air and blood from the heart. These lines serve both to decompress the ventricle and to reduce the possibility of air emboli escaping into the aorta and traveling to the brain.

Percutaneous cardiopulmonary bypass systems are available for patients with circulatory collapse as a result of acute myocardial infarction, failed angioplasty, hypothermia, or massive pulmonary emboli (Phillips and others, 1989). They are not recommended for multisystem trauma because of the large amounts of heparin required before insertion (Brown, 1990). Large-bore cannulas are inserted into the femoral artery and one or both femoral veins and are connected to a portable pump oxygenator. These systems can be used in the cardiac catheterization laboratory, the intensive care unit, the emergency department, or any other area where a patient may benefit from temporary, emergency extracorporeal circulation (see Chapter 11).

Circulatory Assist Devices

The extracorporeal heart-lung machine is the prototype of assisted circulation. It takes over the functions of oxygenating and pumping blood, and by diverting venous return to the pump, it also decompresses the heart. This decreases the work normally performed by the volume- and pressure-loaded ventricles.

In cases where prolonged support of the myocardium is indicated, however, the pump oxygenator is not an optimal choice because of the trauma to the blood and the need for systemic heparinization. Thus in the presence of low cardiac output due to myocardial dysfunction, a number of other assist devices are used to reduce the workload of the heart and to improve organ perfusion. These range from systems that offer temporary relief to the myocardium to devices that support a heart that has suffered irreversible damage and is awaiting transplantation.

The intraaortic balloon pump (IABP) and the Hemopump are two devices used to support patients with postoperative left ventricular failure who have not responded to fluid or pharmacologic therapy (Quaal, 1984). They work on the principle of volume displacement to propel blood into the systemic and coronary circulations (see Chapter 17).

Ventricular assist devices (VADs) may be used when the IABP or Hemopump fails to produce improvement. VADs are extravascular, volume-capturing devices that augment the existing circulation (Frazier and Colon, 1988). The devices may use a roller pump, a centrifugal pump, or a pneumatic or electric pump to propel the blood (Frazier and others, 1990). The roller pump and the centrifugal pump maintain unidirectional blood flow; the other devices require prosthetic valves to achieve one-way flow (see Chapter 17).

Pacemakers

Manipulation of the heart, suturing of the myocardium, hypothermia, electrolyte imbalances, trauma to conduction tissue, and underlying conduction disturbances contribute to the appearance of dysrhythmias in cardiac surgery patients. Bradydysrhythmias are frequent in patients undergoing myocardial revascularization. Atrial dysrhythmias are often seen in patients with valvular heart disease, and temporary or permanent heart block can occur during surgery involving the atrial or ventricular septum.

Temporary pacing leads are routinely inserted to optimize cardiac output by preventing bradydysrhythmias or maintaining normal sinus rhythm (see Chapter 11). Epicardial leads are attached to the atrium when atrioventricular (AV) conduction is unimpaired. Ventricular leads are used in the presence of heart block when atrial beats are not conducted to the ventricle consistently. When AV conduction is delayed, both atrial and ventricular leads may be attached. The distal ends of the leads are inserted into a temporary pacemaker generator, and the patient is paced at a rate of 90 to 100 beats per minute to optimize cardiac output.

Permanent pacing leads are indicated in the presence of impulse formation or conduction disorders leading to complete heart block, bradydysrhythmias, and tachydysrhythmias. Various screw-in or stab leads are available for epicardial attachment to the atrium, ventricle, or both. Pulse generators are attached to the leads, programmed, and tested before being inserted into a subcutaneous pocket. Newer pacemakers offer antitachydysrhythmia functions and rate-responsive modes to change the heart rate as needed to meet demands for increased cardiac output (see Chapter 19).

Implantable Cardioverter Defibrillators

Unlike pacemaker electrodes, which sense asystole or slow heart rates, the internal cardioverter defibrillator (ICD) senses malignant ventricular dysrhythmias such as ventricular fibrillation and ventricular tachycardia. When these conditions are not amenable to pharmacologic or surgically ablative therapy, the ICD is implanted for the purpose of defibrillating the patient. Components include a generator, myocardial patches, and sensing electrodes. These devices often have pacing capabilities (see Chapter 19).

Additional Equipment

Monitoring devices are found in all cardiac ORs to provide a continuous flow of information about the patient's hemodynamic status (see Chapter 9). Doppler devices may be available to assess blood flow where palpation is difficult or does not provide sufficient information about blood flow.

Additional equipment found in the cardiac suite includes "blood refrigerators" for storing packed red blood cells or whole blood. These refrigerators are specially designed to maintain the blood at the proper temperature and to trigger an alarm if the temperature becomes too warm or too cold. Blood refrigerators must have a system to identify which blood belongs to the patient; blood for one patient should be separated from that for another patient.

Also commonly available are standard refrigerators for solutions and medications requiring cold storage, as well as ice machines to provide ice for chilling cardioplegia solutions and blood gas samples.

Blanket warmers keep blankets a comfortable temperature and can be used to warm saline or water. Occasionally these warmers are used to store medications that would crystallize at room temperature. Devices are also available to warm and maintain the desired temperature of saline for irrigation; these devices can be attached to the side of some cooling units.

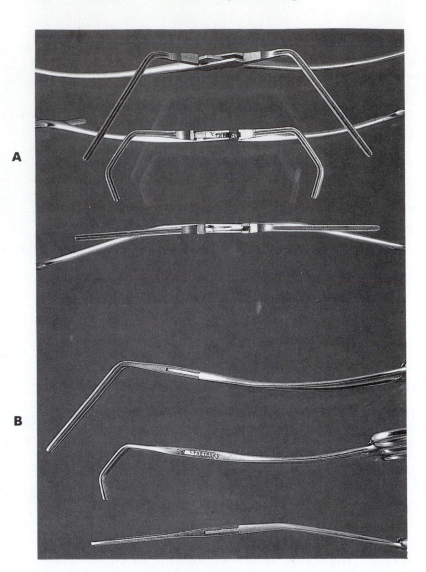

Fig. 5-21 Vascular clamps for occluding blood vessels. **A,** *Top to bottom:* DeBakey multipurpose vascular clamp tip (total occluding); Beck aorta clamp tip (partial occluding); Glover patent ductus clamp tip (total occluding). **B,** *Top to bottom:* DeBakey multipurpose vascular clamp, 60-degree obtuse angle; Beck aorta clamp; Glover patent ductus clamp, straight. (From Brooks-Tighe SM: *Instrumentation for the operating room: a photographic manual,* ed 3, St Louis, 1989, Mosby.)

Blood test results may be transmitted to the OR from the laboratory over a facsimile (FAX) machine if there is no facility adjacent to the operating room for analyzing blood samples. Computer terminals may be located in the room where patient lab results, charges, documentation of care, and other information may be put into or received from the system. One or two (or more) telephone lines are a valuable resource for contacting personnel, giving reports, and receiving information about the patient; extra-long extension cords enable the circulating nurse to remain close to the operating field.

A machine for reviewing coronary cineangiograms prior to surgery also may be available within the suite.

INSTRUMENTS

Instruments used in cardiac surgery are designed for specific purposes and selected according to the weight of the patient, anatomic requirements, and surgeon preference. They must be capable of securely grasping and holding blood vessels, cardiac structures, and other tissue without injury. And they must be available in an array of sizes and shapes to meet the needs of a 2 kg neonate or a 90 kg adult.

Sturdy instruments are required for procedures such as reapproximating sternal bone, and fine instruments must be available for sewing arteries that may be 2 mm or less in diameter and often the consistency of cooked spaghetti. Of particular interest are the vascular clamps (Fig. 5-21). Their atraumatic jaw serrations are specially designed for occluding, or partially occluding, blood vessels without damaging their walls (Box 5-4). Fig. 5-22 illustrates two common jaw patterns used for forceps and occluding clamps. Clamps are constructed with multiple rachets that allow the surgeon to adjust the clamp according to the blood pressure inside the blood vessel. Rachets also enable the surgeon to release the clamp gradually, thereby avoiding a sudden increase or decrease in vascular volume.

Standard self-retaining retractors for exposing the mediastinum are shown in Figs. 5-23 through 5-25. Some are constructed to meet different needs (Figs.

Box 5-4 *Comments about vascular instruments*

William Merz
Consultant and Master Instrument Maker
Baxter Healthcare Corporation
V. Mueller Division
Chicago, Illinois

The important parts on the forceps are the teeth in the jaw sections. These teeth, or longitudinal serrations, must come together and fit nicely into each jaw section. They must hold the tissues firmly without overlapping or scissoring.

The jaw sections must have the proper shape and thickness to hold the tissue without crushing.

The box lock is important; the male piece should not wobble. The thickness of the male piece is important in order to avoid overlapping and scissoring of the distal jaw sections. All sharp edges must be rounded in the box lock area. When the instrument is closed, it must have a slight opening between the two shafts near the box lock area. The shafts should be balanced according to the shape of the instrument. The ratchets must engage properly into the opposite teeth section. The shafts must be set so that the surgeon and the nurse can open the instrument without exerting too much energy.

The instrument must be polished. It must be stamped or etched stainless steel. Then it must be hardened, tempered, and set properly. The final polishing of the instrument should be a bright, shiny finish or a nonglare, satin finish.

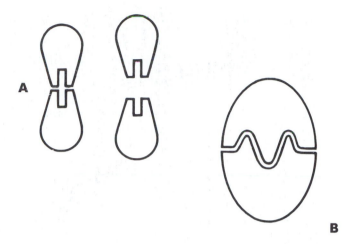
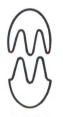

Fig. 5-22 Types of jaws in vascular clamps. **A,** Cooley jaws have two opposing rows of serrated teeth, closed and open. **B,** DeBakey jaws have a single row of serrated teeth opposing a double row of teeth, closed and open. (Courtesy Pilling Co., Fort Washington, Pa.)

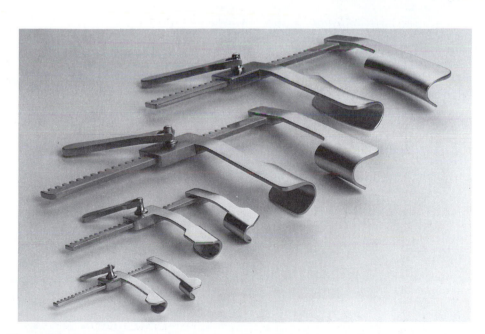

Fig. 5-23 Cooley sternal retractors in various sizes. (Courtesy Pilling Co., Fort Washington, Pa.)

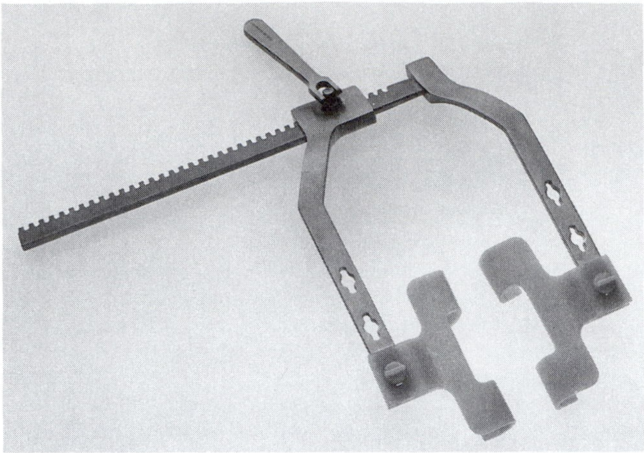

Fig. 5-24 Collins sternal retractor with disposable, radiopaque blades. (Courtesy Codman & Shurtleff, Inc., a Johnson & Johnson Co., Randolph, Mass.)

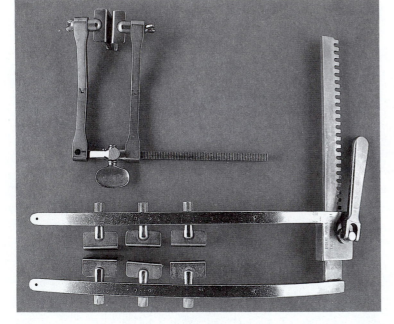

Fig. 5-25 Himmelstein sternal retractor *(top)* and Ankeney sternal retractor *(bottom).* (From Brooks-Tighe SM: *Instrumentation for the operating room: a photographic manual,* ed 3, St Louis, 1989, Mosby.)

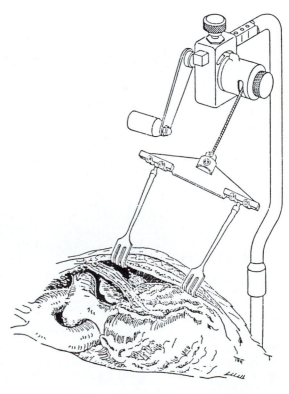

Fig. 5-26 Retractor used to elevate the sternal border for exposure of the internal mammary artery. (Courtesy Rultract, Inc., Cleveland, Ohio.)

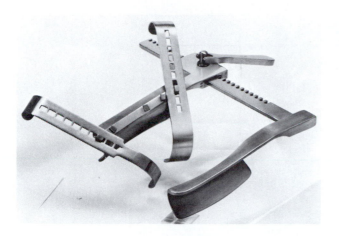

Fig. 5-27 Sternal self-retaining retractor with attachments for left atrial retraction during mitral valve replacement. (Courtesy Pilling Co., Fort Washington, Pa.)

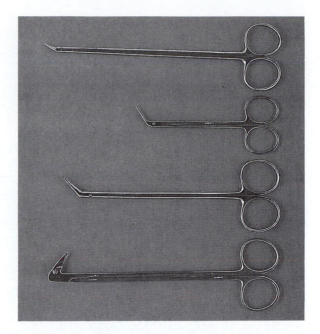

Fig. 5-29 Dietrich and Potts-Smith scissors in an array of forward and backward cutting angles (frequently used to incise coronary arteries). (From Brooks-Tighe SM: *Instrumentation for the operating room: a photographic manual*, ed 3, St Louis, 1989, Mosby.)

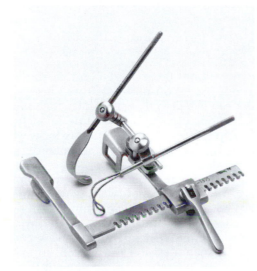

Fig. 5-28 Pediatric cardiac self-retaining retractor with detachable blades. The retractor can be used for midline sternotomy or lateral thoracotomy. (Courtesy Pilling Co., Fort Washington, Pa.)

5-26 through 5-28). Cardiac valves also can be exposed with hand-held retractors.

A variety of scissors and needle holders should be available. Potts-type scissors (Fig. 5-29) are frequently used to incise blood vessels. Castroviejo needle holders (Fig. 5-30) are popular for delicate anastomoses. Instrument kits for pediatric procedures and internal mammary artery procedures (Fig. 5-31) can be added to complement basic sets.

Vascular instruments can be made of tungsten carbide, stainless steel, or titanium. Titanium is stronger, yet lighter, than stainless steel, and these properties make it popular for some microsurgical instruments.

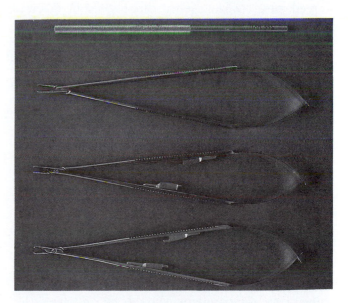

Fig. 5-30 Castroviejo needle holders with and without locks are used for delicate anastomoses. Some surgeons prefer fine standard needle holders with rachet locking mechanisms for performing anastomoses. (From Brooks-Tighe, SM: *Instrumentation for the operating room: a photographic manual*, ed 3, St Louis, 1989, Mosby.)

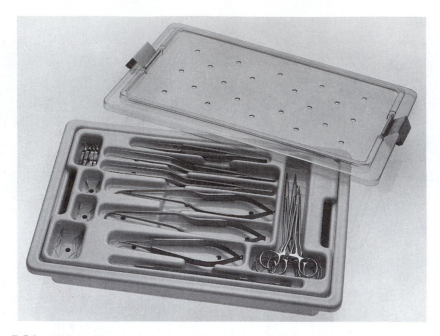

Fig. 5-31 Codman internal mammary artery (IMA) kit. (Courtesy Codman & Shurtleff, Inc., a Johnson & Johnson Co., Randolph, Mass.)

Appropriate use, careful handling, and proper cleaning will prolong the life of instruments and minimize costly repairs and replacements. Most instrument damage is due to misuse and abuse. Scissors constructed to incise coronary arteries should not be used to cut heavy suture; delicate needle holders and forceps should not be used to remove knife blades. Instruments should not be dropped, stacked, or forced into sterilizing pans; care should be taken to avoid placing heavy pans on top of delicate instruments.

Before surgery check instrument jaws for burrs by running them over a sponge. Vascular clamps, especially the cross-clamp, which is likely to be used, should be checked for proper alignment and a secure grip. If they are damaged or not working properly, the instrument(s) should be removed from the setup immediately and a replacement(s) obtained. During and after the procedure keep instruments clean of blood and debris; this will help to prevent damage from hardening of the material in the jaws and box locks, as well as reduce the possibility of introducing dried blood into blood vessels.

At the end of an operation, the instruments should be thoroughly cleaned and decontaminated. A nonmetallic brush should be used to clean them. A soft-bristled toothbrush or scrub brush is good for cleaning micro-size instruments and those with serrated vascular jaws. Instruments should be inspected for cracked, chipped, broken, worn, or otherwise damaged parts. In particular, vascular forceps and clamps should be inspected for bent tips, burrs, or misaligned jaws that could damage vascular structures. Damaged instruments should be sent out for repair immediately.

Instruments should be arranged so that the heavier ones are not placed on more delicate ones. Fine instruments can be placed in separate containers for their protection. Placing instruments in instrument milk will help to keep the jaws and box locks working properly. A regular schedule for sharpening scissors is recommended.

Basic sternotomy sets that are too heavy to place in one pan can be divided into two separate parts. One method is to arrange those instruments needed to open the chest and cannulate on a Mayo tray, and to place the remaining instruments in a back pan. The advantage of such a system is apparent in an emergency when the Mayo tray can be opened to provide its own sterile field, with the instruments made available for rapid institution of cardiopulmonary bypass. The Mayo tray should contain knife handles, wire cutters, a chest retractor, dissecting instruments, tubing clamps, needle holders, and vascular clamps needed for putting a patient on bypass. Additional instruments should be placed in the second pan.

Special sets can be developed for valve surgery, coronary bypass, and thoracic aneurysms. The list in Box 5-5 outlines a variety of instruments that can be selected to create these sets. Included are cutting, retracting, holding, clamping, suturing, and miscellaneous instruments. Because personal preference and training are so critical in the selection of needle holders, forceps, clamps, and other items, nurses should first confer with the surgeon (or the surgeon's former perioperative nursing colleagues) to determine which instruments to purchase. This will help to avoid the unnecessary expense of buying instruments that will not be used.

Box 5-5 *Cardiac instrumentation (partial listing)*

Basic Sternotomy Instruments

Cutting Instruments

No. 3 Bard-Parker knife handles: No. 10 blade
No. 4 Bard-Parker knife handles: No. 20 blade
No. 7 Bard-Parker knife handles: No. 15 blade, No. 15c blade, No. 11 blade
Beaver handles and blades
Sternal wire cutter
Temporary epicardial pacing wire cutter
Lebsche knife and mallet
Cooley "My" scissors: 7¼-inch
Bladder scissors
Metzenbaum scissors: 7-inch (and longer)
Straight Mayo scissors: 6¾-inch
Curved Mayo scissors: 6¾-inch
Potts forward-cutting scissors
Potts backward-cutting scissors
Tenotomy scissors: 7-inch
Bandage/tube–cutting scissors

Retractors

Cooley sternotomy retractor
Ankenney retractor
Himmelstein retractor
Codman retractor
Weitlaner retractors
Gelpi retractors
Richardson retractors, assorted sizes
Army-Navy retractors
Rake retractors
Semb retractors
Vein retractors
Ribbon retractors

Holding Instruments

Regular towel clips: blunt and sharp
Baby towel clips
Kocher clamps with teeth: 7¼-inch
Cooley vascular forceps: 7¾-inch, 9½-inch
DeBakey vascular forceps: 7¾-inch, 9½-inch
Russian forceps: 10-inch
Adson forceps with teeth
English Bonney forceps
Cooley "gold" forceps: 7¾-inch
Dressing forceps: 9½-inch
Geralt forceps: 7-inch, 9¼-inch
Sponge stick forceps
Allis clamps

Clamping Instruments

Hemostats, straight and curved
Criles, curved
Mosquito clamps, straight and curved
Right-angle clamps, assorted lengths
Mixter clamps
Tonsil clamps
Kelly (Pean) clamps, assorted lengths
Tube-occluding clamps

Vascular Clamps

Total-occluding clamps
    Fogarty cross-clamp, straight and angled
    Femoral artery clamps
    Cooley aortic aneurysm clamp
    Crafoord coarctation clamp
    Iliac clamp
    Bulldog clamps
    Patent ductus clamps
    DeBakey multipurpose clamps
Partial-occluding clamps
    Glover clamp
    Derra clamps
    Kay aorta clamp
    Kay-Lambert clamps
    Weck-Beck clamps
    Statinsky clamps
    Beck aorta clamps
    Cooley aorta clamps
    Cooley curved and angled clamps
    Auricular appendage clamp
    DeBakey tangential occlusion clamps

Suturing Instruments

Sarot needle holders
Mayo-Hegar needle holders
Wire needle holders
Vascular needle holders, assorted sizes
Castro-Viejo needle holders

Accessory Items

Cooley vena caval occlusion clamps
Suction tips, assorted sizes
Rumel tourniquet stylets
Ligating clips and appliers
Nerve hook
Freer elevator
Bypass tubing holder
Banding gun (to tighten cannulas to tubing connectors)
Fogarty clamp inserts
Instrument stringers
Rubbershods

Coronary Artery Bypass Instrument Extras

Cutting Instruments

Castro-Viejo micro scissors, forward- and backward-cutting
Dietrich scissors
Potts micro scissors, forward- and backward-cutting
Aortic punch

Retractors

Favalaro internal mammary artery retractor
Rultract internal mammary artery retractor
Parsonnett epicardial retractor
Balfour retractor (for exposure of gastroepiploic artery)

Holding Instruments

Delicate vascular forceps

Continued.

Box 5-5 *Cardiac instrumentation—cont'd*

Vascular Clamps
Micro bulldog clamps

Suturing Instruments
Castro-Viejo micro needle holders
Ryder needle holders
Microvascular needle holders

Accessory Items
Fine suction tips
Coronary dilators: 0.5 to 5.0 mm
Small clip appliers and clips
Radiopaque graft markers
Endarterectomy spatulas
Blunt internal mammary artery infusion needle
Vein irrigation cannulas

Valve Instrument Extras

Cutting Instruments
Curved mitral scissors
Long Bard-Parker No. 3 knife handles: No. 10 blade,
   No. 15 blade

Retractors
Hand-held right and left atrial retractors
Hand-held aortic root retractors
Self-retaining sternal retractors with atrial retraction ac-
   cessories

Holding Instruments
Curved Allis clamp
Long smooth forceps

Clamping Instruments
Baby tubing clamps
Carmalt clamps with rubbershods
Long right-angle clamp

Suturing Instruments
Long needle holders
Suture holder

Accessory Items
French-eye needles
No. 3 dental mirror
Culture tubes
Mitral hook
Sizing obturators and handles
Prosthesis handles
Hand-held coronary perfusion tips
Tubbs dilator
Hegar dilators, assorted sizes
Pituitary rongeurs: up, down, straight
Debridement suction tip

Thoracotomy Instrument Extras

Cutting Instruments
Rib cutters
Nelson scissors, curved: 10-inch
Periosteal elevators

Retractors
Finochietto rib spreader
Burford retractor
"T" malleable lung retractors
Scapular retractor
Bailey rib approximators

Holding Instruments
Duval lung clamps
Rumel thoracic clamps

Clamping Instruments
Bronchus clamps
Right-angle clamps

Vascular Clamps
Crafoord coarctation clamps
Patent ductus clamps, angled and straight

Suturing Instruments
Long hemaclip appliers, assorted sizes
Bronchus, vascular staplers
Long needle holders

Pediatric Instrumentation
Most of the instrumentation listed above is also used for
pediatric procedures. The size of the child and the patient
position determine which instruments are most appropriate. The working end of the instrument may be finer,
but often it is of standard length to allow the surgeon's
and assistants' hands to remain outside the relatively confined surgical field. The following also may be used:

Retractors
Finochietto rib retractor, infant/child sizes
Cooley sternal retractor, infant/child sizes
"T" malleable lung retractors, assorted sizes
Silicone-coated brain retractors

Vascular Clamps
Down-sized and proportionally balanced for smaller ves-
   sels
Cooley pediatric clamps
Castaneda pediatric clamps

Box 5-6 *Sutures for selected procedures**

Pericardial retraction: 2-0 braided polyester, nylon, or silk

Cannulation for cardiopulmonary bypass:
   Aortic pursestring: 2-0 braided polyester (with or without pledget)
   Right atrial pursestring: 2-0 braided polyester or nylon

Cardioplegia infusion
   Aortic vent/antegrade cardioplegia infusion pursestring: 4-0 polypropylene (with or without pledget)
   Right atrial retrograde cardioplegia infusion pursestring: 3-0 polyester

Temporary epicardial pacemaker leads: lead wire attached with 5-0 silk

Chest tubes: 0, 2-0 silk

Sternum: 5 chest wire; polyester (children)

Linea alba: 0, 2-0 polyester

Fascia, subcutaneous tissue: 2-0 absorbable suture

Skin: 3-0, 4-0 absorbable suture or polypropylene, nylon; skin staples (legs)

Coronary anastomoses
   Distal anastomosis:

   Saphenous vein: 6-0, 7-0 polypropylene
   Internal mammary artery: 7-0, 8-0 polypropylene
Proximal anastomosis
   Saphenous vein to aorta: 5-0, 6-0 polypropylene

Valve replacement/repair
   Aortic: 2-0 polyester, alternately colored (blue or green and white)
   Closure of aorta: 4-0 polypropylene
   Mitral: 2-0 polyester, alternately colored
   Closure of left atrium: 3-0 polypropylene
   Tricuspid: 3-0 polyester or polypropylene
   Closure of right atrium: 4-0 polypropylene

Closure of left ventricular aneurysm: 0, 2-0 polyester (with felt strips)

Closure of atrial septal defect: Patch/primary repair: 4-0 polypropylene

Coarctation of aorta (child): Primary repair: 5-0, 6-0 absorbable suture

Thoracic aortic aneurysms
   Ascending aorta: 2-0, 3-0 polyester, polypropylene
   Descending aorta: 3-0, 4-0 polyester, polypropylene

*The sutures listed vary depending on the patient's size and surgeon's preference.

The sterility of the instruments should be maintained until the patient has left the operating room; they can then be used to reopen the sternum if chest tube drainage is excessive, to insert an additional chest tube, or to secure an intravascular line.

SUTURE

Various types and sizes of cardiovascular sutures and needles are used on the heart, surrounding tissue, and blood vessels. Box 5-6 lists sutures commonly used for a number of procedures

In performing vascular anastomoses, surgeons are concerned with creating a patent and leakproof vessel lumen. The development of inert synthetic suture materials such as nylon, polyester, and polypropylene has reduced the incidence of tissue reaction and thrombus formation, which in the past were frequently the cause of failed anastomoses.

Sutures may be constructed as a multifilament or a monofilament. Multifilament polyester sutures allow clotting to occur within the interstices and thereby reduce leaking from the suture line. This factor, as well as the tensile strength of the material, makes these sutures popular for the fixation of vascular grafts and heart valves. They are also frequently used for pursestring stitches used with tourniquets to anchor bypass cannulas or venting catheters. Monofilament sutures may be more desirable than multifilament sutures in the presence of sepsis or trauma because there are no interstices in the suture to harbor bacteria.

The use of swaged needles with tapered tips has also minimized vessel trauma. Cardiovascular suture is often made with needles at each end of the filament. Double-ended stitches allow the surgeon to perform half of an anastomosis with one end of the stitch and then use the other end to complete the anastomosis (Fig. 5-32).

Vessel anastomoses are commonly performed using a continuous suturing technique with polypropylene, a monofilament material. Tension around the circumference of the suture line is distributed evenly with this method and helps to avoid constricting the lumen. When tying polypropylene, surgeons will find the process easier if their hands are first moistened with saline.

When sewing on friable tissue or tissue that does not hold sutures well (such as the myocardium), felt pledgets can be used to buttress the sutures and avoid tearing or cutting of tissue (Fig. 5-33). Pledgets are available precut, or they can be made by cutting a larger piece of felt material. Strips of felt are used to buttress the myocardium for resection of left ventricular aneurysms; these can be prepared at the field by cutting a patch of felt into strips.

Suture is available in single packs or multipacks. Multipacks (Fig. 5-34) of polypropylene suture are helpful during coronary artery bypass procedures where several anastomoses are anticipated. Alternately colored polyester suture within multipacks (green/white or blue/white) are helpful for avoiding confusion in procedures such as valve replacements, which require numerous interrupted stitches to be placed and tied.

Made-to-order suture packs (Fig. 5-35) contain a variety of sutures arranged in a predetermined order to meet the requirements of a particular surgeon or

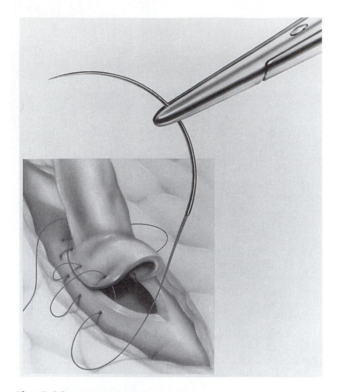

Fig. 5-32 End-to-side vascular anastomosis with double-ended (also called double-armed) suture. (Courtesy Davis & Geck, Danbury, Conn.)

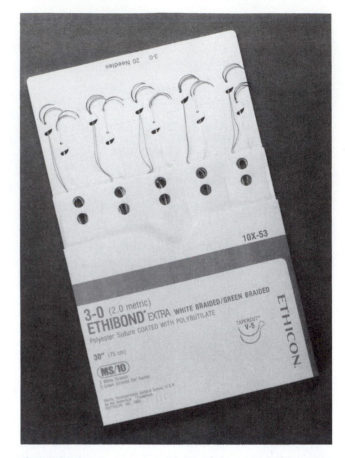

Fig. 5-34 The suture multipack can be used for valve procedures, coronary artery bypass procedures, or other procedures that require multiples of a single type of suture. (Courtesy Ethicon, Inc., a Johnson & Johnson Co., Somerville, N.J.)

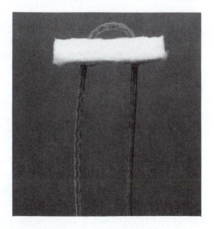

Fig. 5-33 Pledgeted suture. The suture should be placed in the central part of the pledget. (Courtesy Ethicon, Inc., a Johnson & Johnson Co., Somerville, N.J.)

a specific procedure (Zokal, 1990). Packs may be developed for opening and cannulation procedures, coronary artery bypass grafting, and/or valve procedures. Because 80 or more needles may be used, much time can be saved by opening one or two packs versus numerous individual packs. Inventory space is reduced, and there is less waste. If cost savings are to be realized, however, the packs should contain only those sutures that will be used routinely. When ad-

ditional sutures are needed, individual packs should be provided to the scrub nurse. If premade suture packs are not available, it is helpful to have the individual sutures already collected and placed in a bag so that if an emergency arises, the sutures need not first be retrieved from the storage area.

SUPPLIES

Numerous supplies are used during cardiac surgery, and among the most common are those listed in Box 5-7. Specific items depend on surgeon preference, as well as on purchasing agreements that many hospitals have with distributors and vendors.

Because of the large number of items that must be opened for surgery, many cardiac services work with vendors to develop custom trays (Fig. 5-36). These kits may include items used for basic sternotomy procedures (such as rubbershods [Fig. 5-37]) or specialty trays for valve or coronary artery bypass surgery (such as coronary graft markers [Fig. 5-38], bulldog clamps [Fig. 5-39], or aortic punches [Fig. 5-40]). The user determines what items to include. Like the suture packs discussed above, custom trays are cost-effective

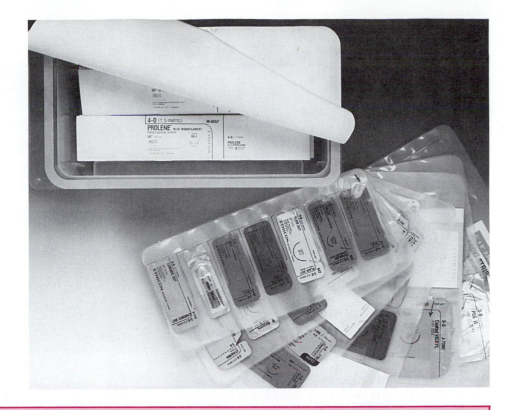

Fig. 5-35 Customized suture packs save turnover time and setup time. (Courtesy Ethicon, Inc., a Johnson & Johnson Co., Somerville, N.J.)

Box 5-7 Supplies commonly used in a cardiac service

Adaptors, connectors, stopcocks
Aortic punches
Autotransfusion supplies
Bulb syringes
Cannulas and catheters for cardiopulmonary bypass
Chest tubes, chest drainage system
Coronary graft markers
Cotton gloves (for retracting the heart)
Disposable drapes, gowns, gloves
Disposable towels
Disposable vascular (bulldog) clamps
Dressing supplies
Electrosurgical pencils: foot-control and hand-control
Graduated pitchers, cups, emesis basins, rinsing bowls
Guidewires
Hypodermic and venting needles

Knife blades
Marking pens
Needle counters
Polyvinylchloride or Silastic tubing in various sizes
Pressure tubing
Rubbershods
Solutions, medications
Sponges (lap tapes, peanuts, radiopaque 4 × 4's)
Suction tips, tubing
Syringes and needles for injections, infusions, and blood samples
Tourniquet catheters
Trash bags
Urinary drainage system (catheters, urine meters, lubricant)
Vascular clamp inserts

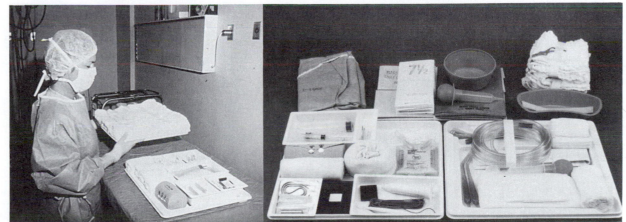

Fig. 5-36 Customized supply kits reduce the time needed to gather and set up items for cardiac procedures. **A,** After the circulating nurse opens the pack on a table, the sterile nurse arranges the contents of the pack. **B,** Sample tray contents of a customized pack. (Courtesy Johnson & Johnson Medical, Inc., Arlington, Tex.)

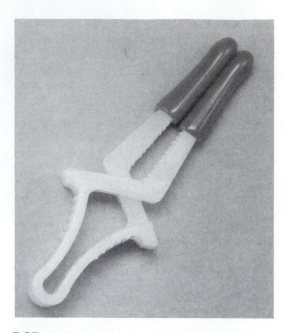

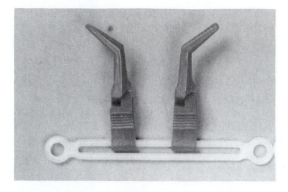

Fig. 5-39 Disposable bulldog clamps. These come in a variety of sizes and angles. (Courtesy Scanlan International, St. Paul, Minn.)

Fig. 5-37 Rubbershods applied to the tips of a bulldog clamp. (Courtesy Scanlan International, St. Paul, Minn.)

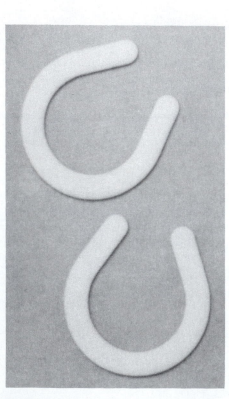

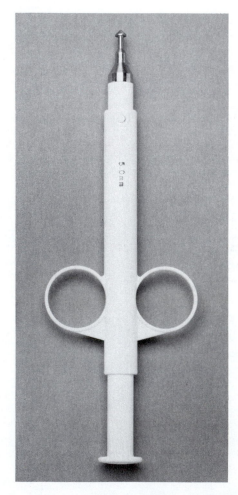

Fig. 5-38 Radiopaque coronary graft markers enable the clinician to identify the site of proximal anastomoses postoperatively. (Courtesy Scanlan International, St. Paul, Minn.)

Fig. 5-40 Disposable aortic punches are used to create the aortotomy for proximal coronary anastomoses. A smaller punch can also be used to create an opening in a vein graft for a side-to-side anastomosis. (Courtesy Scanlan International, St. Paul, Minn.)

Table 5-2 ■ *Sources of graft materials for repair or reconstruction*

Type	Definition	Examples
Synthetic	Made from artificial sources	
Teflon	Fluorocarbon fiber	Felt pledgets for suture
Dacron	Polyester fiber	Straight or bifurcated tube grafts
		Patch material
PTFE	Polytetrafluoroethylene	Tube or patch grafts
Biologic	Made from living, or previously living, tissue	
Autograft	Tissue from one part of a person's body placed in another part	Saphenous vein graft
Heterograft	Tissue from another species placed in a person's body	Porcine valve
		Bovine pericardial patch
Allograft/homograft	Tissue from one person's body placed in another person	Transplant donor heart
		Cadaver aortic valve
		Human umbilical vein

when they include only those items that will be used on all procedures for which the pack is intended. Such consistency may be difficult to achieve when there are many surgeons with differing supply needs.

PROSTHETIC IMPLANTS

In addition to the items listed in Box 5-7, numerous materials are used to replace or repair cardiovascular structures. These prosthetic materials may be synthetic or biologic (Table 5-2) and include intracardiac patches, tube grafts, and heart valves. They should be stored in a clean, dry, protected environment. Care in handling helps to prevent damage or contamination of the implant.

Synthetic Grafts

Synthetic prostheses are available in a variety of meshes, fabrics, felts, tapes, and sutures (Fig. 5-41). Many synthetic materials can be resterilized by steam autoclaving or by using ethylene oxide with adequate aeration unless otherwise advised by the manufacturer (follow manufacturer's instructions). However, numerous resterilization cycles (e.g., greater than three or four times) can jeopardize the integrity of the fibers, so a record should be kept of the number of times a graft has been resterilized. Unused grafts that have been in contact with blood or tissue should be discarded.

Synthetic tube and patch grafts made of Dacron are either woven or knitted; tube grafts may be straight or bifurcated (Fig. 5-42). (Knitted materials can be compared to the construction of a sweater, whereas woven grafts are more comparable to the tighter weave of a shirt.) The decision to use a woven or a knitted graft is based primarily on whether the patient is fully heparinized (such as required for cardiopulmonary bypass) and the speed of tissue ingrowth. **Woven grafts** are less porous than knitted grafts (Table 5-3) because their fibers are closer together. They are indicated when the patient is fully heparin-

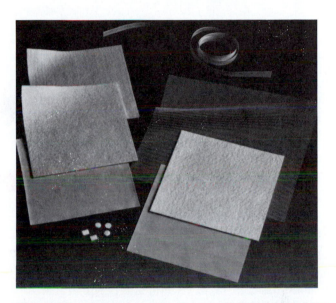

Fig. 5-41 Assorted prosthetic materials to repair intracardiac and extracardiac defects: tapes, Teflon and Dacron patches, and felt pledgets. (Courtesy Meadox Medicals, Inc., Oakland, N.J.)

ized, because there is less bleeding through the interstices of the fabric. Bleeding can be further reduced with preclotting methods (see Chapter 16). Woven grafts may fray at the cut edges, and an eye cautery should be used to heat-seal the edges.

Tube grafts are used to resect a portion of a blood vessel, bypass obstructions, or create an alternative route for blood flow. Woven patch material can be used to repair a portion of a blood vessel, replace the wall of a cardiac chamber, or close a ventricular septal defect. When flat patch material is unavailable, a patch can be cut from a piece of tube graft.

Knitted grafts have a higher porosity and thus allow more bleeding between the fibers. Tissue ingrowth is more rapid when the fibers are farther apart, which facilitates the creation of a new endothelial lin-

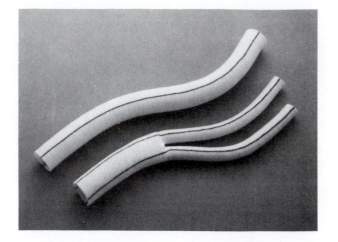

Fig. 5-42 Straight and bifurcated arterial tube grafts. (Courtesy Meadox Medicals, Oakland, N.J.)

Table 5-3 ■ Porosity of prosthetic grafts*

Fabric	Mean porosity
Woven Fabric (Dacron)	
Low-porosity woven (Cooley)	(Less than) 50 ml/min/cm²
Fabric patch	
Tube graft	
Intraaortic (ringed) graft	
Woven (Cooley)	(Less than) 100 ml/min/cm²
Tube graft	
Knitted Fabric (Dacron)	
Meadox knitted (Cooley)	2000 ml/min/cm²
Fabric patch	
Tube graft	
Velour Fabric (Dacron)	
Single-velour	3000 ml/min/cm²
Double-velour	4750 ml/min/cm²
Felt (Dacron)	
Patch graft	Not measured
Pledgets	Not measured

Data from Meadox Medicals, Inc., Oakland, NJ, 1988.
*Porosity is measured as the flow of distilled water through the fabric, at a pressure of 120 mm Hg, expressed in milliliters per minute per square centimeters.

ing. This process can be enhanced with a textured surface made of filamentous loops ("velour"), which attract and provide a structure for cells that form the neointima. Knitted prostheses are also available as straight or bifurcated tubes or patch grafts.

Knitted grafts are generally preclotted with unheparinized autologous venous blood, or they may be precoated by the manufacturer with albumin or collagen to retard bleeding. When preclotting the graft with blood, the surgeon will aspirate enough blood to moisten the graft (approximately 5 to 10 ml). This blood must be withdrawn before the patient receives heparin.

Advantages of knitted grafts are their ease of handling and less fraying at the cut edges as compared with woven grafts. They are used predominantly in the abdominal aorta, in visceral and peripheral arteries, and for patch repairs of endarterectomized carotid arteries. In cardiac repairs knitted patches are used to close atrial septal defects because they are easier to handle, fray less when cut, and endothelialize quickly once heparin is reversed. Temporary residual bleeding through the graft from one atrial chamber to the other causes little problem. The use of unaltered knitted materials outside of the heart in patients fully heparinized, however, is avoided because there would be excessive bleeding into the pericardium, causing tamponade. However, some newer knitted (and woven) grafts that are impregnated with collagen to prevent interstitial bleeding can be used in these situations.

Most tube grafts are crimped to reduce the possibility of compression. Some grafts are externally supported with plastic rings. Grafts made of polytetrafluoroethylene (PTFE) are not crimped but also may be reinforced with external plastic coils. Such grafts can be used to replace a segment of thoracic aorta or vena cava or to provide a conduit for blood flow from one vessel or cardiac chamber to another (such as the creation of a shunt from a systemic artery to a pulmonary artery in pediatric patients who have inade-

quate pulmonary blood flow). The appropriate-size tube graft diameter may be determined with the use of graft sizers. Sizing of PTFE grafts to the appropriate length as well as diameter is critical, because these grafts do not stretch, as crimped grafts do.

Occasionally a small-diameter straight-tube graft will be needed. If one is unavailable, the nurse can scan the bifurcated graft inventory for an appropriately sized "leg." This can be cut from the bifurcated graft and implanted.

Intraluminal Devices

Tube grafts reinforced at one or both ends with metal rings (Fig. 5-43) are used in surgery for thoracic and abdominal aneurysms. These intraaortic devices are anchored in place with nylon tapes tied around the rings. Some surgeons may elect to insert a few interrupted stitches to further secure the prosthesis. If one end of the graft has no ring or the ring has been cut, routine anastomotic techniques are used. Graft sizers are also available for these grafts.

Biologic Grafts

Biologic prostheses can be derived from human tissue or the tissue of another species (see Table 5-2). Human tissue grafts may be one of two types: autografts (the patient's own tissue) or allografts, also called homografts (tissue from another human). Autografts include the saphenous vein segments used during cor-

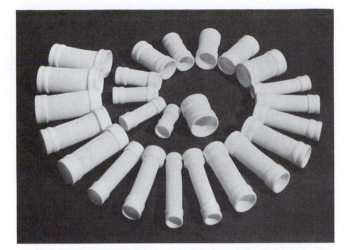

Fig. 5-43   Double-ended, ringed aortic intraluminal devices for emergency repair of thoracic aortic dissections. (Courtesy Bard Vascular Systems Div., Billerica, Mass.)

onary artery bypass surgery and pericardium, a portion of which may be excised and used for patch repairs (it may be first immersed in glutaraldehyde to toughen it, then rinsed in saline, and implanted). Heterografts are obtained from other species and include bovine pericardium and porcine heart valves. Heterografts are stored in sterile solutions and placed in sealed containers. Prior to implantation the storage solution is removed by rinsing with normal saline.

Prosthetic Heart Valves

The era of prosthetic valve replacement began over three decades ago. Various designs and materials have been used as substitutes for native cardiac valves, but the ideal valve prosthesis has yet to be created (Box 5-8).

Cardiac valve prostheses are of two types: mechanical and biologic. Each has advantages and disadvantages (see Chapter 13). The major advantage of mechanical valves is their durability. However, mechanical valves are thrombogenic, requiring patients to undergo chronic anticoagulation postoperatively. This is the major disadvantage of these prostheses.

Biologic valves (Figs. 5-44 through 5-51) have the advantage of not being inherently thrombogenic, thus obviating the need for chronic anticoagulation in the absence of other thromboembolic risk factors, such as atrial fibrillation or a history of transient ischemic attacks. Their disadvantage is that they are less durable than their mechanical counterparts and may need to be replaced, with the attendant risks associated with reoperations.

Other selection criteria include anatomic factors (such as the size of the aortic root or the left ventricle), blood flow and residual pressure gradients, ease of

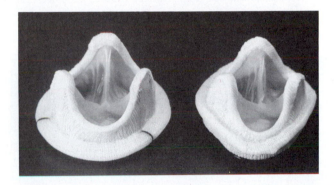

Box 5-8   *The ideal prosthetic heart valve*

Good blood flow
Durable
Nonthrombogenic
Atraumatic to blood
Biocompatible/nonreactive
Easy to insert
Silent
Acceptable to the patient

Modified from Bonchek LI: The basis for selecting a valve prosthesis. In McCauley KM, Brest AN, McGoon DC: *McGoon's cardiac surgery: an interprofessional approach to patient care*, Philadelphia, 1985, FA Davis.

Fig. 5-44   Carpentier-Edwards porcine mitral *(left)* and aortic *(right)* valve prostheses. Note that the aortic sewing ring is narrower than the mitral ring. (Courtesy Baxter Healthcare Corp., Edwards CVS Div., Santa Ana, Calif.)

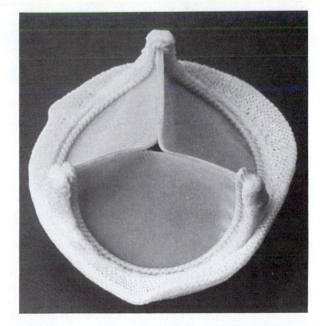

Fig. 5-45   Carpentier-Edwards bovine pericardial aortic valve prosthesis, Model 2700. (Courtesy Baxter Healthcare Corp., Edwards CVS Div., Santa Ana, Calif.)

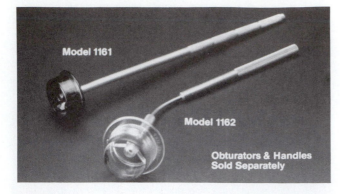

Fig. 5-46 Sizing obturators and handles for Carpentier-Edwards aortic *(top)* and mitral *(bottom)* porcine and bovine pericardial valves. The malleable mitral handle facilitates insertion into the mitral annulus of the left atrium. (Courtesy Baxter Healthcare Corp., Edwards CVS Div., Santa Ana, Calif.)

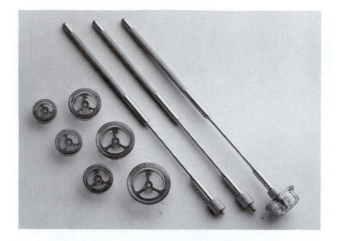

Fig. 5-48 Sizing obturators and handles for Hancock aortic porcine valve. (Courtesy Medtronic, Inc., Minneapolis, Minn.)

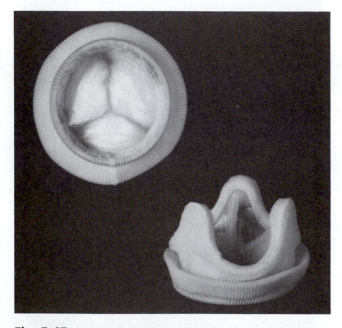

Fig. 5-47 Hancock aortic modified orifice porcine valve prosthesis. (Courtesy Medtronic, Inc., Minneapolis, Minn.)

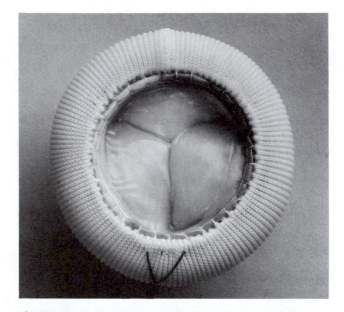

Fig. 5-49 Hancock mitral porcine valve prosthesis. (Courtesy Medtronic, Inc., Minneapolis, Minn.)

insertion, intensity of valve noise, patient preference, and (in the case of homografts) ease of procurement (Austin, 1989).

Obturators specific to each kind of prosthesis are available for determining the appropriate-size valve. Valve holders facilitate suturing and placement (seating) of the prosthesis.

Currently available mechanical prostheses use a ball-and-cage (Figs. 5-52 through 5-54) or tilting disk design (Figs. 5-55 through 5-58) and are made of a variety of materials. These include Silastic for ball-and-cage poppets; pyrolytic carbon for disks; titanium, Stellite alloy, or pyrolytic carbon for orifice rings; and Dacron or Teflon fabric for sewing cuffs.

The valves allow closure with slight regurgitation to prevent stasis of blood. Care should be taken to avoid scratching or injuring the prosthesis.

Biologic valves approved for sale are made from porcine aortic valves or bovine pericardium cut into leaflets and sutured to Dacron or Teflon cloth-covered stents. They are treated and preserved in a glutaraldehyde solution, which must be rinsed off for 2 minutes in each of three separate baths of normal saline (for a total of 6 minutes [Fig. 5-59, p. 98]). This required preparation time may influence the surgeon's suture technique for implanting bioprostheses. One method is to place stitches into the native valve annulus while the prosthesis is being rinsed. When the

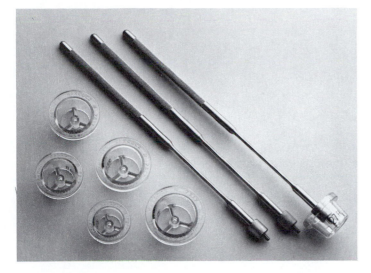

Fig. 5-50 Sizing obturators and handles for Hancock mitral porcine valve. (Courtesy Medtronic, Inc., Minneapolis, Minn.)

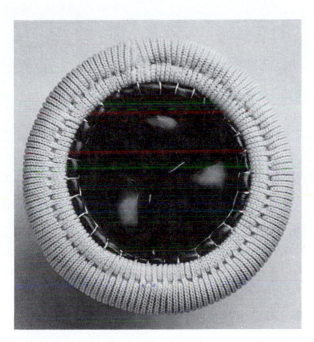

Fig. 5-51 Medtronic Intact porcine valve prosthesis with toluidine blue to retard calcium formation. Hancock sizing obturators are used to size the prosthesis. (Courtesy Medtronic, Inc., Minneapolis, Minn.)

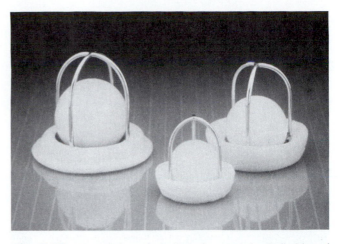

Fig. 5-52 Starr-Edwards ball-and-cage mitral *(left)* and aortic *(center, right)* valve prosthesis. (Courtesy Baxter Healthcare Corp., Edwards CVS Div., Santa Ana, Calif.)

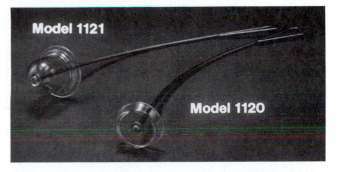

Fig. 5-53 Sizing obturators for Starr-Edwards mitral *(top)* and aortic *(bottom)* valve prostheses. (Courtesy Baxter Healthcare Corp., Edwards CVS Div., Santa Ana, Calif.)

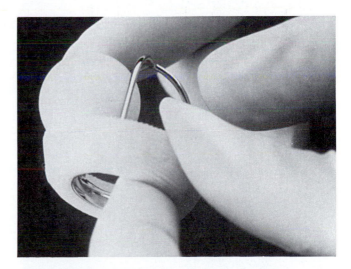

Fig. 5-54 The poppet from the Starr-Edwards aortic valve can be removed to facilitate sewing the suture ring. It is inserted once the prosthesis is seated and the stitches are tied. (The poppet from the mitral valve prosthesis is not removable). (Courtesy Baxter Healthcare Corp., Edwards CVS Div., Santa Ana, Calif.)

valve is ready, sutures are then placed in the prosthetic sewing ring.

When the use of a biologic valve is anticipated, a sterile team member should be available to function as a valve rinser before the valve size is determined. It is recommended that even when the surgeon intends to use a mechanical prosthesis, a person should be ready to rinse a bioprosthesis in the event that circumstances favor its use. Delays in preparing the

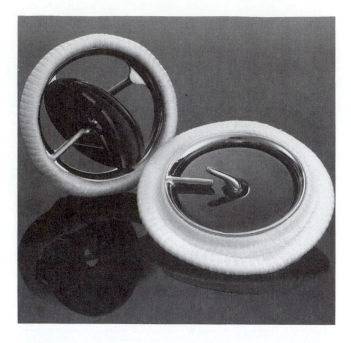

Fig. 5-55 Medtronic-Hall aortic *(left)* and mitral *(right)* tilting disk valve prostheses. (Courtesy Medtronic, Inc., Minneapolis, Minn.)

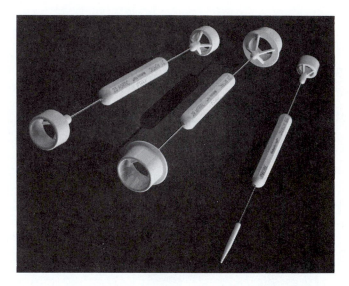

Fig. 5-56 Medtronic-Hall double-ended sizing obturators *(left, center)* and probe *(right)* used to test leaflet movement. (Courtesy Medtronic, Inc., Minneapolis, Minn.)

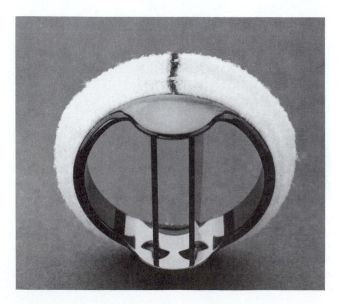

Fig. 5-57 St. Jude Medical bileaflet tilting disk valve prosthesis. (Courtesy St. Jude Medical, Inc., St. Paul, Minn.)

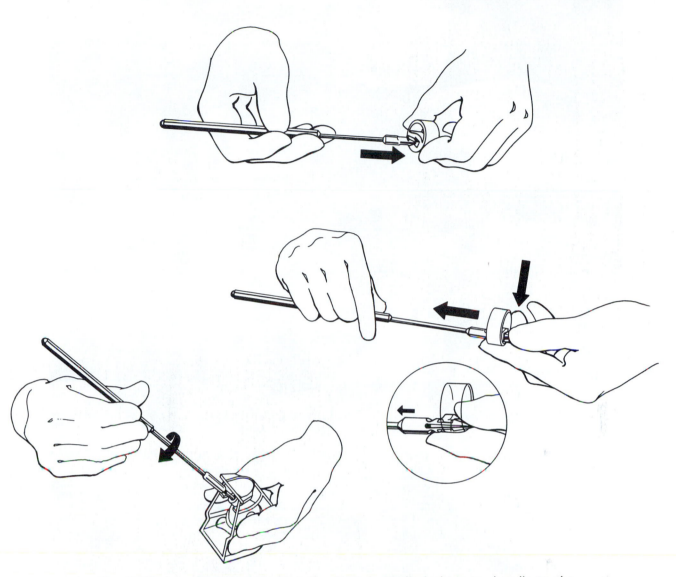

Fig. 5-58 Procedure for attaching the St. Jude Medical obturator handle to the obturator. Prosthesis handle is screwed into valve holder (*bottom*). (Courtesy St. Jude Medical, Inc., St. Paul, Minn.)

valve should be avoided in order to minimize cross-clamp time. During insertion, the prosthesis should be kept moist with saline to avoid drying of the tissue.

Aortic and Pulmonary Allografts (Homografts)

Aortic and pulmonary allografts from cadaver donors (see Chapter 14) are used with increasing frequency for acquired and congenital lesions. A number of advantages have fostered their increasing popularity: little or no risk of thromboembolism, optimal hemodynamic function, no need for anticoagulant medications, and minimal risk of sudden catastrophic failure. They also demonstrate a lower incidence of infective endocarditis than do mechanical or biologic valves, and their long-term durability is superior to that of bioprostheses (Yankah and others, 1988). Allografts may be fresh, but more frequently they are cryopreserved (frozen) and must be thawed according to strict protocol prior to implantation. Aortic homografts include the entire ascending aorta or the valve alone (Fig. 5-60). The graft is trimmed, and the valve alone or the valve and attached aortic wall are implanted.

Pulmonary allografts have become increasingly popular for use in children as conduits or patches for right ventricular outflow tract reconstruction, coarctation of the aorta, and hypoplastic left heart syndrome. The pulmonary tissue is much more pliable, provides better hemostasis, and is less prone to early calcification than is the aortic allograft.

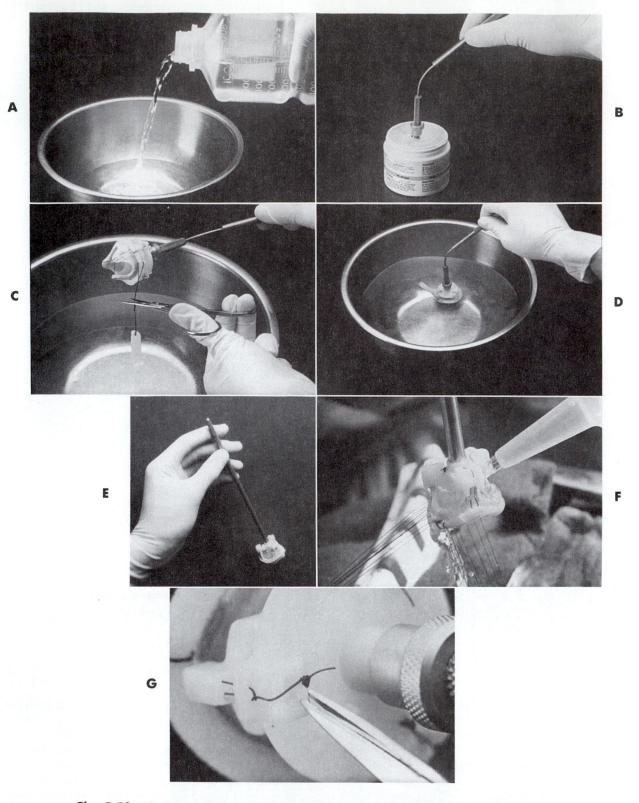

Fig. 5-59 Rinsing procedure for bioprostheses. **A,** A sterile field is prepared with three basins of normal saline. **B,** After the circulating nurse opens the container, the sterile nurse screws the prosthesis handle into the valve holder, which is attached to the prosthesis, and removes the valve. **C,** The circulating nurse and the sterile nurse check the size, type, and serial number on the tag, which the sterile nurse then cuts and removes before rinsing the prosthesis. **D,** The prosthesis is placed in the first basin of saline and gently agitated for a minimum of 2 minutes. The procedure is repeated in the second and third basins of saline. **E,** The valve with the holder and handle still attached is ready for insertion. It should not be allowed to dry out. **F,** The prosthesis is kept moist with frequent saline irrigation using a bulb syringe. **G,** The valve holder is removed by cutting the fixation stitch and pulling away the holder. (Courtesy Baxter Healthcare Corp., Edwards CVS Div., Santa Ana, Calif.)

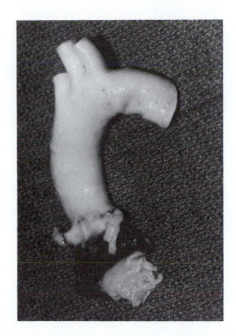

Fig. 5-60 Aortic allograft (homograft) with the aortic valve and arch vessels attached. (Courtesy CryoLife, Inc., Marietta, Ga.)

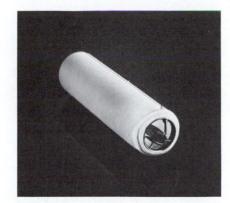

Fig. 5-61 Aortic graft-valve prosthesis containing a Medtronic-Hall disk valve prosthesis. (Courtesy Medtronic, Inc., Minneapolis, Minn.)

Aortic Graft Valve Prostheses

Conduits consisting of mechanical (Fig. 5-61) or biologic (Fig. 5-62) valves attached to a tube graft are used in procedures that require replacement of the native aortic valve and ascending aorta. If vein grafts must be inserted into the conduit during concomitant coronary artery bypass surgery, or if a direct coronary ostial anastomosis is required, an eye cautery can be used to make the opening into the graft. In neonates conduits with valves interposed between tube graft material can be used to reconstruct right ventricle–pulmonary artery continuity if, for example, there is an absent pulmonary valve. Pulmonary homograft valves have been used for these procedures as well.

When sizing graft valve conduits, one needs to remember that in the manufacturing process, the addition of the graft to the valve prosthesis adds 2 mm to the size of the valve sewing ring. For instance, a 25 mm valve sewing ring would contain a 23 mm valve prosthesis. When using the sizers specific for the valve incorporated into the conduit, the sizer with the best fit determines the size of the aortic graft valve prosthesis (e.g., the sewing ring annulus), not the size of the valve within the conduit (which would be 2 mm smaller). Thus if a 27 mm St. Jude Medical sizer fit best into the native annulus, a 27 mm conduit (containing a 25 mm valve) would be selected and implanted.

Annuloplasty Rings

The complications associated with replacement of the mitral and tricuspid valves in particular have fostered

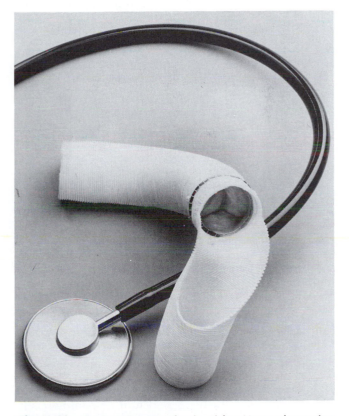

Fig. 5-62 Graft-valve prosthesis with a Hancock porcine valve within the tube graft. (Courtesy Medtronic, Inc., Minneapolis, Minn.)

widespread use of reparative techniques with or without prosthetic devices. Moreover, the use of intraoperative echocardiography to assess valve function has taken much of the guesswork out of evaluating mitral and/or tricuspid repairs (Cosgrove and Stewart, 1989). The prosthetic devices include annuloplasty

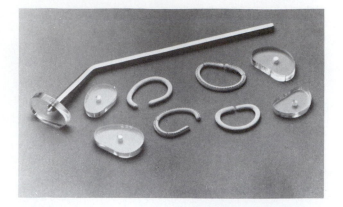

Fig. 5-63 Carpentier-Edwards tricuspid and mitral annuloplasty rings and sizing obturators and holder. Note the gap in the tricuspid rings *(left)* that correlates to the area in the heart containing bundle of His conduction tissue; this helps the surgeon to avoid placing sutures in the area. (Courtesy Baxter Healthcare Corp., Edwards CVS Div., Santa Ana, Calif.)

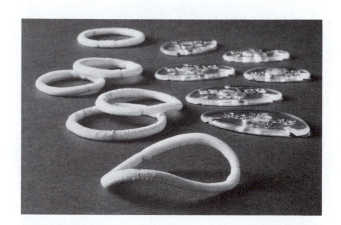

Fig. 5-64 Duran annuloplasty rings *(left)* and sizing obturators *(right)*. (Courtesy Medtronic, Inc., Minneapolis, Minn.)

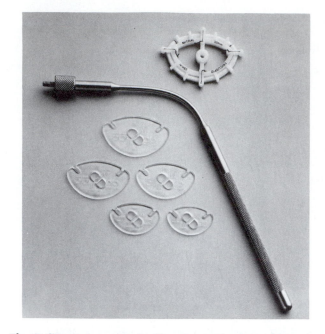

Fig. 5-65 Accessories for Duran annuloplasty rings: ring holder *(top)*, handle for holder *(middle)*, and sizing obturators *(bottom)*. A handle can be made for the sizing obturator by grasping the central portion of the sizer with a tonsil or Kelly clamp. (Courtesy Medtronic, Inc., Minneapolis, Minn.)

rings (Figs. 5-63 through 5-65), which are used in patients with dilated annuli and symptoms of valvular regurgitation. Sizers and handlers are available and specific to mitral or tricuspid procedures.

Patch repairs of valve leaflets can be performed with the patient's own pericardium or commercially available tissue. Autologous tissue may be treated by being soaked for a few minutes in glutaraldehyde, but the glutaraldehyde must be rinsed off before the treated tissue is implanted.

CONCLUSION

Structural standards guide the perioperative nurse in organizing and administering the cardiac OR. Consideration must be given to the wide array of equipment and supplies, the complexity of patient care, and the demands placed on a hospital's human, fiscal, and material resources.

REFERENCES

American College of Cardiology/American Heart Association (ACC/AHA) Task Force: Guidelines and indications for coronary artery bypass graft surgery, *J Am Coll Cardiol* 17(3):543, 1991.

American Nurses Association/American Heart Association: *Standards of cardiovascular nursing practice*, Kansas City, Mo, 1981, ANA.

Association of Operating Room Nurses: *Standards and recommended practices for perioperative nursing*, Denver, 1993, AORN.

Austin WG: Choosing a heart valve substitute. In Grillo HC and others: *Current therapy in cardiothoracic surgery*, Toronto, 1989, BC Decker.

Baue AE, Geha AS, O'Kane H: Organization of a cardiac surgical unit, *Angiology* 25(1):31, 1974.

Bojar RM: *Manual of perioperative care in cardiac and thoracic surgery*, Boston, 1989, Blackwell Scientific Publications.

Brown CV: Portable extracorporeal circulation: a new standard in myocardial infarction care? *J Emerg Nurs* 16(p 2):226, 1990.

Cooley DA: *Techniques in cardiac surgery*, ed 2, Philadelphia, 1984, WB Saunders.

Cosgrove DM, Stewart MJ: Mitral valvuloplasty, *Curr Prob Cardiol* 14(7):355, 1989.

Department of Health, Education, and Welfare: *Minimum requirements of construction and equipment for hospitals and medical facilities*, DHEW Pub No (HRA) 79-14500, Washington, DC, 1978, US Government Printing Office.

Firkins VL, Joy S: The neonate in surgery, *AORN J* 50(6):1193, 1989.

Frazier OH, Colon R: Assisted circulation. In Miller TA, editor: *Physiologic basis of modern surgical care*, St Louis, 1988, Mosby.

Frazier OH and others: First human use of the Hemopump, a catheter-mounted ventricular assist device, *Ann Thorac Surg* 49:299, 1990.

Girard NJ, Morgan RG, Orr MD: Autologous salvage of blood, *AORN J* 47(2):492, 1988.

Huddleston KR: Patent ductus arteriosus ligation: performing surgery outside the operating room, *AORN J* 53(1):69, 1991.

Hyperthermia devices and skin injury, *Med Dev Surveill* 4(1):S8, 1990.

Inter-Society Commission for Heart Disease Resources: Optimal resources for cardiac surgery: guidelines for program planning and evaluation, *Am J Cardiol* 36:836, 1975.

Inter-Society Commission for Heart Disease Resources: Optimal resources for examination of the chest and cardiovascular system, *Circulation* 53(2):A-1, 1976.

Joint Commission on Accreditation of Healthcare Organizations: Accreditation manual for hospitals (vols I and II), Oakbrook Terrace, Ill, 1993, JCAHO.

Kirklin JW, Barratt-Boyes BG: *Cardiac surgery,* ed 2, New York, 1993, Churchill Livingstone.

Kirklin JK, Kirklin JW: Cardiopulmonary bypass for cardiac surgery. In Sabiston DC, Spencer FC: *Surgery of the chest,* ed 5, vols 1 and 2, Philadelphia, 1990, WB Saunders.

Levine PA and others: Electrocautery and pacemakers: management of the paced patient subject to electrocautery, *Ann Thorac Surg* 41(3):313, 1986.

Martin E and others: Autotransfusion systems (ATS), *Crit Care Nurse* 9(7):65, 1989.

Pierson MA: Design of the surgical suite. In Meeker MH, Rothrock JC: *Alexander's care of the patient in surgery,* ed 9, St Louis, 1991, Mosby.

Phillips SJ and others: Percutaneous cardiopulmonary bypass: application and indication for use, *Ann Thorac Surg* 47:121, 1989.

Quaal SJ: *Comprehensive intra-aortic balloon pumping,* ed 2, St Louis, 1993, Mosby.

Regas ML: Surgery outside the OR: when the patient cannot be moved, *AORN* 52(6):1187, 1990.

Scannel JG and others: Optimal resources for cardiac surgery: guidelines for program planning and evaluation, *Am J Cardiol* 36:836, 1975.

Stellar JJ: Pediatric surgery. In Meeker MH, Rothrock JC: *Alexander's care of the patient in surgery,* ed 9, St Louis, 1991, Mosby.

Sympson GM: CATR: a new generation of autologous blood transfusion, *Crit Care Nurs* 11(4):60, 1991.

Yankah AC and others, editors: *Cardiac valve allografts 1962-1987,* New York, 1988, Springer-Verlag.

Zipes DP: Management of cardiac arrhythmias. In Braunwald E, editor: *Heart disease,* ed 4, Philadelphia, 1992, WB Saunders.

Zokal F: Made-to-order suture packs: increasing OR efficiency, *AORN J* 51(3):817, 1990.

SUGGESTED READING

Moura P, Shinn SJ: Planning for operating room design and construction. In Spry C: *The manual of operating room management,* Rockville, Md, 1990, Aspen.

6

Preoperative Assessment

Nurses today . . . are assuming a more collaborative role in the care of their patients. They are, therefore, interested in knowing why certain manifestations of disease appear and why a specific therapeutic regimen is chosen rather than simply observing these events passively.

Jeanette Kernicki, RN, Barbara L. Bullock, RN, and Joan Matthews Register, RN, 1970 (preface)

Assessment, diagnosis, outcome identification, planning, implementation, and evaluation represent standards of clinical practice that form the foundation for clinical decision making. In assessing the cardiac surgery patient, the perioperative nurse is guided by the process and outcome standards developed by the Association of Operating Room Nurses (AORN) (1993) and the *Standards of Cardiovascular Nursing Practice,* jointly developed by the American Nurses' Association (ANA) and the American Heart Association (AHA) Council on Cardiovascular Nursing (1981).

Information concerning the present illness may be abundant or relatively scarce, depending on the nature of the problem and how long it has affected the patient. This information can be obtained from the hospital record, the preoperative interview, and other sources such as professional colleagues, technicians from diagnostic laboratories, and the patient's family and friends. In many instances, before the perioperative nurse conducts the preoperative interview, the patient will have had diagnostic studies to identify the problem and laboratory tests to measure various physiologic parameters pertinent to the surgical management. Based on the results of these tests and the findings from prior assessment interviews (conducted by the patient's physicians and admitting nurses), the perioperative nurse interviews the patient to formulate a plan of care that promotes physiologic and psychologic homeostasis. Intraoperatively, the nurse continues to assess the patient by monitoring the clinical status and comparing it with preoperative baseline data; interventions can be adjusted or modified depending on the patient's response to surgery. During the postoperative evaluation, the perioperative nurse can apply significant findings to future patient assessments.

This chapter describes commonly performed diagnostic and laboratory tests and presents a format for interviewing the patient before surgery based on functional health patterns and nursing diagnoses (Carpenito, 1993; Gordon, 1994; Guzzetta and others, 1989; Roy, 1987). It is not within the scope of this chapter to present a fully detailed assessment as might be performed on admission to the hospital. For a more detailed review, the reader is referred to the references listed at the end of this chapter.

BACKGROUND INFORMATION

The hospital record (i.e., the patient's chart) is especially valuable as a source of historical and diagnostic information. Progress notes from primary and referring physicians, reports of diagnostic and laboratory tests, and nursing admission assessments can be reviewed by the perioperative nurse in preparation for the preoperative patient interview. The record usually includes an entry by the patient's internist or cardiologist describing the events and the symptoms that initially prompted the patient to seek treatment. The perioperative nurse should review this entry (which may have a variable amount of patient details), as well as the assessment by the admitting nurse.

The patient with heart disease commonly will have complained about symptoms such as dyspnea, chest pain or discomfort, syncope, palpitation, edema, cough, and excessive fatigue (Braunwald, 1992). The clinician determines whether or not these symptoms are caused by heart disease by eliciting the patient's history and performing a physical examination.

The history provides information about the patient, the illness, and the impact of the disorder on the functional status (Box 6-1) of the patient. Often there is a subjective component in the evaluation of the patient, and direct contact between physician and patient, or nurse and patient, enables the clinician to arrive at a more complete and accurate assessment.

Box 6-1 *New York Heart Association functional classification system*

Class I
Patients with cardiac disease do not display symptoms of syncope, fatigue, dyspnea, palpitation, or anginal pain with ordinary physical activity. Infants do not demonstrate fatigue with feedings, prolonged feedings, undue respiratory distress or cyanosis after crying or straining, or undue delayed motor development.

Class II
Patients with cardiac disease are comfortable at rest but display the above symptoms during ordinary physical activity.

Class III
Patients with cardiac disease, although comfortable at rest, are markedly limited functionally and display symptoms with less than ordinary exercise.

Class IV
Patients with cardiac disease are unable to engage in any physical activity without discomfort and may have symptoms of cardiac insufficiency even at rest.

Modified from The New York Heart Association, Inc.

and environmental interactions (Friedman, 1992). The clinician will inquire about the prenatal history of infants including maternal viral illnesses (such as rubella) or alcohol and drug use during the first trimester. Maternal diabetes mellitus or parental congenital heart disease is associated with a higher incidence of congenital heart disease in children (Driscoll, 1990). Some congenital malformations may not require surgery until adulthood (i.e., atrial septal defect or bicuspid aortic valve).

Once the history is completed, a review of the patient's systems is performed to determine cardiovascular involvement and other systemic illnesses that may affect the heart. Among these are muscular dystrophies that can cause cardiomyopathies, metabolic disorders that can produce heart failure and conduction disturbances, and inherited connective tissue disorders associated with aortic dissection and mitral valve prolapse (Braunwald, 1992).

Based on the findings from the history and physical examination, a preliminary diagnosis is formulated. To confirm the medical diagnosis and guide treatment, the physician orders specific diagnostic tests.

DIAGNOSTIC PROCEDURES

In addition to confirming the diagnosis, specific diagnostic tests are selected to evaluate the degree of injury or extent of the disorder and select the most appropriate intervention. Some of the most common diagnostic procedures are described here.

Not all of the following tests are performed on every patient; generally, only those needed to confirm the diagnosis or to provide additional data for the selection of the appropriate therapy are ordered (Table 6-1). Given the current emphasis on quality improvement, cost containment, and professional peer review, physicians are increasingly being asked to justify the selection of tests based on whether the data provided by the particular procedure are worth the cost, inconvenience, and risk to the patient (Patterson and Horowitz, 1989).

Previous illnesses are important in the history taking. A history of rheumatic fever or frequent tonsillitis as a child is significant because the sequelae of rheumatic fever and streptococcal infections can lead to damage of the cardiac valves. Other significant illnesses include thyroid disease, venereal disease, and recent dental disease requiring manipulation or extraction. Neurologic, endocrine, and rheumatologic disorders may influence the cardiovascular system as well.

Congenital malformations may be present. These are thought to be the result of multifactorial genetic

Table 6-1 ■ *Diagnostic tests commonly performed for cardiovascular disorders*

	Coronary artery disease	Valvular heart disease	Conduction disturbance	Thoracic aneurysm	Congenital heart disease
Resting ECG	X	X	X	X	X
Exercise ECG (stress test)	X		X		X
Chest x-ray film	X	X	X	X	X
Aortography				X	X
Echocardiogram	X	X	X	X	X
Resting MUGA	X				
Exercise thallium	X				X
CT scan				X	
PET scan with stress	X				
MRI				X	X
Electrophysiology			X		
Cardiac catheterization	X	X	X	X	X

CT, computed tomography; *ECG*, electrocardiogram; *MRI*, magnetic resonance imaging; *MUGA*, multiple uptake gated acquisition; *PET*, positron emission tomography.

Diagnostic studies requiring arterial (or central venous) puncture are characterized as invasive; noninvasive studies do not require arterial access. Occasionally the technique may be semiinvasive, such as radiographs with the intravenous injection of dye. Noninvasive studies include the electrocardiogram (ECG), stress testing, radiography, echocardiography, cardiac Doppler studies, and nuclear imaging. Invasive tests, such as electrophysiology studies, cardiac catheterization, or endomyocardial biopsy, require the insertion of intravascular catheters, electrodes, or bioptomes.

Test results are usually in the patient record and can be reviewed by the perioperative nurse. Patients electively scheduled for surgery may have had cardiac catheterization and other tests performed during a previous hospitalization. The old chart should be available so that these test results can be reviewed preoperatively by the surgical team. Hospitalized patients requiring urgent or emergent surgery are tested as needed to prepare for surgery.

Electrocardiogram

A resting 12-lead ECG provides baseline information about the electrical activity of the heart. It can detect abnormal cardiac rhythms, conduction defects, and signs of ischemia (ST segment changes) or infarction (Q waves), as well as provide information about the position of the heart and the size of the cardiac chambers (Figs. 6-1 and 6-2). QRS complex, ST segment, T wave, and P wave changes may also be due to effects of drugs or electrolyte imbalances. Hypertrophy of the right and left ventricles can also be identified. Results of the ECG are correlated to clinical data obtained from the history and physical examination.

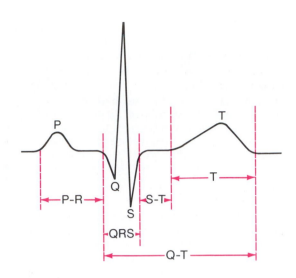

Fig. 6-1   ECG waveform components. **P wave**—electrical activity associated with SA (sinoatrial) node impulse and depolarization of the atria (absent with atrial fibrillation or flutter). **PR interval**—the time the impulse takes to travel through the atria to the AV (atrioventricular) node, the His-Purkinje system, and the ventricles; interval between the onset of the P wave and the onset of the QRS complex (normal duration: 0.12 to 0.20 second). **QRS complex**—electrical depolarization and contraction of the ventricles (normal duration: 0.04 to 0.12 second). **QT interval**—from the onset of the QRS complex to the end of the T wave. **ST segment**—period between completion of depolarization and the beginning of repolarization of the ventricles; interval between the end of the QRS complex and the beginning of the T wave. Displacement of 0.5 mm or more (up or down) is generally indicative of inadequate myocardial perfusion. **T wave**—recovery, or repolarization, phase of the ventricles. (From Canobbio MM: *Cardiovascular disorders*, St Louis, 1990, Mosby.)

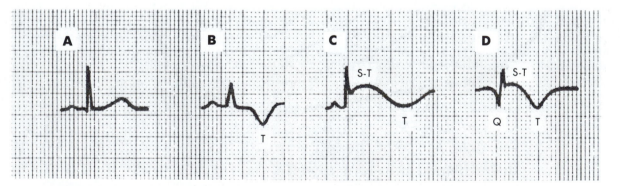

Fig. 6-2   ECG wave changes indicative of ischemia, injury, and necrosis of the myocardium. **A,** Normal left ventricular wave pattern. **B,** Ischemia indicated by inversion of the T wave. **C,** Ischemia and current of injury indicated by T wave inversion and ST segment elevation. The ST segment may be elevated above or depressed below the baseline, depending on whether the tracing is from a lead facing toward or away from the infarcted area and depending on whether epicardial or endocardial injury occurs. Epicardial injury causes ST segment elevation in leads facing the epicardium. Intraoperatively ST segment changes may indicate temporary or permanent ischemic injury resulting from the presence of air in the coronary arteries, a vascular clamp placed too close to a coronary ostium, or incomplete surgical revascularization. **D,** Ischemia, injury, and myocardial necrosis. The Q wave indicates necrosis of the myocardium. (From Andreoli KG and others: *Comprehensive cardiac care*, ed 6, St. Louis, 1987, Mosby.)

The ECG may be normal at rest in the presence of coronary artery disease (CAD), with abnormal changes becoming apparent only with exercise. These patients may undergo continuous electrocardiography with a Holter monitor. This is worn by the patient for 24 to 48 hours, after which the recorded ECG is scanned for abnormalities. Patients with periodic "spells" may be attached to event recorders that are activated when the patient feels dysrhythmias or symptoms such as syncope, palpitations, or chest pain.

Exercise Stress Test

The exercise stress test is used to uncover myocardial dysfunction and other signs of ischemia that become apparent only with the increased metabolic demands created by exertion (or strong emotion). The exercise treadmill test is used to "stress" the heart of patients who are asymptomatic at rest. It may also be ordered for those who have atypical chest pain or who, on occasion, have angina pectoris (Walker, 1988). This test is contraindicated in patients with aortic valve stenosis or other left ventricular outflow tract obstructions because of the danger of cardiac arrest occurring suddenly (probably as a result of ventricular fibrillation).

Patients walk on a gradually inclining treadmill until they reach a target heart rate or demonstrate symptoms of hypotension, ventricular dysrhythmias, ST segment changes, or chest pain. The degree of the ST segment changes and the level of exercise at which they occur provide an indication of the severity of CAD (Sutherland, 1991). They also provide an indication of the patient's functional status. A positive stress test may warrant cardiac catheterization with coronary arteriography. Patients who are unable to exercise may be pharmacologically "stressed" through the administration of dipyridamole followed by thallium scintigraphy.

By quantifying the functional capacity of patients with CAD, stress tests contribute information about the optimum timing for surgery or percutaneous transluminal coronary angioplasty (PTCA). The test may be repeated after surgery to compare preoperative and postoperative functional capacity.

Stress testing in children is performed to assess functional capacity and provide objective guidelines for activity or rehabilitation. Complications of exercise testing in children are similar to those in adults. These include chest pain, syncope, reduction in blood pressure, dysrhythmias, and death (Christiansen and Strong, 1989).

Radiography

Posteroanterior (PA) and lateral chest radiographs (see Fig. 4-5) provide information about the size of the heart, thoracic aorta, and pulmonary vasculature, including signs of pulmonary artery or pulmonary venous hypertension. The clinician also looks for pulmonary disease, such as chronic obstructive pulmonary disease (COPD), effusion, or cancerous lesions, which might contraindicate or change the timing of surgery. Tumors or other mediastinal masses may be apparent and, if present, should also be investigated before the planned cardiac procedure is done.

Cardiac size in adults and children is determined by assessing the cardiothoracic ratio. The cardiac diameter is normally 50% or less of the thoracic diameter on inhalation; a ratio greater than 50% indicates cardiac enlargement. Chest x-ray films may also show the presence of calcium in the cardiac valves, coronary arteries, and aorta. Implants and wires or catheters may be visualized as well (Table 6-2).

The most recent, as well as previously taken, chest x-ray films should be available for review at the time of surgery. In patients with prior sternal operations, the lateral chest x-ray film demonstrates chest wires, the proximity of the heart to the sternum, and possibly the extent of pericardial adhesions. In patients with coarctation of the aorta, rib notching may be evident on the left side of the thorax because of the tortuous path of hypertrophied intercostal arteries.

In patients with suspected thoracic aneurysms, computed tomography or arteriography with injection of radiopaque material is performed in the radiology suite to determine the site and location of the aneurysm and the site of the intimal tear in an aortic dissection (Fig. 6-3). Clearer images are now available with digital subtraction angiography (DSA). This technique involves taking two images, one before the contrast media is injected and one afterward. A computer subtracts one from the other, thereby removing undesired tissue images and leaving an arterial image of high contrast (Pagana and Pagana, 1990).

Echocardiography

One of the fastest growing and most widely used diagnostic techniques for the study of cardiac structure and function is echocardiography, which uses high-frequency sound waves transmitted from a probe (the transducer) to the heart and surrounding structures. These ultrasound waves bounce off the internal or-

Table 6-2 ■ *X-ray densities of intrathoracic structures*

Metal or bone (white)	Structures or fluid (gray)	Air (black)
Ribs, clavicle, sternum, spine	Blood	Lung
Calcium deposits	Heart	
Surgical wires or clips	Veins	
Prosthetic valves	Arteries	
Pacemaker, ICD*	Edema	
Pacemaker wires		

Modified from Thelan LA, Davie JK, Urden LD: *Textbook of critical care nursing: diagnosis and management,* St Louis, 1990, Mosby.
*ICD, Internal cardioverter defibrillator.

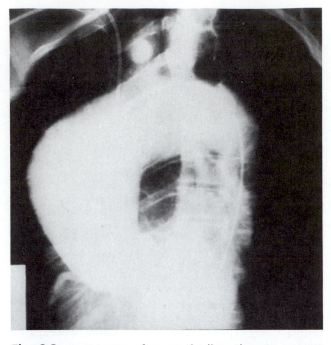

Fig. 6-3 Aortogram of an aortic dissection. (Courtesy Edward A. Lefrak, MD.)

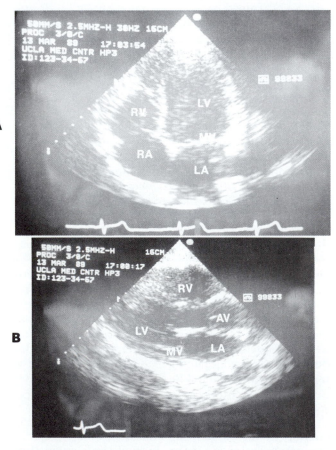

Fig. 6-4 Two-dimensional echocardiography. Labels have been added to identify the structures. **A,** Short-axis view. **B,** Long-axis view. *RA,* Right atrium; *RV,* right ventricle; *LA,* left atrium; *LV,* left ventricle; *MV,* mitral valve. (From Canobbio MM: *Cardiovascular disorders,* St. Louis, 1990, Mosby.)

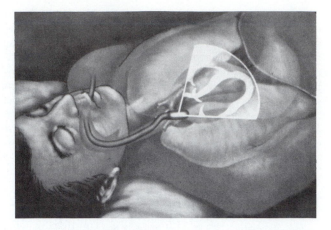

Fig. 6-5 Transesophageal echocardiography (TEE) is performed with the probe positioned in the esophagus; this allows a view of the cardiac chambers that is unobstructed by the sternal bone. (Courtesy Hewlett-Packard Co.)

gan, echo back to the transducer, and are electronically converted into images that are displayed on a monitor or videotape. The transducer may be positioned over the sternum (transsternal), over the exposed heart (epicardial), or inside the esophagus (Fig. 6-4) behind the cardiac structures (transesophageal). When placed directly on the heart, the transducer is placed in a sterile plastic sheath and kept on the operative field.

Because it is noninvasive and does not require the use of ionizing radiation, echocardiography is especially attractive for the evaluation of many conditions in seriously ill children and adults (Popp, 1990a, 1990b). The family of echocardiographic tests include M-mode, 2-dimensional, Doppler, and color flow imaging techniques. M-mode recordings display one-dimensional time-motion (*M* for motion) studies of the heart. Systolic time intervals can be quantified, as well as ventricular wall thickness, aortic or mitral stenosis, cardiac tumors, and valvular vegetations. M-mode techniques are used less frequently because of improvements in the two-dimensional and Doppler technology but are still a valuable source of information (Meyer, 1989).

Two-dimensional echocardiograms visualize more of the heart and provide cross-sectional images along numerous planes (Fig. 6-5), most commonly the precordial sagittal plane (long-axis view of the heart and great vessels) and the transverse plane (short-axis view of the heart and great vessels). Spatial anatomic relationships between cardiac chambers, wall motion abnormalities, valvular movement, anatomic alterations, and the dynamic geometry of cardiac contractions can be seen (Popp, 1990a, 1990b).

With the addition of Doppler ultrasound, sound waves echo back from red blood cells, allowing blood flow to be heard as well as visualized. Information is provided on pulmonary and intracardiac blood pressures, transvalvular gradients, septal shunts, and valvular stenosis and/or regurgitation. The addition of

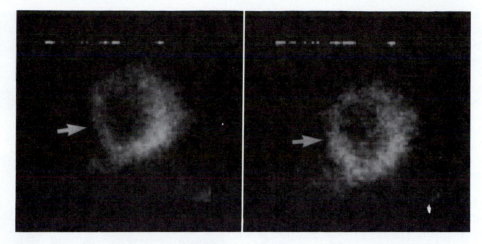

Fig. 6-6 Thallium images (left anterior oblique [LAO] view) demonstrating septal *(arrow)* hypoperfusion during stress that redistributes with rest, consistent with septal ischemia. (From Kinney MR and others: *Comprehensive cardiac care,* ed 7, St Louis, 1991, Mosby.)

color—blue and red—demonstrates the direction and velocity of blood flow. Flow moving toward the transducer is seen as red (or sometimes orange), and flow away from the transducer is seen as blue. Color Doppler is especially useful for diagnosing acquired and congenital abnormalities of cardiac structures and hemodynamic function.

Duplex scanning is a combination of pulsed Doppler and spectral analysis of the Doppler signal with real-time brightness mode (B-mode) ultrasound. Spectral analysis reveals the movement of red blood cells at different speeds (the greater the width of the spectrum, the more turbulent the flow), thereby providing information about blood flow through stenosed vessels and estimations about the degree of stenosis (Fahey and Riegel, 1989).

Transesophageal echocardiography (TEE) is commonly used to evaluate cardiac valves and to assess the need for repair versus replacement of a valve at operation. Intraoperatively TEE is used to test repairs of congenital defects, as well as regurgitant valves, and to assess ventricular function. A baseline preoperative study is performed before the incision is made; the completed repair is then studied and compared with the preoperative findings.

Because air bubbles, as well as blood flow, are visualized, TEE can also be used to detect the presence of residual air (seen as large white specks) in the left ventricle during surgery. The surgeon can then perform additional maneuvers to vent the heart if necessary.

Cardiac Nuclear Scanning

Nuclear studies are used to test myocardial tissue damage, myocardial perfusion, and myocardial function. When the result of a stress test does not conform to the clinical picture, radionuclide studies provide additional information about the presence, location, and extent of CAD (Massie and Sokolow, 1991).

Radioactive materials (such as thallium-201, technetium-99m pertechnetate, and technetium-99m pyrophosphate) are injected intravenously. A scintillation camera is placed over the heart to detect areas of the radionuclide concentration and to record and photograph the images.

Technetium angiography is performed by labeling the red blood cells with the radionuclide, which enters only irreversibly damaged myocardial cells, creating "hot spots." The study is performed to detect infarcted myocardium or tissue that has suffered burns or contusions.

Computer-assisted technetium scanning of the ventricle in motion is performed with multiple uptake gated acquisition (MUGA) studies. Sequential photographs are taken during systole and diastole and synchronized to the ECG. The ejection fraction can be calculated with this technique, and regional and global ventricular wall motion can be evaluated.

Other studies use thallium, which enters the cell like its analogue, potassium, and is distributed throughout the myocardium, reflecting regional blood flow (Fig. 6-6). Thallium is injected into the bloodstream after vigorous exercise, which is continued to stress the heart and circulate the thallium. The heart is scanned for perfusion defects ("cold spots"), indicating the absence of blood flow. If there are no defects, the test is negative. If a defect is present, the patient is scanned again within a few hours. If at that time the defect has taken up thallium, the area is considered to be ischemic; if the defect persists, infarction is thought to have occurred. In patients with a persistent defect but without a known prior infarction or electrocardiographic evidence of infarction, delayed thallium scanning may be performed 24 to 48 hours later to differentiate between stunned and scarred myocardium. Because it may not be feasible to perform another test a day or more later, thallium may be reinjected just after redistribution imaging is performed (Dilsizian and others, 1990). The purpose is to differentiate between viable but jeopardized myocardium. The distinction is important to physicians who may be considering the appropriateness of myocardial revascularization, because coronary artery bypassing is effective for ischemic, but not infarcted, myocardium (Lavie, Ventura, and Murgo, 1991).

When patients are unable to tolerate exercise during ECG or thallium stress tests, a pharmacologic thallium test may be performed with dipyridamole or adenosine (coronary vasodilators), which simulates the exercise portion of the test. Administration of these drugs increases perfusion to myocardium supplied by coronary arteries without significant stenosis but does not increase the blood supply to areas supplied by an obstructed coronary artery. After administration of the drug and the thallium tracer, myocardial perfusion is scanned.

Analysis of coronary perfusion has been enhanced with newer nuclear studies such as single photon emission computed tomography (SPECT) and positron emission tomography (PET). SPECT uses the tomographic technique of creating computer-assisted cross-sectional images from many parts of the body. Single photon–emitting radionuclides (such as thallium) are used to create images of great clarity and precision. PET measures biologic processes by recording the activity of radionuclides in specified tissue; a computer reconstructs the spatial distribution of the radionuclide to determine regional metabolism of the heart and to measure infarct size (Pagana and Pagana, 1990).

Computed Tomography

Computed tomography (CT), also referred to as computed axial tomography (CAT), is a method of scanning the density of tissue with multiple narrow x-ray beams. These beams are blocked by the tissue in proportion to the density of the tissue. A three-dimensional image is formed by computer analysis and transferred to x-ray film (Fig. 6-7). Contrast material may be added to enhance the clarity of the images. Scans are taken at multiple levels to provide "slices" of tissue (Taubman, 1991).

CT scanning with or without the injection of radioactive substances is used to identify aneurysms of the thoracic, abdominal, and distal aorta, and conditions such as tumors, pleural effusions, and other pathologic changes. The test is minimally invasive, and when used for these purposes, CT images are superior to those obtained by conventional radiography. CT scanning to evaluate the native coronary arteries or bypass vein grafts is not widely used, because the process is not yet sufficiently developed to image these structures with precision.

Magnetic Resonance Imaging

Magnetic resonance imaging (MRI) acts on the magnetic field created by spinning atomic particles within the body. A powerful external magnetic field is ap-

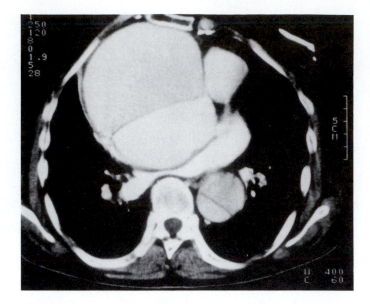

Fig. 6-7   CT scan of thorax. (From Karp RB, Laks H, Wechsler AS: *Advances in cardiac surgery,* vol 4, St. Louis, 1993, Mosby.)

plied, which aligns these particles. When the magnetic field is removed, the particles return to their former position. MRI measures these changes and thereby provides details about anatomy and flow (Fahey and Riegel, 1989). The technique has been used to evaluate the heart and great vessels, as well as the abdominal aorta, in patients with congenital and acquired cardiovascular disease.

Neither contrast media nor ionizing radiation is needed, making MRI especially advantageous. One disadvantage is the need to remain very still during the procedure, which may be difficult in the very young and in the highly anxious patient, both of whom may require sedation. Metallic implants may be a contraindication for MRI.

Cardiac Catheterization

Cardiac catheterization remains the definitive preoperative diagnostic test for CAD to which all others are compared. Although less-risky procedures, such as echo Doppler imaging, are gaining wider acceptance in the diagnosis of simple congenital cardiac lesions (such as atrial septal defect), cardiac catheterization with cineangiography and selective coronary arteriography remains the gold standard for complex congenital lesions and valvular heart disease, as well as CAD. These disorders require visualization of coronary artery perfusion and valve performance, precise measurement of intracardiac blood flow and pressures (Table 6-3), recognition of abnormal shunts, and computation of ratios between pulmonary and systemic blood flow (Spencer, 1989).

In addition to its diagnostic capabilities, cardiac catheterization with coronary arteriography also offers an increasing array of therapeutic interventions

Table 6-3 ■ *Cardiac catheterization data*

Hemodynamic data	Normal values		
Flow			
Cardiac output (CO)	4.0-8.0 L/min		
Cardiac index (CI)	2.5-4.0 L/min/m²		
Ejection fraction (EF)	60%-70%		
Left ventricular end-diastolic volume (LVEDV)	90-180 ml		
Stroke volume (SV)	60-130 ml/beat		
Stroke volume index (SVI)	35-70 ml/beat/m²		
Pressures (mm Hg)	Systolic	Diastolic	Mean
Venae cavae			0-5
Right atrium (RA)			2-6
Right ventricle (RV)	20-30	0-5	
Pulmonary artery (PA)	20-30	10-20	10-15
Pulmonary artery wedge pressure (PAWP)			4-12
Left atrium (LA)			4-12
Left ventricle (LV)	120	0-5	
Left ventricular end-diastolic pressure (LVEDP)			5-12
Aorta	120-140	60-80	70-90
Brachial artery	120	70	
Femoral artery	125	75	
Resistances			
Systemic vascular resistance (SVR)	800-1400 dynes/sec/cm^{-5}		
Pulmonary vascular resistance (PVR)	100-250 dynes/sec/cm^{-5}		
Shunts (Qp/Qs)			
Pulmonary flow/systemic flow	1:1		
Oxygen Saturations			
Venae cavae	70%		
Right atrium	70%		
Right ventricle	70%		
Pulmonary artery	70%		
Pulmonary veins	97%		
Left atrium	97%		
Left ventricle	97%		
Aorta	97%		
Valve Orifices (Adult)			
Aortic	2-4 cm²		
Mitral	4-6 cm²		
Tricuspid	10 cm²		
Angiographic Data	**Findings**		
Coronary arteries	Anatomy/function coronary vascular bed; distal coronary flow; AV fistula; atherosclerosis; anomalous origin of coronary arteries		
Ventriculography	Anatomy/function of ventricles and associated structures; LV aneurysm; congenital abnormalities; valvular stenosis/regurgitation; shunts		
Valvular angiography	Intact mitral/tricuspid complex; valvular incompetence/stenosis/regurgitation		
Pulmonary angiography	Pulmonary embolism; congenital abnormalities		
Aortography	Patency of aortic branches; normal mobility, competence, and anatomy of aortic valve; aneurysms: saccular, fusiform; dissections; origin of aortic dissection; shunts or anomalous connections; congenital defects or obstructions		

Modified from Seifert PC: Cardiac Surgery. In Meeker MH, Rothrock JC: *Alexander's care of the patient in surgery,* ed 9, St. Louis, 1991, Mosby; and from Sabiston DC, Spencer FC: *Gibbon's surgery of the chest,* 2 vols, ed 4, Philadelphia, 1983, WB Saunders.

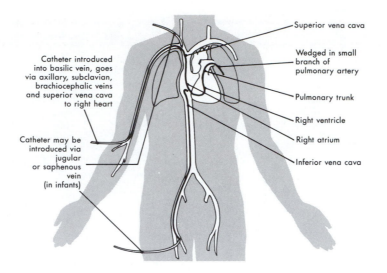

Fig. 6-8   Right-sided heart catheterization. The heart is approached from the basilic vein (Sones technique) or the femoral vein (Judkins technique). (From Kern MJ: *The cardiac catheterization handbook,* St Louis, 1991, Mosby.)

such as lysis of acute coronary thrombosis, PTCA, stent placement, coronary atherectomy (Good and Gentzler, 1991), and balloon, umbrella, or coil occlusion of an atrial or ventricular septal defect or persistent patent ductus arteriosus (Bridges and others, 1991). Other procedures include blade or balloon atrial septostomy to allow mixing of oxygenated and unoxygenated blood for cyanotic conditions such as transposition of the great vessels. Balloon dilatation of stenotic valves or blood vessels is available for a variety of acquired and congenital problems (Radtke and Lock, 1990; Zeevi and others, 1988).

Catheterization is performed by inserting catheters into arteries or veins and threading them to the heart to obtain x-ray movies (cineangiograms) of cardiac chambers and coronary arteries and to measure intracardiac and intravascular pressures. Various insertion sites may be used depending on the age of the patient, the anatomy, and the information required. Among these are the femoral artery or vein in the groin (Judkins technique); the median basilic vein and brachial artery in the antecubital fossa (Sones technique); the subclavian, saphenous, or jugular vein; and, in neonates, the umbilical artery and vein (Freed, 1989; Kern, 1991). The femoral artery is generally the preferred entry site because of the ease of insertion and relatively few complications, but aortoiliac disease or other lower-extremity vascular problems may necessitate the use of arm veins.

Right-sided heart catheterization (Fig. 6-8) is indicated for patients with intracardiac shunts, pulmonary disease, a history of dyspnea, or right-sided cardiac valve disorders. The catheter is inserted percutaneously (or via cutdown when necessary) into the femoral or basilic vein, threaded to the respective vena cava, and passed into the right atrium. Contrast media may be injected to opacify defects or shunts, and pres-

sures are recorded. Blood samples from the venae cavae and right atrium may be taken to measure oxygen saturations when atrial septal defects, anomalous pulmonary venous return, or other shunts are suspected. The catheter is advanced into the right ventricle and the outflow tract, and then through the pulmonary valve to the proximal and distal pulmonary arteries. Anatomic information and hemodynamic data, including blood pressures, blood oximetry, and cardiac output, are recorded.

Left-sided heart catheterization (Fig. 6-9) is performed to study CAD, cardiomyopathy, pericardial constriction, left-sided valvular lesions, and congenital abnormalities. The catheter is inserted into the femoral or brachial artery and threaded retrogradely to the ascending aorta. Coronary arteriograms and left ventriculograms can then be performed.

Coronary arteriography is performed by selectively injecting dye into the right and left coronary ostia. Obstructions, flow, and distal perfusion ("run-off") are evaluated. To maximize clarity, each vessel is viewed from several angles and recorded so that arteries overlapping one another in one position may be clearly visualized from a different angle. The right anterior oblique (RAO) projection provides good visualization of the left main coronary artery (Fig. 6-10). This projection at 30 degrees also offers a clear view of the left anterior descending (LAD) coronary artery, LAD septal perforators, and the circumflex system. A 45-degree RAO demonstrates the right coronary artery and posterior descending (interventricular) coronary artery (Fig. 6-11). The left anterior oblique (LAO) projection at 55 to 60 degrees is used to study the mid and distal LAD coronary artery, as well as the diagonal branches of the LAD. Depending on the lesion, cranial and caudal projections may also be recorded.

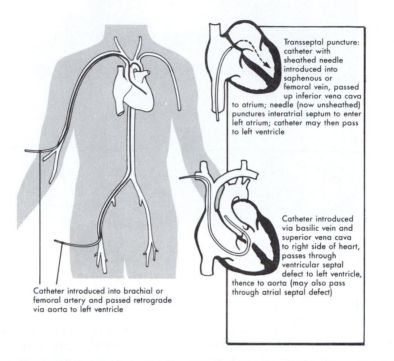

Fig. 6-9 Left-sided heart catheterization. The heart is approached from the brachial (Sones technique) or femoral (Judkins technique) artery. The left side of the heart can also be approached via the right side with the catheter passed through an atrial or ventricular septal defect. (From Kern MJ: *The cardiac catheterization handbook*, St Louis, 1991, Mosby.)

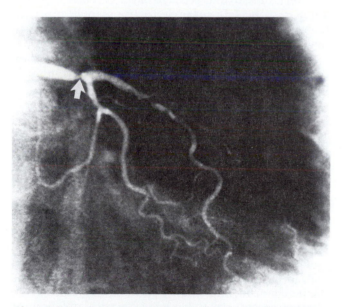

Fig. 6-10 Cineangiographic (moving picture) frame showing left main coronary artery stenosis *(arrow)* in the right anterior oblique (RAO) projection. (From Kern MJ: *The cardiac catheterization handbook*, St Louis, 1991, Mosby.)

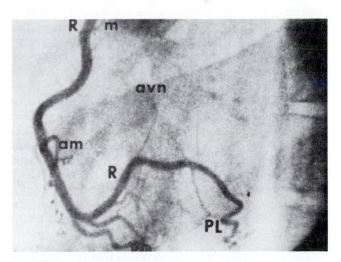

Fig. 6-11 Coronary angiogram of a normal right coronary artery in the RAO position. *R (top),* Proximal right coronary artery; *m,* main right artery; *am,* acute marginal coronary artery; *avn,* atrioventricular nodal artery; *R (bottom),* distal right coronary artery; *PL* posterior lateral coronary artery. (From Canobbio MM: *Cardiovascular disorders*, St Louis, 1990, Mosby.)

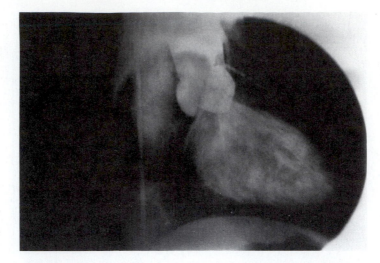

Fig. 6-12 Left ventriculogram in the RAO position. Note opacification of the aortic valve and the sinuses of Valsalva. (From Kern MJ: *The cardiac catheterization handbook,* St Louis, 1991, Mosby.)

Coronary anomalies may be identified, such as the left main coronary artery arising from the right sinus of Valsalva (instead of its normal take-off from the left sinus), the right coronary artery arising from the left sinus of Valsalva, or the presence of only one main coronary artery arising from the aorta. Such anomalies are significant for a variety of reasons, among them that patients with proximal obstructions of a single large coronary artery are at increased risk of myocardial infarction, and pediatric patients being considered for arterial switch procedures to repair transposition of the great arteries may need to undergo an alternative operation.

Left ventriculography is performed by passing a catheter through the aortic valve into the left ventricle. Rarely, the left ventricle may also be approached through a transseptal puncture from the right atrium. When congenital atrial or ventricular septal defects are present, the physician may use these openings to enter the left heart from the right side.

Blood sampling and pressure measurements are performed. Ventricular wall motion is studied by injecting dye into the ventricular chamber (Fig. 6-12); this demonstrates regional and global wall motion and displays areas that may be hypokinetic (weakly contractile), akinetic (not contractile), or dyskinetic (paradoxical motion such as that seen with left ventricular aneurysms). Shunts and regurgitating blood are revealed. The cardiac output and ejection fraction are estimated.

Cardiac valves (most commonly the aortic and mitral) are studied to determine their structure and function. The cardiologist can assess valvular orifice size, impedence to flow (stenosis), and/or reflux (regurgitation), as well as the structural integrity of the valvular components. Valves that have become stenotic often demonstrate some degree of regurgitation as well.

Differences in pressure behind and in front of primarily stenotic valves (the pressure gradient) can be calculated for aortic valve stenosis by simultaneously measuring the systolic blood pressure in the ascending aorta and the left ventricle. The difference in pressure (which is normally equal when the aortic valve is open) provides an indication of the severity of the stenosis. When cardiac failure is present, however, the ventricle may be too weak to generate a high intraventricular pressure and the gradient may be considerably diminished. This may be apparent on the left ventriculogram as hypokinesis of the ventricular wall. Occasionally stenosis of the aortic valve may be too severe to allow transvalvular passage of the catheter from the aorta into the left ventricle; a transseptal approach from the right side may then be used, or the test is deferred.

Stenotic mitral valve gradients can be similarly computed. Left atrial tumors, such as myxomas, may be detected when contrast material is injected.

Electrophysiology Studies

Electrophysiology studies involve procedures similar to cardiac catheterization and are performed to study cardiac rhythms. Of particular concern are recurrent ventricular tachydysrhythmias and ventricular fibrillation. These are often associated with coronary artery disease, but other etiologic factors include cardiomyopathy, ventricular dysplasia, and congenital abnormalities (Teplitz, 1991).

The goal of the studies is to confirm the dysrhythmia, locate its origin and path of conduction, define the mechanism, and assess treatment modalities (e.g., pharmacologic, cryothermic or electrical ablation, or surgical excision or implantation of a device) (Kern, 1991).

The procedure is similar to right-sided heart catheterization. Multiple electrode catheters are placed high in the right atrium (to study sinus node impulses), in the coronary sinus (to study the bundle of His and bundle branches), and in the right ventricle (to study the Purkinje system). Occasionally catheters are placed in the left side of the heart. Ventricular tachydysrhythmias are induced by electrical stimulation of different areas of the heart that have been "mapped," and dysfunctional areas are identified. Numerous drugs may be tested for their antidysrhythmic effects at the site of the pacing stimulus. Patients considered suitable for ablative treatment or insertion of antidysrhythmia devices are referred as necessary. Direct mapping and stimulation of the epicardium and the endocardium may be performed as part of a surgical procedure.

Thoracoscopy

Thoracoscopy is an endoscopic diagnostic and therapeutic technique that uses percutaneous insertion of the scope into one or both pleural cavities. It is used mainly for thoracic disorders but may be used for treatment of mediastinal problems. Originally described in 1922, thoracoscopy was infrequently used until it regained popularity in the 1970s. Improvements in endoscopic instrumentation and video capability have provided the impetus for the use of this technique for the diagnosis of pleural effusion and pleural masses. Mediastinoscopes, laparoscopes, and thoracoscopes have been used for this procedure. Attachments for cautery and manipulation of tissue are available.

Therapeutic thoracoscopy has been performed for peripheral lung resection, pleural biopsy, and closure of leaking blebs. Wider application of thoracoscopy for pericardial drainage, pericardial biopsy, and pericardiectomy is under investigation (Miller, 1991; Page, Jeffrey and Donnelly, 1989).

LABORATORY TESTS

The referring physician who first evaluated the patient will have ordered a number of blood and urine studies in association with the initial history and physical examination (H & P). The laboratory tests described below are those commonly ordered on admission (or a few days before admission) in preparation for surgery. Some of these tests (i.e., coagulation studies, blood gases, electrolyte levels, and complete blood counts) are performed at regular intervals during surgery to monitor physiologic function (Table 6-4). Laboratory values commonly vary from institution to institution; nurses should familiarize themselves with their laboratory's normal and abnormal values.

A complete blood count is performed to determine the number, percentage, and oxygen-carrying capacity of red blood cells (RBCs), and to count the total number and percentage of each type of white blood cell (WBC). This provides baseline data for comparison intraoperatively and postoperatively. A low he-

matocrit preoperatively (normal: 42% to 52% for males, 35% to 47% for females) may require infusion of packed RBCs. Intraoperatively and immediately postoperatively, a hematocrit of 25% (or less) in adults may be well tolerated and not require infusion if intravascular volume is adequate for perfusion (NIH, 1988). A hematocrit of 60% or higher (polycythemia) may be seen in patients with chronic hypoxia (e.g., tetralogy of Fallot), who compensate by increasing the percentage of oxygen-carrying RBCs. These patients may undergo preoperative phlebotomy to lower the hematocrit, thereby reducing blood viscosity and the risk of thromboembolism (Hazinski, 1992).

Blood is tested for viral contamination, including the human immunodeficiency virus (HIV) and hepatitis. Increasingly, patients are donating their own blood preoperatively ("autologous predonation") to avoid the risks of homologous blood transfusions. Blood is also tested for the presence of cold antibodies, which could cause agglutination of the patient's blood when the patient is cooled intraoperatively to hypothermic temperatures.

Hematologic tests provide a detailed coagulation profile to uncover bleeding tendencies or disorders that could affect the operative course. This information creates a baseline for future comparison and enables the clinician to treat the disorder appropriately. In addition, the medication history should be reviewed, because certain drugs prolong the clotting time or interfere with coagulation function. Aspirin and dipyridamole block the effectiveness of circulating platelets, thrombolytic agents (streptokinase or tissue plasminogen activator) break down clots, and warfarin (Coumadin) and heparin prolong bleeding time. Effective hemostastis can be further hindered as a result of the destruction of platelets and clotting factors that occurs intraoperatively from the trauma to blood contacting plastic bypass tubing and suctioning devices. A low platelet count is notable and alerts the nurse to anticipate possible replacement of this blood product.

Determination of electrolyte levels is important because of their effects on cardiac function. In particular, low potassium (K+) levels may trigger dysrhythmias on induction of anesthesia and throughout the perioperative period. When possible, replacement therapy is initiated before surgery to bring electrolyte levels into the normal range.

Cardiac enzymes are markers of myocardial damage. The most common are lactic dehydrogenase (LDH) and creatinine kinase (CK). CK has three isoenzymes, one of which, CK-MB (*MB* refers to myocardial bands), is found primarily in cardiac muscle. Elevations of these CK-MB bands provide a unique marker of myocardial damage. Depending on how elevated the isoenzyme is, it can be considered indicative of myocardial injury or infarction (Pagana and Pagana, 1990). Patients who have suffered a myocardial infarction preoperatively may not be able to withstand the stress of surgery; these patients may undergo more conservative treatment (e.g., coronary care monitoring, rest, antidysrhythmia medications).

Table 6-4 ■ *Laboratory data*

Test	Normal values	Test	Normal values
(ABGs)		1 week old	$3.9\text{-}6.3 \times 10^6/\mu l$
pH	7.38-7.44	3-6 months old	$3.1\text{-}4.5 \times 10^6/\mu l$
Po₂	95-100 mm Hg	2-6 years old	$3.9\text{-}5.3 \times 10^6/\mu l$
Pco₂	35-40 mm Hg	Adult	
Blood chemistry		Male	$4.6\text{-}6.2 \times 10^6/\mu l$
Glucose (fasting)	70-110 mg/100 ml	Female	$4.2\text{-}5.4 \times 10^6/\mu l$
Protein (total)	6.8-8.5 g/100 ml	White blood cells	
Blood urea nitrogen	8.0-25 mg/100 ml	(WBCs)	
(BUN)		1 day old	$9.4\text{-}34.0 \times 10^3/\mu l$
Uric acid	3.0-7.0 mg/100 ml	1 month old	$5.0\text{-}19.5 \times 10^3/\mu l$
Cardiac enzymes		Adult	$4.5\text{-}11.0 \times 10^3/\mu l$
Creatine kinase (CK)	5-75 mU/ml	Creatinine (urine, 24-hr)	
CK-MB (isoenzyme)	0%	Male	20-26 mg/kg/24 hr
Lactic dehydrogenase		Female	14-22 mg/kg/24 hr
(LDH)		Electrolytes	
LDH₁ (isoenzyme)	17%-27%	Potassium (K)	3.8-5.0 mEq/L
LDH₂ (isoenzyme)	27%-37%	Sodium (Na)	136-142 mEq/L
Coagulation profile		Chloride (Cl)	95-103 mEq/L
Platelet count	150,000-400,000/μl	Magnesium (Mg)	1.5-2.0 mEq/L
Prothrombin time (PT)	Depends on thromboplastin reagent used: typically 9.5-12.0 sec	Lipids	
		Cholesterol	<200 mg/dl
Thrombin time	Depends on concentration of thrombin reagent used; typically 20-29 sec	Triglycerides	10-190 mg/dl
		Phospholipids	150-380 mg/dl
		Free fatty acids	9.0-15.0 mM/L
Partial thromboplastin time (PTT)	Depends on phospholipid reagent used; typically 60-85 sec	Liver function	
		Albumin (serum)	3.5-5.0 g/dl
		Alkaline phosphatase	20-90 IU/L
Activated PTT	Depends on activator and phospholipid reagents used; typically 20-35 sec	Globulin (serum)	2.3-3.5 g/dl
		Serum bilirubin (total)	0.2-1.4 mg/dl
		Pulmonary function	
Fibrinogen	200-400 mg/dl	*Normal values vary depending on the patient's age, sex, weight, and race. The following are generally calculated:*	
Fibrinogen split products	10 mg/L		
Complete blood count		Residual volume (RV)	
(CBC)		Tidal volume (TV)	
Hemoglobin (Hgb)		Expiratory reserve volume (ERV)	
1-3 days old	14.5-22.5 g/dl	Inspiratory reserve volume (IRV)	
2 months old	9.0-14.0 g/dl		
6-12 years old	11.5-15.5 g/dl	Total lung capacity (TLC)	
Adult		Vital capacity (VC)	
Male	13.5-18.0 g/dl	Urinalysis	
Female	12.0-16.0 g/dl	Color	Amber, yellow
Hematocrit (Hct)		Clarity	Clear
2 days old	48%-75%	pH	4.6-8.0
2 months old	28%-42%	Specific gravity (SG)	1.002-1.035
Adult		Protein	0.0-8.0 mg/dl
Male	42%-52%	Sugar, ketones, RBCs, WBCs, casts	Negative
Female	35%-47%		

Modified from Pagana KD, Pagana TJ: *Mosby's diagnostic and laboratory test reference*, St Louis, 1992, Mosby.

Some elevation of these enzymes is seen in the postoperative patient as a result of the intraoperative trauma caused by median sternotomy, atrial cannulation, and other maneuvers performed on the heart. The clinician evaluates the degree of elevation of the CK-MB and LDH levels, in addition to other clinical signs, such as new Q waves, to determine whether perioperative myocardial infarction has occurred or whether the elevation is due to surgical trauma (Graebner and others, 1985).

Liver and kidney function tests results may be abnormal in patients with chronic heart failure, possibly because of congestion related to right-sided failure in the former case and reduced cardiac output in the latter case. Occasionally, kidney function is affected by the injection of contrast media during cardiac cathcterization. Surgery may be delayed to allow the kidneys to recover so that the anticipated additional stress from cardiopulmonary bypass does not aggravate the injury.

Renal function is assessed by testing blood urea nitrogen and creatinine levels. Renal failure may produce electrolyte imbalances of potassium and calcium, both of which are important for cardiac conduction and contractility. Elevated potassium levels (hyperkalemia) decrease the rate of ventricular depolarization and repolarization and depress atrioventricular conduction. Potassium levels in excess of 10 to 14 mEq/L can lead to cardiac standstill. The effects of hyperkalemia are evident during surgery when cardiac standstill (evidenced by a flat-line ECG) is purposely induced by the infusion of hyperkalemic cardioplegia solutions.

Low potassium levels (hypokalemia) prolong the period of ventricular repolarization, allowing supraventricular and ventricular dysrhythmias to occur (Thelan, 1990). Low potassium levels are commonly caused by diuretic therapy, which promotes potassium excretion.

Liver disease can affect the synthesis of clotting factors and thereby prolong bleeding times. The liver also produces enzymes, proteins, and other products vital to maintaining homeostasis, detoxifies and breaks down many endogenous and exogenous substances, and metabolizes and stores carbohydrates, proteins and fats (Pagana and Pagana, 1990).

PREOPERATIVE PATIENT INTERVIEW

Before the preoperative patient interview, the perioperative nurse can review the admission nursing assessment in the patient's chart for background information about the patient's physical, psychologic, and social status. Because the format of the assessment questionnaire will influence the data collected, the admission assessment form should reflect a holistic view of the patient, facilitate identification of nursing diagnoses, and assist the nurse in predicting patient outcomes (Guzzetta and others, 1989). The assessment form should reflect a systematic, logical, and ordered process that incorporates observation, interviewing, and physical assessment and communication skills.

Some perioperative nurses may be unaccustomed to performing a holistic evaluation of the patient. In this era of cost containment, when many patients are admitted on the morning of surgery, the perioperative clinician may be the only nurse to see the patient before surgery and to assess the patient's needs. For most patients, emotional and social needs are as important as physical needs. An assessment based on human response patterns (NANDA, 1986; Roy, 1984) or functional health patterns (Gordon, 1994) can assist the perioperative nurse in identifying all of these needs and problems. Box 6-2 lists human response patterns and possible cardiac-related diagnoses that fall under each pattern. When the perioperative nurse uses a similar format based on these patterns, infor-

mation is elicited that provides insight not only into the patient's physiologic condition, but also into how the illness has affected psychologic and social aspects of the patient's life.

Assessing the physical, mental, and emotional needs of neonates and children should be familiar to perioperative nurses, even if their cardiac programs focus only on adults with acquired lesions (or congenital lesions becoming apparent in adulthood). When a pediatric cardiac program is not available, many heart centers that perform adult surgery may operate on babies requiring ligation of a persistent patent ductus. The procedure does not require cardiopulmonary bypass and can be performed in the operating room (OR) or neonatal intensive care unit (NICU). Although pediatric considerations are not described in detail, some guidelines are offered in this and subsequent chapters that may assist the perioperative nurse in caring for these patients and their significant others.

The order of the following patterns and the guidelines for obtaining information within each may be altered according to the perioperative nurse's judgment about the patient's condition. The initial interview can take place in the OR suite, physician's office, surgical inpatient unit, diagnostic laboratory, or some other location. In urgent or emergent situations, priority sections of the assessment form (e.g., physiologic data within the exchanging pattern) are completed first and other sections are completed at a later time (Guzzetta and Seifert, 1991). A patient who is very young or elderly may be unable to verbalize information, and the perioperative nurse may need to depend on significant others for information about the patient's psychosocial status.

Communicating

The nurse assesses the patient and, whenever possible, the family's ability to communicate verbally and nonverbally. Does the patient understand, speak, read, and write English? If not, and if the patient is alert and oriented, is a translator available? If speech is impaired, it should be determined whether the cause is physiologic or psychologic (e.g., stroke, oral anatomic defect, severe anxiety). With very young children, the parents are interviewed, and their ability to communicate is assessed; elderly patients may have children or significant others who can contribute information.

The patient may be intubated, comatose, severely short of breath, or premedicated. Nonverbal communication, such as restlessness, wanting to hold the nurse's hand, or clinging to a religious object, may be the only indicator that the patient is in distress, is anxious, or is fearful.

Perceiving

Sensory deficits may result from physical and/or emotional factors and may be related or unrelated to the

Box 6-2 *Selected nursing diagnoses for the cardiac surgery patient: classification by human response patterns*

Communicating: A Human Response Pattern Involving the Sending of Messages

Communication, impaired verbal

Perceiving: A Human Response Pattern Involving the Reception of Information

Body image disturbance
Hopelessness
Personal identity disturbance
Powerlessness
Self-esteem, chronic low
Self-esteem disturbance
Self-esteem, situational low
Sensory/perceptual alterations: visual, auditory, kinesthetic, gustatory, tactile, olfactory

Feeling: A Human Response Pattern Involving the Subjective Awareness of Information

Anxiety
Fear
Grieving, anticipatory
Grieving, dysfunctional
Pain
Pain, chronic

Knowing: A Human Response Pattern Involving the Meaning Associated with Information

Knowledge deficit (specify)
Thought processes, altered

Moving: A Human Response Pattern Involving Activity

Activity intolerance
Activity intolerance, high risk for
Diversional activity deficit
Fatigue
Growth and development, altered
Home maintenance management, impaired
Mobility, impaired physical
Peripheral neurovascular dysfunction, high risk for
Self-care deficit, bathing/hygiene
Self-care deficit, dressing/grooming
Self-care deficit, feeding
Self-care deficit, toileting
Sleep pattern disturbance
Swallowing, impaired

Exchanging: A Human Response Pattern Involving Mutual Giving and Receiving

Airway clearance, ineffective
Aspiration, high risk for
Body temperature, altered, high risk for
Breathing pattern, ineffective
Cardiac output, decreased

Dysreflexia
Fluid volume deficit
Fluid volume deficit, high risk for
Fluid volume excess
Gas exchange, impaired
Hyperthermia
Hypothermia
Infection, high risk for
Injury, high risk for (specify) (electrical, physical, chemical hazards, positioning, retained foreign objects)
Nutrition, altered: less than body requirements
Nutrition, altered: more than body requirements
Nutrition, altered: high risk for more than body requirements
Oral mucous membrane, altered
Skin integrity, impaired
Skin integrity, impaired, high risk for
Tissue integrity, impaired
Tissue perfusion, altered (specify) (renal, cerebral, cardiopulmonary, gastrointestinal, peripheral)
Urinary retention
Ventilation, spontaneous, inability to sustain
Ventilatory weaning response, dysfunctional

Relating: A Human Response Pattern Involving the Establishing of Bonds

Caregiver role strain
Family processes, altered
Parental role conflict
Parenting, altered
Parenting, altered, high risk for
Role performance, altered
Sexual dysfunction
Sexuality patterns, altered
Social interaction, impaired
Social isolation

Valuing: A Human Response Pattern Involving the Assigning of Relative Worth

Spiritual distress (distress of the human spirit)

Choosing: A Human Response Pattern Involving the Selection of Alternatives

Adjustment, impaired
Coping, defensive
Coping, family: potential for growth
Coping, ineffective family: compromised
Coping, ineffective family: disabling
Coping, ineffective individual
Decisional conflict (specify)
Denial, ineffective
Health-seeking behaviors (specify)
Noncompliance (specify)
Therapeutic regimen (individual), ineffective management of

Modified from Seifert PC: Cardiac Surgery. In Rothrock JC: *Perioperative nursing care planning*, St Louis, 1990, Mosby; and from Kim MJ, McFarland GK, McLane AM: *Pocket guide to nursing diagnoses*, ed 5, St Louis, 1993, Mosby.

illness. Information should be elicited about changes in vision, hearing, movement, smelling, and tasting.

It should be determined how the patient or significant others perceive the effects of the illness and the proposed surgical intervention. The functional restrictions often imposed by cardiovascular disease can influence the individual's self perception. Self-esteem, body image, and personal identity may be affected. The inability to perform activities of daily living may lead to feelings of hopelessness and powerlessness with the realization that activities once taken for granted can no longer be accomplished. The perceived loss of control may be a source of frustration and anger in patients such as business executives who are used to making their own decisions.

Elderly patients may be accompanied by family members or other caretakers who should be included in the preoperative preparations. This also applies to children who may have separation anxiety and a fear of being abandoned by their parents. Parents and other members of the family may demonstrate feelings of inadequacy or guilt about the child's illness.

Feeling

The human response pattern of feeling relates to both physical and emotional feelings. Patients often have a history of pain. Pain may be chronic (e.g., angina pectoris), or acute and unrelieved (e.g., aortic dissection). Patients with ischemic heart disease may complain of chest pain with or without radiation to the neck, jaws, and arm(s); patients with valvular heart disease may complain of shortness of breath, syncope, fatigue, and anginal or upper abdominal pain. Postoperatively, pain and altered comfort are commonly related to the incision(s), positioning, and restrictions imposed by tubes, drains, and monitoring devices.

The nurse asks the patient about pain or discomfort, including the onset, duration, quality, location, radiation, associated symptoms, precipitating factors, and relieving factors of each symptom. Does the patient have palpitations or other cardiac rhythm disturbances? Objective manifestations of pain, such as guarding, and protective behaviors, such as moaning, crying, grimacing, or withdrawal, should be looked for. The patient's muscle tone or nervous system responses, such as changes in blood pressure, respiratory rate, pulse, and pupils, are evaluated. Diaphoresis, if present, is noted. The patient may complain of being cold. Patient complaints about any of these discomforts are significant because pain and the shivering that accompanies chilling elevate the metabolic rate and increase the workload of the heart.

Children may have unique words or expressions that denote pain and discomfort. Some children perceive themselves as feeling well. They should not be told that the surgery will make them feel better, because immediately postoperatively they will feel worse as a result of incisional pain, monitoring lines, and drainage tubes (Hazinski, 1992). They can be told that within a few days they will have less discomfort.

Emotional responses should be elicited as well. Fear and anxiety can affect both psychologic and physical well-being. Mental stress has been implicated in the development of myocardial ischemia (Rozanski, 1988). The nurse elicits the expression of fears and unspecified threats from the patient, answers questions, and communicates reassurance through body language and tone of voice. Specific questions about morbidity or mortality should be directed to surgeons or attending physicians.

Occasionally patients express extreme fear that they will die during surgery. The nurse should not tell the patient that this is an unfounded fear. Rather, the nurse should allow the patient to discuss the concern. The surgeon should be informed in order to discuss the fear with the patient; a consultation with psychiatric or social services may be requested. Although unusual, surgery has been cancelled when such a situation arises.

Knowing

The nurse may briefly assess what the patient (or family member) knows about the planned surgical intervention. Misconceptions may be uncovered that can be clarified, and expectations can be correlated to the planned interventions and outcomes. Patients are normally anxious, which may interfere with eliciting necessary information. Psychologic reactions to stress are often seen in the form of coping mechanisms such as denial or withdrawal. By alleviating fears and providing comfort measures, the nurse may be able to reduce the patient's overall anxiety and obtain a more accurate description of the patient's past experiences.

The level of consciousness and orientation to person, place, and time are assessed to determine the patient's ability to understand instructions and ask questions. Assessment of knowledge and learning needs may be complicated by the patient's unreadiness to learn or the lack of adequate time to complete the evaluation. If an abbreviated assessment must be performed, learning needs should be documented so that they can be met at a later date by another member of the cardiac team. Many hospitals have a nurse who performs preoperative patient teaching; specific details about the OR can be communicated by the perioperative nurse. Communicating with the patient also allows a relationship to develop between the perioperative nurse and the patient. Knowing one of the surgical team members may allay some of the patient's fears about the unknown and fearful OR environment.

The presence of risk factors for coronary artery disease (Table 6-5) and the patient's perception and level of knowledge about these risk factors can influence the long-term results of surgery. What the patient knows and how he or she has responded to illnesses and problems in the past can provide some indication of teaching needs and future adherence to prescribed therapeutic regimens.

Table 6-5 ■ *Risk factors for coronary artery disease*

Nonmodifiable	Modifiable
Age	Elevated serum cholesterol
Sex	Hypertension
Family history	Cigarette smoking
Race	Obesity
	Elevated serum lipids
	Diabetes mellitus
	Psychologic stress
	Personality type

Modified from Murdaugh CL: The person with coronary artery disease risk factors. In Guzzetta CE, Dossey BM: *Cardiovascular nursing: holistic practice*, St Louis, 1992, Mosby.

Information about recent medications and the patient's response to them may be elicited or reviewed in the chart. Among those of particular interest are cardiotonics, diuretics, myocardial depressants (such as antidysrhythmics, calcium channel blockers, and beta-adrenergic blockers), antibiotics, anticoagulants, immunosuppressants, antihypertensives, and corticosteroids. This information is pertinent during surgery because medications can have many effects. For example, they may alter coagulation, pose an increased risk of infection, signal the potential development of dysrhythmias, influence tissue healing, and produce toxicity, sensitivity, or allergic reaction.

Information pertinent to discharge planning may require an optimum teaching environment, which is difficult to create in the immediate preoperative period. This has become more of a challenge in the era of cost containment, when patients are admitted on the day of surgery. Patient teaching may need to be performed during the preoperative screening that generally occurs a few days before surgery. It may be done via telephone, or in some cases it can take place in the physician's office or in the patient's home. The Mended Hearts, Inc., a support group for patients who have had cardiac surgery, has had to modify its visiting program as a result of these changes, and their suggestions for patient teaching include those just described, as well as establishing day or evening teaching sessions at the hospital and developing a referral system with cardiologists and surgeons (Conley, 1992). When preoperative teaching cannot be performed, the perioperative nurse can communicate the need for education on life-style and risk factor modifications or prescribed postoperative therapeutic regimens to the nurses caring for the patient after surgery.

To prioritize teaching needs, the nurse should distinguish between what the patient knows, what the patient does not know, what the patient needs to know, and what the patient wants to know. Patients are often unaware of the technical details of a procedure, and many do not want vivid descriptions of sternal splitting, saphenous vein excision, or chest wiring. The nurse respects the patient's desire to remain ignorant of those details. Conversely, some individuals are able to cope by gaining extensive knowledge of a procedure. These patients have done their "homework" and inquire about cardiopulmonary bypass and the long-term patency of saphenous vein grafts versus internal mammary artery conduits. These patients can achieve a greater sense of control with knowledge about their condition and treatment plan.

Preoperatively patients need to have information that facilitates a positive experience. Patients will be less frightened and more cooperative (and release fewer endogenous catecholamines) if they are aware of the sequence of events that will take place immediately before anesthesia induction and surgery. The nurse can describe the transportation to the OR, explain the preinduction area and insertion of intravascular lines, and comment on what the patient will see, hear, and feel in the OR. The patient should be told how many people are in the room and what they do. Many patients are aware that a urinary drainage catheter is inserted, and they may ask when the catheter is inserted, if it hurts, and if they are awake when it is inserted.

Postoperatively family members may be reassured to know that they will be able to see, talk to, and touch the patient, even though the patient may be heavily sedated. They should be aware that the patient will appear pale and feel cool and clammy. They should also be prepared for the array of tubes, lines, and drains that are used to monitor the patient and provide access for medications and blood samples.

In some cases family members or significant others may not want to see the patient in the intensive care unit (ICU). They can be reassured that there is no correct or incorrect protocol for visiting. It may be too stressful for some individuals and will only increase their (and the patient's) anxiety (Seifert, 1990).

Patients appreciate forewarning about being intubated and unable to talk. Recovered patients often mention the frustration of being alert but unable to speak. The nurse can assure the patient that alternative methods of communication will be available in the ICU.

Moving

Cardiovascular disease can have an impact on the patient's ability to move, perform activities of daily living and self-care, sleep, and play. These alterations are often associated with symptoms of varying severity that affect the patient's functional status (see Box 6-1).

The nurse can investigate the presence and the effects of fatigue, pain, and dyspnea on sleep patterns and self-care regarding hygiene, grooming, feeding, and diversional activity. Impaired physical mobility, activity intolerance, and inability to manage a home are not uncommon in patients with a cardiac output that is insufficient to meet exercise-induced demands.

Children with severe congenital anomalies may demonstrate altered growth and development and feeding difficulties. Elderly patients frequently have joint problems that impair mobility. Postoperatively, patients will have some impairment of mobility due to pain, and to the effects of positioning and immobility of 3 to 4 hours or more during surgery.

Exchanging

The human response pattern of exchanging relates to the patient's physical condition and includes most of the physiologic diagnoses and collaborative problems commonly encountered during surgery. The exchanging pattern also reflects many of AORN's (1993) patient outcome standards that pertain to injury, skin integrity, fluid and electrolyte balance, infection, and physiologic responses to surgery. Data within this category take priority if the patient's condition is unstable and immediate surgical intervention is indicated. Many of the findings associated with the patient's physiologic status can be anticipated by reading the H & P in the chart. On occasion this may be the only way to obtain sufficient information about the patient.

During surgery and the first few hours postoperatively, assessment of the physiologic parameters enables the nurse to anticipate alterations in cardiovascular function and act on those changes to restore physiologic stability. In assessing the patient, the nurse should identify whether the patient's condition and the presenting signs and symptoms are acute or chronic (Weeks, 1986). In addition, the preoperative data should be distinguished from intraoperative and postoperative data so that the clinician can evaluate the significance of any changes or new events.

General appearance

Initial inspection of the patient should focus on the ABCs of basic life support: airway, breathing, and circulation. Is the patient intubated or wearing a nasal cannula for oxygen? Does the patient's facial expression (signs of apprehension and pain) or body posture (sitting upright or leaning forward) indicate dyspnea, shortness of breath, or labored breathing? Are the neck veins distended? Is chest expansion symmetric and rhythmic? Is there nasal flaring or use of accessory respiratory muscles? Is cyanosis present? The bluish discoloration of cyanosis reflects a decreased oxygen saturation of circulating hemoglobin and may be a result of right-to-left intracardiac shunting, impaired pulmonary function, or hypoxia from any cause. Clubbing of the nail beds (spongy or swollen nail bases with an angle of greater than 180 degrees between the nail and the nail base) is also associated with cyanosis and is a sign of chronic oxygen deficiency (Thelan, Davie, and Urden, 1990).

What is the color of the skin, lips, tongue, nail beds, conjunctiva, and mucous membranes: cyanotic, pale, dusky, or jaundiced? The color may be an indication of hypotension or low cardiac output, or of hepatic congestion related to right ventricular heart failure.

Skin integrity

It should be determined whether the patient has any allergies to medications, antimicrobial solutions, dressing tape, or other substances. The presence of rashes, abrasions, lacerations, bruises, petechiae, varicosities, nodules, or other lesions are noted, as well as signs of hydration, edema, elasticity, texture, turgor, mobility, and thickness. Does the skin feel cool or warm? Does the patient have a fever? Fever is significant because of the increased workload that it places on the heart.

Are there percutaneous intravascular lines? Are they patent? Is there swelling, redness, or pain at the insertion site? Are there stomas or drains that should be covered during surgery?

Past surgical incision sites should be looked for. Is there a bulge in the abdomen or chest indicating the presence of a pacemaker or internal defibrillator? Is there evidence of greater saphenous vein stripping or removal from previous surgery that will require the use of alternative conduits in the patient scheduled for coronary bypass grafting? Patients who have undergone a previous median sternotomy will have mediastinal adhesions that obscure anatomic landmarks; these adhesions must be cautiously dissected to avoid injury to the right ventricle or major blood vessels. Adhesions are less of a problem in patients with previous lateral thoracotomies who are scheduled for a procedure using a median sternotomy incision. These can include adults who have previously undergone closed mitral commissurotomy via a lateral incision or children who have received palliative shunts through a thoracotomy prior to median sternotomy for repair of the congenital defect.

The skin over dependent areas of the body, such as the heels, buttocks, sacrum, back, and occipital area of the head, is assessed, and any existing marks, lesions, or areas of breakdown are noted. Elderly or very young patients may be at increased risk for skin breakdown because their skin is less sturdy than the integumentary system of adults. Additional padding may be indicated for surgery that may last 3 or 4 hours or more. The site(s) where the dispersive pad(s) is (are) to be applied should be checked. Dispersive pads are generally applied to the buttocks, thereby avoiding bony prominences and the sacrum.

Respiratory status

It should be determined whether the patient has had anything to eat prior to the scheduled surgery; food or fluid in the stomach is an anesthetic risk for aspiration. The patient's respiratory rate, rhythm, and depth, as well as chest wall expansion and symmetry with respiration, are noted. Normally, the adult breathes 16 to 20 times per minute; children under 1 year of age may have rates of up to 40 breaths per minute. Is the depth of breathing shallow, moderate, or deep? Neonates are obligatory nose breathers. Children are normally diaphragmatic muscle breathers; anything that compromises air flow or the movement of the diaphragm can be a source of rapid respiratory failure and lead to cardiac dysrhythmias and arrest (Joy, 1990).

Does the patient complain of dyspnea, and is it a

chronic problem or sudden in onset? Labored breathing accompanies a number of cardiac conditions; it often occurs with exertion and may be affected by position. When it occurs at rest, it is almost certainly a manifestation of congestive heart failure.

Paroxysmal nocturnal dyspnea occurs at night, with the patient awakening with a frightening sense of suffocation. Patients with orthopnea have difficulty breathing when lying flat and may require two or more pillows for sufficient elevation to be able to sleep. These patients may become extremely anxious in the OR if left in the supine position without the head elevated. They should be offered pillows, or the bed can be elevated to facilitate breathing.

If the patient has a cough, is it productive or nonproductive? Is it weak or strong? The color, amount, odor, and consistency of the sputum are noted. Coughing up of blood may be a sign of pulmonary edema or acute pulmonary embolus. A history of tuberculosis is also noted.

The nurse listens to breath sounds and notes if they are diminished or if abnormal sounds such as crackles are heard. Rales occur when air passes through bronchi that contain fluid of any kind, and they may be found in patients who are fluid overloaded, who have mitral stenosis, or who are in left ventricular failure with pulmonary edema.

The patient's arterial blood gasses (Table 6-4) are evaluated for the level of oxygen and carbon dioxide, and the acid-base balance of the arterial blood. The method of oxygen delivery (i.e., endotracheal tube or nasal cannula) is noted, as well as the percentage of oxygen delivered and the flow rate or setting. Pulse oximetry monitors may be attached to the foot, finger, earlobe, or nose by a finger clip or by an adhesive to measure arterial blood oxygen saturation (SaO_2). Transcutaneous patches may be applied to very young patients to measure oxygen and carbon dioxide levels.

Pulmonary function testing may be ordered for patients at risk for postoperative acute respiratory failure, such as those with mitral or aortic valve disease.

Cardiovascular status

In addition to dyspnea, common symptoms of heart disease are chest pain, palpitations, syncope, and fatigue. Their severity will affect the functional capacity of the patient (see Box 6-1). In addition to these symptoms, children may demonstrate feeding difficulties, lack of weight gain, frequent respiratory infections, or irritability.

Pain. The most common cause of chest pain in the cardiac surgery patient is myocardial ischemia, which is generally described as an uncomfortable sensation of pressure, tightness, or squeezing. It may be dull or aching rather than sharp or spasmodic. The pain may radiate to the throat, jaw, shoulders, arms, abdomen, or back, but it almost always also involves the sternal region (Massie and Sokolow, 1991). The discomfort associated with myocardial ischemia, angina pectoris, is commonly triggered by exertion, strong emotion,

eating a large meal, or exposure to cold. It usually subsides with the administration of nitroglycerin and cessation of exertional activity. Acute onset of chest pain should be reported immediately to the surgeon and/or anesthesiologist for treatment.

The pain accompanying myocardial infarction is more severe and prolonged and is unrelieved by rest or medications. Some patients have variant (Prinzmetal) angina—by definition, pain that occurs at rest. These patients may have evidence of coronary artery spasm with or without fixed coronary artery obstruction (Magilligan and Ullyot, 1991).

Ischemic pain may accompany hypertrophy of either ventricle or aortic valve disease. Pain may also be produced by pulmonary hypertension, pericarditis, myocarditis, and mitral valve prolapse. Aortic dissection produces tearing or stabbing pain of great intensity that often radiates to the back.

Palpitations. Patients may complain of palpitations or an awareness of the heartbeat. This may or may not be hemodynamically significant.

Premature ventricular contractions may be felt as missed beats, and ventricular tachycardia may be sensed as fluttering. Atrial fibrillation is often seen in patients with valvular disease (and postoperatively in patients who have undergone coronary artery bypass surgery). These findings are significant when there is a decline in left ventricular filling and cardiac output that leads to reduced perfusion of the brain. This can produce momentary dizziness, blurring of vision, or loss of consciousness (syncope), especially when the patient is in the upright position. Syncope may also occur in patients with aortic valve stenosis or hypertrophic obstructive cardiomyopathy and is usually exertional or postexertional.

Fatigue. Fatigue is common in patients with cardiovascular disease, but it is nonspecific (Braunwald, 1992). The patient may complain of muscle weakness as a consequence of reduced cardiac output. Or the fatigue may be a result of diuresis, excessive blood pressure reduction in hypertensive patients, or the use of beta-adrenergic blocking agents.

Edema. Edema may be present in the lower extremities in ambulatory patients or in the dependent parts of the body in patients on bed rest (i.e., the back and sacral regions). It is characteristic of bilateral chronic venous insufficiency (which may be significant if the saphenous vein is to be used as a conduit in coronary artery bypass surgery) or heart failure. When edema is cardiac in origin, fluid collection results from elevated right atrial pressure secondary to right ventricular failure, left ventricular failure, or pulmonary hypertension.

Blood pressure. Systemic blood pressures in the arms and legs are checked bilaterally and noted to be equal or unequal, high, normal or low. Hypertension can produce a chronically increased afterload, which predisposes the heart to develop left ventricular hypertrophy.

Unequal pressures in the arms may be a contraindication to the use of the internal mammary artery as

Table 6-6 ■ *Physiologic features of the very young and the very old (compared with young or middle-aged adults)*

	Very young	Very old
Cardiovascular		
Myocardium	Less contractile tissue Less compliant CO increased by faster heart rate	Increased subendocardial fat Increased heart weight Reduced resting CO
Valves	Less tension created by papillary muscle	Fibrous thickening, calcification of leaflets and annulus
Coronary arteries	Anomalies of coronary arteries	Coronary arteriosclerosis, atherosclerosis; tortuous epicardial arteries
Conduction system	Impulse conduction faster	Impulse conduction slower
Blood volume	Total circulating amount small; volume per kilogram of body weight relatively greater	Reduced plasma volume Reduced blood water content
Respiratory	Inadequate cough reflex Increased chest wall compliance, decreased pulmonary compliance Higher oxygen consumption Short, narrow airway obstructed easily	Decreased ability to eliminate secretions Increased chest wall rigidity, decreased lung compliance Reduced vital capacity, maximum ventilation volume
Renal	Glomeruli small and immature Tubular concentration of fluids and electrolytes diminished Unable to excrete increased amount of electrolytes and hydrogen ions (acids)	Fewer functional glomeruli Reduced renal blood flow and glomerular filtration rate Impaired ability to excrete increased amount of water and electrolytes; reduced ability to excrete hydrogen ions.
Other		
Temperature control	Immature regulating system; rapid heat loss	Decreased control
Metabolic rate	Higher	Lower
Stress response	Decreased phagocytic capability of leukocytes Immature immunoglobulin synthesis	Limited capability to retain homeostasis Decreased adrenal activity

Modified from Fairman R, Rombeau JL: Physiologic problems in the elderly surgical patient. In Miller TA, editor: *The physiologic basis of modern surgical care*, St Louis, 1988, Mosby; and Hazinski MF: *Nursing care of the critically ill child*, ed 2, St Louis, 1992, Mosby.
CO, Cardiac output.

a bypass graft, because the perfusion pressure could be suboptimal. Patients with coarctation of the aorta may demonstrate higher blood pressures in the upper extremity as compared with the lower extremity, and patients with aortic dissections may have unequal bilateral carotid, femoral, brachial, or radial artery blood pressures when the dissection occludes one or more of these vascular branches. Physiologic differences between the very young and the elderly should be integrated into the assessment when appropriate (Table 6-6). The patient may have a radial artery pressure line. Preoperatively the nurse can palpate the carotid pulse for comparison and correlate the readings to the arterial waveform displayed. Intraoperatively the femoral pulse can be palpated to compare central pressures with peripheral (radial) pressures.

Pulses. Carotid, femoral, brachial, radial, ulnar, popliteal, dorsalis pedis, and posterior tibial pulses may be palpated preoperatively to determine a base-line for future comparison. This information is especially important to nurses caring for patients in the postoperative period who have had the femoral artery cannulated for cardiopulmonary bypass or the insertion of an intraaortic balloon.

It should be noted whether the pulses are symmetric, regular or irregular, bounding or thready, and fast or slow. The following values should be assigned:

Absent	0
Thready	1+
Diminished	2+
Normal	3+
Bounding	4+

Heart sounds. Heart sounds are auscultated and correlated with other data. The first heart sound (S_1) is associated with changes in flow related to the closing of the mitral and tricuspid valves at the beginning of ventricular systole and is almost simultaneous with the carotid impulse and QRS complex of the ECG. The second heart sound (S_2) reflects changing flow patterns associated with the closure of the aortic and pulmonic valves at the beginning of ventricular diastole. Both S_1 and S_2 are normal sounds.

The presence of a third heart sound (S_3), creating a "gallop" rhythm, is abnormal in adults and is related to the filling of a distended or noncompliant ventricle. A fourth heart sound (S_4) reflects the vibrations of the ventricular wall with the influx of blood from atrial contraction. A distinctly audible S_4 is considered abnormal (Braunwald, 1992).

Bruits and murmurs. Are there bruits (turbulent blood flow around obstructions) in the carotid or femoral arteries or in the abdominal aorta that could be a sign of vascular disease? Significant carotid stenosis increases the risk of stroke in patients undergoing cardiac surgery; this increased risk is a result of the brief periods of hypotension that are necessary during cardiac operations (for instance, when flow is momentarily decreased to allow the aortic cross-clamp to be applied without excessive tension on the vessel). Carotid endarterectomy may be performed before or concurrently with the cardiac procedure in patients with significant, symptomatic carotid disease.

Murmurs are sounds produced by turbulent blood flow into a cardiac chamber or through a heart valve. They are classified as systolic, diastolic, or continuous. They are further described according to their location, radiation, intensity, configuration, duration, and quality. Patients with valvular stenosis, regurgitation, or a combination of the two commonly have murmurs, as do patients with some intracardiac shunts. Other sounds that may be heard with a stethoscope include pericardial and pleural friction rubs. These are signs of inflammation and produce characteristic leathery or scratchy sounds, respectively.

Patients may also have thrills, vibratory sensations felt over the location of the ascending aorta in patients with aortic stenosis. The narrowed valve orifice produces a jet of squirting blood against the aortic wall, which can be palpated.

Cardiac rhythm. Assessment of the cardiac rhythm enables the nurse to evaluate the baseline rhythm, obtain information about myocardial oxygen supply and demand, and use the information as an indication of myocardial ischemia, injury, or infarction. Coronary artery disease, ventricular hypertrophy, drug toxicity, and electrolyte imbalances are among the conditions that may produce changes in rhythm, although these conditions are not always reflected on the ECG.

Many of the dysrhythmias have a deleterious effect on the oxygen supply/demand balance, because they produce inefficient contractions. For instance, ventricular tachydysrhythmias shorten the diastolic period during which the ventricles fill and most myocardial blood flow occurs; if this rhythm persists, cardiac output and myocardial perfusion are jeopardized, and the heart is at increased risk for ventricular fibrillation. In atrial fibrillation atrial activity is disorganized and ineffective. With the loss of atrial contractions the atrial contribution to diastolic ventricular filling is absent, eventually resulting in a reduction of stroke volume.

Alterations in the heart rate include tachydysrhythmias (100 to 160 beats per minute) and bradydysrhythmias (40 to 60 beats per minute). The origin of the dysrhythmia—the atrium, the atrioventricular junction, or the ventricle—is noted. It should be determined whether alterations are new in onset, and the patient's ability to tolerate the dysrhythmia is assessed.

Is there atrioventricular heart block (indicating damage to the conduction tissue from ischemia, infarction, drug effects, or other causes)? Are the ST segments elevated (see Fig. 6-2) or depressed (which can indicate myocardial ischemia)? Other signs and symptoms associated with dysrhythmias include low urinary output, dizziness, transient ischemic attacks, hypotension, weakness, and confusion.

Hemodynamic data. The patient's systemic blood pressure and cardiac output (normal for adults is 5 L/min) are noted. Large patients may have higher outputs. To determine if the cardiac output is appropriate for the body size, the cardiac index is noted, which is derived by dividing the cardiac output by the body surface area (normal for adults ranges from 2.5 to 4.0 L/min/m^2).

The central venous pressure and the pulmonary artery systolic, diastolic, and wedge pressures are assessed (see Table 6-3). These values provide information about right and left ventricular function and volume status, and can alert the nurse to changes in cardiac status before clinical signs of failure become apparent.

Peripheral vascular status

It should be determined whether previous vein harvests, vein stripping, or varicosities will preclude the use of saphenous vein as a bypass conduit. Atherosclerotic aortoiliac disease may create problems if femoral access is required for blood pressure monitoring or insertion of an intraaortic balloon. It should also be noted if abdominal aortic or lower-extremity arterial bypass graft surgery has been performed, since this could also preclude the insertion of invasive catheters. When blood pressure monitoring lines are inserted into the radial artery, the nurse should be aware that ulnar artery patency is necessary to prevent ischemic injury to the hand. This can be ascertained by performing Allen's test (Box 6-3).

Neurologic status

The patient's level of consciousness and orientation to person, place, and time are assessed. Pupillary size, shape, and equality are noted. Is the reaction to light brisk, sluggish, or nonreactive? The patient is assessed preoperatively for signs of confusion, restlessness, slurred speech, weakness, numbness, or paralysis that could signal impaired perfusion, abnormal blood glucose concentrations in diabetic patients, or the effects

---

Box 6-3 Allen's test

Allen's test is performed to determine the adequacy of collateral (ulnar) blood flow to the hand when the radial artery is cannulated for blood pressure monitoring.

1. Elevate the patient's arm above the heart.
2. Press one thumb on the patient's radial artery and the other thumb on the ulnar artery while the patient clenches the fist (this squeezes the blood from the palm and fingers).
3. Release pressure on the ulnar artery while maintaining pressure on the radial artery.
4. If the blood returns rapidly (within 3 to 5 seconds) to the palm and fingers when the patient opens the hand, ulnar patency is present.
5. To determine the patency of the radial artery, repeat the test and release the radial artery.

Modified from Daily EK: Hemodynamic monitoring. In Guzzetta CE, Dossey BM: *Cardiovascular nursing: holistic practice*, St Louis, 1992, Mosby.

---

of preoperative medications. The perioperative nurse should report changes in neurologic function to the surgical intensive care nurses, who will want to compare preoperative and postoperative findings.

The presence of carotid disease (history of transient ischemic attacks or stroke, documented diagnostic findings) is noted. Impaired cerebral perfusion increases morbidity and mortality in the cardiac surgery patient. Inducing hypotension during surgery (e.g., lowering bypass flow rates to reduce bleeding at a coronary anastomotic site) is especially risky in patients with obstructions within one or both carotid arteries.

Urinary/renal status

Has the patient had problems urinating that may suggest a urinary tract infection or some form of obstruction? In male patients with a history of benign prostatic hypertrophy or prostate surgery, residual scar tissue could make urinary catheterization difficult and require the use of sounds to dilate the urethra. In both males and females, if urethral narrowing is severe, insertion of a suprapubic catheter may be necessary.

The kidneys are acutely sensitive to cardiac output. The results of urine studies, including the amount, color, clarity, and odor, are noted, and laboratory data are reviewed for creatinine level, blood urea nitrogen (BUN), and specific gravity to assess kidney function (see Table 6-4). During surgery, urinary output is monitored continuously and calculated at least every 30 minutes. Urinary output measurements before, during, and after cardiopulmonary bypass are documented for comparison and to reflect kidney perfusion and function.

Patients with chronic renal failure who require hemodialysis must be managed perioperatively with consideration given to their altered excretory function. A dialysis catheter may be inserted in the OR for later use. Cardiac medications, anesthetic agents, and muscle relaxants that are excreted through the kidneys should be avoided when possible or used cautiously and monitored closely. Also, the danger of sepsis is high in patients with renal failure (Legler, 1987), and additional precautions may be warranted in perioperative management. Renal failure hampers calcium excretion, resulting in increased serum calcium levels; this may be a contraindication to the use of bioprostheses because of the accelerated calcification of the prosthesis in these patients.

Acute renal failure may be related to a decrease in circulating blood volume, hypotension, and/or the effects of cardiopulmonary bypass. In the absence of underlying renal disease, acute renal failure generally is reversible if it is diagnosed and treated quickly.

Nutritional status

The patient's nutritional status is assessed to determine increased risk for skin breakdown, infection, or poor healing. Patients who are obese or very thin may be at risk. Patients with cardiac cachexia have muscle wasting and a marked reduction in tissue mass, as well as a negative nitrogen balance, resulting from reduced caloric intake and increased caloric expenditure.

Ears, eyes, nose, mouth, and throat

It should be determined whether the patient has difficulty hearing, seeing, smelling, tasting, or swallowing. Tracheobronchial problems may make intubation difficult. Patients may require the use of their eyeglasses or hearing aids in the immediate preoperative period, but these and other removable prostheses (such as dentures) should be removed and given to a family member or placed in a safe location prior to surgery.

Patients with colds, as well as those with loose or carious teeth, have a higher risk of infection. Surgery may be cancelled and rescheduled at a later date once these problems are corrected.

Gastrointestinal system

Laboratory results from liver function tests, if performed, are noted, as well as serum albumin levels, which, if reduced, may indicate a protein deficit that can affect wound healing and the maintenance of vascular oncotic pressure. Low gamma globulin levels may also pose an increased risk of infection for the patient.

It should be determined whether there is a history of stomach or duodenal ulcers, gastrointestinal bleeding, or other bleeding tendencies, which could be a concern perioperatively. A bleeding history is usually a contraindication to mechanical heart valves that require chronic anticoagulation postoperatively.

Bowel preparation may or may not be ordered prior to surgery. If stool is present, rectal temperature probes will not accurately reflect core body temperature. Esophageal and bladder temperature probes can obviate this problem.

Endocrine system

The endocrine system affects the chemical and energy activities associated with metabolism. The function of the thyroid, pancreatic, adrenal, pituitary, and other hormone-producing glands affects aerobic and anaerobic energy production, which is vital to cardiac function. If these disorders are present, the most recent laboratory results are checked and abnormal findings reported.

Cardiopulmonary bypass induces hyperglycemia, which in diabetic patients will require adjusting insulin dosages. NPH (Neutral Protamine Hagedorn) insulin–dependent patients may also demonstrate a reaction to the protamine sulfate infusion for reversal of heparin and should be monitored closely for swelling, redness, hives or blisters, and other skin changes that may signal anaphylaxis.

Relating

The relating pattern is assessed to determine how the patient relates to others in terms of role performance, and sexual and social relationships. The marital status of the patient is determined, as well as the presence of a spouse, children, extended family, and friends. If these individuals will be present for the surgery, it should be noted where they will be waiting, and information should be provided about the time frame for surgery and plans for perioperative communication. If surgery has been delayed, family members will appreciate being told so that they can anticipate a longer wait (and not automatically assume that the delay is due to intraoperative problems).

Also included in this pattern is the establishment and maintenance of bonds that are frequently affected by heart disease and the profound physical and psychologic effect it has. The heart is associated with love and other emotions; the physical consequences of cardiovascular disease affect the patient's ability to maintain personal, professional, and societal roles. Pain and fatigue, two common symptoms, make interpersonal relationships and the performance of familial roles more difficult. Sexual dysfunction may also be attributed to discomfort, fatigue, or the fear of recurring anginal attacks, or it may be the result of poor perfusion.

Valuing

When companionship is denied or compromised by debilitating symptoms, patients may be in spiritual distress. Their religious preference should be determined, as well as whether they desire to have access to a spiritual counselor. Not infrequently, patients have a heightened fear of death before surgery, and religious services or articles may provide comfort. An attempt should be made to elicit whether any treatments are prohibited by the religion. Jehovah's Witnesses' refusal of blood transfusions should be communicated to the surgeon, anesthesiologist, and other appropriate personnel. The nurse needs to check that the necessary documentation forms are available and signed.

The valuing category also refers to cultural orientation. The nurse identifies the patient's cultural background or heritage and practices, including how the culture defines responses to pain, enactment of the sick role, and the behavior of the family with regard to the illness.

Choosing

Choosing relates to the patient's coping abilities, judgment, participation, and wellness behavior. Both the patient's and the family's ability to cope with and adjust to the health problem are assessed. Difficulties may be experienced by both patients and families as the disease progresses and its impact is increasingly felt. Responses such as denial, disbelief, anger, regression, lack of cooperation, or acceptance may be evident.

The assessment should include an evaluation of the patient's willingness to comply with past and proposed future therapeutic regimens, which may necessitate life-style changes. Is the patient aware of the implications of the insertion of a mechanical heart valve (which requires chronic anticoagulation)? Will the family understand and support life-style changes related to diet, medication, exercise, and follow-up laboratory tests? Patients demonstrating a willingness to make life-style changes can be expected to have a successful recuperative and rehabilitative course, and to be open to teaching by clinicians. Difficulty in following prescribed behaviors may point to a diagnosis of noncompliance, but the nurse should investigate whether failure to adhere to recommendations is purposeful or a result of inadequate knowledge and support.

Ideally, preparation for home care begins on the patient's admission. The perioperative nurse can reinforce, review, clarify, and add to information and instructions the patient and significant others need to have in order to plan for discharge. Misconceptions should be clarified and questions answered.

CONCLUSION

The extensive array of diagnostic and laboratory tests enables the clinician to identify anatomic and functional disorders of the heart with greater precision. Interviews with patients and professional colleagues produce additional data, and ongoing monitoring systems provide a continuous source of information that must be interpreted and integrated into the clinical picture.

The perioperative nurse must be selective in assessing this information during the perioperative period (see Box 6-4 for some critical preoperative as-

Box 6-4   *Preoperative assessment "pearls"*

Anne P. Weiland, RN, MSN, ANP
Washington Hospital Center
Washington, D.C.

Always look at the chest x-ray [film] specifically for signs of cancer or other intrathoracic problems that may require modification of the operative plan or preclude it altogether.

Make sure that coagulation status is known. Even if technically abnormal lab values are accepted, know *why* they are abnormal, so that if the patient bleeds excessively, this problem can be treated appropriately and promptly.

Note the preoperative hematocrit and creatinine. These values, even if technically abnormal, provide a baseline for the intraoperative and postoperative periods.

Make sure that the potassium (K^+) level is 4.0 or close to that value to avoid problems during induction.

Look for occult peripheral and cerebrovascular disease, especially carotid artery and abdominal aorta disease, since these conditions threaten morbidity and mortality. Know the vascular history, particularly any previous vein harvests or strippings, and potential problems with large-vessel (femoral) access.

Know the preoperative cardiac medicines, especially antiarrhythmics; if the patient's heart becomes irritable, it will be important to know which drug works best and most promptly.

sessment factors) and focus on the most pertinent actual or potential problems that exist. When there are changes in the patient's status, either gradual or sudden and life-threatening, priorities are adjusted, diagnoses modified, and plans altered accordingly.

REFERENCES

American Nurses' Association and American Heart Association Council on Cardiovascular Nursing: *Standards of cardiovascular nursing practice*, Kansas City, MO, 1981, ANA.

Association of Operating Room Nurses: *Standards and recommended practices for perioperative nursing*, Denver, 1993, AORN.

Braunwald E: The history: the physical examination. In Braunwald E, editor: *Heart disease*, ed 4, Philadelphia, 1992, WB Saunders.

Bridges ND and others: Preoperative transcatheter closure of congenital muscular ventricular septal defects, *N Engl J Med* 324(19):1312, 1991.

Carpenito LJ: *Nursing diagnosis: application to clinical practice*, ed 5, Philadelphia, 1993, JB Lippincott.

Christiansen JL, Strong WB: Exercise testing. In Adams FH, Emmanouilides GC, Riemenschneider TA, editors: *Heart disease in infants, children, and adolescents*, ed 4, Baltimore, 1989, Williams & Wilkins.

Conley JE: President's message, *Heart Beat* 41(4):2, 1992.

Dilsizian V and others: Enhanced detection of ischemic, but viable myocardium by the reinjection of thallium after stress-redistribution imaging, *N Engl J Med* 323(3):141, 1990.

Driscoll DJ: Evaluation of the cyanotic newborn, *Pediatr Clin North Am* 37(1):1, 1990.

Fahey VA, Riegel BJ: Advances in diagnostic testing for vascular disease, *Cardiovasc Nurs* 25(3):13, 1989.

Freed MD: Invasive diagnostic and therapeutic techniques. 1. Cardiac catheterization. In Adams FH, Emmanouilides GC, Riemenschneider TA, editors: *Heart disease in infants, children, and adolescents*, ed 4, Baltimore, 1989, Williams & Wilkins.

Friedman WF: Congenital heart disease in infancy and childhood. In Braunwald E, editor: *Heart disease*, ed 4, Philadelphia, 1992, WB Saunders.

Good LP, Gentzler RD: Coronary atherectomy: an alternative to balloon angioplasty, *AORN J* 53(1):32, 1991.

Gordon M: *Nursing diagnosis: process and application*, ed 3, St. Louis, 1994, Mosby.

Graebner GM and others: Creatine kinase and lactate dehydrogenase in the muscles encountered during median sternotomy and in the myocardium of the cardiac chambers, *J Thorac Cardiovasc Surg* 89:700, 1985.

Guzzetta CE and others: *Clinical assessment tools for use with nursing diagnosis*, St Louis, 1989, Mosby.

Guzzetta CE, Dossey BM: *Cardiovascular nursing: holistic practice*, St Louis, 1992, Mosby.

Guzzetta CE, Seifert PC: Cardiovascular assessment. In Kinney MR and others: *Comprehensive cardiac care*, ed 7, St Louis, 1991, Mosby.

Hazinski MF: *Nursing care of the critically ill child*, St Louis, 1992, Mosby.

Joy C: Pediatric surgery. In Rothrock JC: *Perioperative nursing care planning*, St Louis, 1990, Mosby.

Kern MJ, editor: *The cardiac catheterization handbook*, St Louis, 1991, Mosby.

Kernicki J, Bullock BL, Register JM: *Cardiovascular nursing: rationale for therapy and nursing approach*, New York, 1970, GP Putnam's Sons.

Lavie CJ, Ventura HO, Murgo JP: Assessment of stable ischemic heart disease, *Postgrad Med* 89(1):45, 1991.

Legler DC: Uncommon diseases and cardiac anesthesia. In Kaplan JA, editor: *Cardiac anesthesia*, ed 2, vol 2, Philadelphia, 1987, WB Saunders.

Magilligan DJ, Ullyot DJ: The heart. I. Acquired disease. In Way LW, editor: *Current surgical diagnosis and treatment*, ed 9, Norwalk, Conn, 1991, Appleton & Lange.

Massie BM, Sokolow M: Heart and great vessels. In Schroeder SA and others, editors: *Current medical diagnosis and treatment*, Norwalk, Conn, 1991, Appleton & Lange.

Meyer RA: Echocardiography. In Adams FH, Emmanouilides GC, Riemenschneider TA, editors: *Heart disease in infants, children, and adolescents*, ed 4, Baltimore, 1989, Williams & Wilkins.

Miller JI: Therapeutic thoracoscopy: new horizons for an established procedure, *Ann Thorac Surg* 52:1036, 1991.

NIH (National Institutes of Health), Office of Medical Applications of Research: Perioperative red cell transfusion, *JAMA* 260(18):2700, 1988.

North American Nursing Diagnosis Association: Twenty-one new nursing diagnoses and a taxonomy, *Am J Nurs* 86:1414, 1986.

Pagana KD, Pagana TJ: *Diagnostic testing and nursing implications*, St Louis, 1990, Mosby.

Page RD, Jeffrey RR, Donnelly RJ: Thoracoscopy: a review of 121 consecutive surgical procedures, *Ann Thorac Surg* 48:66, 1989.

Patterson RE, Horowitz SF: Importance of epidemiology and biostatistics in deciding clinical strategies for using diagnostic tests: a simplified approach using examples from coronary artery disease, *J Am Coll Cardiol* 13(7):1653, 1989.

Popp RL: Echocardiography, part 1, *N Engl J Med* 323(2):101, 1990a.

Popp RL: Echocardiography, part 2, *N Engl J Med* 13(3): 165, 1990b.

Radtke W, Lock J: Balloon dilatation, *Pediatr Clin North Am* 37(1):193, 1990.

Roy C: Framework for classification systems development: progress and issues. In Kim MJ, McFarland GK, McLane AM, editors: *Classification of nursing diagnoses: proceedings of the fifth conference,* St Louis, 1984, Mosby.

Rozanski A and others: Mental stress and the induction of silent myocardial ischemia in patients with coronary artery disease, *N Engl J Med* 318:1005, 1988.

Seifert PC: Cardiac surgery. In Rothrock JC: *Perioperative nursing care planning,* St Louis, 1990, Mosby.

Spencer FC: Congenital heart disease. In Schwartz SI, editor: *Principles of surgery,* ed 5, New York, 1989, McGraw-Hill.

Sutherland L: Patient assessment: diagnostic studies. In Kinney MR and others: *Comprehensive cardiac care,* St Louis, 1991, Mosby.

Taubman MR: Advances in diagnostic testing. In Wingate S, editor: *Cardiac nursing: a clinical management and patient care resource,* Gaithersburg, Md, 1991, Aspen.

Teplitz L: Surgical treatment of ventricular arrhythmias: historical and current perspectives, *Crit Care Nurs Q* 14(2):41, 1991.

Thelan LA, Davie JK, Urden LD: *Textbook of critical care nursing: diagnosis and management,* St Louis, 1990, Mosby.

Walker WE: Acquired cardiac disorders. In Miller TA: *Physiologic basis of modern surgical care,* St Louis, 1988, Mosby.

Weeks LC: Initial nursing assessment and management of the critically ill cardiovascular patient. In Weeks LC, editor: *Advanced cardiovascular nursing,* Boston, 1986, Blackwell Scientific Publications.

Zeevi B and others: Interventional cardiac procedures in neonates and infants: state of the art, *Clin Perinatol* 15(3):633, 1988.

SUGGESTED READINGS

Canobbio MM: *Cardiovascular disorders,* St. Louis, 1990, Mosby.

Dellasega C, Rothrock JC: The aging patient. In Rothrock JC: *Perioperative nursing care planning,* St Louis, 1990, Mosby.

Underhill SL and others: *Cardiac nursing,* ed 2, Philadelphia, 1989, JB Lippincott.

7

Nursing Diagnoses

The idea of nursing diagnosis broke the link between information collection and care planning. Clinical judgment was inserted as a recognized responsibility.

Marjory Gordon, RN, 1982 (p. 1)

Quality patient care is the degree to which patient care services increase the probability of desired patient outcomes and reduce the probability of undesired outcomes, given the current state of knowledge.

Joint Commission on the Accreditation of Healthcare Organizations, 1989 (p. 1)

Review and analysis of the assessment data results in the identification of patient problems, needs, and health status. Many of these problems are related to medical diagnoses, necessitating physician-prescribed orders and collaborative interventions (Carpenito, 1993). Collaborative problems (potential complications), as well as nursing diagnoses, require judgment and critical thinking by the nurse. Nursing considerations can be found in subsequent chapters that discuss specific cardiac disorders.

Nursing diagnoses (see Box 6-2) reflect judgments about the patient's responses to health problems that are amenable to nursing interventions. These problems may already exist, or the patient may be at high risk for these problems to develop. For instance, most patients demonstrate some anxiety, which can be modified with nursing interventions. Most patients do not have an infection as their presenting problem, but because of the risk of contamination and the high mortality associated with infection, the diagnosis of "high risk for infection" is commonly made so that nursing actions aimed at reducing the risk are integrated into the plan of care.

Problems must be resolved and undesirable outcomes avoided. This is achieved by identifying expected outcomes that reflect the unique physical and psychosocial needs of patients. When possible, outcomes should be formulated with the patient, significant others, and health care providers. Nationally recognized standards of patient care are reflected in the patient outcomes identified by the Association of Operating Room Nurses (AORN) (1993), listed in Box 7-1.

Validation by the patient of the diagnoses selected and the outcomes desired provides the necessary information to select an appropriate plan of care and facilitates a positive surgical experience. Patient and nurse goals that are congruent are more likely to be achieved; the patient with contradictory goals will probably perceive the care received to be substandard and unsatisfactory (Seifert and Grandusky, 1990).

Congruence between the expected outcomes and the patient's present and potential physical capabilities and behavioral patterns is also important for establishing realistic expectations of the disease and the consequences of treatment (AORN, 1993). Outcomes research (Agency for Health Care Policy and Research [AHCPR]; Joint Commission on the Accreditation of Healthcare Organizations [JCAHO], 1989; Rothrock, 1990) has further delineated factors that must be considered. These include "patient-based factors" (the severity of the illness or co-morbid conditions), "practitioner-based factors" (professional competence), and "organization-based factors" (availability of material resources). Distinguishing between these factors promotes monitoring and more precise measurement of quality improvement efforts. It also highlights the interdependent nature of health care activities.

HUMAN RESPONSE PATTERNS AND ASSOCIATED DIAGNOSES

The profound impact of cardiovascular disease on the physical and emotional integrity of the patient suggests a number of nursing diagnoses (Seifert, 1990). Identification of problems is facilitated by a holistic assessment based on the human response patterns (described in Chapter 6) developed by the North American Nursing Diagnosis Association (NANDA) (1986; Guzzetta and Seifert, 1991). When assessing the patient, the nurse clusters the signs and symptoms to determine whether the diagnosis within that pattern is applicable.

Box 7-1   *Patient outcome standards for perioperative nursing*

Standard 1

The patient demonstrates knowledge of the physiologic and psychologic responses to surgical intervention.

Standard 2

The patient is free from infection.

Standard 3

The patient's skin integrity is maintained.

Standard 4

The patient is free from injury related to positioning, extraneous objects, or chemical, physical, and electrical hazards.

Standard 5

The patient's fluid and electrolyte balance is maintained.

Standard 6

The patient participates in the rehabilitation process.

From Association of Operating Room Nurses: Patient outcome standards for perioperative nursing. In *Standards and recommended practices for perioperative nursing,* Denver, 1993, AORN.

Communicating

The communicating pattern of human responses includes **impaired verbal communication** and may be related to the inability to speak or understand the dominant language. The etiology may also be cardiovascular insufficiency, sedation, dyspnea, reduced level of consciousness, or physical barriers such as endotracheal tubes.

Perceiving

Impaired functional status often affects how individuals perceive themselves. **Disturbances in body image** and self-concept are related to the functional restrictions imposed by disease. **Self-esteem** and **personal identity** are similarly affected, and feelings of **hopelessness** and **powerlessness** may become apparent with the realization that activities once taken for granted can no longer be accomplished. As the disease progresses in severity, **sensory/perceptual alterations** may be evident that affect vision, hearing, movement, smelling, and tasting.

Feeling

Anxiety is a common diagnosis in this patient population and may be accompanied by the **fear** of more specific threats to the patient. Fear and anxiety may aggravate physical discomfort, or **pain.** Pain may be produced by the disease, or it may be the result of uncomfortable procedures or positions requested of the patient.

Knowing

Knowledge deficits are common in heart disease because of the complexity of the disorder and its treatment. Patients may also purposely avoid learning more about the disorder because of the perceived threat to their physical or emotional well-being. Coping mechanisms such as denial often play a role. The nurse must assess the patient's ability and readiness to learn, and distinguish between what the patient knows and wants to know, what the patient chooses not to know, and what the patient needs to know to maximize the benefits of the recommended or prescribed therapy. **Thought processes** may be affected by the underlying disease or by disturbances in self-esteem.

Moving

Functional status not only affects self-concept but also impairs **mobility** and the performance of activities of daily living. Intraoperatively immobility itself impairs movement postoperatively and can aggravate preexisting musculoskeletal problems.

Fatigue may be a problem and in association with pain and dyspnea can produce **activity intolerance** and restrict **diversional activities** and **home maintenance management. Self-care deficits** related to hygiene, grooming, feeding, and toileting are not uncommon in these patients. **Sleep patterns** may be disturbed, particularly in patients with paroxysmal nocturnal dyspnea or orthopnea.

Children with congenital heart disease often demonstrate **altered growth and development,** as well as many of the diagnoses already listed within this pattern. In addition to physical parameters, mental and emotional development may be delayed. Siblings, parents, and other caregivers may display regressive behaviors.

Exchanging

The exchanging pattern includes most of the physiologic diagnoses that are commonly encountered during the perioperative period. It also reflects many of AORN's (1993) outcome standards that pertain to injury, skin integrity, fluid and electrolytes, infection, and the physiologic response to surgery.

The circulatory system is the focal point for cardiac surgery patients, and the most common nursing diagnoses are **decreased cardiac output** and **altered tissue perfusion.** Patients with impaired cardiac function have, or are at risk for, a reduction in cardiac output, which in turn jeopardizes adequate perfusion of organ systems. Alterations in cardiac output may be related to electrical factors (conduction disturbances), mechanical factors (preload, afterload, contractility), or structural factors (valve disease, ventricular abnormalities, congenital anomalies).

Diagnoses related to oxygenation and breathing include **ineffective airway clearance, high risk for aspiration, ineffective breathing pattern,** and **impaired gas exchange.** These diagnoses reflect the duration of surgery, the patient's immobility and subsequent retention of secretions, the respiratory effects of anesthesia, and underlying cardiac and pulmonary pathologic conditions.

Regulation of the patient's temperature is common during surgery. Hypothermia during surgery is a method of protecting the heart, but it becomes a problem when it occurs preoperatively or postoperatively. In the preoperative period the shivering that accompanies chilling should be avoided because of the increased metabolic demands on the heart that accompany shivering. Actions are implemented to keep the patient warm before the induction of anesthesia and the use of neuromuscular blocking agents that reduce shivering.) Postoperatively some residual **hypothermia** is often encountered, and rewarming of the patient is performed gradually so that the body is able to adjust to the shifting of blood from central organs to the periphery as rewarming and vasodilatation occur.

Other diagnoses include **high risk for injury, impaired skin integrity,** and **impaired tissue integrity.** Patients with compromised cardiac function requires special precautions to avoid skin and tissue injury, especially those who are very young or very elderly, or those who are obese **(altered nutrition, more than body requirements)** or cachectic **(altered nutrition, less than body requirements).** These dangers may be potentiated by the use of equipment such as electrosurgical units, defibrillators, powered equipment, and chemical agents.

The **high risk for infection** is ever present, and the diagnosis is routinely applied to cardiac surgery patients. The diagnosis of **altered protection** is also applicable to these patients and is related to a reduction in the ability to protect oneself from internal or external threats.

Fluid volume excess and **fluid volume deficit** are related to factors such as blood loss, fluid shifts, dehydration or overhydration, immobility, and the inability to maintain appropriate fluid status as a result of congestive heart failure or renal failure.

Relating

Establishing and maintaining bonds may be affected by heart disease. The functional restrictions often affect the patient's ability to engage in personal, professional, and societal roles. **Social interaction, role performance,** and **family processes** are more difficult when pain, fatigue, and other symptoms are present. **Sexual dysfunction** may accompany these problems as well.

Valuing

When companionship is denied or restricted by debilitating symptoms, patients may be in **spiritual distress.** They may be unable to participate in religious ceremonies or benefit from the spiritual support of religious counselors. Religious beliefs may affect certain interventions, such as the refusal of Jehovah's Witnesses to receive blood transfusions. Religious and emotional aspects of the heart (e.g., as "the seat of the soul"), combined with the fear of death or disfigurement, warrant investigating this diagnosis.

Choosing

Problems of **adjustment** and **coping** are not unusual in patients and families as the disease progresses and its impact becomes increasingly apparent. **Conflicts** between patient and health care professionals or between patient and significant others may arise. Adaptive behaviors may be developed, or denial, anger, disbelief, regression, and lack of cooperation may become evident.

Consideration must be given to the ability or desire of the patient to engage in **health-seeking behaviors** and to follow prescribed therapeutic regimens. The nurse should distinguish between a patient's refusal to comply with recommendations and the inability to follow orders because of insufficient information and emotional support. These considerations are significant for patients who are expected to make life-style changes such as risk factor modification, adherence to a precise medication schedule, or long-term laboratory follow-up testing.

SELECTED NURSING DIAGNOSES FOR THE CARDIAC SURGERY PATIENT

The previous discussion addresses the many possible diagnoses found in the perioperative cardiac surgery patient. The following selected diagnoses (not all of which are NANDA approved) are listed with the patient outcomes that can be derived from them. Patient outcomes with an asterisk (*) are based on AORN's (1993) Patient Outcome Standards for Perioperative Nursing (see Box 7-1).

1. Nursing Diagnosis
Knowledge deficit related to the physiologic effects of the cardiac disorder, proposed surgical procedure, and/or immediate postoperative events.
Patient Outcome*
The patient demonstrates knowledge of the physiologic responses to the cardiac disorder (at his or her level of understanding), the proposed surgical treatment, and immediate postoperative events as evidenced by verbalization of the disease state, purpose of surgery, and recovery process.

2. Nursing Diagnosis
Knowledge deficit related to the psychologic responses to the cardiac disorder, the proposed surgical treatment, and/or immediate postoperative events.
Patient Outcome*
The patient demonstrates knowledge of the psychologic responses to the cardiac disorder (at his or her level of understanding), the proposed surgical treatment, and immediate postoperative events as evidenced by verbalization of the perception of the cardiac disorder, surgery, and postoperative events; identification of concerns or fears; and communication of data relevant to planning.

3. Nursing Diagnosis
Anxiety related to apprehension about the surgery and/or perioperative events.
Patient Outcome
The patient's anxiety is reduced; manifestations of anxiety (increased heart rate, elevated blood pressure, increased respiratory rate, diaphoresis, restlessness, agitation, crying, poor eye contact) are reduced or absent.

4. Nursing Diagnosis
High risk for injury related to the surgical position.
Patient Outcome*
The patient is free from injury related to the surgical position as evidenced by the absence of neuromuscular impairment and tissue necrosis.

5. Nursing Diagnosis
High risk for injury related to retained foreign objects.
Patient Outcome*
The patient is free from injury related to retained foreign objects as evidenced by correct counts or unremarkable x-ray films when necessitated by incorrect counts.

6. Nursing Diagnosis
High risk for injury related to chemical hazards.
Patient Outcome*
The patient is free from injury related to chemical hazards as evidenced by the absence of allergic reactions (and tissue necrosis) to solutions and medications.

7. Nursing Diagnosis
High risk for injury related to physical hazards.
Patient Outcome*
The patient is free from injury related to physical hazards as evidenced by the availability and proper functioning of appropriate instruments, equipment, and supplies.

8. Nursing Diagnosis
High risk for injury related to electrical hazards.
Patient Outcome*
The patient is free from injury related to electrical hazards as evidenced by the absence of redness or blistering of skin at the conclusion of the surgical procedure.

9. Nursing Diagnosis
High risk for injury related to thermal hazards.
Patient Outcome*
The patient is free from injury related to thermal hazards as evidenced by the absence of tissue damage secondary to hyperthermia or hypothermia.

10. Nursing Diagnosis
High risk for wound infection related to surgical incision(s), catheters and intravascular lines, and/or altered cardiac function.
Patient Outcome*
The patient is free from infection related to breaks in aseptic technique during surgery as evidenced by the absence of redness, edema, purulent incisional drainage, or untoward elevation of temperature postoperatively.

11. Nursing Diagnosis
High risk for impaired skin integrity.
Patient Outcome*
The patient's skin integrity is maintained as evidenced by the absence of bruises, skin breakdown, discoloration, open skin lesions, or excoriation during the perioperative period (Rothrock, 1990).

12. Nursing Diagnosis
High risk for impaired myocardial, peripheral, and cerebral tissue integrity related to surgery, hypothermia, cardiopulmonary bypass, and/or surgical particulate or air emboli.
Patient Outcome
The patient's myocardial, peripheral, and cerebral tissue integrity is adequate or improved as evidenced by the absence of new electrocardiographic manifestations of infarction and by the presence of palpable peripheral pulses and a clear or improving sensorium postoperatively (American Association of Critical-Care Nurses [AACN], 1990).

13. Nursing Diagnosis
High risk for fluid volume deficit and/or electrolyte imbalance related to blood loss, blood reaction, and/or use of hyperkalemic cardioplegia solution.
Patient Outcome*
The patient's fluid volume and electrolyte balance is maintained as evidenced by a hematocrit within the acceptable range, and electrolytes, arterial blood gasses, urinary output, and blood pressures within normal limits.

14. Nursing Diagnosis
High risk for decreased cardiac output related to emotional or physiologic (electrical, mechanical, or structural) factors.
Patient Outcome
The patient's cardiac output is maintained or improved as evidenced by a reduction in the patient's emotional stress level; the availability of supplies, equipment, and medications to foster optimal cardiac output; and the absence of injury to cardiovascular structures.

15. Nursing Diagnoses
High risk for altered participation (ineffective) in rehabilitation (Rothrock, 1990).
Patient Outcome*
The patient will participate in rehabilitation as evidenced by verbalizing or participating in planning for discharge, identifying knowledge deficits related to potential complications or referral services requiring patient education, and demonstrating ability to perform activities related to postoperative care (Rothrock, 1990).

CONCLUSION

Nursing diagnoses and patient outcomes guide the perioperative nurse in selecting the appropriate interventions to achieve stated goals. The following chapter provides a generic care plan that reflects some common patient problems and outcomes related to cardiac surgery.

REFERENCES

Agency for Health Care Policy and Research: *Quick reference guide for clinicians: acute pain management in adults: operative procedures,* Rockville, MD, 1992, AHCPR.

American Association of Critical-Care Nurses: *AACN outcome standards for nursing care of the critically ill,* Laguna Niguel, Calif, 1990 AACN.

Association of Operating Room Nurses: Patient outcome standards for perioperative nursing. In *Standards and recommended practices for perioperative nursing,* Denver, 1993, AORN.

Carpenito LJ: *Nursing diagnosis: application to clinical practice,* ed 5, Philadelphia, 1993, JB Lippincott.

Gordon M: *Nursing diagnosis: process and application,* New York, 1982, McGraw-Hill.

Guzzetta CE, Seifert PC: Cardiovascular assessment. In Kinney MR and others: *Comprehensive cardiac care,* ed 7, St Louis, 1991, Mosby.

Joint Commission on the Accreditation of Healthcare Organizations: National forum spotlights clinical indicators and cultural change, *Agenda for Change Update* 3(2):1, 1989.

North American Nursing Diagnosis Association: Twenty-one new nursing diagnoses and a taxonomy, *Am J Nurs* 86:1414, 1986.

Rothrock JC: *Perioperative nursing care planning,* St Louis, 1990, Mosby.

Seifert PC: Cardiac surgery. In Rothrock JC: *Perioperative nursing care planning,* St Louis, 1990, Mosby.

Seifert PC, Grandusky R: Nursing diagnoses: their use in developing care plans, *AORN J* 51(4):1008, 1990.

8

Perioperative Nursing Care Planning

The ideal way to manage complications is to avoid them, which is best accomplished with a carefully conducted care plan.

Robert S. Litwak, MD, and Simon Dack, MD, 1982, p. 22

The purpose of planning is to identify and implement actions necessary to achieve the desired patient outcomes. Planning is also critical to avoiding or reducing injury or complications. Safety considerations have been identified among the nursing diagnoses in the previous chapter. Other problems exist that are clearly medical: ventricular fibrillation, hemorrhage, infarction, cerebral vascular accident, and anaphylactic reactions. Whether diagnoses are nursing or medical, the nurse must be aware of the various potential problems and complications and the expected patient response, anticipate their occurrence, observe for the expected patient responses, and be prepared to act quickly in a collaborative manner should problems or complications arise. Thus the nurse must constantly reassess which needs have the greatest priority and rearrange or modify interventions accordingly. These considerations should be reflected in the plan of care, whether it is written or unwritten. When they are documented, care plans can serve as written evidence of the nurse's knowledge and judgment.

GENERIC CARE PLANS

Care plans based on the diagnoses and patients outcomes identified in Chapter 7 are outlined below. Patient outcomes with an asterisk (*) are based on the Association for Operating Room Nurse's (AORN's) (1993) Patient Outcome Standards for Perioperative Nursing (see Box 7-1). The interventions are generic to the cardiac surgery patient and are not meant to be all-inclusive. The perioperative nurse must incorporate the unique physical and psychosocial needs of the patient and place them in order of priority to implement care appropriately (Seifert, 1990).

Perioperative considerations related to specific surgical procedures are listed in subsequent chapters related to those topics.

1. Nursing Diagnosis
Knowledge deficit related to the physiologic effects of the cardiac disorder, proposed surgical procedure, and/or immediate postoperative events.

Patient Outcome*
The patient demonstrates knowledge of the physiologic responses to the cardiac disorder (at his or her level of understanding), the proposed surgical treatment, and immediate postoperative events as evidenced by verbalization of the disease state, purpose of surgery, and recovery process.

Interventions
Assess level of consciousness.
Confirm patient's identity.
Confirm that consent for surgery has been granted.
Assess patient's understanding of cardiac disease.
Assess effects of cardiac disorder on physiologic and functional status.
Assess effects of cardiac medications on patient's thought processes.
Determine patient's knowledge of current medication regimen.
Elicit patient's understanding of surgical procedure and possible alternative procedures (e.g., saphenous vein and/or internal mammary artery).
Respect normal level of denial.
Answer patient's and family's questions.
Elicit understanding of prior cardiac procedures; if patient has questions or misunderstandings, provide information or refer to appropriate health care professional as indicated.
Note presence of sternotomy scars; reoperations require longer surgical time and may be accompanied by increased bleeding. Inform patient and family of possible prolonged operative time.
Assess patient's and family's understanding of possible complications: perioperative myocardial infarction, stroke, hemorrhage, renal failure, infection, dysrhythmias, death.

Ascertain where family or significant other will be waiting during surgery; provide communication per institutional protocol.

Describe/explain the following events (use models, diagrams, fact sheets and so forth):

Preoperative

NPO status

Premedication

Time and mode of transport to operating room (OR)

Preinduction (holding) area

Interview by circulating nurse

Insertion of peripheral intravascular lines

Transport to OR, transfer to OR bed

OR environment—what patient will see, hear, feel, smell (e.g., numerous staff, what they are wearing, equipment, sound of people moving, cool temperature, uncomfortable procedures)

Induction of anesthesia

Insertion of nasogastric tube, central vascular lines, urinary catheter

Skin preparation

Intraoperative

Anticipated length of surgery

Surgical procedure, intraoperative events, equipment (as requested)

Postoperative

Surgical intensive care unit (SICU) environment—noises, equipment, protocols

Condition of patient on arrival in SICU—tubes, lines, catheters, patient cool and pale; medicated/anesthetized; unable to talk while intubated

Alternative methods of communication available in SICU

Visiting hours, anticipated length of stay in SICU, step-down unit

(Reassure family/significant other that it is not necessary to visit patient in SICU if the experience is too frightening; staff can keep family informed and communicate information.)

Special pediatric considerations (Joy, 1990)

Determine if patient and family have participated in hospital surgical tour.

Orient patient and family to nursing unit, playroom, and hospital room.

Be honest about painful procedures (e.g., injections, blood tests).

Encourage child to bring a special toy for security.

Show patient and family surgical staff's clothing, particularly face masks; allow child to play with apparel.

Stress to patient that surgery is performed only on the part of the body that has been discussed and specified.

Special geriatric considerations (Dellasega and Rothrock, 1990)

Assess patient's ability to see and hear, and ascertain patient's experience with previous surgery (if any).

Modify teaching plan in accordance with sensory/perceptual alterations; minimize use of audiovisual materials if they create too much confusion for patient.

Use a one-on-one approach in a quiet, private environment.

Include family members and significant others involved in patient care outside the hospital.

Obtain frequent feedback during teaching process.

Use frequent reminders and reinforce learning.

2. Nursing Diagnosis

Knowledge deficit related to the psychologic responses to the cardiac disorder, the proposed surgical treatment, and/or immediate postoperative events.

Patient Outcome*

The patient demonstrates knowledge of the psychologic responses to the cardiac disorder (at his or her level of understanding), the proposed surgical treatment, and immediate postoperative events as evidenced by verbalization of the perception of the cardiac disorder, surgery, and postoperative events; identification of concerns and fears; and communication of data relevant to planning.

Interventions

Elicit patient's feelings about the impact of the disease on activities of daily living.

Encourage verbalization of fears, "silly questions," concerns, perceived threats.

Assess patient's and family's fears, concerns, understanding of procedure.

Determine religious beliefs affecting surgical procedure (e.g., Jehovah's Witnesses' attitude toward blood transfusion).

3. Nursing Diagnosis

Anxiety related to apprehension about the surgery and/or perioperative events.

Patient Outcome

The patient's anxiety is reduced; manifestations of anxiety (increased heart rate, elevated blood pressure, increased respiratory rate, diaphoresis, restlessness, agitation, crying, poor eye contact) are reduced or absent.

Interventions

Assess anxiety level and physiologic response, such as increased blood pressure and heart rate (in children, may also see crying, clinging to parent, restlessness, and trembling).

Assess patient's knowledge of cardiac disease and planned surgery.

Implement perioperative teaching.

Encourage verbalization of concerns, perceived threats, fears.

Orient patient to OR environment; note if patient has taken preoperative tour.

Explain perioperative events as they occur; describe what patient will see, hear, and feel.

Remain with patient on induction; hold patient's hand.

Answer requests for information.

Provide comfort measures, such as warm blankets, religious articles.

In children, note developmental stage and plan interventions accordingly.

4. Nursing Diagnosis
High risk for injury related to the surgical position.
Patient Outcome*
The patient is free from injury related to the surgical position as evidenced by the absence of neuromuscular impairment and tissue necrosis.
Interventions
Assess airway; confirm effective breathing pattern.
Have extra personnel to position patient.
Use patient transfer roller if patient is unable to move.
Avoid shearing forces and friction during patient positioning and transfer; lift patient rather than pulling or sliding (Dellasega and Rothrock, 1990).
Check pulses in extremities (Biddle and Cannady, 1990).
Assess range of motion/mobility before positioning; note physical injuries.
Pad pressure points.
Have available necessary positioning supplies.
Maintain accessibility to groin (e.g., femoral artery)
Assess bony prominences and dependent pressure sites at end of surgery.
Select positioning devices in accordance with skin condition, tissue integrity, and weight (Joy, 1990).
Protect eyes and ears.
In pediatric patients, may need to use body restraints (Joy, 1990).
In elderly patients, be especially cautious positioning joints, notably the hips, knees, and ankles (Dellasega and Rothrock, 1990).
Supine
Maintain proper body alignment.
In patients with reduced range of motion or back problems, place in functional position.
Use extra padding as necessary on arms, hands, feet, back, sacrum, and back of head.
Maintain airway; avoid decreased chin-to-chest angle, especially in children and obese patients; assess respiratory rate and rhythm, chest expansion, and oxygenation; monitor pulse oximetry.
Observe for decrease in blood pressure, heart rate, and peripheral resistance, especially during induction of anesthesia; monitor blood pressure and ECG (Kneedler and Dodge, 1987).
Lateral
If placed on right side, may compress vena cava (especially in obese patients) with subsequent reduction in preload; monitor systemic, pulmonary pressures.
Monitor respiratory rate and rhythm, oxygenation, and ECG; note compromised respiratory function.
Use axillary rolls, pillows between legs; provide padding for arms, elbows, feet, and head.
Attach arm boards, over-arm boards; use stabilizing pillows, sandbags, or other devices anteriorly and posteriorly.

Place adhesive tape across buttocks (if it does not interfere with access to surgical site and/or groin).

5. Nursing Diagnosis
High risk for injury related to retained foreign objects.
Patient Outcome*
The patient is free from injury related to retained foreign objects as evidenced by correct counts or unremarkable x-ray films when necessitated by correct counts.
Interventions
Account for suture and hypodermic needles, knife blades, umbilical tapes, rubbershods, pledgets, vessel loops, bulldog clamps, cannulas, pill sponges, guidewires, stopcocks, connectors for tubing, prosthetic materials, instruments, and other items per institutional protocol.
Remove tissue debris from instruments, such as calcium particles, plaque, thrombus, vegetations.
Remove suture particles from surgical site.
Complete necessary documentation; follow policy for incorrect counts, per institutional protocol.

6. Nursing Diagnosis
High risk for injury related to chemical hazards.
Patient Outcome*
The patient is free from injury related to chemical hazards as evidenced by the absence of allergic reactions (and tissue necrosis) to solutions and medications.
Interventions
Note allergies (especially to skin preparation solutions, depilatories, and dressing materials).
Identify fluids, solutions, irrigations, injectates, medications: heparin injectate, heparin solution, topical "slush," cardioplegia solution, papaverine, epinephrine, thrombin, antibiotic solution, "glue" components, normal saline, lactated Ringer's solution, and other fluids on field.
Follow hospital protocol for allergic/anaphylactic blood reactions.
Inject blood vessels (e.g., saphenous vein) and other tissue with physiologic solutions or prescribed fluids only.
Remove glove powder from outside of gloves after gloving and before handling tissue.
Remove toxic storage solution (e.g., glutaraldehyde) from grafts/prosthetic material with saline before use per protocol.

7. Nursing Diagnosis
High risk for injury related to physical hazards.
Patient Outcome*
The patient is free from injury related to physical hazards as evidenced by the availability and proper functioning of appropriate instruments, equipment, and supplies.
Interventions
Inspect vascular clamps, forceps, needle holders, and

other instruments for malalignment, missing teeth, burs, and malfunctions; replace as necessary.

Avoid overstretching of sternal (or internal mammary artery [IMA]) retractor; remove IMA post(s) after IMA dissection if post is impinging on patient's arm.

Use a minimal amount of nonirritating adhesive tape on skin, especially in patients with frail skin (e.g., very young or old patients [Dellasega and Rothrock, 1990]).

Moisten surgeon's or assistant's hands when they are tying fine suture to prevent snagging, per request.

Visualize entire length of suture before handing to surgeon; discard suture with knots.

Prevent snagging of suture; avoid clamping suture with unprotected metal jaws (use rubbershods or special suture clamps).

Have available chest x-ray films, cardiac catheterization cineangiograms, arteriogram, angiograms, CT scans, and so forth, as requested.

If reoperation: display lateral and anteroposterior chest x-ray films (to note adherence of heart and great vessels to sternum, to count chest wires, to note the presence of prostheses, and so forth); have special supplies and equipment as requested by surgeon (e.g., oscillating saw, topical hemostatic agents).

Have backup supplies or alternative source of supplies available (e.g., grafts, valves, pledgets, special suture); list lot and serial number of all implants.

Have additional sterile instruments, equipment, and supplies (e.g., case carts) available in anticipation of emergency procedures.

When OR is not in use, keep room prepared for cardiac procedures: sterile instrument sets in place, sternal saw power source ready for use, light source available, electrosurgical unit(s) in working order (attachments available), OR table parts attached to bed, defibrillator plugged in, temporary atrioventricular pacemaker available, inventory (supplies, solutions, etc.) stocked.

8. Nursing Diagnosis
High risk for injury related to electrical hazards.
Patient Outcome*
The patient is free from injury related to electrical hazards as evidenced by the absence of redness or blistering of skin at the conclusion of the surgical procedure.
Interventions
Ensure appropriate location of electrosurgical unit dispersive pad site(s); place pad on clean, dry skin over muscular area; avoid bony prominences, scarred or excessively hairy areas; place pad as far from ECG electrodes as possible.

In patients with pacemakers or internal defibrillators, place dispersive pad away from generator sites; minimize use of electrosurgery (may require device programmer).

Check that defibrillator (and fibrillator) and external pacemaker are in proper working order; schedule regular maintenance checks with biomedical engi-neering; report malfunctioning equipment and devices per institutional protocol.

Ensure that the appropriate connector for the anteroposterior paddles/patches is available (some patients scheduled for internal defibrillator insertion may arrive in the OR with disposable external defibrillator patches incompatible with the OR defibrillator).

Insulate proximal tip of electrosurgical pencil when using in deep cavities or in retrosternum (e.g., during IMA dissection); verify with surgeon.

Check epicardial pacing leads and wires for kinks or cracks; if pacing wires are not in use postoperatively, place insulating covers over distal tips of each wire; have external pacemaker generator available (unifocal and bifocal).

Verify defibrillator settings with surgeon.

Have surgeon verbalize when defibrillator is to be discharged.

Have appropriate-size internal paddles; ensure that they fit into defibrillator.

For reoperation, have internal and external paddles; verify setting with surgeon before discharging; in adults with extensive pericardial adhesions, consider using pediatric-size internal paddle(s) until sufficient space is dissected in pericardial cavity to allow insertion of regular-size paddle; coordinate changing over to regular paddle(s) with surgeon (use this technique if paddle tips can be changed).

Apply sufficient electrode paste to external paddles before placing paddles on patient's chest, or use saline sponge (if sterile conducting medium is required for external defibrillation [e.g., intraoperatively]).

9. Nursing Diagnosis
High risk for injury related to thermal hazards.
Patient Outcome*
The patient is free from injury related to thermal hazards as evidenced by the absence of tissue damage secondary to hyperthermia or hypothermia.
Interventions
Check setting of thermia unit; maintain temperature per protocol.

Turn warming unit off when patient is being cooled; turn unit on when patient is being rewarmed.

Cover thermia blanket with sheet or thin blanket; avoid direct contact with skin.

Ensure integrity of thermia blanket; avoid injury from needles or other sharp objects.

In neonates, use radiant heater (per protocol), head covering, plastic blankets or wrappers, or warming bed with heaters; avoid excessive heat.

Expose only skin area required for operation; both the very young and the elderly are more susceptible to temperature changes.

Ensure that temperature of topical solutions is appropriate for use (cold during induced arrest, warm before or after induced arrest).

Have cardiac insulating pads (if surgeon requests them), cold lap tapes, and so forth, available to retain hypothermic temperature during cardiac repair; have sufficient cold topical irrigating solution.

When profound hypothermia is used, protect ears, nose, and other prominences from frostbite with additional padding.

Avoid direct contact of ice or ice chips with skin or tissue (ice chips in the pericardium may cause phrenic nerve injury).

Maintain cool temperature in room during period of induced arrest; increase temperature during closing of incision; verify with surgeon; have warming blankets on SICU bed per protocol.

Provide warm blankets preoperatively (verify with surgeon) and postoperatively.

Monitor patient's temperatures (rectal, esophageal, bladder, ventricular septal, in-line bypass); verify accuracy of monitoring system; report malfunctions; adjust room temperature as needed.

10. Nursing Diagnosis
High risk for wound infection related to surgical incision(s), sites of catheters and intravascular lines, and/or altered cardiac function.
Patient Outcome*
The patient is free from infection related to breaks in aseptic technique during surgery as evidenced by the absence of redness, edema, purulent incisional drainage, or untoward elevation of temperature postoperatively.
Interventions
Use depilatories or electric clippers to shave hair; avoid razors if possible.

Assess risk factors for postoperative infection (e.g., previous cardiac operations, duration of surgery, duration of cardiopulmonary bypass, length of hospitalization [preoperatively and in SICU], blood transfusions, postoperative blood loss, diabetes mellitus).

Dress all incisions and sites of intravascular lines.

Have prescribed topical antibiotic solution available for irrigation.

Ensure that prophylactic antibiotics are given preoperatively.

Use closed urinary drainage system; keep drainage bag off floor and below bladder level.

Routinely perform skin preparation to knees (or feet if leg vein is needed) in anticipation of inserting femoral artery pressure line or intraaortic balloon, and/or instituting femoral artery bypass.

Confine and contain instruments and supplies used in groin or leg; change gown and gloves when contaminated.

If OR bed is elevated or lowered (for IMA dissections), or turned from side to side (to de-air ventricle), take appropriate measures to retain sterility of field, gowns, gloves, and drapes; take precautions to maintain sterility of bypass lines.

Keep setup sterile until patient leaves OR (in case incision needs to be reopened for exploration).

Document lot and serial numbers of all implants, and other information as requested by institutional protocol.

Ensure that handwashing, universal precautions, and appropriate sterilization and decontamination procedures are followed.

11. Nursing Diagnosis
High risk for impaired skin integrity.
Patient Outcome*
The patient's skin integrity is maintained as evidenced by the absence of bruises, skin breakdown, discoloration, open skin lesions, or excoriation during the perioperative period (Rothrock, 1990).
Interventions
Assess skin integrity; note bruises, lesions, discoloration, and/or other problems; assess skin turgor and elasticity (especially in very young and elderly patients).

Pad hands, elbows, and back of head; pad heels and feet when possible.

Keep drapes off lower extremities and head; use anesthesia screen or special drape holders and equipment.

Ensure that SICU bed is prepared with mattress padding.

Prevent pooling of preparation solutions.

12. Nursing Diagnoses
High risk for impaired myocardial, peripheral, and cerebral tissue integrity related to surgery, hypothermia, cardiopulmonary bypass, and/or surgical particulate or air emboli.
Patient Outcome
The patient's myocardial, peripheral, and cerebral tissue integrity is adequate or improved as evidenced by the absence of new electrocardiographic manifestations of infarction and by the presence of palpable peripheral pulses and a clear or improving sensorium postoperatively (American Association of Critical-Care Nurses [AACN], 1990).
Interventions
Minimize or limit activities that increase myocardial oxygen demand (e.g., decrease anxiety, decrease environmental stimulation such as excess noise, direct lighting [AACN, 1990]).

Monitor ECG throughout procedure; note dysrhythmias, ectopic beats for potential cardiac arrest; note bradydysrhythmias and ECG evidence of ischemia (e.g., ST segment changes).

Anticipate need for antidysrhythmic agents if ectopy is noted.

Monitor ECG during induced arrest; if ECG activity is noted, prepare to reinfuse cardioplegia solution.

Maintain extra supply of "slush" to keep heart cold.

Keep instruments clean of blood and particulate matter that could become a source of emboli (tissue debris such as fat, bone fragments, suture pieces, excess bone wax); remove particulate matter remaining in surgical site, and/or notify surgeon.

Check bypass lines before institution of cardiopulmonary bypass; note presence of air in arterial lines and notify surgeon and/or perfusionist; ensure that arterial and venous lines are secure.

Use discard suction at site of heart valve excision to remove particulate debris.

Determine whether single or double venous cannulation is to be used (have caval clamps or tapes available for double cannulation, per surgeon's preference).

Fill/refill venous lines according to protocol and with designated solutions only; avoid excessive air in venous lines (can cause air lock).

Be able to identify inflow lines readily from outflow lines; label if necessary.

Verify that vent/suction lines are suctioning (and not infusing).

If femoral artery bypass is to be instituted, have appropriate supplies and instruments to access femoral artery.

Avoid kinks in bypass tubing; avoid pressure on bypass lines; ensure band connections are secure in bypass tubing (especially arterial and other high-pressure lines).

When venting catheters and lines are used, have appropriate connectors, tubing, and so forth.

Have correct heparin dosage (if given at field); have additional heparin available if emergency reinstitution of bypass is required after heparin reversal (with protamine sulfate); verify that heparin has been given.

Avoid restrictive leg dressings (when vein is excised).

When intraaortic balloon pump (IABP) or other catheter is in femoral artery, avoid bending legs (resulting in kinking of lines or injury to vessel wall).

13. Nursing Diagnosis
High risk for fluid volume deficit and/or electrolyte imbalance related to blood loss, blood reaction, and/or hyperkalemic cardioplegia solution.

Patient Outcome*
The patient's fluid volume and electrolyte balance is maintained as evidenced by a hematocrit within the acceptable range, and electrolytes arterial blood gasses, urinary output, and blood pressures within normal limits.

Interventions
Review patient's record for blood order (type and number of units).

Review laboratory studies: complete blood count, coagulation profile, electrolytes, arterial blood gasses (ABG's).

Monitor intraoperative blood loss; note sudden and/or excessive bleeding.

Ensure that suction is available and working properly.

Monitor intraoperative ABG's, electrolytes, blood laboratory values, ECG.

Monitor pulmonary and systemic blood pressures for indication of volume status.

Have blood (packed red blood cells) immediately available (in OR or directly adjacent to OR); follow protocol for proper blood storage.

Ensure adequate blood and blood product supply via communication with blood bank; verify with surgeon and anesthesiologist.

Use autotransfusion suction before patient is fully heparinized (and cardiotomy suction is available) to conserve blood.

Use sump (cardiotomy) suction only when patient is fully heparinized; suction with sump suction whenever possible to conserve blood and to return it immediately to the bypass pump; avoid using cardiotomy suction after protamine reversal.

Avoid excessive negative pressure with pump sucker to reduce shear stress on red blood cells (Kirklin and Barratt-Boyes, 1993).

Use discard suction for irrigating solutions (to reduce amount of irrigation returning to bypass pump and causing an undesired drop in hematocrit).

Use discard suction to remove topical solutions from pleural cavity (if opened) and pericardial cavity.

Use discard suction for antibiotic solutions.

Ensure that autotransfusion system is working properly; have available additional supplies (suction tubing, cannisters).

Anticipate need for platelets, fresh frozen plasma, "glue" (calcium chloride, thrombin, and cryoprecipitate) with reoperations and/or history of anticoagulation and antiplatelet therapy; have topical hemostatic agents available.

If patient has been receiving warfarin anticoagulants, note if medication has been discontinued and heparin initiated.

Note if patient discontinued antiplatelet therapy preoperatively.

Monitor intraoperative urinary output.

Verify that urine is draining when catheterizing bladder; notify surgeon or anesthesiologist if urine is not visualized; if urethral strictures are present, have available dilators, water-soluble lubricant, large syringe, coudé catheters, and other supplies as requested by surgeon; anticipate possible insertion of suprapubic catheter if other measures fail; have available necessary items.

Have chest tubes available; if pleural cavity is entered, anticipate placement of a tube in the pleural space (during surgery or immediately postoperatively).

Have available additional chest tubes, Y-connectors, and tubing if extra chest tubes are connected; have chest drainage containers and/or cardiotomy reservoirs to collect drainage.

Monitor chest tube drainage closely; alert surgeon if drainage exceeds acceptable amount (e.g., more than 150 ml/hr to 200 ml/hr) or is bright red.

Secure tubes and drains (and connections) before leaving OR.

In addition to standard postoperative report, include information on cardiac status, dysrhythmias, difficulties with defibrillation cardiac medications, baseline pulmonary function, location of pressure monitoring and infusion lines, electrolyte levels (especially potassium), and any other information that will facilitate patient care in the SICU.

14. Nursing Diagnosis
High risk for decreased cardiac output related to emotional or physiologic (electrical, mechanical, or structural) factors.

Patient Outcome

The patient's cardiac output is maintained or improved as evidenced by a reduction in the patient's emotional stress level; the availability of supplies, equipment, and medications to foster optimal cardiac output; and the absence of injury to cardiovascular structures.

Interventions

Institute measures to reduce emotional stress, which can increase myocardial oxygen demand.

Monitor pulmonary and systemic pressures; note drop in systemic pressures, increase in pulmonary pressures indicating myocardial dysfunction; correlate with distended, sluggish heart.

Monitor cardiac output, cardiac index, pulmonary vascular resistance, systemic vascular resistance, and other hemodynamic parameters.

Monitor for fluid volume deficit or excess.

Note reduction in urinary output, which may indicate a reduction in cardiac output.

If pulmonary artery pressure line has not been inserted, anticipate insertion of line immediately postoperatively; left atrial pressure line may be inserted; have appropriate supplies available.

Observe for reaction during protamine infusion (drop in systemic blood pressure).

Monitor ECG rate and rhythm, especially for lethal dysrhythmias (e.g., ventricular tachycardia/fibrillation).

Have epicardial temporary pacing wires ready for insertion.

Have defibrillator ready when fibrillation is seen before induced arrest or immediately after removal of cross-clamp; test defibrillator before start of procedure; have backup defibrillator and internal paddles available.

Have appropriate ECG leads and cables for cardioversion.

Have appropriate ECG leads for use with IABP; have IABP and supplies available.

15. Nursing Diagnosis

High risk for altered participation (ineffective) in rehabilitation (Rothrock, 1990).

Patient Outcome*

The patient will participate in rehabilitation as evidenced by verbalizing or participating in planning for discharge, identifying knowledge deficits related to potential complications or referral services requiring patient education, and demonstrating ability to perform activities related to postoperative care (Rothrock, 1990).

Interventions

Assess patient's ability to deep breathe and cough; teach patient how to use cough pillow and splint.

Assess patient's/family's understanding of procedure performed; clarify misconceptions; if necessary, refer patient to specialist for additional information.

Assess patient's understanding of prescribed life-style modifications; assess feelings of patient/family about these changes; answer questions or refer to appropriate personnel.

Encourage patient/family to clarify misconceptions and seek additional information and support as needed.

Assess family's ability to assist patient in recuperation and rehabilitation; refer as necessary.

Verify patient's/family's knowledge of reportable signs and symptoms related to specific procedure (e.g., bypass graft closure, valve failure, infection).

Verify patient's/family's knowledge of prescribed medications: name, dosage and times, side effects, and signs and symptoms; list medications.

Verify patient's/family's understanding of special considerations related to surgery (e.g., risk factor modification for patients with coronary artery disease; need for laboratory follow-up in patients with prosthetic valves requiring chronic anticoagulation).

CONCLUSION

Planning enables the nurse to identify interventions that will achieve selected outcomes and avoid complications. These interventions are directed by the nursing diagnoses and collaborative problems that have been formulated to reflect particular patient needs (McFarland and McFarlane, 1989), but they should also incorporate an awareness of the potential hazards common to all cardiac surgery patients.

Actions must be continuously reappraised for their appropriateness and effectiveness, and the priority given to their implementation. How successfully this is achieved is determined by the actions that the nurse takes. Successful outcomes are dependent on the nurse's intellectual, interpersonal, and technical abilities (Yura and Walsh, 1988).

REFERENCES

American Association of Critical-Care Nurses: AACN outcome standards for nursing care of the critically ill, Laguna Niguel, Calif, 1990, AACN.

Association of Operating Room Nurses: Outcome standards for perioperative nursing. In *Standards and recommended practices for perioperative nursing*, Denver, 1993, AORN.

Biddle C, Cannady MJ: Surgical positions: their effects on cardiovascular, respiratory systems, *AORN J* 52(2):350, 1990.

Dellasega C, Rothrock JC: The aging patient. In Rothrock JC: *Perioperative nursing care planning*, St Louis, 1990, Mosby.

Joy C: Pediatric surgery. In Rothrock JC: *Perioperative nursing care planning*, St Louis, 1990, Mosby.

Kirklin JW, Barratt-Boyes B: *Cardiac surgery*, ed 2, New York, 1993, Churchill Livingstone.

Kneedler JA, Dodge GH: *Perioperative patient care: the nursing perspective*, ed 2, Boston, 1987, Blackwell Scientific Publications.

Litwak RS, Dack S: Concepts of patient care. In Litwak RS, Jurado RA: *Care of the cardiac surgical patient*, Norwalk, Conn, 1982, Appleton-Century-Crofts.

McFarland GK, McFarlane EA: *Nursing diagnosis and intervention: planning for patient care*, ed 2, St Louis, 1993, Mosby.

Rothrock JC: Generic care planning. In Rothrock JC: *Perioperative nursing care planning*, St Louis, 1990, Mosby.

Seifert PC: Cardiac surgery. In Rothrock JC: *Perioperative nursing care planning*, St Louis, 1990, Mosby.

Yura H, Walsh M: *The nursing process: assessing, planning, implementing, evaluating*, ed 5, Norwalk, Conn, 1988, Appleton & Lange.

9

Perioperative Nursing Care

We're always ready.

Anonymous

Do whatever it takes.

Anonymous

Although the existence of a well-prepared plan is implied when patients achieve successful outcomes, it is the actions themselves that result in the surgical goal being met. A plan of care provides guidelines for nursing actions, but there is no one formula that can replace the nurse's judgment and decision-making skill in a given situation. Cardiac surgery patients are complex and do not always respond in a predictable manner. Perioperative nurses must be alert to unexpected changes in the patient's condition and be prepared to intervene appropriately (Boxes 9-1 and 9-2). New information must be assessed, judged for its significance, integrated into the plan of care, and reflected in the actions taken. Priorities may have to be reordered. Interventions may have to be modified or alternative actions followed based on the knowledge, experience, and skill of the nurse.

Nursing actions include not only performing activities to achieve patient outcomes, but also supervising others in carrying out the plan, monitoring the patient's response to interventions, and documenting nursing actions and patient responses (Davis, Kneedler, and Manuel, 1979). The achievement of patient outcomes provides tangible evidence of the success or failure of the interventions and reflects the nurse's intellectual, interpersonal, and technical ability (Yura and Walsh, 1988). A high degree of communication, cooperation, and collaboration among team members is necessary if successful outcomes are to be achieved.

This chapter reviews the activities of a standard cardiac procedure using cardiopulmonary bypass (CPB) with myocardial protection. Generic care plans outlines in Chapter 8 are applicable to these activities. Specific operative procedures and related nursing considerations are discussed in the following chapters.

ADMISSION TO THE CARDIAC SERVICE

The admission process varies according to the underlying pathologic condition and the condition of the patient. Patients admitted for symptoms of congestive heart failure may already be in the hospital for a diagnostic workup and cardiac catheterization. Patients who are hemodynamically stable but too debilitated to withstand the stress of immediate surgery may require nutritional support before the operative procedure is done. Emergency admissions (for acute derangements such as postinfarction ventricular septal rupture or aortic dissection) often come to the operating room (OR) directly from the coronary care unit or after emergency admission to the cardiac catheterization laboratory or the radiology angiography suite. Patients undergoing an elective procedure may be admitted the day before surgery, although an increasing number of patients arrive on the day of surgery because of reimbursement considerations and cost-containment measures. Typical adult admission orders (Box 9-3) are implemented. Same-day admission patients usually have the preoperative laboratory work and consultations performed during the preadmission screening a day or two before they are admitted.

PREOPERATIVE PATIENT TEACHING

The preadmission screening period is an especially good time to perform patient teaching because there may be less stress at this time as compared with the immediate preoperative period (Hedenkamp and Howell, 1986). Patient teaching performed before admission can decrease the amount of instruction nec-

Box 9-1 *RN first assistant considerations during surgery*

Patient/Family Interactions*

In addition to meeting specific teaching needs of patients and families, also promote psychologic well-being and a sense of security by alluding to staff nurses' competence and complimenting fellow caregivers. If there are complaints about care, listen to the concerns and investigate the problem or report it to the appropriate person(s) as warranted.

Always approach families with a positive expression on your face (this does not necessarily mean a broad smile); a frown may cause them to assume that their loved one is in "trouble" and cause unnecessary stress. When talking to families of patients who may die in the OR, be honest about the seriousness of the situation, but always allow the family to retain some hope for improvement (even if survival seems unlikely).

Do not strongly either encourage or discourage a family's viewing of a deceased patient. There may be guilt feelings, denial, and other emotions that affect the decision. If the family wishes to view the body, remove excess blood, etc., cover the body with a clean sheet (the head may be left uncovered), and transfer to a quiet room. Accompany the family to the room and provide chairs and tissues. Offer coffee or water. Stay with the family if it seems appropriate, and touch the body (the head, the hands) to show the family that this is "acceptable" behavior.

Peer Relationships

Participate in general perioperative duties: setting up for surgery, patient preparation (washing, positioning, etc.), cleaning up after the case.

Share knowledge gained from assisting duties with staff (including assistive personnel) in the OR, nursing units, diagnostic laboratories, etc.

Provide rationales for the surgeon's preferences (e.g., suture, instruments); help to differentiate between changes in the surgeon's routine that are an exception versus permanent alterations due to new technology, research findings, etc.

Participate in inservices and staff meetings.

Assist managers with capital and operational budget considerations.

During emergencies, determine whether it is more important for you to scrub in immediately, or whether assistance to the circulator (e.g., grounding, positioning, skin preparation) to get the patient ready is of greater priority. This will differ with each emergency and must be decided on an individual basis.

Technical Considerations

Develop a "disaster" mentality; anticipate and mentally plan for sudden adverse changes (e.g., acute hemorrhage, ventricular fibrillation) in the patient's hemodynamic status; play "what if?"

Inspect inflow lines for air, especially arterial infusion catheters during cannulation, and cardioplegia infusion lines before each delivery of the solution.

When working on the pericardium: be aware of the location of the phrenic nerve; know the location of the tips of the instruments you are holding to prevent injury to the heart, lungs, and other tissue.

Do not obscure the surgeon's vision with instruments, hands, etc.

Do not bump the surgeon's arms or hands; if the surgeon is leaning on your arm or hand, don't move without giving advance warning.

Know the location of the entire length of the suture and verify that it is not caught on an instrument or other item.

Used curved scissors to cut the suture; use scissor tips for cutting; point the tips up or down depending on what will pose the least risk of injuring surrounding tissue.

Retract the right pleura to provide more room for the surgeon to insert a right atrial cannulation pursestring and to attach atrial pacing wires (if bypass is terminated and the inflated lungs are in the way).

Stabilize the handle of the cross-clamp with a rolled or folded towel to prevent wobbling (and possible injury to a blood vessel).

If using a long, narrow (e.g., coronary) suction tip, stabilize the midshaft of the sucker on sternal edge, retractor, hand, etc., for greater control.

Follow the suture so that there is sufficient length between the portion of the suture held in your hand and the needle end of the stitch so that when the surgeon pulls the needle through the tissue, the suture does not tug at your hand and possibly injure tissue.

Avoid holding too much suture between your hand and the needle, which could result in excess suture obscuring the anastomotic site.

When requested to open the jaws of the cross-clamp, do so slowly and smoothly.

Verbalize the patient's systemic blood pressure to the surgeon (especially drops in pressure) when the surgeon is unable to see the monitors during manipulation of the beating heart to inspect anastomoses, potential bleeding sites, etc.

Suction opened pleural space(s) before completion of the procedure.

Look for bleeders in a systematic manner; suction specific areas rather than wide expanses of tissue; suction after cauterizing, applying hemostatic clips, or suture ligating to confirm control of the bleeding site.

*Applicable to all perioperative nurses.

Box 9-2　*Nursing considerations during surgery*

Gail Kaempf, RN, MSN, CNOR
Presbyterian Medical Center of Philadelphia
Philadelphia, Pennsylvania

Circulator

Prior to incision have:
　Blood in refrigerator
　Atrioventricular sequential pacemaker
　Defibrillator turned on and checked
　Backup internal paddles
　Backup sternal saw
Stay close to defibrillator during initial rewarming.
Avoid leaving room during cannulation, warming, or patient's coming off bypass.
Check prosthetic valve inventory before start of case (preferably enough in advance to be able to borrow or express ship in a replacement in time for surgery).

Scrub Nurse

Have an extra pair of gloves for each size used by scrub team.
Identify entire object (e.g., instrument, laparotomy tape) before removing from operative field to avoid snagging a suture, disturbing a clamp attached to a blood vessel, or otherwise causing an injury.
Do not follow suture unless specifically requested to do so.
Prepare for double cannulation for any surgery to right side of heart.
Keep instruments sterile and in order until patient exits room.
Check temperature of topical irrigating solutions immediately prior to use on a beating heart (if cold, may cause heart to fibrillate).

Circulating and Scrub Nurses

Be honest with surgeon—admit mistakes or errors, make surgeon aware of missing items.
Verify that suture packet is what is needed:
　Prior to placing on field (circulator)
　Prior to loading on needle holder (scrub nurse)

Box 9-3　*Preoperative orders: admission to the cardiac service*

Diagnosis _____
Allergies _____ Activity _____
Diet _____ Fluid intake _____
Vital signs _____
Height and weight (kg) _____
Chest x-ray (PA and lateral)
ECG
Blood chemistry,* CBC, PT, PTT bleeding time
Urinalysis
Type and crossmatch
　4 units packed RBCs
　2 units fresh frozen plasma
　10 units platelets
Pulmonary function test with ABGs
Respiratory consult to teach incentive spirometry
Patient teaching by nurse clinician
Medications
　Hypnotic (e.g., Restoril) PO PRN HS
　Persantine 75 mg PO this HS
Old chart to floor
NPO after midnight
Surgical permit
Hibiclens shower HS before surgery
Mandol 1 g to OR with patient

Courtesy John R. Garrett, MD.
ABGs, Arterial blood gasses; *CBC,* complete blood count; *ECG,* electrocardiogram; *HS,* bedtime; *NPO,* nothing by mouth; *OR,* operating room; *PA,* posteroanterior; *PO,* orally; *PRN,* as needed; *PT,* prothrombin time; *PTT,* partial thromboplastin time.
*Blood chemistry includes the following: glucose, acetone, urea nitrogen, creatinine, CO_2 content, sodium, potassium, chloride, calcium, uric acid, phosphorus, magnesium, alkaline phosphatase, amylase, lipase, total protein, albumin, globulin, bilirubin, cholesterol, and triglycerides.

essary during the abbreviated and usually tense period immediately before surgery. Also, it can ease some of the fear and anxiety caused by the impending surgery, as well as concerns about resumption of functional activities, pain, death, absence from home or work, and recuperation (Carr and Powers, 1986).

The perioperative nurse's initial contact with the patient may occur during the preadmission screening, on the nursing unit, or in the preinduction area of the OR. The patient can also expect preoperative visits by anesthesia personnel, surgeons and their associates, and others involved in the care of the patient.

Preoperative teaching assignments vary with the institution. Formal patient teaching may be provided by the patient's primary nurse on the unit, a cardiovascular clinical specialist, or the perioperative nurse.

Many RN first assistants (RNFAs) include this function in their role (Espersen, 1993). Whether the perioperative clinician visits the patient during the preadmission period or just before surgery, it is important that the nurse collect sufficient information to plan the most appropriate care. The interaction is also helpful to the patient because it can provide the reassurance of meeting someone who will be directly involved in giving care during the operation.

When teaching is done on the unit, the perioperative nurse can reinforce what has been taught and provide information that is uniquely related to the surgical environment. This may be as simple as the sights and sounds that one can expect on entry into the OR or as complex as the principles involved in extracorporeal circulation. (Whereas some patients use denial to cope with stress, others rely on knowledge as a defense mechanism.) No matter what is discussed, the information should be accurate and meet the patient's identified needs.

The surgeon reviews the operative plan and discusses the benefits and risks of the operation in order to obtain an informed consent from the patient. Preoperative communication between the surgeon, the patient, and the patient's significant others educates the patient and family about associated risks and benefits and provides information to the surgeon and nurse about the patient's expectations, fears, concerns, and coping strategies, all of which are important for perioperative patient management. Ensuring that the patient and family are properly informed and know what to expect before, during, and after surgery can facilitate a smooth postoperative experience (Harlan, Starr, and Harwin, 1980).

Any fears of the patient regarding the risks of blood transfusion should be addressed and have prompted some states to enact blood safety laws. These laws require that when blood transfusion may be necessary during surgery, the patient must be informed preoperatively of all available methods of receiving blood transfusions—autologous and homologous. One of the few exceptions for complying with the law is the need for emergency surgery (COBE Laboratories, 1993).

Patients can meet the cardiac surgery critical care nurses and visit the postoperative unit to prepare themselves for their postsurgical experience. However, patients and/or families may not wish to see the intensive care unit (ICU) if it arouses fear and dread. These wishes should be respected, but family members or close friends planning to see the patient in the immediate postoperative period should be prepared for what they will see in the patient: multiple lines and catheters, pallor, cool skin, some facial edema, and unresponsiveness. Even though the patient may not be able to react, visitors should be encouraged to talk to the patient for their own psychologic welfare, and possibly for the patient's as well.

ADVANCE DIRECTIVES

Advances in health care technology and the increase in the number of elderly patients undergoing cardiac surgery has created ethical and legal challenges for health care workers. In particular, there is now the capability of extending life beyond the point where patients are capable of making decisions or expressing wishes about future health needs. To avoid uncertainty about a patient's wishes, advance communication between the patient, family, and health care providers can alleviate some of the problems that may arise during a health care crisis (American Association of Retired Persons [AARP], 1986). The passage of the Patient Self-Determination Act enables patients, on admission to the hospital, to provide instructions about their wishes should they become terminally ill or have little hope of being weaned from life support. Advance directives include living wills, durable powers of attorney, and anatomic gifts.

Living wills are documents concerning treatment that direct others about the care desired by the patient who is terminally ill and unable to provide further instruction. Generally, these documents express a desire not to prolong imminent death; care necessary to maintain comfort and dignity should be provided.

Durable powers of attorney delegate either very broad or specific authority to a proxy, who makes decisions about health care needs. This authority endures if the patient becomes incapable of making his or her own decisions (Reigle, 1992). Often a spouse is the delegated authority (AARP, 1986). If the patient chooses, the authority can be revoked at any time.

Anatomic donations of body tissue and organs may also be arranged in advance. The Uniform Anatomical Gift Act of 1968, as well as the revisions made to the act in 1987, permits the donor to sign a legally valid document authorizing such gifts without the need for additional permission by family members (Hawke, Kraft, and Smith, 1990). In the absence of the patient's documented desire to donate, an anatomic gift may be made by family members in the following order of priority: spouse, adult child, parent, adult brother or sister, or guardian (Reigle, 1992). The Omnibus Reconciliation Act of 1986 was enacted to require hospitals receiving Medicare or Medicaid reimbursement to request organ donation from family members.

ENTRY INTO THE OPERATING ROOM

The cardiac surgery patient's risk for sudden decompensation mandates that unpredictability should be expected. Certain assumptions are warranted. Chief among these are the importance of maintaining the balance between myocardial oxygen supply and demand, and the deleterious effects that a disproportionate increase on the demand side (or decrease on the supply side) has on cardiac function. Nursing actions should be implemented with these assumptions in mind.

The preoperative assessment begins as the nurse approaches the patient: Is the patient sitting up and alert to the surroundings? Are there attending critical care nurses, and monitors and other equipment on the transport stretcher, indicating a more unstable status?

The circulating nurse greets the patient by name and checks the identification band. Patients may feel cold and uncomfortable. Offering a warm blanket is not only a comfort measure, but also reduces the metabolic impact of shivering. The proposed operation is confirmed, and any patient allergies are elicited. Questions and concerns should be answered and clarified; however, patients may be hesitant to initiate a discussion that they feel might heighten their anxiety. Family members may be in attendance, and they should be included in these interactions.

Often the family will have been given an approximate time period for the anticipated length of surgery. The perioperative nurse should ask the family what they have been told. Occasionally the time frame provided by the surgeon (actual surgical time) needs to be expanded to include the activities performed immediately before the incision is made (e.g., insertion of monitoring lines, skin preparation) and actions after the skin is closed (e.g., application of dressings, attachment to portable monitors). These activities can add 1 to 2 hours to the original time estimate relayed to the family. There may be unnecessary concern when the initial time period has passed and the family is still waiting to receive word that the surgery is completed. Another consideration is that once the patient arrives in the ICU, admission procedures (e.g., checking vital signs, connecting monitoring lines and drainage tubes) must be performed. It may be as long as 1 hour before family members can first see the patient. Families tend to watch the clock closely, and offering a simple explanation of the various procedures that are performed in addition to the surgical repair itself can alleviate some of their emotional stress.

Another source of stress may be the cancellation of surgery due to an insufficient number of ICU beds or to another patient's need for emergency surgery taking precedence over the scheduled operation. The increased anxiety and emotional stress accompanying the decision to cancel the operation may produce ischemic discomfort, dyspnea, and shortness of breath, and the nurse should be vigilant in observing the patient for these signs (Bresser, Sexton, and Foell, 1993). Patients and families may be angry and feel a loss of control, but most accept the postponement, realizing that they themselves could be the ones needing an emergency operation. Perioperative nurses can reassure patients and family members that feelings of anger are understandable (and acceptable) and that the decision was made only after careful deliberation.

Chart Review

The perioperative nurse reviews the hospital record for completion of laboratory work, operative permits, results of diagnostic studies, history and physical examination, medications, and other pertinent data. In the case of patients scheduled for coronary artery bypass grafting who underwent cardiac catheterization during a previous hospitalization, the old chart will be needed so that the test results can be reviewed. Special note should also be taken of abnormal laboratory values: prolonged bleeding times, elevated or low potassium levels (normal 3.5 to 5.5 mEq), cardiac enzymes, liver problems, and other results that may have a direct bearing on the surgical procedure.

The most recent chest x-ray films (posteroanterior and lateral) should be available for evaluation of the heart and lungs, especially in patients undergoing repeat sternotomy whose pericardial adhesions may be against the sternum. In addition, the surgeon will want to view the cineangiogram of coronary artery bypass patients to note the location, size, and severity of coronary artery lesions; assess the pattern of coronary blood flow; and evaluate the contractile state of the heart. Portable cine viewers are often located near the OR, and the perioperative nurse may be responsible for obtaining these films before surgery.

MONITORING

Patients usually have peripheral intravenous (IV) lines inserted in the preinduction area; intraarterial blood pressure monitoring lines (A-lines) may also be started at this time or in the OR itself. A local anesthetic may be used at the insertion site(s) and a sedative injected IV to allay the patient's anxiety. Additional central monitoring lines, such as a pulmonary artery catheter, are inserted in the OR (Table 9-1). Whether these are placed before or after anesthesia induction and intubation is decided by the anesthesiologist and varies from institution to institution. The nurse should remain close to the patient during induction and observe the monitors for signs of hemodynamic instability and cardiac rhythm disturbances (Fig. 9-1).

If the patient is intubated first, the nursing staff can apply the electrosurgical dispersive pads, catheterize the bladder, and position and wash the patient while the monitoring lines are being inserted. These nursing activities may have to be halted temporarily if assistance is needed to insert the central lines. The nurse should observe the electrocardiogram (ECG) and blood pressure monitors frequently for signs of hypotension or ventricular irritability, such as ectopy, tachycardia, or fibrillation. The defibrillator should be positioned near the patient so that it is readily available if needed.

In patients who are in cardiogenic shock, there may be no time to establish invasive monitoring lines. The most important consideration for the anesthesiologist is to have a patent IV line so that medications and volume can be infused. Monitoring can be achieved with noninvasive methods: ECG, blood pressure cuff, pulse oximeter for arterial hemoglobin saturation, and capnography for end-tidal carbon dioxide measurements. Intravascular lines can be inserted after the patient has been stabilized (Skeehan and Marshall, 1990).

If the anesthesiologist prefers to introduce the pulmonary (or central venous) pressure catheter before endotracheal intubation, most nursing activities should be delayed until the patient has been anesthetized. Padding of the hands and elbows can usually be performed at any time, but this and other interventions should be done in consultation with anesthesia personnel to prevent unnecessary stimulation of the patient. (Postponing padding of the hands may also enable the nurse to hold the hand of an anxious patient during induction.)

After the patient is intubated, a urinary drainage catheter is inserted to prevent bladder distension and to monitor renal function, especially during and after CPB. The catheter may contain a temperature probe; other temperature monitoring devices may be used in the esophagus, nasopharynx, or rectum. (CPB in-line sensors are used to measure blood temperatures, and ventricular septal temperature probes may be inserted during induced cardiac arrest.)

Transesophageal echocardiography (TEE) has enabled clinicians to make immediate perioperative an-

Table 9-1 ■ *Physiologic monitoring*

Monitoring device	Location	Assesses/measures
Cardiovascular System		
ECG	Electrodes placed on shoulders, hips, and left axillary line	Electrical activity of heart: lead II useful to monitor cardiac rhythm (good visualization of P wave and QRS) and myocardial ischemia (inferior surface); lead V5 useful to detect myocardial ischemia (anterior surface)
Intraarterial catheter	Radial artery (also: femoral artery, aorta, bypass circuit; in children, may use superficial temporal or dorsalis pedis arteries; in neonates, may use umbilical artery)	Direct arterial blood pressure (BP); blood gasses; blood chemistries
Blood pressure cuff	Right or left arm	Indirect BP
Central venous pressure (CVP) line	Right atrium (RA)	RA pressure (CVP); right ventricular (RV) filling pressure; RV preload
Pulmonary artery (PA) catheter	PA (proximal and distal)	PA pressures: systolic, diastolic, mean, wedge; pulmonary vascular resistance; left ventricular (LV) filling pressure; LV preload; cardiac output (CO); assessment of stroke volume, stroke work, systemic vascular resistance; mixed venous saturation (continuous indirect assessment of CO)
Left atrial (LA) catheter (when used)	LA	LA pressure (direct); LV filling pressure; LV preload
Transesophageal echocardiography (TEE)	Esophagus	Valve function before and after repair; LV wall motion, failure; intracardiac air bubbles
Urinary drainage catheter	Urinary bladder	Urinary output, renal perfusion; indirect measure of CO
Respiratory System		
Mass spectrometry	Anesthesia circuit	Inspired/expired O_2, CO_2, and anesthetic gasses; used to avoid hypoxia, hypercarbia, anesthetic overdose
Pulse oximeter	Finger or toe cot; earlobe, nose	Oxygen saturation of arterial hemoglobin; tissue oxygenation
Capnography	Anesthesia circuit	End-tidal CO_2; used to detect integrity of anesthesia circuit; avoid disconnections of monitor, endotracheal tube; detect spontaneous ventilation, rebreathing, obstructive pulmonary disease
Central Nervous System		
Temperature	Esophagus, nasopharynx, urinary bladder, rectum, ventricular septum, bypass circuit, PA catheter	Core and peripheral temperature of heart, brain, and other organs
Electroencephalogram (when used)	Scalp electrodes	Detect cerebral ischemia, embolus; indication of depth of anesthesia
Renal System		
Urinary drainage catheter	Bladder	Urinary output; indirect measure of cardiac output

Modified from Skeehan TM, Marshall WK,: The cardiac operating room. In Hensley FA, Martin DE, editors: *The practice of cardiac anesthesia*, Boston, 1990, Little, Brown.

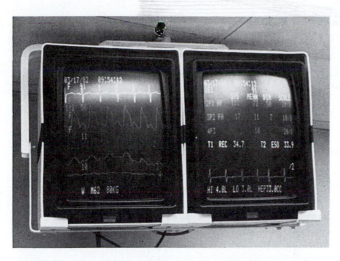

Fig. 9-1 Monitor screens can display ECG; systemic, pulmonary, and central venous pressures and waveforms; esophageal and rectal temperatures; high and low bypass flows; and name (obscured), age, weight, sex, and heparin dose. (Courtesy Doug Yarnold, CRNA.)

atomic and physiologic diagnoses. Not only is TEE frequently used to assess valvular repairs, but it is also increasingly being used to monitor signs of myocardial ischemia, ventricular function, intracardiac air, and maldistribution of cardioplegia (McCloskey, 1991).

INTRAOPERATIVE MEDICATIONS

Numerous medications (Table 9-2) are used during surgery. Among these are drugs to maintain hemodynamic stability, maximize cardiac output, and promote metabolic homeostasis. Anesthesia, perfusion, and nursing services generally have specific patient drug needs, and the creation of individual medication exchange carts, jointly planned with pharmacy personnel, can be efficient and helpful. Nurses may wish to include heparin, topical antibiotics and hemostatic agents, 1% lidocaine (Xylocaine) (for topical anesthesia), calcium chloride, intracardiac epinephrine, papaverine, and other medications that may be needed by the sterile team. Perioperative nursing responsibilities for medications vary and should be reflected in the drug inventory maintained by the OR nursing staff.

Medications used before or during induction are selected with consideration given to their effects on myocardial oxygen supply and demand. In patients with obstructive coronary lesions, the supply of blood is relatively fixed, and interventions are aimed at minimizing or reducing myocardial oxygen demand. Drugs are used to control myocardial contractility, blood pressure and heart rate, ventricular wall tension, circulatory blood volume, and aortic pressure and coronary blood flow. Hypotension unresponsive to volume administration may be treated with vasocon-

Table 9-2 ■ *Medications used in adults during cardiac surgery**

Medication	Purpose/description/delivery
Analgesics and Anesthetics	
Thiopental	Induction, ultrashort-acting barbiturate, intravenous bolus
Fentanyl (Sublimaze)	Synthetic narcotic, intravenous bolus and/or infusion
Sufentanil (Sufenta)	Synthetic narcotic, intravenous bolus and/or infusion
Alfentanil (Alfenta)	Synthetic narcotic, intravenous bolus and/or infusion
Morphine	Narcotic, intravenous bolus
Halothane (Fluothane)	Inhalation anesthetic, maintenance
Enflurane (Ethrane)	Inhalation anesthetic, maintenance
Isoflurane (Forane)	Inhalation anesthetic, maintenance
Muscle Relaxants	
Vecuronium (Norcuron)	Intubation, maintenance of muscle relaxation
Pancuronium (Pavulon)	Maintenance of muscle relaxation
Amnesiacs	
Midazolam (Versed)	Hypnotic; anxiety-reducing sedative
Scopolamine	Sedative; amnesic
Cardiovascular Agents	
Anticholinergics	
Atropine	Decreases vagal tone; treats sinus bradycardia
Glycopyrrolate (Robinul)	Similar to atropine but has less incidence of dysrhythmias than atropine with slower onset
Vasopressors	
Norepinephrine (Levophed)	Increases force and velocity of contraction; increases systemic and pulmonary vascular resistance
Phenylephrine (Neo-synephrine)	Arteriolar and venous vasoconstriction; increases blood pressure and systemic vascular resistance

Modified from Larach DR: Cardiovascular drugs. In Hensley FA, Martin DE, editors: *The practice of anesthesia*, Boston, 1990, Little, Brown. *Continued.*

Table 9-2 ■ *Medications used in adults during cardiac surgery—cont'd*

Medication	Purpose/description/delivery
Vasodilators	
Nitroglycerin (Tridil)	Dilates coronary arteries; reduces preload
Phentolamine (Regitine)	Decreases systemic and pulmonary vascular resistance
Prostaglandin E 1 (Prostin VR)	Vascular smooth muscle dilator, potent pulmonary vascular dilator; used to maintain patency of ductus arteriosus in cyanotic neonates, patients with severe pulmonary hypertension
Nitroprusside (Nipride)	Arteriolar and venous vasodilatation; reduces preload and afterload
Inotropic Agents	
Amrinone (Inocor)	Increases cardiac output, force and velocity of contraction
Calcium chloride	In ionized form, increases cardiac output, BP, and contractility
Dopamine (Intropin)	In low doses, increases renal and mesenteric perfusion; with moderate doses increases heart rate, contractility, and cardiac output; in higher doses increases systemic and pulmonary vascular resistance
Dobutamine (Dobutrex)	Increases contractility with less increase in heart rate than occurs with dopamine; has vasodilatation effect on vascular bed
Ephedrine	Increases contractility, cardiac output, and BP
Epinephrine (Adrenalin)	Increases rate and strength of contraction, BP (effective brochodilator)
Isoproterenol (Isuprel)	Increases heart rate, contractility, cardiac output; decreases systemic vascular resistance
Antidysrhythmics	
Lidocaine (Xylocaine)	Acts on ventricles; decreases automaticity of ischemic ventricular tissue
Bretylium (Bretylol)	Prolongs duration of action potential and refractory period; useful for ventricular dysrhythmias refractory to therapy
Digoxin (Lanoxin)	Decreases ventricular rate in atrial fibrillation or flutter, and other supraventricular dysrhythmias; avoid in patients with Wolff-Parkinson-White syndrome and other accessory atrioventricular pathways
Nifedipine (Procardia)	Calcium channel blocker; reduces coronary artery spasm; produces coronary vasodilatation; extremely light sensitive; must be given PO or via nasal or oral mucosa; antihypertensive
Procainamide (Pronestyl)	Decreases automaticity and conduction in all cardiac tissue (normal and ischemic); stabilizes cellular membranes
Quinidine	Similar to procainamide; atrial and ventricular dysrhythmias
Verapamil (Calan, Isoptin)	Calcium channel blocker; used to treat atrial dysrhythmias; slows ventricular rate in atrial fibrillation or flutter; can be given IV
Adenosine	Supraventricular dysrhythmias
Diuretics	
Furosemide (Lasix)	Decreases renal absorption of sodium and chloride; increases excretion of water and electrolytes, especially potassium, sodium, chloride, magnesium, and calcium
Mannitol	Osmotic diuretic; pulls free water out of organs (reducing cerebral edema); protects kidneys
Anticoagulants/Coagulants	
Heparin	Systemic anticoagulation during CPB; blocks activation of thrombin (and intrinsic clotting cascade)
Protamine sulfate	Heparin antagonist; NPH insulin-dependent diabetic patients may be at increased risk for protamine reaction
Antibiotics	
Cephalosporins (Mandol, Ancef, Keflex, Keflin, Cefadyl)	Broad-spectrum prophylaxis
Tobramycin (Nebcin)	Aerobic gram-negative and gram-positive bacteria
Vancomycin	Severe endocarditis
Bacitracin	Topical irrigation
Miscellaneous	
Lidocaine 1% (plain)	Local anesthesia
Papaverine	Reduces arterial spasm (e.g., mammary artery)
Potassium	Replaces electrolyte loss
Sodium bicarbonate	Corrects acidosis
Insulin (NPH, etc.)	Corrects hyperglycemia in diabetic patients
Topical hemostatic agents	Intraoperative control of bleeding
Desmopressin (DDAVP)	Pharmacologic hemostatic agent

strictors and inotropic drugs; hypertension may respond to additional anesthetic drugs, vasodilators, beta blockers (e.g., propranolol hydrochloride [Inderal]), or a combination of these. Anesthesia is achieved with a combination of agents to provide sleep, amnesia, analgesia, muscle relaxation, and blunting of autonomic nervous system reflexes (Kirklin and Barratt-Boyes, 1993).

POSITIONING AND SKIN PREPARATION
Positioning

The supine position is the most commonly used position for cardiac surgery because it exposes the entire anterior chest, both groins for femoral artery access, and, when needed, the legs for saphenous vein excision. The surgeon can make a median sternotomy incision (see Chapter 11), which provides excellent exposure for surgery of the heart and great vessels and facilitates cannulation for a CPB. Patients in the supine position generally have their arms tucked along the side. Special caution should be taken when tucking the arms to prevent disruption of peripheral IV infusion lines and intraarterial blood pressure monitoring lines (A-lines). The nurse should confirm with anesthesia personnel that IV lines are infusing properly and that the arterial waveform has not been damped or otherwise adversely affected. The A-line is frequently placed in the radial artery; a splint may need to be applied to the wrist to maintain the correct position of the arterial catheter. In obese patients the neck should be slightly extended so that the sternal notch can be incorporated into the field during draping and visualized for sternal splitting.

A left full-lateral or semilateral position in conjunction with a thoracotomy incision is used for operations requiring access to the descending thoracic aorta and for some procedures on the transverse aortic arch (see Chapter 16). Right lateral thoracotomies may be used for repeat mitral valve procedures. When the patient is positioned laterally, access to the legs and groin may be more difficult. With the right leg flexed, the right femoral artery is more easily accessible than the left in patients placed in the left full-lateral position. If femoral artery cannulation for bypass is planned, the nurse should provide an adequate area in which to insert and secure the cannula.

Additional nursing considerations related to positioning for median sternotomy and lateral incisions are given in Chapters 8 and 11. The reader is also referred to perioperative nursing texts for a fuller discussion of positioning techniques.

Skin Preparation

Hair removal is a subject of debate. In the past, cardiac patients often had full body shaves, but this practice has been largely abandoned. Most male patients, however, do have hair removed along the sternal midline from the sternal notch to just above the umbilicus.

Female patients rarely require chest hair removal, and for cosmetic reasons the procedure is avoided. In coronary artery bypass patients, the skin along the inner aspect of the leg (in the path of the greater saphenous vein) is often clipped (or shaved). Hair in the inguinal region is also removed should entry into the femoral artery be required.

Numerous studies have demonstrated an increased incidence of skin damage and postoperative wound infection associated with intraoperative shaving, and the technique is not recommended. When hair removal is considered necessary, the use of depilatories or sterile skin clippers (rather than razors) has been suggested. Ideally, hair removal is done outside of the OR (Rothrock, 1993). However, patients admitted directly for emergency surgery will require hair removal in the OR. Clippers should be immediately available for such occurrences.

Antimicrobial agents are applied to the skin as expeditiously as possible without jeopardizing antisepsis. Povidone-iodine provides antimicrobial activity for up to 8 hours and is widely used for skin preparation. In gel form it can be applied rapidly to the anterior chest, abdomen, groin, legs, and feet. Patients with iodine sensitivity may be prepared with chlorhexidine gluconate, but its antimicrobial activity endures for only about 4 hours (Rothrock, 1993).

Skin preparation to the knees is recommended for all cardiac surgery patients because access to the femoral arteries may be required for intraaortic balloon or pressure monitoring line insertion. If saphenous vein is to be removed, a circumferential leg preparation (to and including the feet) is recommended. The feet can be placed on a "picket fence" (see Chapter 5) to elevate the legs.

It is also recommended that skin preparation solutions or gels routinely be readily available when patients enter the OR. Not infrequently, a patient may suddenly become hemodynamically unstable, and precious time may be wasted organizing a table to wash the skin. In extreme emergencies antimicrobial solutions can be quickly sprayed onto the skin.

DRAPING

General principles are followed for draping the patient (Kleinbeck, 1991), with special consideration given to bypass lines and the multiple surgical sites that may exist (e.g., chest, legs, and groin for femoral access). Goals for draping the cardiac surgical patient include:

- Exposing the surgical site(s)—chest, legs, groin
- Maintaining sterility of the field, including instruments and equipment, and bypass lines
- Ensuring that the sterile end of bypass lines and other items passed off the field are securely attached to the drapes
- Ensuring that suction lines, bypass and cardioplegia infusion lines, electrosurgical pencils, defibrillator paddles, pressure monitoring lines, and pacemaker cables are easily and quickly accessible

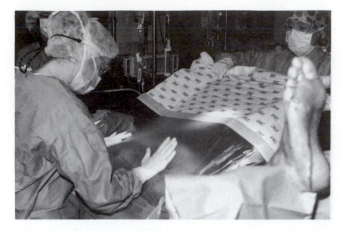

Fig. 9-2 Application of an adhesive, antimicrobial drape to the chest. (Photograph by Howard Kaye.)

- Creating a surface for instruments, such as needle holders, forceps, and suture tags, so that they do not slide off the field (e.g., using a magnetic mat or forming a flat surface with towels)
- Minimizing the potential for suture snagging on drapes, instruments, or other items (e.g., covering retractor handles with a towel or moist laparotomy tape)

Tangling of cords and tubing should be avoided; the nurse can arrange these so that there is an adequate length of cords and/or tubing to reach the area required on the field (e.g., the length of the defibrillator cable on the field should be sufficient for the attached paddle tips to reach the inside of the pericardium without the clinician's having to tug on the cords).

Clear plastic adhesive drapes impregnated with iodophor or other bactericidal agent (Fig. 9-2) are often applied to the chest and occasionally to the legs. Some centers use stockinette to cover the feet and legs; the surgeon can cut through this material to expose the leg. The feet can be wrapped in towels secured with a towel clip.

Adhesive drapes are also useful for covering the exit site of catheters or pressure lines in the groin of patients who come to the OR with these in place. It is difficult to prepare these areas adequately, and they should be draped out of the sterile field. The catheter can be covered with a folded sterile towel, with the adhesive placed over this and the surrounding area to exclude it from the sterile field.

A "belly band" (incorporated into a disposable draping system [Fig. 9-3] or made from towels) can be placed across the umbilicus and attached to either side of the drape. Bypass lines can be securely attached to the band where it meets the side drape. The band should not be positioned so high as to cover the chest tube exit sites or so low as to obscure the common femoral artery.

Side pockets help to keep lines and other items readily available without cluttering the field. Drapes designed for cardiac surgery (see Fig. 9-2) usually have a trough or pockets along each side. Individual pock-

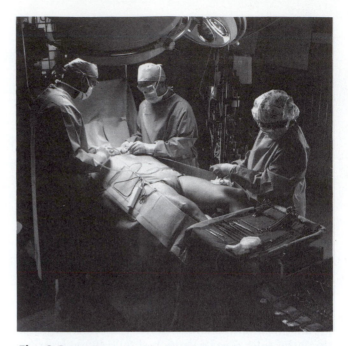

Fig. 9-3 Cardiovascular draping system provides exposure of the chest, groin, and legs. (Courtesy Kimberly-Clark Professional Health Care.)

ets can also be made from towels and attached to the drapes with towel clips. To maintain sterility, nonpenetrating towel clips should be used if they are to be adjusted or removed during the procedure.

Drapes should be waterproof. They should extend below the level of the patient but not touch the floor. Draping of equipment and furniture (e.g., instruments tables, Mayo stand, slush machine, ring stands) should take into consideration their different heights. Drapes should be long enough (without touching the floor) so that if these items come into contact with each other, cross-contamination does not occur.

Many companies make disposable drape packs for cardiac surgery that combine a variety of drapes for the procedure. Customized drape packs can also be put together that include sheets, gowns, towels, and other desired items. Packs are advantageous in that they reduce setup time.

INFECTION CONTROL MEASURES

Planning for infection control is outlined in Chapter 8. Implementing activities to minimize the risk of infection is affected by patient factors, by how team members perform, and by the environment in which they must work. Strict aseptic practices are mandatory, but small, cramped ORs present a challenge to perioperative cardiac nurses interacting with many persons, managing multiple pieces of equipment, and caring for surgical patients whose compromised cardiovascular system places them at risk for infection.

Traffic patterns should be established that reduce movement within the OR, and entering and exiting the room by personnel should be kept to a minimum. The arrangement of furniture and other items needs to be done in a way that protects the sterility of the instruments, supplies, and drapes. Consolidating equipment is one alternative. Carts can be constructed (or purchased) that allow stacking of equipment such as electrocautery devices and the defibrillator. Suspending items from the ceiling (with a handle that allows the nurse to adjust the height) is another option. The motor of an electric sternal saw may be attached to the surgeon's headlight power source; the air tanks of pneumatically powered saws can be moved to a peripheral area of the room once the chest has been opened. Extra-long electrical cords may allow other items (e.g., hypothermia/hyperthermia units) to be positioned farther away from the surgical field and thus provide more room for personnel to move around the operative area without contacting sterile areas.

Patient factors must be considered. In addition to the intrinsic cardiac disease, other physiologic alterations may predispose the patient to infection. Patients with a colostomy or ileostomy require special interventions (e.g., using an adhesive antimicrobial drape) to exclude the stoma or ostomy device from the sterile field. Patients arriving in the OR with femoral artery catheters (intraaortic balloon pumps [IABPs], pressure lines) can be managed in a similar manner. IABPs and ventricular assist devices (VADs) pose challenges in addition to the potential for contamination. The integrity of the lines and catheters must also be protected, and team members must work in unison during transfer to the OR bed, positioning, skin preparation, and draping. Additional personnel may be needed to perform these activities safely.

For patients returning to the OR for control of postoperative bleeding, chest dressings should be removed with aseptic technique to avoid contamination of the incision. Other dressings are removed as necessary. The leg dressing in coronary artery bypass patients may remain and be covered with the sterile drapes. The contralateral groin may or may not be included in the operative site, depending on the surgeon's preference. Skin preparation and draping will be influenced by the anticipated findings, and the nurse should discuss this with the surgeon before the skin is prepared.

Dressings applied to the internal jugular or subclavian venous exit sites for invasive pressure lines should be kept out of the sterile field. These dressings may have to be reapplied or their edges trimmed to achieve this.

Although postoperative cardiothoracic infections are relatively rare, the development of mediastinitis can be a life-threatening complication (Bor and others, 1983). Perioperative antibiotic prophylaxis has proved to be a consistent benefit as an adjunct to aseptic and antiseptic practices in avoiding postoperative wounds. Various antibiotic regimens using first- and second-generation cephalosporins may be followed. Kreter and Woods' (1992) metaanalysis of clinical trials over a 30-year period demonstrated a one-and-one-half-fold reduction in wound infection rates with cefamandole and cefuroxime as compared with cefazolin. Other antibiotics also have specific indications for use. The emergence of methicillin-resistant (gram-positive) *Staphylococcus aureus* has led to prophylaxis with vancomycin in conjunction with an additional agent that can cover gram-negative pathogens.

TRANSFUSION THERAPY AND BLOOD CONSERVATION
Homologous Blood

Although the indications for transfusion of homologous blood and blood products have undergone a change as a result of the risk of blood-borne diseases, blood transfusion can be a lifesaving measure in patients with reduced oxygen-carrying capacity, coagulopathies, or hypovolemia. Alternative measures such as volume expanders and artificial blood may not be suitable for the patient. Blood availability remains a necessary aspect of cardiac surgery. The main indication for transfusion is to enhance the oxygen-carrying capacity of the blood; the decision is based on the hemoglobin and hematocrit count, as well as the clinical status of the patient.

At least four units of packed red blood cells (RBCs) are generally ordered for cardiac surgery patients. The blood should be in the OR before the patient arrives. Many cardiac OR suites have their own blood refrigerator, which permits rapid access to the blood.

The units should be initially checked (e.g., patient's name and hospital record number, blood type, and unit number) when the blood is delivered to the OR and before it is stored in the blood refrigerator. Just before transfusion, it should be checked again by the person hanging the unit and by a witness. In large OR suites, blood refrigerators may contain the blood of more than one patient, and transfusion errors can be greatly reduced by confirming that patients are receiving the blood ordered for them. At the end of the procedure, any remaining units of blood should be promptly returned to the blood bank or sent to the ICU with the patient and stored in the ICU's blood refrigerator.

In addition to units of packed RBCs, fresh frozen plasma, platelets, and other blood products should be available, but these do not need to be prepared (e.g., thawed) and brought to the OR unless they are needed to enhance coagulation. These products, once ready, should not be refrigerated, and there is a time limit for their use. Wasting of blood products can be reduced by assessing the patient's hemodynamic and hemostatic status, and by communication with the surgeon and anesthesia personnel.

Transfusion Reaction

The nurse should be alert to transfusion reactions. An acute hemolytic reaction is the most severe reaction and can be fatal. Bloody urine and hemodynamic al-

Table 9-3 ■ *Cellular composition of autologous blood collected by various methods*

Method of collection	Red blood cells	Platelets	Coagulation factors	Comment
Preoperative deposit	+	−	+ / −	Platelets and labile factors V and VIII decrease rapidly with storage time
Normovolemic hemodilution	+	+	+	High levels of platelet and coagulation factor activities are present if used on day of collection
Intraoperative salvage				
Unwashed	+	+ / −	+	Platelets may be present, but functional activity is unknown
Washed	+	−	−	Platelets and coagulation factors are removed by washing
Postoperative salvage (unwashed)	+	+ / −	+ / −	Platelets and coagulation factors are consumed in the operative wound; levels may be severely reduced and are unlikely to be therapeutic

From Stack G, Snyder EL: Alternative to perioperative blood transfusion. In Stoelting RK, editor: *Advances in anesthesia,* vol 8, St Louis, 1991, Mosby.

terations are notable signs that alert the clinician. Signs and symptoms usually associated with transfusion reactions, such as chills, anxiety, dyspnea, and pain, are of little use in the anesthetized patient. Even skin changes such as hives and rashes may not be readily apparent when surgical drapes cover most of the body. If such a complication occurs, the transfusion should be discontinued immediately and the institutional protocol implemented (American Association of Blood Banks, 1987).

Occasionally, massive blood transfusions are required for severe bleeding. The importance of good working relationships with the blood bank cannot be overemphasized for rapidly acquiring large amounts of blood and having additional units prepared expeditiously. It is helpful if the blood bank is notified as soon in advance as possible as to the blood needs of the patient.

Autologous Blood

Autologous blood salvaging methods (Table 9-3) have enhanced blood conservation and reduced (but not eliminated) the need for homologous bank blood. Autologous blood transfusions are now considered the safest form of transfusion therapy (Council on Scientific Affairs, 1986).

The first autologous transfusions were performed as early as 1921 when Dr. F.C. Grant collected a patient's blood preoperatively and later infused it during surgery. With the increased concern about the transmission of viral diseases, predeposit programs and intraoperative blood-salvaging techniques began to increase (Cobe Laboratories, 1991).

Predeposit donation can be considered in patients undergoing an elective procedure and whose condition allows phlebotomy; blood should not be collected within 72 hours before surgery. Directed donation (by a specific individual known to the patient) is requested

by some patients, but the safety of this technique over standard blood collection methods is questionable.

Another form of autotransfusion can be performed before the start of the operation. Blood is withdrawn from the patient and placed into collection bags to be reinfused later during the procedure. Blood removed is replaced with volume expanders. An advantage of this method is that it provides fresh whole blood with viable platelets and clotting factors. Autotransfusion can also be accomplished with the use of the cardiotomy suction during CPB. Blood from the surgical site is aspirated into the bypass machine and enters the CPB circuit, from where it can be infused back into the body (see Chapter 11).

Blood Salvaging Devices

With autotransfusion devices the patient's blood (and other matter) is aspirated into a sterile collection system, where the blood is washed, concentrated, and reinfused as needed (some systems filter the aspirate and then reinfuse it without including a washing cycle). Anticoagulation is necessary to prevent clot formation in the circuit; heparin or citrate can be used.

Available commercial devices include those using suction cannisters, semicontinuous flow systems (see Chapter 5), or single-use disposable devices. Collected blood that has been heparinized may retain systemic anticoagulation if the blood is not adequately washed. To reduce hemolysis, these devices should be used to aspirate pools of blood rather than skimming tissue surfaces, because this creates a traumatic blood-air interface (Stack and Snyder, 1991).

Blood replacement in Jehovah's Witnesses presents a special challenge. Semiautomated centrifugal systems can be adapted so that the RBCs remain in a continuous circuit within the patient's intravascular space. In addition, present methods of CPB using crystalloid priming solution have been largely successful in avoiding blood transfusions. In most cases patients were able to tolerate the hemodilution and the reduction of circulating RBC mass (Tinker and Roberts, 1987). Pharmacologic and topical hemostatic agents (see later in chapter) can reduce bleeding and the need for transfusion.

DEFIBRILLATION

Current methods of myocardial protection (see Chapter 11), such as those using warm cardioplegia solution for initial and final infusion, have enhanced the global distribution of the solution. This has contributed to better preservation of the myocardial substrates that are necessary for the resumption of cardiac function once the aortic occlusion clamp is removed. Hearts often start to contract spontaneously when the clamp is removed and warm blood enters the coronary circulation (and washes out the residual cardioplegia solution).

Nevertheless, the heart is irritable and may fibrillate if inadvertently touched. If the heart starts to fibrillate, a shock of electrical current is delivered directly to the cardiac surface with internal defibrillator paddles. Both the sterile nurse and the circulating nurse should monitor the ECG for ventricular fibrillation and prepare to defibrillate the patient. (The sterile nurse can also observe the heart directly while the aortic cross-clamp is removed to detect fibrillation.) By monitoring the ECG and observing the sterile team members, circulating nurses will be aware of whether defibrillation will be required and can position themselves near the defibrillator to charge the power source and discharge the current when requested to do so by the surgeon.

The standard level of energy current for internal defibrillation in the adult is 10 to 20 joules; this dose will defibrillate more than 90% of fibrillating hearts. Lower settings often require repeat shocks; higher settings can cause myocardial necrosis (Kerber and others, 1980). The setting and the action of discharging should be confirmed with the surgeon in order to prevent injury to the patient or to staff. Internal paddles do not require additional lubrication, since they are moistened by physiologic fluid. On discharging the defibrillator, the circulating nurse should recharge the machine immediately and then observe the ECG monitor for the return of a regular rhythm. If the patient is still fibrillating, the paddles can be activated without waiting; if the patient has been defibrillated, the energy can be "dumped" (see the individual manufacturer's instructions for performing this safely). Frequent monitoring of the ECG will alert the nurse to the development of fibrillation, which can occur at any time before or after the heart is purposely arrested. (Fibrillation occurring during cardioplegic arrest is treated by reinfusing cardioplegia solution if continued standstill is desired). In some centers an anesthesiologist or anesthetist may be responsible for defibrillation. Some internal paddles contain the control button in the handle; these can be discharged by the surgeon.

Nurses activating the device for defibrillation

Box 9-4   Operator failures during defibrillation

Maintenance

Corrosion of internal paddles due to inappropriate sterilization
Chipped insulation on internal paddles
Battery depletion due to failure to recharge, or incorrect placement in charger base
Unit damage resulting from testing with paddles shorted together
Fluids spilled on units
Dirt, blood on paddles
Inconsistent checking of equipment
Infrequent, periodic preventive maintenance

Use

Loose cable-unit connections
Fires due to arcing sparks
Inappropriate activation of "synchronous" button
Personnel shocked themselves while placing paddles on own chest to check rhythm
Inadequate understanding of device operation

Modified from Cummins RO and others: Defibrillator failures: causes of problems and recommendations for improvement, JAMA 264(8):1019, 1990.

should ensure that the device is in the "asynchronous" and not the "synchronous" mode. In the synchronous mode, the machine looks for an R wave or a QRS complex to synchronize the shock. Because there is no R wave or QRS complex in ventricular fibrillation, the machine will not discharge. It is recommended that the device be kept routinely in the asynchronous mode, and that the other mode be instituted only for specific situations (e.g., converting atrial fibrillation to normal sinus rhythm). Conversely, if the patient requires cardioversion for (recent-onset) atrial fibrillation, then the synchronous mode is used to avoid shocking the patient during a vulnerable period that could produce ventricular fibrillation. To synchronize the shock, the defibrillator must be connected to the patient via ECG cables that are connected directly to the defibrillator. They may also be "slaved" into the anesthesia monitoring system. Without this ECG connection, the defibrillator is unable to detect existing R waves, and the shock cannot be timed properly.

Defibrillator failures can occur. The machine should be checked before every operative procedure, and a backup machine of the same manufacturer, design, and model should be available. The nurse must ensure that the internal paddles will connect into the defibrillator. The internal paddles of defibrillators made by different companies are not interchangeable, and paddles of different models of the same company are frequently not interchangeable. Additional sterile internal paddles should also be kept nearby in the event that those at the surgical field are contaminated.

Operator failures (Box 9-4) can also occur. In one study (Cummins and others, 1990), it was shown that

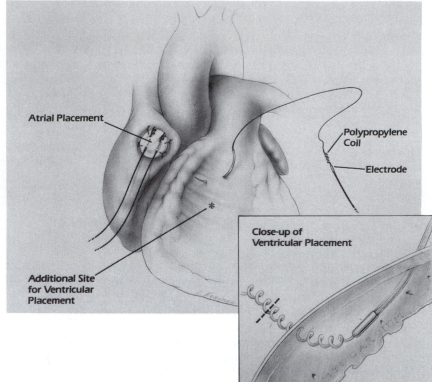

Fig. 9-4 Temporary pacing wires. The fixation coil can be positioned in the atrium or the ventricle. The fixation coil and the electrode are pulled into the myocardium with the needle at the end of the lead. When the electrode and a portion of the coil are in position *(inset),* the remaining coil and needle are cut and removed. For atrial placement, a button *(shown)* can be used to fasten the leads to the heart. (Courtesy Medtronic, Inc. Minneapolis, Minn.)

such failures were related to maintenance and use of the device. Device-related failures were associated with malfunctioning components or poor design. The study concluded that adequate initial training and continuing education to ensure proper use of these devices were important for minimizing errors.

Sterile external paddles are necessary for certain procedures. In patients undergoing repeat sternotomy, pericardial or pleural adhesions can prevent insertion of internal paddles if the adhesions have not yet been dissected. Internal cardioverter defibrillator generator implantation may require external defibrillation (see Chapter 19) if the generator fails to defibrillate the patient during testing of the device. External settings can be from 200 joules up to 360 or more (internal settings are commonly between 10 and 20 joules).

Wall and Clarke (1992) described another method of internal defibrillation in the presence of sternal adhesions. One paddle was placed on the anterior surface of the heart; the second paddle was placed through the peritoneum at the inferior end of the sternal incision and held against the cardiac portion of the diaphragm and above the left lobe of the liver. A single countershock of 50 joules successfully defibrillated the patient.

Familiarity with various defibrillation methods can help the perioperative nurse to anticipate and prepare for alternative maneuvers. Because energy settings vary with the method used and the amount of tissue to be traversed, double-checking the setting and confirming it with the surgeon is an important safety consideration.

TEMPORARY EPICARDIAL PACING

Temporary pacing is used to maintain an optimal heart rate and atrioventricular (AV) synchrony in order to achieve an adequate cardiac output. (In patients with chronic atrial fibrillation, only ventricular pacing wires are inserted, because atrial pacing is ineffective.) Pacing wires can also be used to suppress some dysrhythmias; atrial dysrhythmias may be treated with rapid atrial pacing (Manion, 1993).

Pacing wires are generally inserted before the termination of bypass so that they will be available if needed to maintain a heart rate (e.g., 90 to 100 beats per minute) that will provide an adequate cardiac output. (Insertion is also easier during CPB when the lungs are deflated and out of the way of the right atrium.)

The electrode (bare wire) end of the wire is sutured to the epicardial surface of the right atrium for atrial pacing (Fig. 9-4). A second wire is attached in a similar manner near the first wire (but should not touch the first wire). A second pair of wires is sutured to the right ventricle for ventricular pacing (Fig. 9-5, *A*); in some cases one ventricular wire may be placed on the ventricle for pacing and a second (ground) wire sewn to the skin. All but the electrode end of each wire is insulated with plastic. A scored Keith needle at the other end of the wire is used to bring the wire out through the chest wall. (Some wires are positioned to exit at the base of the sternotomy skin incision.) The needle is broken at the scored section (Fig. 9-5, *B*), and that end of the wire is inserted directly into an

A

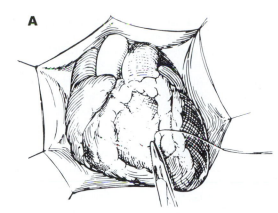

B

C

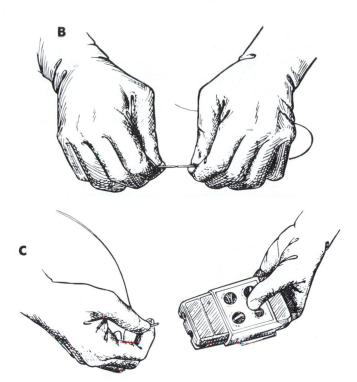

Fig. 9-5 **A,** A pacing wire is attached to the myocardium with the needle tip of the electrode. The wire is pulled until the electrode contacts the ventricle; the needle is then cut and removed. The electrode is fixed to the heart with a fine silk suture. A straight needle at the other end of the lead is used to bring the lead out through the chest wall. **B,** The straight needle is snapped at the scored portion and, **C,** inserted into the temporary pacemaker generator. (Courtesy Ethicon, Inc., a Johnson & Johnson Co., Somerville, N.J.)

external pacemaker generator (Fig. 9-5, *C*) or into a connecting cable that is then connected to the generator.

The needle tips are broken off at the scored portion and connected to the temporary pacer generator (Fig. 9-6). AV sequential generators have four openings for the two pairs of wires from the patient. Single-chamber generators (two openings for wires) are available, but dual-chamber pacing is performed when possible to maximize cardiac efficiency. By stimulating both the atrium and the ventricle to contract, AV sequential pacing enables the atrium to contribute to ventricular filling, thereby increasing stroke volume and cardiac output (Osborn and Leonard, 1989). Patients with rate-dependent cardiac output also benefit from temporary pacing at about 100 beats per minute.

Because pacing obscures some ECG changes, pacing may need to be temporarily interrupted to assess ST segment elevations suggestive of myocardial ischemia. Occasionally pacemakers complete with the native heart rate, at which time the pacer can be discontinued. Not all patients require pacing during surgery, but postoperative dysrhythmias amenable to pacemaker therapy warrant the insertion of temporary leads. When not pacing, the wires should be wrapped with the bare wire/electrode end covered; these can be taped to the chest during transport. When external generators are in use, the box and attached cables and wires should also be secured with tape. Extreme caution should be taken when moving patients who are connected to a pacemaker generator to prevent disruption of connections or dislodgment of the wires.

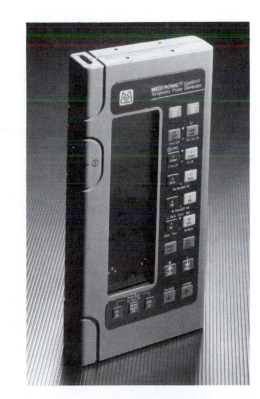

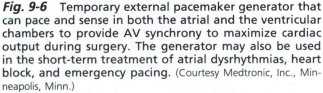

Fig. 9-6 Temporary external pacemaker generator that can pace and sense in both the atrial and the ventricular chambers to provide AV synchrony to maximize cardiac output during surgery. The generator may also be used in the short-term treatment of atrial dysrhythmias, heart block, and emergency pacing. (Courtesy Medtronic, Inc., Minneapolis, Minn.)

The wires are removed on the fourth or fifth post-operative day (or earlier). The wires are firmly grasped and gently tugged to disengage the lead from the heart and pull it out through the chest wall. If there is resistance, pulling should be stopped and the surgeon notified. In such cases the wire may be cut where it exits the skin; this usually does not cause a serious problem (Manion, 1993).

HEMOSTASIS

Hemostasis and blood salvaging have become even more important in recent years because of the risks involved with blood transfusions. Achieving hemostasis in cardiac surgery is influenced by a variety of factors. The patient assessment should include risk factors for increased intraoperative bleeding, such as a history of abnormal bleeding, liver dysfunction, aspirin ingestion, or heparin or coumadin therapy. CPB damages blood components and decreases or alters clotting factors; hypothermia retards clotting mechanisms; heparin inhibits coagulation; and tissue dissection injures blood vessels. Anastomoses on fibrotic or calcified sections of aorta may require adjunctive measures to ensure hemostasis.

Laboratory tests to screen for potential coagulation

Table 9-4 ■ Topical hemostatic agents

Generic name (trade name)	Mode of action	How used	Special precautions
Thrombin (Thrombostat, Thrombogen)	Facilitates conversion of fibrinogen to fibrin (clot) through catalytic process.	Spray, powder, or in combination with Gelfoam.	Of bovine origin; may cause allergic reaction. Never inject into or allow to enter large vessels.
Absorbable gelatin sponge (Gelfoam, Gelfilm)	Provides physical matrix for clot formation through capillary action.	Dry sponge moistened with saline or thrombin solution. Cut sponge to desired size. Also available as a powder, film, or prostatectomy cone.	Do not use in the presence of infection or intestinal spillage. Do not use on skin edges. Possible increased incidence of wound infection if left in place. Increase in size of product due to absorption of blood could cause unwanted pressure in confined space. Not to be used with menorrhagia or postpartum bleeding.
Microfibrillar collagen sheet hemostat (Avitene)	Provides web-type surface for aggregation of platelets.	Loose powder or compacted form.	Of bovine origin; may cause allergic reaction. Can provide focal point for infection. Do not moisten with saline or thrombin. Do not use with cell saver devices. Not for injection.
Absorbable collagen sheet hemostat (Instat)	Platelets aggregate on sheet and release coagulation factors, which combine with plasma factors to form a clot.	Collagen sheet; applied to bleeding site with pressure.	Of bovine origin; may cause allergic reaction. Do not use in contaminated wounds; may enhance infection.
Absorbable collagen sponge (Helistat)	Same as absorbable collagen sheet hemostat.	Sponge applied to bleeding site with pressure.	Of bovine origin; may cause allergic reaction. Not to be used in skin closure.
Oxidized cellulose (Oxycel); oxidized regenerated cellulose (Surgicel, Surgicel Nu-Knit)	Clotting process is initiated physically; forms gelatinous mass, which aids in clot formation and absorbs seven to eight times its weight in blood.	Surgicel: sheet. Oxycel: pad, strips, pledgets. Nu-Knit: sheet. All of the above products work best when applied dry.	May be left in situ, but advisable to remove after clot forms (may dislodge and migrate). Remove from confined spaces, because swelling of product may exert unwanted pressure on surrounding tissue. Do not use to wrap around vascular anastomotic sites. Do not implant in bone defects.
Epinephrine	Topical; induces vasoconstriction.	Added to local anesthetic agent.	Be alert for systemic effects.
Bone wax	Physical action.	Smeared on oozing bone surface.	Remove excess bone wax.

From Moak E: Hemostatic agents: adjuncts to control bleeding, *Todays OR Nurse* 13(11):6, 1991.

problems include the platelet count, prothrombin time (PT), and partial thromboplastin time (PTT). Deficiencies should alert the nurse to the possible need for platelets, fresh frozen plasma, or other blood products necessitated by the specific deficiency. Patients receiving coumadin (e.g., for prosthetic heart valves) often have the medication stopped 4 to 5 days before surgery and heparin substituted until the night before the operation. PT and PTT are monitored during this period.

In the absence of preexisting bleeding disorders, hemostasis is related to the type of vascular injury and to the technical performance of the operation. (Reoperation requiring extensive dissection of adhesions is also associated with increased bleeding.) Constant surveillance of the operative field will enable the sterile nurse to recognize sudden hemorrhage and be prepared to institute emergency measures. Depending on the situation, suction may be required first in order to expose the origin of the bleeding; direct pressure may be applied for temporary control of hemorrhage. Vascular clamps should be immediately available; their size and configuration will depend on the size and location of the bleeding vessel. Sutures and pledget material to repair vessels are used once the bleeding site has been determined. Smaller, discrete bleeding structures may be cauterized, clamped and tied, or suture ligated. (Cautery should not be used in close proximity to anastomoses sewn with polypropylene!) Bleeding from nonvascular sources may require other methods of hemostasis, such as pressure and topical hemostatic agents.

Persistent, generalized oozing may occur on raw surfaces (e.g., pericardial adhesions) or in vascular beds where extensive dissection has been performed (e.g., internal mammary artery [IMA] retrosternal bed). A number of topical hemostatic agents are available for use in those areas where capillary and small-blood vessel bleeding persists (Table 9-4). These agents should be kept in a cup or towel and handled with clean, dry instruments. They should not be allowed to enter the bloodstream through opened, large blood vessels (which could lead to extensive intravascular clotting) and should not be aspirated into blood salvaging (autotransfusion) systems.

The use of epinephrine for hemostasis is not recommended for cardiac patients because of its sympathetic effects on the cardiovascular system. Bone wax, made from refined beeswax, is applied to the sternal edge to control bleeding from the marrow (Fig. 9-7). It is pressed along the cut edge of the sternum, and excess wax is removed. Bone wax should be used sparingly.

Fibrin "glue" is another agent that has been widely used in Europe for hemostasis. It is made by combining 20 ml of cryoprecipitate (or autologous plasma) with a mixture of thrombin (500 IU/ml) and 10% calcium chloride (20 ml). (Additional batches are made by doubling the ingredients.) The cryoprecipitate and the thrombin–calcium chloride mixture must be placed in separate syringes (Fig. 9-8), because combining the ingredients will rapidly produce a fibrin

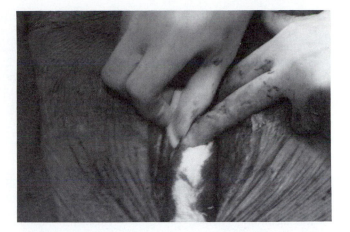

Fig. 9-7 Bone wax is applied to the sternal edge. (Courtesy John R. Garrett, MD; Howard Kaye, photographer.)

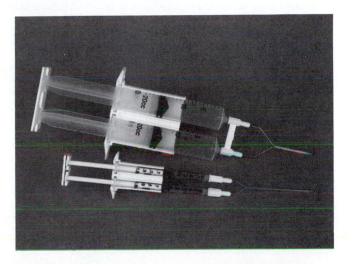

Fig. 9-8 Fibrin glue syringes contain cryoprecipitate in one syringe and a thrombin–calcium chloride mixture in another; a dual dispensing tip is used to prevent clogging within the tips. (Courtesy Micromedics, Inc., Eagan, Minn.)

clot. When the contents of each syringe are sprayed onto the area desired, a coagulum forms that controls oozing. There is some concern that bank blood cryoprecipitate can transmit viral disease; also, sensitivity to bovine material should be determined before bovine-derived thrombin is used. Few problems have been reported in the literature (Oz and others, 1992; Rousou and others, 1989).

Pharmacologic agents are being increasingly used as alternatives or adjuncts to transfusion (Table 9-5). These are categorized as hemostatic agents (to reduce bleeding), platelet protective agents (to conserve clotting elements), and recombinant human erythropoietin (to stimulate the production of new RBCs). One of the hemostatic agents, desmopressin (1 deamino-8-D-arginine vasopressin, or DDAVP), induces transient increases in factor VIII and von Willebrand fac-

Table 9-5 ■ *Pharmacologic blood conservation agents*

Compound	Chemical structure	Mechanism
Hemostatic agents		
Desmopressin	Antidiuretic hormone analogue	Stimulates secretion of factor VIII and von Willebrand factor
ε-Aminocaproic acid	Lysine analogue	Blocks plasmin; stabilizes clots
Tranexamic acid		
Platelet protective agents		
Aprotinin	Bovine polypeptide	Serine protease inhibitor; inhibits platelet aggregation; inhibits plasmin
Dipyridamole	Pyridopyrimidine	Inhibits platelet aggregation
Prostacyclin	Arachidonic acid metabolite	Inhibits platelet aggregation
Recombinant human erythropoietin	Recombinant protein	Stimulates erythropoiesis
Red blood cell substitutes		
Modified human hemoglobin	Polymerized, pyridoxylated stroma-free hemoglobin	Transports chemically bound oxygen
Perfluorochemicals	Emulsified perfluorocarbon compounds	Transports dissolved oxygen
Volume expanders	Hydroxyethyl starch; dextran polymers	Osmotically active agents increase intravascular volume and blood flow

From Stack G, Snyder EL: Alternative to perioperative blood transfusion. In Stoelting RK, editor: *Advances in anesthesia,* vol 8, St Louis, 1991, Mosby.

tor. It has been used to shorten prolonged bleeding times and decrease blood loss in patients with or without intrinsic coagulopathies. Desmopressin does not always produce a consistent effect in hemostatically normal patients whose blood loss is not excessive, but it does offer some benefit where blood loss is greater.

Additional methods of achieving hemostasis are specific to the type of surgery performed. For instance, operations on the thoracic aorta (Chapter 16) may require interventions such as preclotting grafts to minimize interstitial bleeding, or anastomotic wraps made with small-caliber (e.g., 8 or 10 mm) tube grafts. Other techniques are described in subsequent chapters.

CHEST TUBE INSERTION

Chest tube insertion during cardiac surgery has two purposes: (1) to remove fluid (e.g., blood) from the pericardial cavity in order to reduce the risk of cardiac tamponade and (2) to remove fluid and air from the pleural cavity in order to prevent pneumothorax, which would compromise ventilation and gas exchange. Although mediastinal drainage tubes are routinely inserted in patients who have had heart surgery via a median sternotomy, not all of these patients require pleural tubes unless the pleural space has been entered. This commonly occurs with IMA dissection, but it can also occur during sternal splitting if the lungs have not been sufficiently deflated.

One straight mediastinal tube is positioned in the midline, and a second tube, straight or angled, may be placed as well. The tube size is often 36 French, which allows good drainage and a lesser chance of occlusion as compared with a smaller size. The tube is inserted by making a stab wound in the epigastrium, placing the tip of a Kelly or tonsil clamp through the

skin wound into the mediastinum, and pulling the tube out through the skin (Fig. 9-9). The exiting portion of the tube is sutured to the skin. When the chest is being closed (and hand-held suction devices can no longer be used to aspirate blood from the pericardium), the drainage tube must be connected to suction to remove accumulating blood and fluid in order to

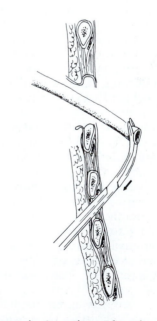

Fig. 9-9 Chest tube insertion. After the clamp has been passed through the skin incision into the pericardium, the distal end of the tube is grasped and pulled out through the skin until the desired length of tube remains in the pericardium. (From Gregory BS: Thoracic surgery. In Meeker MH, Rothrock JC: *Alexander's care of the patient in surgery,* ed 9, St Louis, 1991, Mosby.)

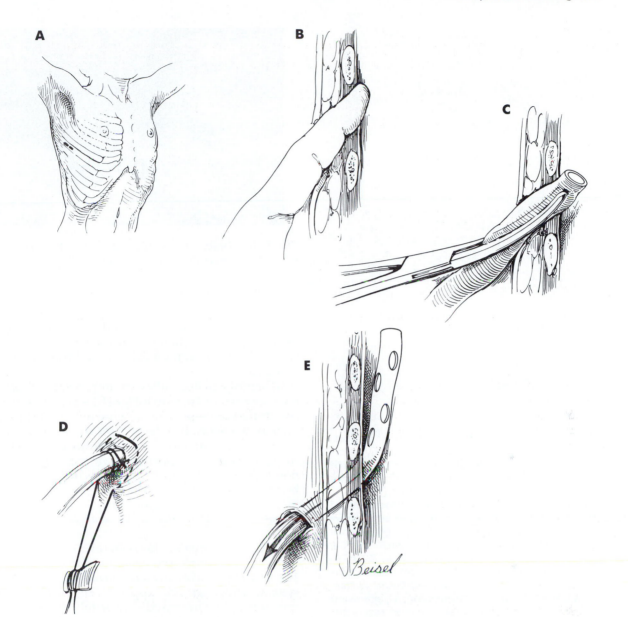

Fig. 9-10 Postoperative insertion of a right pleural chest tube. **A,** Incision. **B,** Finger dilatation. **C,** Tube insertion with a clamp. **D,** Suture fixation of tube to skin. **E,** Completed procedure. (From Waldhausen JA, Pierce WS: *Johnson's surgery of the chest,* ed 5, St Louis, 1985, Mosby.)

avoid compression on the heart, which could lead to tamponade. An endotracheal suction (18-French) catheter attached to a suction line can be inserted into the chest tube to remove intrapericardial fluid quickly. Pleural tubes are inserted in a similar manner intraoperatively. The skin exit site is more lateral (under the breast), and the tube is often angled to conform to the anatomy and to drain behind the lung. The location of the pleural tube(s) depends on whether the right or left (or both) pleura has been opened.

Postoperative pleural chest tube insertion (Fig. 9-10) is accomplished by inserting the internal end of the tube through a skin incision into the pleural cavity. This may be performed in the ICU.

If blood in the pleural space(s) has not been aspirated intraoperatively, the nurse can expect initially to see approximately 100 ml of blood (or more if irrigating solutions have spilled into the cavity) drain from the pleural tube once it has been connected to suction. Within a short period of time, however, this drainage should be significantly reduced. Persistent drainage from a pleural tube may be indicative of IMA bleeding and may require open exploration. This is generally performed only if other possible causes (such as coagulation deficiencies) have not been implicated.

The chest tubes are attached to a collecting chamber that collects and reinfuses shed mediastinal blood

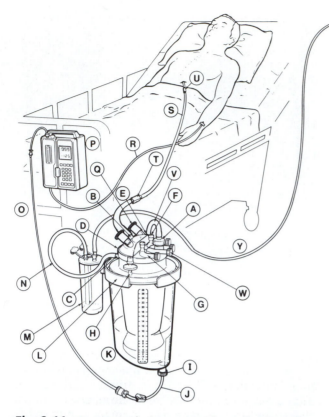

Fig. 9-11 Autotransfusion system for collection of postoperative shed mediastinal blood. The cardiotomy reservoir is converted to a blood collection chamber from which blood can be reinfused into the patient. *A*, Quick prime connector; *B*, chest drainage inlet connectors (three); *C*, vent connector; *D*, deep-vacuum/low-level pressure relief valve; *E*, shunt line connector; *F*, inside Luer connectors (two); *G*, cardiotomy inlet connectors (four); *H*, Luer connector and low-level vacuum relief valve with filter; *I*, blood outlet connector; *J*, Quick-Loc outlet line; *K*, CATR-3500 autotransfusion reservoir; *L*, CATR-H holder; *M*, Sorenson Receptaseal water seal/vacuum regulator; *N*, vacuum line for reservoir/regulator connection; *O*, extension line; *P*, infusion pump; *Q*, chest drainage inlet connector caps; *R*, blood administration set tubing; *S*, chest drainage tubing; *T*, "straight line" connector; *U*, chest cannula; *V*, Quick-Loc shunt line; *W*, CATR-3500 blood inlet connector Quick-Loc caps; *X*, Y-connector (not shown); *Y*, vacuum line for regulator/vacuum source connection. (Courtesy Baxter Healthcare, Inc., Bentley Laboratories Div., Irvine, Calif.)

(Fig. 9-11). This system was first described by Schaff and his associates (1978) and has become a standard method of salvaging postoperative shed blood. The patient's chest tubes are connected to the sterile drainage system. Anticoagulation is not required, because the blood is mechanically defibrinated by the action of the heart and lungs against the blood cells.

When a cardiotomy reservoir is converted into a chest tube drainage system, the perfusionist removes the cardiotomy reservoir from the CPB circuit and modifies it to accept the chest tubes and be connected to wall suction. The distal end of the chest tube(s) is inserted into the appropriate port. Prior to the pa-

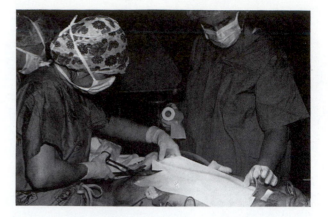

Fig. 9-12 Dressings are applied to the chest and other incisional sites. (Photograph by Howard Kaye.)

tient's transfer to the surgical ICU, the reservoir is attached to the patient's bed and suction is discontinued; the patient is then transported. On admission to the ICU, suction is reestablished and transfusion initiated as indicated.

When three chest tubes are in place, a second collecting chamber (such as a PleurEvac) can be used for the third tube—preferably a pleural rather than a mediastinal tube. It is important to ensure that the system is connected to suction once the chest is closed, so that blood accumulating in the pericardium does not tamponade the heart. Suction is discontinued just before the patient leaves the OR.

COMPLETION OF THE PROCEDURE

After CPB termination, heparin reversal, and achievement of hemostasis, the chest is closed (see Chapter 11) and chest tubes are connected to the drainage system. Dressings are applied (Fig. 9-12). Before transferring the patient, the nurse telephones a report to the ICU; special concerns or fears verbalized by the patient preoperatively should be included, as well as operative details and physiologic alterations (Box 9-5). Perioperative documentation follows the standard protocol. It should include a complete description of the operation performed, the names of the surgical team members, identification of medications and prosthetic implants (with lot and serial numbers), the postoperative skin condition, and other pertinent data.

If there is a delay in transporting the patient to the ICU (e.g., because of sudden increased chest tube drainage or hemodynamic instability), the perioperative nurse can notify the unit and, if possible, revise the anticipated time of arrival. If arrival cannot be estimated at the time of the call, the OR nurse can call after the patient has been stabilized. Delays should also be communicated to waiting family members; the nurse should explain the delay honestly but in a reassuring manner so that the family's concern is not unnecessarily heightened.

Box 9-5 *Patient transfer report*

Procedure (include source of autogenous grafts): ___

___

Monitoring devices
CVP _____ Arterial line _____
Swan _____ Peripheral lines _____

___

Intraoperative occurrences
Blood loss _____ BP _____
Dysrhythmias _____ Bypass problems _____
Defib × _____ Lo temp _____
Setting _____ Hi temp _____
Cross-clamp time _____ Pump time _____
CO _____ CI _____ Urine _____

Blood: Given _____ Available _____
Autotransfusion totals: _____ ml _____ Units
Components: FFP _____ Platelets _____ Cryo _____
Additional ordered (type) _____

Medications
Neo _____ Dopamine _____ Dobutamine _____
Lidocaine _____ Nitro _____ Levophed _____
Epinephrine _____ Nitroprusside _____ Inocor _____
DDAVP _____ Other _____

Tubes/drains: Mediastinal _____ Pleural _____

Epicardial leads: Atrial _____ Ventricular _____
Pacing: Yes/No Rate _____

Labs: K⁺ _____ Na⁺ _____ Glu _____
Hgb _____ Hct _____ Other _____

Patient concerns _____
Additional information _____
ICU bed No. _____ ETA _____ Reported by _____
To _____ Time _____

BP, blood pressure; *CI*, cardiac index; *CO*, cardiac output; *cryo*, cryoprecipitate; *CVP*, central venous pressure line; *DDAVP*, 1-deamino-8-D-arginine vasopressin (desmopressin); *defib*, defibrillation; *ETA*, estimated time of arrival; *FFP*, fresh frozen plasma; *glu*, glucose; *Hct*, hematocrit; *Hgb*, hemoglobin; *hi/lo temp*, high and low temperatures; *K⁺*, potassium; *Na⁺*, sodium; *neo*, neosynephrine; *nitro*, nitroglycerin; *Swan*, Swan-Ganz pulmonary artery catheter.

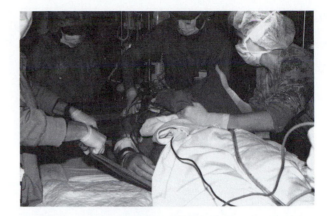

Fig. 9-13 Patient transfer to the bed is performed in unison, under the direction of the anesthesiologist. It should be performed slowly and smoothly, with caution taken to avoid disrupting intravascular lines and catheters, urinary drainage systems, and pacemaker wires. (Photograph by Howard Kaye.)

attached to an oxygen tank and is monitored during transport; a portable defibrillator accompanies the patient. The patient will remain intubated and mechanically ventilated in the ICU for a number of hours in order to reduce the metabolic demands imposed by breathing.

POSTOPERATIVE MANAGEMENT

Postoperative management focuses on maintaining adequate cellular perfusion. Continuous monitoring of cardiac output, heart rate, systemic and pulmonary pressures, oxygen saturation of arterial hemoglobin, and mixed venous blood is performed. Chest drainage, urinary output, blood gasses, temperature, and level of consciousness are assessed frequently (Box 9-6).

An important difference between a cardiac surgery patient and other patients in the ICU who have undergone surgery is that the former is also recovering from the effects of CPB. Postoperative management focuses on the temporary physiologic derangements that surgery and CPB produce. Box 9-7 lists some of the considerations of postoperative care. These emphasize the importance of assessing the patient directly and not relying solely on the display monitors. Perioperative nurses accompanying the patient to the ICU should be familiar with these considerations so that they can anticipate changes in the patient's status that may indicate a need for surgical exploration.

Communication between ICU and OR nurses, especially during the first few hours postoperatively is also encouraged, particularly if the patient becomes unstable as a result of excessive blood loss or tamponade.

For additional information on postoperative management, the reader is referred to the Suggested Readings.

Before the patient is moved to the ICU bed for transfer (Fig. 9-13), hemodynamic stability is reconfirmed and chest tube drainage (from mediastinal and pleural tubes, if present) assessed. Early drainage of 200 to 400 ml/hr is almost always "surgical" and requires exploration (Waldhausen and Orringer, 1991). Because of the possibility of having to reopen the chest, instruments, back tables, and internal defibrillator paddles should be kept sterile until the patient has reached the ICU, or at least left the operating room. The patient is ventilated with an Ambu bag

Box 9-6 *Postoperative orders: admission to the cardiac intensive care unit*

Admit to the cardiac ICU _____
Status/post _____
Condition _____
Allergies _____
Vital signs q 15 min until stable, then q 1 hr
Continuous cardiac output
Hypothermia/hyperthermia blanket until temperature 36° C (96.8° F)
Pacemaker: A _____ V _____ wires
Pacemaker settings _____
Ventilator settings _____
Suction q 2-4 hr and PRN
Splint chest when suctioning and coughing
Chest tubes to 20 cm suction
    Location _____
Record chest tube drainage q 1 hr
Autotransfusion protocol
Nasogastric tube to low continuous suction
Urinary drainage catheter to gravity with q 1 hr output
IV: D_5 Ringer's lactate at 20 ml/hr
Strict I & O
Daily weights
Labs: STAT Blood chemistry panel,* coagulation panel,† WBCs, platelets, PT/PTT, CPK, creatinine, BUN, calcium
ABGs q 4 hr and 30 min after ventilation setting changes
Check K^+ and H & H q 4 hr × 24 hr
Portable chest x-ray on admission
ECG on admission
Keep 4 units of packed RBCs on hold in blood bank
Meds: Mandol 1.0 g IV q 6 hr × 2 days
        Tylenol 650 mg rectally/PO if temperature greater than 38.3° C (101° F)
        Morphine 1-2 mg IV q 2 hr PRN for pain

Courtesy John Rf. Garrett, Md.
A, atrial; *ABGs,* arterial blood gasses; *BUN,* blood urea nitrogen; *CBC,* complete blood count; *CPK,* creatinine phosphokinase; *ECG,* electrocardiogram; *ETCO₂,* end-tidal carbon dioxide; *H & H,* hematocrit and hemoglobin; *I & O,* intake and output; *K,* potassium; *PRN,* as needed; *PT,* prothrombin time; *PTT,* partial thromboplastin time; *RBCs,* red blood cells; *SAO₂,* oxygen saturation of arterial hemoglobin; *V,* ventricular; *WBCs,* white blood cells.

*Blood chemistry panel includes the following: pH, PCO_2, PO_2, Hct, Na, K, Cl, glucose, Hgb, base excess/bicarbonate, O_2 saturation, ionized calcium, and osmolality.
†Coagulation panel includes the following: PT, PTT, fibrinogen, fibrin split products, thrombin time, platelets, and CBC.

Box 9-7 *Postoperative assessment "pearls"*

Anne P. Weiland, RN, MSN, ANP
Washington Hospital Center
Washington, D.C.

Always treat the *patient*, not the *numbers*. Laboratory and hemodynamic values are meaningful only in the face of the overall clinical impression.

If the toes are warm and the patient is making urine, peripheral perfusion is adequate.

Always *ensure* that the patient is being ventilated properly if a hemodynamic problem occurs abruptly. Never trust the ventilator.

Tolerate a lower hematocrit in the immediate postoperative period. It generally will rise as the patient diureses, and transfusion may be avoided.

Watch the potassium level (K^+) carefully, particularly in the face of brisk diuresis, and do not get behind with volume and electrolyte replacement therapy.

Coagulation abnormalities should be corrected promptly in order to avoid excessive blood loss, unless there is suspicion that the laboratory values are incorrect.

Platelet replacement may be necessary in the face of a normal number of circulating platelets because of the effects of preoperative aspirin therapy.

Make sure the chest tubes are open and draining.

Small increments of furosemide (Lasix) may be needed to stimulate urine output, in the face of steady volume replacement, until high levels of antidiuretic hormone engendered during CPB dissipate.

REFERENCES

American Association of Retired Persons: *A matter of choice: planning ahead for healthcare decisions,* Washington, DC, 1986, AARP.

American Association of Blood Banks: *Blood transfusion therapy: a physician's handbook,* Arlington, Va, 1987, AABB.

Bor D and others: Mediastinitis after cardiovascular surgery, *Rev Infect Dis* 5:885, 1983.

Bresser PJ, Sexton DL, Foell DW: Patients' responses to postponement of coronary artery bypass graft surgery, *Image J Nurs Sch* 25(1):5, 1993.

Carr JA, Powers MJ: Stressors associated with coronary bypass surgery, *Nurs Res* 35:243, 1986.

COBE Laboratories: *Educational guide to autotransfusion using the COBE Baylor Rapid Autologous Transfusion (BRAT) system,* Lakewood, Colo, 1991, COBE Laboratories.

COBE Laboratories: User's forum, *COBE BRAT Clin Notes* 7(1):1, 1993.

Council on Scientific Affairs: Council report: autologous blood transfusions, *JAMA* 256:17, 1986.

Cummins RO and others: Defibrillator failures: causes of problems and recommendations for improvement, *JAMA* 264(8):1019, 1990.

Davis DL, Kneedler JA, Manuel BJ: *The nursing process series. IV. Implementation,* Denver, 1979, Association of Operating Room Nurses.

Esperson C: The RN first assistant in cardiac surgery. In Rothrock JC: *The RN first assistant: an expanded perioperative nursing role,* ed 2, Philadelphia, 1993, JB Lippincott.

Harlan BJ, Starr A, Harwin FM: *Manual of cardiac surgery,* vol 1, New York, 1980, Springer-Verlag.

Hawke D, Kraft J, Smith SL: Tissue and organ donation and recovery. In Smith SL: *AACN tissue and organ transplantation: implications for professional nursing practice,* St Louis, 1990, Mosby.

Hedenkamp EA, Howell LH: Preoperative and postoperative care of the cardiac surgical patient. In Weeks LC, editor: *Advanced cardiovascular nursing,* Boston, 1986, Blackwell Scientific Publications.

Kerber RE and others: Open chest defibrillation during cardiac surgery: energy and current requirements, *Am J Cardiol* 46:393, 1980.

Kirklin JW, Barratt-Boyes BG: *Cardiac surgery,* ed 2, New York, 1993, Churchill Livingstone.

Kleinbeck SVM: Principles and procedures of surgical asepsis. In Meeker MH, Rothrock JC: *Alexander's care of the patient in surgery,* ed 9, St Louis, 1991, Mosby.

Kreter B, Woods M: Antibiotic prophylaxis for cardiothoracic operations: metaanalysis of thirty years of clinical trials, *J Thorac Cardiovasc Surg* 104(3):590, 1992.

Manion PA: Temporary epicardial pacing in the postoperative cardiac surgical patient, *Crit Care Nurse* 13(2):30, 1993.

McClosky G: Echocardiography in the operating room. In Stoelting RK, editor: *Advances in anesthesia,* vol 8, St Louis, 1991, Mosby.

Osborn MJ, Leonard PF: Cardiac pacemakers and anesthesia. In Tarhan S: *Cardiovascular anesthesia and postoperative care,* ed 2, St Louis, 1989, Mosby.

Oz MC and others: Autologous fibrin glue from intraoperatively collected platelet-rich plasma, *Ann Thorac Surg* 53:530, 1992.

Reigle J: Preserving patient self-determination through advance directives, *Heart Lung* 21(2):196, 1992.

Rothrock JC: Perioperative patient preparation. In Rothrock JC: *The RN first assistant: an expanded perioperative nursing role,* ed 2, Philadelphia, 1993, JB Lippincott.

Rousou J and others: Randomized clinical trial of fibrin sealant in patients undergoing resternotomy or reoperation after cardiac operations: a multicenter study, *Thorac Cardiovasc Surg* 97:194, 1989.

Schaff HV and others: Autotransfusion of shed mediastinal blood after cardiac surgery, *J Thorac Cardiovasc Surg* 75:632, 1978.

Skeehan TM, Marshall WK: The cardiac operating room. In Hensley FA, Martin DE, editors: *The practice of cardiac anesthesia,* Boston, 1990, Little, Brown.

Stack G, Snyder EL: Alternatives to perioperative blood transfusion. In Stoelting RK, editor: *Advances in anesthesia,* vol 8, St Louis, 1991, Mosby.

Tinker JH, Roberts SL: Management of cardiopulmonary bypass. In Kaplan JA, editor: *Cardiac anesthesia,* ed 2, Philadelphia, 1987, WB Saunders.

Waldhausen JA, Orringer MB: *Complications in cardiothoracic surgery,* St Louis, 1991, Mosby.

Wall MJ, Clarke DR: Intraabdominal paddle placement for internal defibrillation during cardiac reoperation, *Ann Thorac Surg* 53:914, 1992.

Yura H, Walsh MB: *The nursing process: assessing planning, implementing, evaluating,* ed 5, Norwalk, Conn, 1988, Appleton & Lange.

SUGGESTED READINGS

Guzzetta CE, Dossey BM: *Cardiovascular nursing: holistic practice,* St Louis, 1992, Mosby.

Kinney MR and others: *Comprehensive cardiac care,* ed 7, St Louis, 1991, Mosby.

Thelan LA, Davie JK, Urden LD: *Textbook of critical care nursing: diagnosis and management,* St Louis, 1990, Mosby.

Underhill SL and others: *Cardiac nursing,* ed 2, Philadelphia, 1989, JB Lippincott.

Weeks LC, editor: *Advanced cardiovascular nursing,* Boston, 1986, Blackwell Scientific Publications.

10

Evaluating Outcome Achievement

Cardiac surgical nursing is challenging and demanding. The rapid progress being made in the medical and surgical treatment of heart disease makes constant evaluation of nursing care mandatory.

Maryann Powers, RN, and Frances Storlie, RN, 1969 (preface)

Evaluation is performed to judge the patient's progress toward the attainment of outcomes and to appraise the effectiveness of nursing interventions in achieving those outcomes (Association of Operating Room Nurses [AORN], 1993). The evaluation process is systematic and ongoing; it supplies data for quality improvement efforts, enhances future planning, fosters more effective interventions, and establishes greater accountability for the nurse (McGurn, 1981). When specified outcomes are not met, the nurse attempts to determine the reasons why. The nursing diagnosis may have been inaccurate, the plan incomplete, or the actions inappropriate or insufficient. Or, the outcomes were unrealistic because the patient, family, and significant others were not involved in their development. Additional underlying patient factors, such as left ventricular dysfunction or multisystem organ failure, may have contributed to less than optimal outcomes.

In some situations a problem may not be attributable to poor patient care management or preexisting patient factors. It may be created by existing structures or policies (McGurn, 1981). Nurses may have difficulty meeting the Standards of Clinical Practice to provide nursing care or the Standards of Professional Performance to engage in professional role activities because of inadequate environmental resources and support (AORN, 1993). A common impediment cited by many nurses is the lack of sufficient time (or encouragement) to interview patients preoperatively and postoperatively; this problem is becoming particularly evident with the increasing number of patient admissions occurring on the morning of surgery.

Another consideration is the multidisciplinary nature of cardiac care, necessitating cooperation and collaboration between members of the health care team. Rarely can the achievement of outcomes be attributed solely to the interventions of one person. A more comprehensive and accurate evaluation of patient outcomes is likely when there are formal and informal joint reviews by nurses, physicians, and other members of the cardiac team.

Although collaborative working relationships often reflect the interdependent nature of many nursing activities, the importance of sound nursing judgment is no less critical when actions are generated from medical orders or are directly supervised by physicians. Preparing a patient for emergency surgery and performing in the RN first assistant (RNFA) role are just two examples of interdependent practice that require the nurse to have well-developed critical thinking skills.

Changes in the health care system have also had an impact on the nurse's role in evaluating patient care. Reimbursement issues and regulatory mandates have increased the nurse's accountability for the human, material, and fiscal resources used in the delivery of care. Factors related to safety, effectiveness, efficiency, environmental concerns, and cost are now an integral part of the evaluation process (AORN, 1993). Nurses must be able to demonstrate the cost-effectiveness of their interventions and the cost-benefit derived from the services provided.

RESEARCH

Evaluation techniques can also be used to identify problems amenable to the research process. Problems may include something that seems wrong, a situation that needs a solution, or an area that needs improvement or modification. If the problem is to become a researchable question, the "who" and "what" must be clearly delineated so that information specific to the problem can be obtained (Rothrock, 1989b).

Not all perioperative nurses develop and implement research studies, but they can base their practice on research findings and support scientific investigations by serving as study participants and/or expert reviewers of content areas. When nursing interventions are based on research results, perioperative nursing becomes a planned process rather than one based on assumptions or hunches (Spry, 1989).

Managers and administrators benefit from research activities because these can provide accurate information for developing clinical and administrative policy. Joint efforts by members of health care facilities and educational institutions combine operational and theoretical expertise to promote access to ideas and resources. Nursing managers can facilitate this process by nurturing an environment that welcomes questions from practicing nurses and fosters critical thinking (Smeltzer and Hinshaw, 1993). In the perioperative arena research activities can be used by managers to study not only patient-related needs, but also other factors such as calculation of the staffing and supply costs of surgical procedures, determination of the most efficient scheduling system, and evaluation of new products.

PATIENT CARE MANAGEMENT

The primary objective of patient care management is to assist the patient in achieving optimal surgical outcomes (see Chapter 7). Goal attainment is demonstrated by the patient's progress toward the expected outcome (and the absence of injury or other complications) during the preoperative, intraoperative, and postoperative periods. The evaluation process can be concurrent or retrospective, objective or subjective. Concurrent evaluation is performed while the activities are being performed and the patient responses can be continuously monitored. Retrospective reviews provide a cumulative picture of nursing care and can be used to measure the overall effectiveness of nursing interventions in achieving patient outcomes (AORN, 1991). Objective evaluations of outcomes are based on data collection; subjective evaluations rely on observation of patient responses (Kleinbeck, 1990). Regardless of the type of process, information should be communicated to appropriate team members and documented in a retrievable form (AORN, 1993). The nurse can evaluate responses from patients themselves (Box 10-1) or solicit information from significant others, clinical colleagues, and others directly or indirectly involved in providing care. Among the indicators supporting goal achievement are expected physiologic signs and symptoms, expected psychologic and emotional responses, behavioral expectations, patient statements, and laboratory and diagnostic test results (Willis, 1990).

As a result of the review process, the nurse identifies opportunities to improve care that can be incorporated into future patient situations. The nurse investigates whether outcomes identified by the caregiver were congruent with the patient's expectations and whether the goals of patient care were realistic (Rothrock, 1990).

To evaluate interventions and outcomes, the nurse should possess the knowledge and skill to develop individualized outcomes and criteria to measure their

Box 10-1 *Comments to nurses from a patient who has undergone coronary artery bypass surgery*

Leo Rosenbaum
Sebring, Florida 1993

Establish a *personal* relationship with the patient before surgery to give the patient confidence in your ability.

In establishing the personal relationship before surgery, explain to the patient what he or she might expect after surgery. This is a confidence builder. Also, explain in detail what the procedure will be just before surgery: in particular, the necessity for the cooling down period and the fact that the patient could feel very cold. When the patient wakes up in recovery, visit to say that all went well.

Explain the importance of coughing and turning (postoperatively) while in the recovery room and the fact that it may be difficult (painful) at first. Please know that the patient is in pain and try to handle him or her with a gentle but firm hand.

Briefing the patient on what he or she should be doing on discharge is a given, but explaining the consequences of doing or not doing what is suggested is also important.

Probably most important, don't forget why you became a nurse. A little TLC (tender loving care) personally administered goes a long way toward making patients recover more quickly than they otherwise might.

achievement. Data must be collected to provide consistent measurement of responses and analyzed to determine whether the outcomes were met. Additional or alternate nursing actions that are necessary can be identified, and the status of goal achievement communicated appropriately (Willis, 1990).

Evaluation activities can be performed at any time during the perioperative period, but certain outcomes may require review specifically in the preoperative, intraoperative, or postoperative period, depending on the time frame established for their accomplishment. Outcomes related to knowledge and emotional well-being, for example, may be evaluated preoperatively and postoperatively when patient communication is necessary for confirmation. Outcomes affected by intraoperative variables, but appearing (or absent) in the postoperative period, such as infection, are evaluated after the completion of surgery. Outcomes related to more immediate physiologic responses, such as those relating to patient safety, are likely to be monitored continuously throughout the perioperative period.

Preoperative Period
Anxiety

Anxiety reduction during the preoperative period is a common goal of nursing care. Feelings of anxiety are aroused by generalized, nonspecific fears of the unknown, in contrast to specific fears of death, pain, or body image disturbances. Interventions to reduce fear focus on the provision of information that addresses the known threat, and on the creation of a supportive environment that allows the patient to benefit from the information.

The vague, undefined sense of apprehension or uneasiness that characterizes the feeling of anxiety can range from mild to panic level (Jones and Jakob, 1984). Some degree of anxiety is common in most if not all patients awaiting cardiac surgery, and a moderate degree of anxiety may be adaptive and even therapeutic when arousal is appropriate to the situation (Vidor, 1990). In its more severe form, however, anxiety provokes a powerful adrenergic response that can create additional stress for an already-jeopardized myocardium. Studies have shown that either low or high levels of anxiety produce poorer outcomes (Jamison, Winston, and Maxson, 1987).

Including family members in preoperative interviews is beneficial because they can have a positive effect on the patient's recovery. The family (or significant others) often provides the primary support for the patient and can enhance patient coping mechanisms. If family members themselves have unmet needs, unrealistic expectations, or excessive fear and anxiety, transference of these feelings to the patient may increase the patient's own stress level. Thus meeting the family's needs may be closely linked to meeting the patient's needs (Leske, 1986).

In a study by Dockter and colleagues (1988), the investigators recommended better preparation of family members prior to their witnessing the condition and appearance of the patient. Immediately postoperatively, for example, families should be aware that the patient may be intubated and sedated, appear pale, feel clammy, and have multiple indwelling lines and catheters.

The informational needs of families of critically ill patients have been studied by a number of researchers (Leske, 1986; Molter, 1979; Reeder, 1991), and the findings have been consistent in demonstrating the importance of the following:

- To feel there is hope
- To receive information about the patient once a day
- To be called at home about changes in the patient's condition
- To know why things are being done for the patient
- To be assured that the best care possible is being given to the patient
- To know exactly what is being done for the patient
- To have questions answered honestly

The implications for perioperative nurses are that, whenever possible, family members should be included in the interactions between perioperative nurse and patient. These can provide an opportunity to explain or clarify what the planned treatment is, and why and how it will be implemented. In addition, periodic communication with family members or significant others during the intraoperative period can foster feelings of hope, provide reassurance, and enhance coping mechanisms, which in turn can help family members to support and encourage the patient during recuperation.

To determine the effectiveness of interventions for anxiety, the nurse compares the physiologic and psychologic characteristics of the anxious behavior with the patient's responses to interventions. Physiologic manifestations often include rapid breathing and increased heart rate; successful outcome achievement could be measured in terms of (1) respiratory rate within 5 breaths of the patient's normal respiratory rate and (2) heart rate within 10 beats of the patient's normal pulse. Psychologic cues to anxiety may include withdrawal, crying, poor eye contact, increased muscle tension, and urinary frequency (Becket, 1989). Interventions that help the patient to recognize the presence of cues to anxiety and enhance the use of coping strategies (Jones and Jakob, 1984) can assist the patient in being more relaxed and cooperative during preoperative activities. However, sufficient time to discuss concerns may not always be available, and patients may continue to worry about the anticipated surgery (Rothrock, 1989a, 1989b). The support of family members and friends can often ease some of the stress felt by patients.

Restlessness and agitation may also be present, but the nurse should first determine whether these are signs of emotional or physiologic distress (such as hypoxia or some other physical alteration). The appropriate intervention is then instituted and evaluated.

The nurse can also judge patient needs and identify a variety of possible interventions by discussing anxiety-reducing techniques (and the educational needs of patients) with members of The Mended Hearts, Inc., a support group for patients who have undergone cardiac surgery. Members make preoperative and postoperative visits, or communicate by telephone, to provide moral support and education about the impending surgery. Because they have experienced cardiac surgery, The Mended Hearts members have great insight into patient needs; they are a valuable resource to nurses and to patients (especially patients displaying excessive levels of anxiety preoperatively).

Evaluation can be performed postoperatively as well. The nurse can solicit suggestions from the patient (and significant others) about which interventions were most effective and apply these to future situations.

Knowledge

Knowledge about the physiologic and psychologic responses to the cardiac disorder and its treatment helps patients to cope with the disease, participate in the therapy and recuperation, and promote healthy behaviors that contribute to a successful outcome with fewer complications. Preoperatively the patient should have a sufficient understanding of the effects of the illness and the treatment to participate in preoperative activities (such as intravascular catheter insertion and application of electrocardiographic electrodes). Postoperatively, outcome achievement will also be evaluated with regard to recovery and rehabilitation (see later section).

Studies by Miller and Shada (1978) revealed that cardiac surgical patients participating in structured teaching programs consistently identified the need for more information about mechanical ventilation, suctioning procedures, use of an endotracheal tube, deep breathing and coughing, and chest tube removal. Patients may not fully appreciate the type, degree, and location of pain and discomfort postoperatively. This may be related to insufficient time for comprehensive teaching or to differing expectations between nurses and patients as to which information should be provided (Rothrock, 1989a).

Intraoperative Period

Injury

Intraoperatively the patient is at risk for injuries related to positioning, retained foreign objects, and physical, chemical, electrical, and thermal hazards. For example, immediately after positioning, the nurse should determine that pressure areas are properly padded. When arms and hands are tucked along the side of a supine patient, the nurse and anesthesia personnel jointly ensure that intraveneous solutions are infusing properly and that intraarterial monitoring lines have not been disturbed and are recording the blood pressure accurately. Patients in the lateral position are evaluated to ensure that circulation of dependent body parts is not jeopardized, that ventilation of the dependent lung is adequate, that musculoskeletal injury is avoided, and that pressure points are protected. Patients with limited range of motion, back problems, or joint pain require special precautions during positioning.

When the arms must be flexed, the nurse should consider the potential risk of neuropathy. Nerve injury tends to occur in the arms more frequently than in the legs. Ulnar motor and sensory nerve conduction during different elbow positions was studied by Harding and Halor (1983). Their findings showed that increased elbow flexion was associated with decreased nerve conduction velocity; their conclusion was that ulnar nerve compression neuropathy may occur with extreme elbow flexion and that the longer the elbow was maintained in that position, the more likely it was that injury would occur (Bailes, 1989).

Brachial plexus nerve injury during cardiac surgery was studied by Hickey and colleagues (1993), who used somatosensory evoked potential (SEP) monitors to measure ulnar and median nerve SEPs. The authors demonstrated nerve deficits in one fifth of the study group during the first 24 hours postoperatively. They associated this finding with retraction of the sternum and retraction of the chest wall for internal mammary artery exposure and concluded that the use of SEP monitoring may be valuable in predicting peripheral nervous system injury. Using this technique may provide an early warning to the surgeon to modify the surgical technique.

In the immediate postoperative period and a few hours after surgery, the effects of positioning can be evaluated when the patient is awake and able to describe symptoms of neuromuscular discomfort. The nurse will want to confirm that joint problems were not aggravated by the positioning techniques and that patients with fragile skin or little adipose tissue were adequately protected against pressure sores or tissue necrosis.

Occipital skin breakdown and hair loss following cardiopulmonary bypass (CPB) have been reported and may be related to systemic hypothermia, immobility, bypass effects, and pharmacologic therapy. The problem was investigated in a descriptive study by Huffman and colleagues (1992). Intrinsic (age, diagnosis, hematocrit, hemoglobin, pitting edema) and extrinsic (intraoperative temperatures, head pressure, CPB variables, medications) factors associated with skin integrity disturbances were monitored. No occipital skin problems were observed in the study group. Huffman (1993) speculated that the results of this study could not be attributed to any one type of pillow or padding material. CPB factors (for example, pulsatile versus nonpulsatile flow) or some other undetected variable may be associated with the condition.

Injury can also be caused by retained foreign bodies; their absence is usually confirmed by documentation of correct counts. When needles or other small objects are missing, an x-ray film is taken, and review of the film should rule out the presence of the missing object. When counts are incorrect, it may be helpful to review the method used to keep track of these objects during surgery. For example, anchoring bulldog clamps and free needles not in use can help to avoid their misplacement; pill (Kittner) sponges can be kept in a container or placed in a clamp; hypodermic needles can be placed in a cup or a needle boat, or attached to a syringe. Inattentiveness or feeling pressured to hurry may be the cause of misplaced items in the majority of cases, but how one arranges supplies and instruments may also increase the possibility of missing items.

Chemical injury is best prevented by instituting preventive measures such as avoiding known patient allergy–producing substances, labeling fluids, and placing only physiologic solutions near the surgical site. Toxic substances (such as glutaraldehyde valve storage solution) should be kept away from topical solutions. Allergic reactions or tissue injury should be absent throughout the intraoperative period. Exposure to ethylene oxide can be another hazard to both patients and staff. Ethylene oxide should be limited to sterilization of items that cannot be steam sterilized, and adequate aeration of ethylene oxide–sterilized supplies should be confirmed (Kneedler and Purcell, 1989). If items have not been fully aerated, they should not be used. In dire emergencies, such as the immediate need for internal defibrillation devices (requiring ethylene oxide sterilization), institutional policy should be followed.

Physical hazards include malfunctioning or missing instruments (that result in prolonging ischemic time), supplies, or equipment. For example, malaligned jaws on vascular clamps can tear blood vessels and cause severe bleeding; torn vessels are also more difficult to repair than those that are surgically incised. Unsafe medical devices are another concern; nurses more than any other health care professionals encounter the majority of problems. Because they provide direct patient care, nurses may be among the first to detect a malfunction in a medical device. A pilot study by George and Boruch (1989), designed to investigate the nurse's role in medical device surveillance, showed that most of the subjects were not familiar with the requirements of the Food and Drug Administration (FDA) for reporting malfunctioning devices. Clearly, patient safety could be enhanced with greater understanding and implementation of the regulations.

Electrical injuries producing redness, blistering, and other signs of burning are another potential hazard. Misuse of electrical equipment can also place the patient at risk for developing lethal dysrhythmias and conduction disturbances. Evaluation should demonstrate absence of these signs of injury.

Absence of thermal injuries from excessive heat is confirmed by the absence of reddened or burned areas. Mechanical warming pads, blankets from a warming unit, and heated solutions should all be tested before being placed in contact with the patient's skin or internal organs. Heat lamps should be kept a safe distance from the patient to avoid injury.

Cold injuries are also a potential problem. The very young and the elderly are at increased risk because of immature and less-efficient internal temperature regulatory mechanisms, respectively. To generate heat, the body shivers. Shivering increases the metabolic rate and oxygen consumption, which, in cardiac patients with depressed ventricular function, can compromise cardiac output. Although neuromuscular blocking medications will prevent shivering, the patient is at risk for sudden cardiac decompensation during the period before administration of the paralyzing agent. Inadvertent hypothermia can become a problem again after the termination of cardiopulmonary bypass (when the patient has been made normothermic). If the temperature drifts down significantly, it can impair coagulation processes and predispose the patient to irregularities in the heartbeat. Interventions such as increasing the room temperature, using warm topical solutions, and reactivating the thermia blanket can retard this process.

Some patients have "cold allergies" that cause red blood cell agglutination at low temperatures. The presence of this allergy should be communicated to the cardiac team by the blood bank; intraoperatively the patient's temperature may not be reduced as much as it would be in other patient's undergoing similar surgery. It is especially important to avoid delays during the period of cross-clamping, when higher temperatures pose a risk of ischemic injury. Another cold-related injury can result from ice in contact with the phrenic nerve. Nerve injury can impair movement of the diaphragm and affect breathing; this would become apparent when the patient attempts to breathe independently.

Fluid and electrolyte status

Preoperatively the nurse assesses the patient's status: mental state, skin turgor, blood pressure, pulses, temperature, renal status, intravenous (IV) infusion rate, and laboratory results—especially hematocrit and potassium (K^+) level. Intraoperatively fluid and electrolyte status is commonly evaluated by frequent monitoring of urinary output, volume status via intravascular pressure catheters, and pulmonary and systemic blood pressures, and by laboratory tests to determine arterial blood gasses, blood counts, and electrolyte levels. In addition, the electrocardiogram (ECG) is used to detect rhythm disturbances associated with electrolyte imbalances, particularly potassium. Perioperative nursing interventions focus on preparation (e.g., having blood and blood products available, being aware of preexisting bleeding disorders), implementation (e.g., using suction devices safely and appropriately, salvaging blood), communication (e.g., with surgical team members and blood bank personnel), and monitoring (e.g., laboratory results, ECG, blood loss, intravascular pressures, urinary output). Volume status can change suddenly, as when acute hemorrhage occurs, and the importance of planning becomes evident in these situations.

Although decisions relating to replacement therapy are generally not within the scope of the perioperative nurse (AORN, 1993) monitoring fluid and electrolyte balance, instituting safety mechanisms (e.g., avoiding excessive aspiration of either topical crystalloid solutions or hyperkalemic cardioplegia solutions into the CPB circuit), and anticipating therapeutic interventions (e.g., blood administration for a low hematocrit) are important nursing considerations. During cardiac surgery fluctuation of K^+ levels is common and should alert the nurse to the possible development of cardiac dysrhythmias.

Although electrolyte imbalance has not been a nursing diagnosis approved by the North American Nursing Diagnosis Association (NANDA), the importance of maintaining electrolyte balance, especially in the cardiac surgery patient, does warrant its consideration by nurses. Cullen (1992) noted this in a study of the defining activities of critical care nurses related to fluid and electrolyte balance. Among the most commonly stated nursing interventions applicable to the perioperative nurse were those related to monitoring and observing for signs and symptoms of fluid and electrolyte imbalance, having replacement therapy available, consulting with physicians about the fluid and electrolyte status of the patient, teaching patients about therapy, and promoting a positive body image (Cullen, 1992).

Perioperative nurses should also be aware that banked blood stored for more than 3 days has elevated plasma K^+ concentration levels because the electrolyte leaks out of the red blood cells over time. Multiple transfusions of old blood may produce significantly elevated K^+ levels, which can lead to intraoperative cardiac arrest. Whenever possible, the perioperative nurse should ensure that patients at high risk (e.g., trauma patients, patients undergoing repeat sternotomy) receive fresh blood. Hypokalemia is another potential risk that can result from induced hypothermia, CPB, and intraoperative diuresis. In a survey by Felver and Pendarvis (1989), it was shown that perioperative nurses desire more information about perioperative electrolyte imbalances. In addition to discussing electrolyte physiology and possible causes of imbalance, the authors recommend assessment of risk factors and communication of their presence to postoperative nurses who will be caring for these patients.

Skin integrity

Freedom from skin breakdown or alteration during surgery is affected by multiple factors. Immobility during surgery is a major risk factor, but patients who are obese, malnourished, dehydrated, diabetic, infected, very old or young, and/or who have circulatory impairment have an even greater risk of skin impairment (American Association of Critical Care Nurses [AACN] 1990). Studies have shown that body pressure enduring for more than 1 to 2 hours may cause pathologic changes leading to tissue necrosis; retained moisture under dependent skin areas can cause maceration of the epidermis (Berecek, 1975; Mock and Swiech, 1989).

Because positioning changes and direct skin care are unfeasible during surgery, the perioperative nurse relies on preventive measures so that the effects of body pressure and immobility do not result in impairment or worsen preexisting conditions. Careful removal of residual adhesives (e.g., from previously applied ECG electrodes or dressing tape) can reduce direct trauma to the skin, as can the use of nonallergenic skin preparation solutions. Skin preparation fluids should not be allowed to drip down under the buttocks and other dependent body areas. Adequate padding of dependent and peripheral areas of the body, patient transfer onto and off of the OR bed without shearing trauma, and nonreactive dressings and adhesive tape are among the interventions that can reduce the incidence of impaired skin integriy. After surgery, the nurse evaluates the skin, giving special attention to the site(s) of dispersive pads and bony prominences. Patient teaching interventions include proper wound care, signs and symptoms of incisional disruption or infection, the need for proper nutrition and adequate rest, and notification of health care personnel when problems arise (Kim, McFarland, and McLane, 1993). Documentation of a patient's skin condition should reflect the preoperative and postoperative status, interventions, and the patient outcome (Edel, 1990).

Tissue integrity

Maintaining the integrity of various organ systems depends on their being adequately perfused and on reducing ischemic injury from particulate and air emboli, as well as preventing avoidable delays during surgery. Body organs require sufficient oxygen, nutrients, and other metabolic substrates for cellular metabolism. The delivery and use of these substances is affected by preexisting conditions, notably the cardiac disease, and induced circulatory alterations such as CPB, hypothermia, and cardioplegic arrest. Perioperative nursing interventions that decrease myocardial oxygen demand, protect myocardial integrity, enhance the safety of extracorporeal circulatory techniques, and promote wound healing can minimize renal, cerebral, cardiopulmonary, gastrointestinal, and peripheral tissue impairment.

Pharmacologic manipulation of vasomotor tone with vasoconstrictors and vasodilators is one method of enhancing organ perfusion. Hypothermia and cardioplegic arrest reduce metabolic needs and conserve energy resources. Among the nursing interventions are assessing the patient's clinical status and comparing it with baseline values. For example, preexisting neurologic deficits should be included in the report to the surgical intensive care unit (SICU) nurses so that postoperatively the SICU nurse can distinguish between prior deficits and those acquired perioperatively.

Intraoperatively the nurse monitors the patient's status (e.g., assessing urinary output as an indicator of kidney perfusion) and institutes measures to promote a safe CPB run (e.g., using bypass circuit components appropriately). Preparation for and implementation of defibrillation, cardioversion, cardiac pacing, and antidysrhymia therapy are activities related to protecting and maintaining cardiac function. Keeping surgical debris off of instruments and supplies is another important action that can reduce tissue injury related to embolization of particulate matter.

Cardiac output

A decreased cardiac output can be caused by a variety of mechanical (e.g., preload, afterload, contactility), structural (e.g., valve dysfunction), or electrical (alterations in heart rate and/or rhythm) factors that affect the pumping ability of the heart. Decreased cardiac output may also be due to an inadequate circulating blood volume (e.g., hypovolemia). To implement the most appropriate therapy, it is helpful to differentiate between cardiogenic and hypovolemic etiologies (Lazure and Cuddigan, 1987), but often these factors are interrelated, making precise identification of the problem difficult. In addition, the diagnosis of decreased cardiac output itself requires further clarification, because the term has different meanings among nurses. In an effort to specify the diagnosis, Kern and Omery (1992) validated six subcategory labels for the diagnosis of decreased cardiac output: dysrhythmias, decreased preload, myocardial ischemia, increased afterload, cardiovascular drug effects, and cardiac surgery alteration. Independent and collaborative nursing actions, as well as monitoring activities, were listed for each.

Among the independent nursing activities for the subcategory "cardiac surgery alterations" are a number that apply to perioperative nurses. (Similar activities identified in the other subcategories would also be applicable.) These include monitoring the hemodynamic status, promoting rest, providing pain relief, positioning for comfort and ease of breathing, instituting warming measures to prevent shivering, teaching patients and families, and monitoring pacemaker activity. Applicable collaborative interventions include assisting with insertion and monitoring of an intraaortic balloon pump and a ventricular assist device. Performing these activities can help prevent myocardial ischemia or depression and promote a cardiac output equal to patient needs (Kern and Omery, 1992).

Specific perioperative interventions can also focus on problems caused by cardiogenic or hypovolemic factors. Instituting safety measures to minimize myocardial injury is covered earlier in this section under the subheading Injury. Treatment for bradydysrhythmias includes having pacemaker leads and generators available and assisting with their insertion; tachydysrhythmias, can be treated by defibrillation or cardioversion and by correcting underlying problems (e.g., ischemia, hypovolemia).

When a decreased cardiac output is due to hypovolemia (e.g., from bleeding or fluid shifts), correction of the volume deficit and control of the bleeding site (if indicated) can increase preload and the subsequent cardiac output. Using autotransfusion devices and ensuring an adequate supply of blood and blood products are collaborative activities that contribute to a successful outcome.

The performance of RNFA activities can also have a direct impact on cardiac function and surgical outcome. Collaborative RNFA-surgeon interactions not only enhance the technical results of surgery, but also foster greater cohesiveness among cardiac team members (Seifert, 1993). RNFAs can enhance the knowledge and skill of fellow staff members by sharing what has been learned at the field about specific anatomic factors, instrument use, surgeon preferences, and specific operative techniques. Avoiding injury and promoting patient safety are fundamental RNFA concerns. For example, the RNFA can reduce the risk of myocardial injury by using instruments appropriately and cautiously and by avoiding overzealous manipulation of tissue. Archie's (1992) study comparing MD first assistants and RNFAs during abdominal aortic aneurysm surgery, showed that equally satisfactory surgical repair was achieved with either first assistant and that morbidity and mortality were independent of the type of assistant.

Postoperative Period
Knowledge and rehabilitation

Outcomes related to knowledge may be evaluated preoperatively, especially when they pertain to learning needs that lessen the patient's fear and anxiety, and enhance intraoperative care. In the postoperative period patient teaching activities are directed toward maximizing recovery and rehabilitation. Confirmation that outcomes have been achieved can be made by patient observation, chart review, consultation with colleagues, demonstration of activities that have been taught (such as deep breathing and coughing, use of incentive spirometry, leg exercises), and verbalization of what has been learned by the patient (AORN, 1991; Willis, 1990).

Patients with coronary artery disease (CAD), valvular heart disease, and other cardiovascular disorders have specific learning needs that should be addressed. Teaching can be performed by the cardiac perioperative nurse, but often critical care nurses, unit nurses, and others participate in the educational process. Teaching protocols vary among institutions, but the perioperative nurse can provide valuable information directly to the patient or indirectly by providing inservices to patient educators about the short-term and long-term implications of surgery.

In patients with CAD, the nurse needs to confirm that the patient is aware of the progressive nature of the atherosclerotic process, the purpose of surgery, and possible life-style modifications that can have both a physical and a psychologic impact on the patient. In patients with valve disease, implantation of a mechanical prosthesis that requires chronic anticoagulation may have a substantially different impact on the patient's life-style as compared with reparative procedures that do not subject the patient to the risks of bleeding complications associated with warfarin therapy.

The nurse can assess patient outcomes by using the criteria established (or other measurable indicators) to determine the degree of goal attainment. The nurse can appraise the level of patient satisfaction, identify occurrences that posed risk management concerns, and determine whether there were areas that could have been strengthened or improved. Monitoring these areas and making necessary adjustments based on the findings contribute to quality improvement efforts (Gregory, Lewis, and Ward, 1992).

Differences between women and men during recovery may also be a factor in evaluating outcomes. Rankin's (1990) study suggested that male patients were more at risk for high levels of depression, anger, and anxiety during the postoperative period, whereas women were more at risk for biophysical problems and tended to have a longer length of stay in the intensive care unit. By the third postoperative month, however, recovery was similar for men and women. These findings may be significant in planning individualized care during the patient's recuperation and rehabilitation.

Infection

Surgical wound infections make up a significant portion of nosocomial infections. In the cardiac surgery patient infections can be deadly, especially if mediastinitis develops. Aseptic technique and infection control practices are critical interventions, but they are only as effective as the level of compliance demonstrated by team members. Controlling the movement of personnel and supplies in and out of the OR has been shown by Ferrazzi and colleagues (1986) to reduce infection in their study of patients undergoing coronary artery bypass grafting (CABG). Complete hair covering was recommended in a study by Simmons (1978), because bacteria harbored in the hair can be a source of contamination.

Preoperative skin preparation agents and the length of time required to prepare the skin have been the subject of investigation. Because so much skin area needs to be prepared in the majority of cardiac procedures, agents that reduce the time are popular. Howard (1991) compared the effectiveness of a 10-minute water-soluble iodophor scrub and paint procedure to a 2-minute iodophor-in-alcohol procedure. No significant differences in surgical wound infections were found between the two groups.

Other factors can contribute to a successful outcome. Classen and associates (1992) found that prophylactic antibiotics given 0 to 2 hours prior to the surgical incision, compared with infusion more than 2 hours before or after skin incision was made, led to a decrease in the incidence of postoperative wound infections. The perioperative nurse can help to ensure that the antibiotic has been given by reviewing the patient's record to verify infusion of the medication. If it has not been given, the anesthesiologist and surgeon should be notified and the antibiotics ordered and infused before the start of the operation (Johnson, 1992).

HUMAN RESOURCE MANAGEMENT

The process of evaluation can also be used to assess how effectively human resources have been used and how well individual team members have performed.

Evaluation of Nursing Care

Performance reviews identify the current level of practice and particular areas of strength and weakness. The level of intellectual and technical skill is appraised in light of the complexity and demands of the patient population and the surgical procedures. As a result of the appraisal process, teaching/learning opportunities can be provided to strengthen deficient areas.

The evaluation of a nurse's performance includes the supervisor's review, peer review, preceptor appraisal, and self-assessment; patients and medical colleagues may also contribute to the assessment process. Methods of evaluation include verbal reports, needs assessments, and written appraisals (deBlois, 1989).

Evaluation is commonly accomplished through direct observation of the nurse's clinical performance based on competency-based skills (see Chapter 2) and standards of practice. However, limited staffing or time may necessitate supplemental or alternative options such as written examinations. The staff should participate in deciding how evaluations are to be performed. If the decision is to use a written examination, it should be comprehensive and include material from the unit competency skills list, as well as from articles, lectures, standards and recommended practices, and audiovisual materials. A passing grade should be established. Basic competencies may require a 100% passing grade because the stated skills are essential for safe patient care (Watson, 1992). Tests used to evaluate nurses being considered for promotion would measure advanced nursing practice and would not necessarily require a 100% passing grade. Based on the test results, additional learning needs may become apparent.

Peer review evaluations are performed by perioperative colleagues with the same role expectations and job descriptions as the nurse being evaluated (AORN, 1991). One way to implement the process is for the supervisor to select two or three colleagues who demonstrated knowledge, skill, and objectivity and then allow the nurse being evaluated to select his or her evaluator from this group. Self-assessments are also useful, because they can provide an opportunity for the nurse to identify personal strengths and weaknesses, specify learning needs, set goals, and confirm (or deny) that expectations of performance are congruent with those of the supervisor.

Interpersonal Relationships

Labor-management relations and the stress of the cardiac surgical environment can affect performance and, subsequently, patient outcomes. Excessive staff turnover and increased use of sick time may be an indication of low staff morale affecting the cohesiveness of the team. Dissatisfaction among team members impedes communication and productive working relationships. Staff nurses may need to ventilate frustrations or discuss concerns that affect the group in an open and honest manner. Albrecht and Halsey (1991) showed that nurse managers who listened to employees ventilate frustrations and offered advice were perceived by the staff nurses as supportive. These interventions eased fears of insecurity and helplessness and provided needed reassurance (Diomede, 1992).

If team members become physically and emotionally drained, particularly after prolonged periods of long workdays and/or multiple emergencies, they may require additional support and consideration in the form of time off and/or formal recognition of their efforts. Visiting recuperating patients can be an especially gratifying experience for the perioperative nurse because, in addition to providing an opportunity for patient evaluation, the patient's comments often reaffirm the important contribution that the nurse has made to the patient's well-being.

Interpersonal relationships between nurses, physicians, technologists, and others can be evaluated. If the interactions are constructive and reflective of respect for one another, and if there is cooperation among the team members, team function is more likely to be efficient and mutually rewarding. Collaboration enhances job satisfaction, which in turn promotes retention and reduces turnover costs (Seifert, 1993). Cooperation among perioperative nurses and nurses in other specialty units is another factor that can impact communication and patient care.

EVALUATION OF FISCAL AND MATERIAL RESOURCES

Patient outcomes have become increasingly tied to the cost of achieving those outcomes. The most beneficial nursing interventions are being perceived as those that provide quality care in the most cost-effective manner. Consideration of cost has become an integral component of care, and the nurse must be able to justify the expenses, as well as the clinical benefits, of care.

A study by Takes (1992) demonstrated that perioperative nurses wanted to learn about cost-effectiveness and had positive feelings about saving the hospital money. However, nurses also expressed their concern that too much emphasis on cost considerations could have adverse effects (Diomede, 1992).

Cost-containment measures affect the availability, amount, and use of instruments and supplies. No longer can nurses afford to replace vascular clamps at will or increase the prosthetic valve inventory "just in case." Instruments must be treated with care to prolong their use. Prosthetic grafts and valve supply levels should be determined according to projected caseloads and in consultation with the surgeon. Rarely used sizes of valves and grafts should be kept to a minimum. In the event of emergencies, alternate sources for prostheses should be available (e.g., from colleagues in other institutions with whom an agreement to share has been established).

When surgeons verbalize a preference for a different or newer prosthesis (or other supply item), the nurse responsible for purchasing and/or maintaining the inventory can discuss possible options for using up existing models to reduce shelf stock; when an old item is used, it can be replaced with the new, preferred model. The nurse can also investigate the possibility of an exchange program or consignment options with the manufacturer of the new model so that capital expenditures for the newer item can be minimized.

The use of supplies is another area where efficiency and cost-effectiveness are important factors. Cardiac procedures require numerous items, and significant cost savings can be realized with the use of custom packs. Rusynko and Schall (1984) described methods of selecting and evaluating open heart packs that considered cost and storage factors. Kinney and Lutjen's (1986) study showed that the use of custom packs resulted in significant cost savings, as well as a 25% reduction in staff time needed to clean and prepare the OR for an upcoming procedure.

Minimal amounts of suture should be opened, and other cost-containment measures should be taken. Because nurses are most familiar with the material resources required, they are the best qualified to assume a proactive role in cost-containment efforts. RNFAs can also contribute to cost-savings, because their familiarity with surgeons' preferences and rationales for the use of specific supplies and equipment can enhance more judicious use of material resources. If perioperative nurses themselves do not initiate and develop expense-reduction measures, it is likely that externally imposed restraints will be established for them by those without an understanding of the clinical aspects of care.

ADDITIONAL METHODS OF EVALUATION

Patient satisfaction questionnaires and the interaction with colleagues, administrators, and professional and community organizations provide additional opportunities to evaluate patient care and human and material resources. Members of the health care team, such as surgeons, perfusionists, anesthesiologists, nurses in other specialty areas, and cardiologists, are important sources of information and opinion concerning the patient's response to surgery. Whether formally (as in grand rounds) or informally (as in private discussion), members of the health care team can provide valuable insights into patient needs and offer additional or alternative interventions. National organizations such as the American Heart Association* and The Mended Hearts† and their local affiliations can be important allies in helping patients to achieve desired outcomes.

CONCLUSION

Meeting the needs of patients undergoing cardiac surgery is as challenging and demanding today as it was a quarter of a century ago when Powers and Storlie (1969) wrote about the care of these patients. As technology has become more complex, a greater variety of methods have become available to evaluate patient care; these can enhance a deeper and fuller understanding of the impact that cardiac surgery has on patients and identify opportunities to continually improve care.

---

*7272 Greenville Ave., Dallas, TX 75231.
†7320 Greenville Ave., Dallas, TX 75231.

REFERENCES

Albrecht TL, Halsey J: Supporting the staff nurse under stress, *Nurs Manage* 22:60, July 1991.

American Association of Critical-Care Nurses: *Outcome standards for nursing care of the critically ill,* Laguna Niguel, Calif, 1990, AACN.

Archie JP: Influence of the first assistant on abdominal aortic aneurysm surgery, *Tex Heart Inst J* 19(1):4, 1992.

Association of Operating Room Nurses: *Perioperative nursing process* (revised by Diomede B), Denver, 1991, AORN.

Association of Operating Room Nurses: *1993 standards and recommended practices,* Denver, 1993, AORN.

Bailes BK: Perioperative nursing research. IV. Intraoperative phase, *AORN J* 49(5):1397, 1989.

Becket N: Anxiety. In McFarland GK, McFarlane EA: *Nursing diagnosis and interventions: planning for patient care,* St Louis, 1989, Mosby.

Berecek KH: Etiology of decubitus ulcers, *Nurs Clin North Am* 10:157, 1975.

Classen DC and others: The timing of prophylactic administration of antibiotics and the risk of surgical wound infection, *N Engl J Med* 326:281, 1992.

Cullen L: Interventions related to fluid and electrolyte balance, *Nurs Clin North Am* 27(2):569, 1992.

de Blois CA: Preceptors in the OR: learning to evaluate others, *AORN J* 49(5):1387, 1989.

Diomede B: Research review: cost effectiveness, *AORN J* 56(2):347, 1992.

Dockter B and others: Families and intensive care nurses: comparisons of perceptions, *Patient Educ Couns* 12:29, 1988.

Edel EM: Impaired skin integrity, *Todays OR Nurse* 12(7):40, 1990.

Felver L, Pendarvis JH: Electrolyte imbalance, *AORN J* 49(4):992, 1989.

Ferrazzi P and others: Reduction of infection after cardiac surgery: a clinical trial, *Ann Thorac Surg* 42:321, 1986.

George VD, Boruch RF: Medical device reporting: a pilot study of nurses, *AORN J* 49(3):815, 1989.

Gregory B, Lewis J, Ward S: *Quality improvement in perioperative nursing MILS,* Denver, 1992, AORN.

Harding C, Halor E: Motor and sensory ulnar nerve conduction velocities, *Arch Phys Med Rehabil* 65:227, 1983.

Hickey C and others: Intraoperative somatosensory evoked potential monitoring predicts peripheral nerve injury during cardiac surgery, *Anesthesiology* 78:29, 1993.

Howard RJ: Comparison of a 10-minute aqueous iodophor and 2-minute water insoluble iodophor in alcohol preoperative skin preparation, *Complications Sur* 10:43, 1991.

Huffman M: Personal communication, 1993.

Huffman M and others: *Identification of perioperative risk factors in the development of skin integrity problems post cardiopulmonary bypass* (poster abstract). Presented at the Conference on Nursing Quality Assessment and Improvement, New Orleans, Oct 22-24, 1992.

Jamison RN, Winston CV, Maxson WS: Psychological factors influencing recovery from outpatient surgery, *Behav Res Ther* 25(1):31, 1987.

Johnson JH: Research review: prophylactic antibiotics, *AORN J* 56(2):347, 1992.

Jones PE, Jakob DF: Anxiety revisited—from a practice perspective. In Kim MJ, McFarland GK, McLane AM, editors: *Classification of nursing diagnoses: proceedings of the fifth national conference,* St Louis, 1984, Mosby.

Kern L, Omery A: Decreased cardiac output in the critical care setting, *Nurs Diagn* 3(3):94, 1992.

Kim MJ, McFarland GK, McLane AM: *Pocket guide to nursing diagnosis,* ed 5, St Louis, 1993, Mosby.

Kinney GJ, Lutjens LR: Cost accountability in the OR: a case for custom-designed, procedure ready packs, *AORN J* 43(6):1306, 1986.

Kleinbeck SV: Introduction to the nursing process. In Rothrock JC: *Perioperative nursing care planning,* St Louis, 1990, Mosby.

Kneedler JA, Purcell SK: Perioperative nursing research. II. Intraoperative chemical and physical hazards to personnel, *AORN J* 49(3):829, 1989.

Lazure LL, Cuddigan J: Clinical validation of decreased cardiac output: differentiation of defining characteristics according to etiology. In McLane AM, editor: *Classification of nursing diagnoses: proceedings of the seventh conference,* St Louis, 1987, Mosby.

Leske JS: Needs of relatives of critically ill patients: a follow-up, *Heart Lung* 15(2):189, 1986.

McGurn WC: Evaluation and evaluation research. In McGurn WC: *People with cardiac problems,* Philadelphia, 1981, JB Lippincott.

Miller SP, Shada EA: Preoperative information and recovery of open heart surgery patients, *Heart Lung* 7:486, 1978.

Mock VL, Swiech K: Impaired skin integrity. In McFarland GK, McFarlane EA: *Nursing diagnosis and interventions: planning for patient care,* St Louis, 1989, Mosby.

Molter NC: Needs of the relatives of critically ill patients: a descriptive study, *Heart Lung* 8:332, 1979.

Powers M, Storlie F: *The cardiac surgical patient,* New York, 1969, Macmillan.

Rankin SH: Differences in recovery from cardiac surgery: a profile of male and female patients, *Heart Lung* 19(5):481, 1990.

Reeder JM: Family perception: a key to interpretation. In Leske JS, editor: Family Interventions, *AACN Clin Issues Crit Care Nurs* 2(2):188, 1991.

Rothrock JC: Preoperative psychoeducational interventions, *AORN J* 49(2):597, 1989a.

Rothrock JC: The researchable question. In Kleinbeck SV: *Reading and reviewing research: a guide for the perioperative nurse,* Denver, 1989b, AORN.

Rothrock JC: Measuring outcomes of care planning. In Rothrock JC: *Perioperative nursing care planning,* St Louis, 1990, Mosby.

Rusynko BS, Schall B: Custom open heart packs, *AORN J* 40(3):379, 1984.

Seifert PC: The RN first assistant and collaborative practice. In Rothrock JC: *The RN first assistant: an expanded perioperative nursing role,* ed 2, Philadelphia, 1993, JB Lippincott.

Simmons N: Hair in the theatre, *Br Med J* 149:111, 1978.

Smeltzer CH, Hinshaw AS: Integrating research in a strategic plan, *Nurs Manage* 24(2):42, 1993.

Spry CC: Overview of nursing research. In Kleinbeck SV: *Reading and reviewing research: a guide for the perioperative nurse,* Denver, 1988, AORN.

Takes KL: Cost-effective practice: do OR nurses care? *Nurs Manage* 23:96Q, 1992.

Vidor KK: Anxiety related to impending surgery, *Todays OR Nurse* 12(9):36, 1990.

Watson DS: Developing a competency-based education program for nurse-monitored sedation, *Semin Perioper Nurs* 1(4):224, 1992.

Willis C: Evaluate effectiveness of the plan of care. In Kneedler JA, editor: *CNOR Study Guide,* Denver, 1990, National Certification Board: Perioperative Nursing.

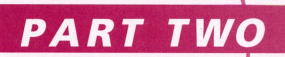

PART TWO

Surgical Interventions

11

Generic Procedures

The ultimate object of my work in this field has been to be able to operate inside the heart under direct vision. From the beginning, I have not only been interested in the substitution of a mechanical device for the heart, but also for the lung.

John H. Gibbon, Jr., MD 1954 (p. 171)

Safe and effective cardiac surgery is possible because of the technologic developments that have enabled surgeons to work on the heart without injuring it or the other major organs of the body. The use of endotracheal anesthesia in thoracic surgery, first described by Elsberg in the early twentieth century, allowed surgeons to enter the thorax without causing a pneumothorax, with its accompanying pulmonary collapse and asphyxia (Crawford and Kratz, 1990). Cardiopulmonary bypass (CPB), introduced into clinical use by Gibbon (1954), provided a method for operating on a quiet, bloodless field, unobscured by the lungs, while at the same time perfusing the brain and the rest of the body. And methods to protect the heart itself—reported by Melrose and others (1955); Sealy, Brown, and Young (1958); Gay and Ebert (1973); Conti and others (1978); Buckberg (1979); and others—helped to minimize the dangers associated with intraoperative induced cardiac arrest. This chapter describes the types of incisions used to expose the heart and other thoracic structures, CPB, and methods to protect the myocardium during cardiac procedures.

THORACIC INCISIONS

The incision should allow adequate and proper exposure of the operative site. Depending on the particular anatomic and physiologic problem, a variety of incisions are available to expose the heart and other thoracic structures (Table 11-1).

Median Sternotomy

Median sternotomy is the most commonly used incision for acquired cardiac disorders because it provides the best access to the heart and mediastinum, as well

as optimum exposure for the institution of CPB. It is also the incision of choice for pericardiectomy, thymectomy, and anterior mediastinal tumors (Waldhausen and Pierce, 1985).

Sternotomy also produces the least respiratory impairment and causes less discomfort for the patient than do other thoracic incisions (Harlin, Starr, and Harwin, 1980). Unlike the various lateral thoracotomy incisions, sternotomy requires no muscle division, and the sternal bones can be closed firmly together. Postoperatively coughing and deep breathing do not create the same degree of pain encountered by patients with thoracotomy due to moving ribs and incised chest muscles (McLaughlin, 1991). This facilitates the performance of postoperative breathing exercises, which enhance pulmonary function.

Injury to the brachial plexus has been reported. Originally thought to be related to the position of the arms and stretching of the brachial plexus from sternal retraction, more recent studies have shown that this complication is most likely due to injury to the first rib (Crawford and Kratz, 1990). Preventive measures include opening the sternum as little as possible and positioning the retractor as caudally as possible (Baisden, Greenwald, and Symbas, 1984).

Sternal incision

The skin incision is made from the sternal notch to the xiphoid process. Waldhausen and Pierce (1985) have stressed the importance of not extending the incision into the suprasternal space for physiologic, as well as cosmetic, reasons. For instance, if tracheostomy is anticipated, the tracheal opening should be placed as far from the sternotomy incision as possible because of the risk of cross-contamination and infection.

The sternal bone is divided with an air-driven or electrically powered saw (Fig. 11-1). Battery-powered

Table 11-1 ■ *Thoracic incisions*

Incision	Position	Indications	Special needs
Median sternotomy: incision down center of sternum	Supine	Most adult cardiac procedures except those on branch pulmonary arteries, distal transverse aortic arch, and descending thoracic aorta	Padding for hands, elbows, feet, back of head, dependent bony prominences
Anterolateral thoracotomy: curvilinear incision along subpectoral groove, right or left side	Supine with a pad or pillow under operative site; arm supported in sling or overarm board; arm on unaffected side may be tucked along side	Trauma to anterior pericardium and left ventricle	Padding for extremities; pillow or other device to elevate affected side; armboard or sling for arm on affected side
Lateral thoracotomy: curvilinear incision along costochondral junction anteriorly to posterior border of scapula	Placed on side with arms extended and axilla and head supported; knees and legs protected	Lung biopsies; first-rib resection; lobectomy	Armboard, overarm board, axillary roll, padding for extremities, pillow between legs; tapes, sandbags, straps or other devices to support torso
Posterolateral thoracotomy: curvilinear incision from subpectoral crease below nipple extended laterally and posteriorly along ribs almost to posterior anterior midline below scapula (location of intercostal incision depends on surgical site)	Lateral with arms extended and axilla and head supported; knees and legs protected	Descending thoracic aortic aneurysms; distal transverse aortic arch; pulmonary and esophageal resection	Similar to needs for lateral thoracotomy
Transsternal bilateral thoracotomy: submammary incision from one anterior axillary line to the other across sternum at fourth interspace	Supine	Used to extend either right or left anterolateral thoracotomy (rarely used)	Same as median sternotomy
Subxiphoid incision: vertical midline incision from over xiphoid process to about 10 cm inferiorly (may divide lower portion of sternum to enhance exposure)	Supine	Pericardial drainage, pericardial biopsy, attachment of pacing or defibrillator electrodes	Same as median sternotomy
Thoracoabdominal incision: low curvilinear incision on left side extended to anterior midline, continued vertically down abdomen	Anterior thoracotomy with chest at 45-degree angle to table; abdomen supine	Thoracoabdominal aneurysm	Same as anterolateral thoracotomy

Data from McLaughlin (1991); Edmunds, Norwood, and Low (1990); Waldhausen and Pierce (1985); and Crawford and Kratz (1990).

saws are also available. Manual sternotomy with a Lebsche knife and mallet is rarely performed (see Chapter 5). The saw should be checked and tested before it is needed, and a backup saw should be readily available. RN first assistant (RNFA) considerations are listed in Box 11-1.

Operative procedure: median sternotomy

1. The skin incision is made from the sternal notch to the linea alba, 1 to 2 cm below the xiphoid process.
2. The periosteum along the manubrium and the sternal body is coagulated to mark the midline (Fig. 11-2). The fibrous bands between the two clavicular heads are divided, and the xiphoid process is cut in the middle. The distal retrosternal space is bluntly dissected with the finger (Edmunds, Nor-

wood, and Low, 1990; Harlan, Starr, and Harwin, 1980). Bleeding points are coagulated.
3. The sternum is divided along the midline with a reciprocating saw (Fig. 11-3) or an oscillating saw. The anesthesiologist may deflate the lungs momentarily just before the sternum is divided to reduce the risk of opening the pleural spaces.

Depending on surgeon preference, the bone is incised from the upper end of the incision to the lower end, or the reverse. A hand-held retractor (such as an Army-Navy or rake retractor) can be placed along the sides and at the upper end of the incision to protect the skin and subcutaneous tissue.
4. The upper and lower edges of the sternal periosteum are cauterized to control bleeding from the marrow (Fig. 11-4). Bone wax may be applied to

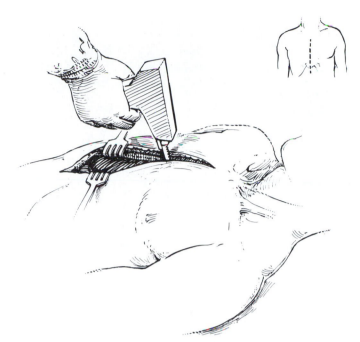

Fig. 11-1 Median sternotomy with a power saw. (From Walhausen JA, Pierce WS: *Johnson's surgery of the chest,* ed 5, St Louis, 1985, Mosby.)

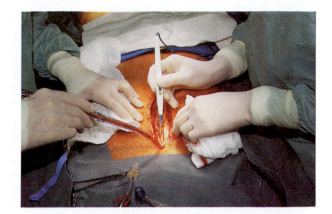

Fig. 11-2 Incision and cautery of the periosteum. The RN first assistant *(left)* retracts the skin edges, and aspirates and retracts with the suction tip. (Courtesy John R. Garrett, MD; Howard Kaye, photographer.)

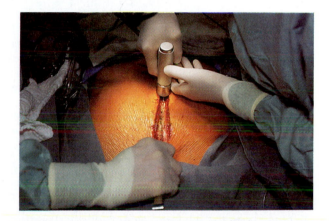

Fig. 11-3 Sternal division with a saw; the RN first assistant is holding a retractor at the upper end of the incision *(bottom of picture)*. (Courtesy John R. Garrett, MD; Howard Kaye, photographer.)

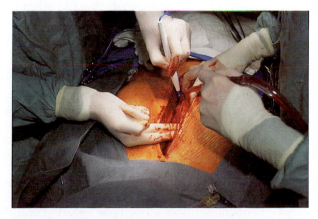

Fig. 11-4 While the RN first assistant elevates the sternal bone, the surgeon cauterizes to control bleeding. (Courtesy John R. Garrett, MD; Howard Kaye, photographer.)

Box 11-1   *RN first assistant considerations related to the incision*

Retract skin edges manually with a laparotomy pad to expose subcutaneous and periosteal bleeders; after sternum is divided, a hand-held retractor can be used to expose retrosternum and upper end of incision.

Suction cautery plume when chest is being opened.

Avoid retracting sternum too vigorously during repeat sternotomy to prevent tearing the heart and/or great vessels.

If sudden, copious bleeding is seen during repeat (or initial) sternotomy, follow surgeon's orders; for example, RNFA may be requested to suction (autotransfusion and discard suction both may be necessary to clear field adequately) or to compress both sides of the chest together to tamponade bleeding while surgeon accesses femoral artery for CPB cannulation.

Look for bleeding vessels at upper end of incision before sternal retractor is inserted (once retractor is opened, it may stretch tissue and close bleeders, concealing their presence and making it harder to find them later after retractor is removed).

After initial incision into pericardium is made, place a suction tip under pericardium to elevate off the heart and prevent injury to underlying myocardium (or, the surgeon may do this with the fingers).

Provide countertraction during insertion of chest wires.

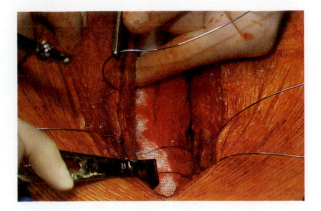

Fig. 11-5 The RN first assistant provides countertraction while the surgeon inserts wire sutures into the sternum. (Courtesy John R. Garrett, MD; Howard Kaye, photographer.)

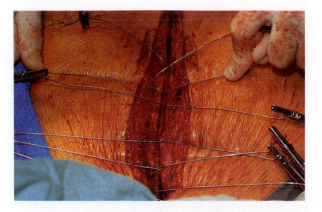

Fig. 11-6 The sternal wires are crossed and then twisted manually. Note the Kocher clamps attached to the ends of the wires to facilitate their manipulation. (Courtesy John R. Garrett, MD; Howard Kaye, photographer.)

the sternal edges for excessive bleeding, but it is used sparingly as a result of reports noting impaired wound healing and possible embolization of the wax to the lungs (Robicsek and others, 1981).

Additional bleeding points along the incision are cauterized. Occasionally, bilateral suture ligatures are required for large venous bleeders at the upper end of the incision; this is more common in patients with systemic venous hypertension.

5. The sternal retractor is inserted and opened gradually to avoid sternal fractures. Prior to insertion of the retractor, the sternal edges may be covered with laparotomy pads or surgical towels (Gay, 1990).

Sternal closure

1. After hemostasis has been achieved, stainless steel wire sutures (No. 5 or 6) are passed around or through the bone (Fig. 11-5). Generally, five or six wires are inserted. A simple or a mattress suture technique, or a combination technique, may be performed. Countertraction on the sternum by the assistant may make passage of the wire through the bone easier.
2. The surgeon and assistant evaluate the sternum for bleeding from branches of the internal mammary artery or other blood vessels, and hemostasis is achieved.
3. The wires are twisted closed tightly enough to immobilize the sternum (Figs. 11-6 through 11-8). Excess wire is cut, and the ends are buried into the periosteum. Some surgeons prefer a wire closure device (Fig. 11-9) that uses locking plates and a crimper to close the wires. When this is used, it is important to avoid entangling temporary pacing wires and drapes in the device.
4. Linea alba fascia is closed with nonabsorbable suture in an interrupted stitch. Subcutaneous tissue and skin are closed with absorbable suture (Fig. 11-10); occasionally staples may be used on the skin (a staple remover must accompany the patient).

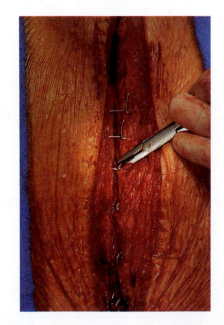

Fig. 11-7 After excess wire is cut, the wire needle holder is used to completely tighten the wires. The wire ends are then buried into the subcutaneous tissue. (Courtesy John R. Garrett, MD; Howard Kaye, photographer.)

Weak sternums

In osteoporotic or otherwise weak, unstable sternums, additional methods may be employed to bolster the closure. Nylon bands (Parham bands) may be passed around the sternum and secured with metal plates. Another technique is to thread extra-long sternal wires vertically down and back along the lateral sternal borders (Fig. 11-11). The transverse wires are then inserted around the vertical wires so that when the sternum is approximated, the transverse wires do not cut through the sternum, because they are buttressed by the vertical wires (Robicsek, Daugherty, and Cook,

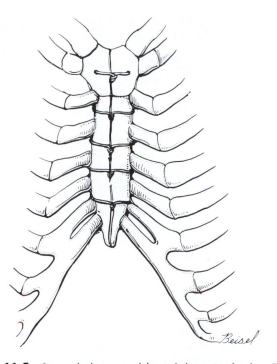

Fig. 11-8 Sternal closure with stainless steel wire. The first wire is placed through the manubrium, and remaining wires are placed around the sternal body. Wires may also be placed through the sternum. (From Walhausen JA, Pierce WS: *Johnson's surgery of the chest,* ed 5, St Louis, 1985, Mosby.)

1977; Sutherland, Martinez, and Guynes, 1981). A third technique to reduce the possibility of cutting through the bone is to place two or more heavy (No. 5) polyester sutures between the wires. (If these patients require emergency sternotomy, scissors, as well as wire cutters, will be necessary to open the sternum.)

Delayed sternal closure

Occasionally, delayed sternal closure is necessary in patients whose impaired clotting mechanisms may

pose a significant risk of cardiac tamponade in the early postoperative period. In these cases the patient is transferred to the surgical intensive care unit with the sternum left open and just the skin closed. Anterior mediastinal tubes drain the pericardium. Once volume replacement and correction of the bleeding diathesis is achieved, the patient is returned to the operating room and the chest is closed as described above.

Delayed sternal closure may also be indicated in patients with a distended heart that is unable to tolerate compression, causing hypotension and reduced cardiac output. After cardiac function improves and the heart size decreases, the sternum can be closed (Cooley, 1984).

Operative procedure: repeat sternotomy

Repeat sternotomy is becoming more frequent, especially in patients who have undergone coronary artery bypass grafting (CABG) but whose progressive coronary atherosclerosis and vein graft disease have caused recurring angina (Loop and others, 1983). Reoperation is associated with an increased morbidity and mortality, and this is due in part to the dangers that are encountered during reopening of the sternum.

As part of the healing process after initial sternotomy, dense adhesions form between the pericardium, the great vessels, the retrosternum, and, in CABG patients, the bypass conduits. The severity of these adhesions is usually apparent on the lateral chest x-ray film (which should be available in the operating room for review by the surgeon). Occasionally there is a retrosternal space that will allow passage of a sternal saw such as that shown in Fig. 11-1, but very often dense adhesions necessitate the use of an oscillating saw to divide the sternum from the anterior table down to the posterior table. Another technique used by some surgeons anticipating repeat operation (e.g., in young patients undergoing open mitral commissurotomy) is partial closure of the pericardium at the

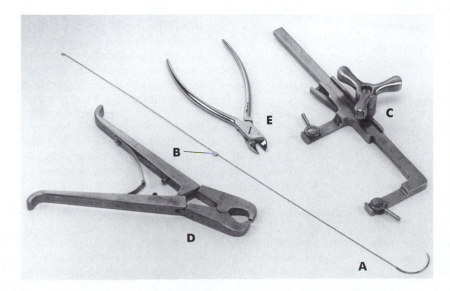

Fig. 11-9 Pilling-Wolvek sternal approximator and fixation system. The sternal wire *(A)* is inserted into each side of the sternum, and the needle is removed with the wire cutters *(E).* Each end of the wire is placed through a locking plate *(B)* so that the wires are crossed over the outer sternum. The ends of the wires are then separately secured into an arm of the approximator *(C).* As the knob is turned clockwise, the arms move wider apart, tightening the wire around the bone. The crimper *(D)* is applied to the locking plate and closed tightly to crimp the plate and secure the wires. The excess wire is removed with the wire cutters. (Courtesy Pilling Co., Fort Washington, Pa.)

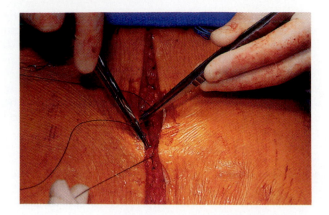

Fig. 11-10 Subcutaneous tissue closure with absorbable suture. (Courtesy John R. Garrett, MD; Howard Kaye, photographer.)

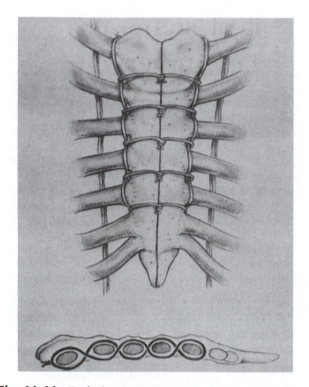

Fig. 11-11 Technique to prevent, or correct, sternal separation. Sternal wires are threaded along each side of the sternum. Transverse wires are placed around the vertical wires, which act as a bolster to prevent the transverse wires from cutting through the bone. (From Robicsek F, Daugherty HK, Cook JW: The prevention and treatment of sternum separation following open heart surgery, *J Thorac Cardiovasc Surg* 73:267, 1977.)

time of the first operation. This technique can reduce the amount of adhesions that form without obstructing pericardial drainage.

Procedural considerations. Because there is a risk of massive hemorrhage from laceration of the structures below the sternum (in particular, the right ventricle, great vessels, and patent bypass grafts), both sides of

the groin should be prepared and draped as part of the sterile field. The surgeon may then expose the femoral vessels for cannulation. Bypass lines should be ready so that CPB can be instituted quickly if necessary. If extensive bleeding is encountered, the patient can be placed on femoral bypass (described later in this chapter). The patient must be heparinized before CPB is instituted. Femoral bypass can reduce blood loss and the risk of myocardial ischemia and allow shed blood to be reinfused; it also decompresses the heart and facilitates dissection of the pericardial adhesions.

Procedure

1. The skin incision is made along the previous incision; scar tissue may be excised.
2. Cautery is used to dissect the subcutaneous tissue and to expose the sternal wires. The lower fascial closure is reopened, and the retrosternal area is evaluated.
3. The exposed wires are cut or untwisted.
4A. The wires are removed with a wire twister (or Kocher clamp). A reciprocating saw (see Fig. 11-1) or an oscillating saw is used to divide the sternum.
4B. The wires are not removed, and the free ends of the wire are retracted upwardly to elevate the sternum away from mediastinal structures (Garrett and Matthews, 1989), An oscillating saw is used to divide the sternum; the retained wires serve as a barrier to the saw blade as it cuts through the posterior table of the sternum (Macmanus and others, 1975). The wires are removed after the bone is divided.
5. After the bone is cut, the sternal edges are gently retracted with rakes (or other preferred retractors), and the tissue between the retrosternum and the pericardium is divided with a knife or scissors. The sternal retractor is not inserted until the heart is freed from the sternum to lessen the risk of tearing attached cardiac structures.
6. Once the heart is freed from the sternum, dissection proceeds along the diaphragmatic surface of the heart, where a relatively free plane may be found. Dissection then continues around the right atrium, over the right ventricle, and over the aorta and pulmonary artery (Harlin, Starr, and Harwin, 1980). If serious bleeding is encountered, CPB can be instituted.
7. After the heart is freed sufficiently, the surgeon can cannulate for CPB) see later section). After CPB is instituted and the heart is decompressed, left ventricular adhesions can be dissected more easily.

Sternal infection

Infection of the sternum may range from suprasternal soft tissue infection, which is usually responsive to debridement, drainage, and superficial wound care, to deep wound infection causing mediastinitis and requiring more extensive treatment. Wound complications occur in approximately 1% to 5% of patients undergoing sternotomy and are related to repeat sternotomy, surgical technique, reoperation for bleeding, external cardiac massage, and prolonged mechanical ventilation (Ottino and others, 1987). Other predisposing factors that have been reported include diabetes mellitus, age over 60 years, postoperative low cardiac output syndrome, chronic pulmonary insufficiency, duration of operation, excessive use of cautery, and prolonged CPB (Craver and others, 1991).

Sternal instability with or without purulent drainage should be treated promptly with reoperation. Cultures are obtained, and appropriate antibiotic therapy is instituted. Chest closure must be secure; the method shown in Fig. 11-11 is often used.

The presence of purulent drainage and mobile sternal fragments often signal deep mediastinal infection (Craver and others, 1991; Culliford and others, 1976). Mediastinitis may occur within the first postoperative week, or 2 weeks or more after the initial operation. Signs and symptoms include sternal pain, fever, leukocytosis, erythema, tenderness, and wound drainage.

Treatment for mediastinitis has changed over the years. In the past it was limited to surgical debridement, healing by primary closure, and closed mediastinal catheter irrigating systems. In severe cases of infection, use of these techniques alone demonstrated a morbidity and mortality greater than 25% in some series. Current therapy reflects a modification of these methods, which may be helpful in less severe cases of sternal infection. In more severe cases, therapy is staged. Initial care includes drainage of the wound by opening the soft tissues, infusion of parenteral broad-spectrum antibiotics, and wound cleaning and dressing changes. At this point, minimal manipulation of the sternum is recommended to avoid systemic showering of infected debris, and most or all of the chest wires are retained to help stabilize the sternum. Once the infection is controlled, definitive wound closure is accomplished by reoperation to debride the sternum and perform muscle or omental flap closure (Craver and others, 1991). Mortality for postcardiotomy mediastinitis has been reduced with these procedures (Pairolero, Arnold, and Harris, 1991).

Tissue flap wound closure. The pectoralis and rectus abdominis muscles and the omentum have been used as flaps individually or in combination to eradicate mediastinal dead space and to close sternal wounds. The pectoralis muscle may be the only suitable graft in patients who have had abdominal surgery involving the rectus muscles and omentum. The use of one or both internal mammary arteries (IMAs) for CABG also affects the choice of muscle flaps.

Operative procedure: flap closure of the sternum *(Craver and others, 1991)*

1. The patient is placed in the supine position with the arms at the sides.
2. The entire chest and abdomen are prepared.
3. Skin edges and subcutaneous tissue are de-

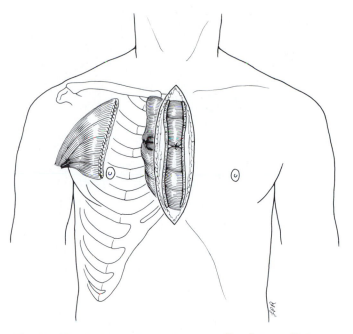

Fig. 11-12   Right pectoralis turnover flap (see text). (From Craver JM and others: Management of postcardiotomy mediastinitis. In Waldhausen JA, Orringer MB: *Complications of cardiothoracic surgery*, St Louis, 1991, Mosby.)

brided, and approximately 1 to 2 mm of tissue along the edges is excised.
4. Sternal bone edges are debrided with rongeurs and curettes until bleeding is encountered. Exposed costal cartilages are widely resected to prevent their becoming a nidus for infection.
5. Fibrinous exudate is removed from the surface of the heart.
6. The wound is irrigated, and hemostasis is achieved.
7. The surgical team changes gowns and gloves, and a new set of instruments replaces those used during the first part of the procedure.
8A. **Pectoralis muscle flap** (Fig. 11-12):

The skin and subcutaneous tissue is elevated digitally and with cautery off the pectoralis major muscle from medial to lateral aspects.

The thoracoacromial pedicle, which provides the primary blood supply to the pectoralis major, is ligated and divided.

The clavicular attachment is taken down to mobilize the flap, and the muscle is turned over to reach the midline. IMA perforators are spared so that they can perfuse the flap.

The flap is then split in the direction of its fibers to allow it to reach the upper and lower portions of the wound.

If more coverage is needed, the pectoralis can be rotated (see Fig. 11-6), rather than turned over; the rotation flap can be used when the ipsilateral IMA has been harvested. A rectus abdominis flap also can be used.

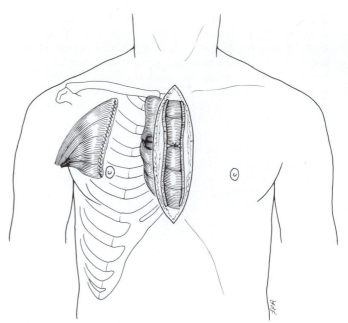

Fig. 11-14 Right rectus abdominis flap in place (see text). (From Craver JM and others: Management of postcardiotomy mediastinitis. In Waldhausen JA, Orringer MB: *Complications in cardiothoracic surgery*, St Louis, 1991, Mosby.)

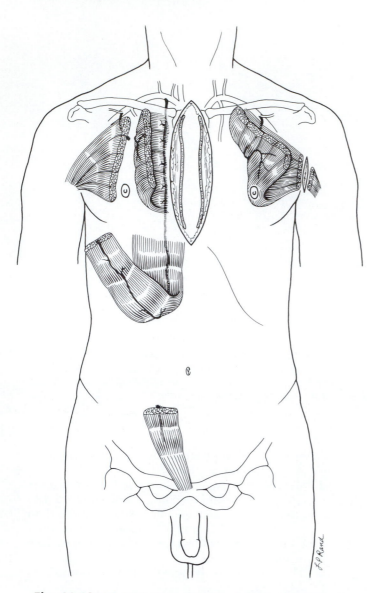

Fig. 11-13 Multiple muscle flaps: right pectoralis turnover flap; left pectoralis rotation advancement flap; right rectus abdominis muscle flap being elevated up to the chest (see text). (From Craver JM and others: Management of postcardiotomy mediastinitis. In Waldhausen JA, Orringer MB: *Complications in cardiothoracic surgery*, St Louis, 1991, Mosby.)

8B. **Rectus abdominis flap** (Figs. 11-13 and 11-14):
The midline sternal incision is extended inferiorly over the rectus muscle to be harvested.
The anterior rectus sheath is divided and peeled back to expose the rectus muscle. The muscle is digitally elevated from the posterior sheath, and the inferior epigastric pedicle is ligated and divided.
The inferior portion of the muscle is brought up to the chest; intercostal bundles are ligated as encountered.
The flap is attached to the wound, and the rectus sheath is closed.

8C. **Omental flap:**
This flap is useful when both IMAs have been used and when the sternal wound is extensive.
The midline sternal incision is extended, and the omentum is mobilized. Omental attachments to the transverse colon are divided with ties. Gastroepiploic artery continuity is maintained to provide a blood supply to the flap.
The flap is transferred subcutaneously or transdiaphragmatically into the mediastinum.
A nasogastric tube is kept in place for 3 to 4 days to decompress the stomach and duodenum and avoid compression of the pedicle.
9. The subcutaneous tissue of the chest wall is elevated, and the flaps are secured in position with absorbable interrupted sutures.
10. Soft drainage tubes are placed above and below the flaps in the midline and in the donor bed.
11. The skin is closed primarily. Occasionally skin grafting may be necessary to close the incision.

Other Thoracic Incisions

Although the median sternotomy is the most widely used incision, other thoracic approaches are necessary for certain lesions (see Table 11-1). These include the anterolateral (Fig. 11-15), lateral, posterolateral (Fig. 11-16), subxiphoid, and thoracoabdominal incisions (see Chapter 16 on surgery for the thoracic aorta). Exposure of the distal portion of the transverse aortic

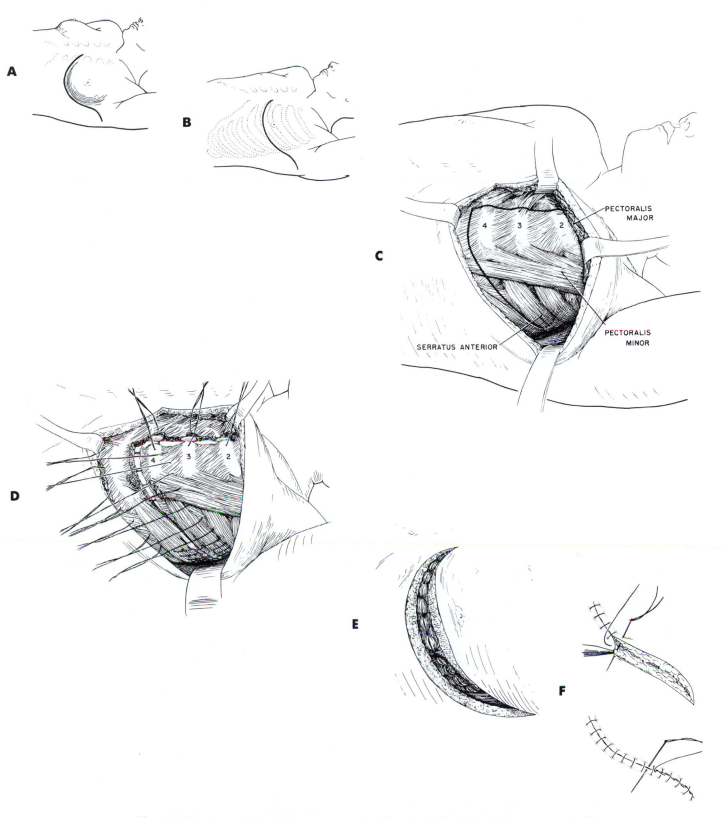

Fig. 11-15 Anterolateral thoracotomy. **Incision: A,** In females a submammary incision is preferable in order to avoid breast scars. **B,** In males the incision is made over the interspace to be entered. **C,** The major muscles and the ribs (numbered) are shown. **Closure: D,** Approximation of the pectoralis major is performed with interrupted or running sutures. **E,** Superficial fascia and subcutaneous tissue are closed. **F,** The skin is closed with a running (shown) or a subcuticular technique. (From Walhausen JA, Pierce WS: *Johnson's surgery of the chest,* ed 5, St Louis, 1985, Mosby.)

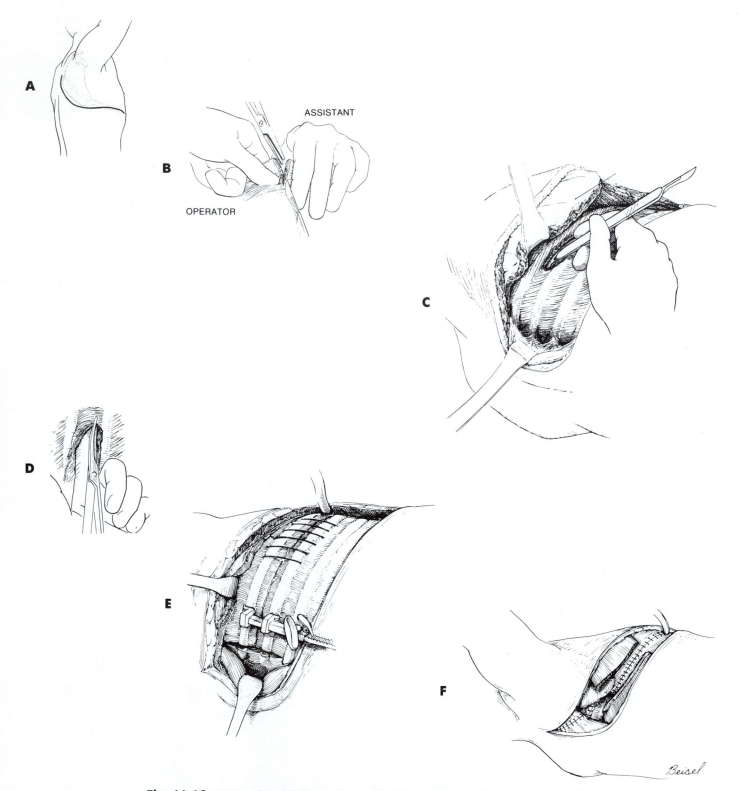

Fig. 11-16 Posterolateral thoracotomy. **Incision: A,** Line of incision. **B,** Manual pressure is used to control bleeding while the surgeon incises through the chest muscles. **C,** The chest is entered through the fourth or fifth intercostal space. **D,** Scissors are used to open the interspace. The index finger is inserted to protect the lung. **Closure: E,** An anterior chest tube is inserted to drain air, and a posterior tube is inserted to drain fluid. A rib approximator can be used to assist with tying of the pericostal sutures. **F,** The chest wall muscles are closed in layers. (From Walhausen JA, Pierce WS: *Johnson's surgery of the chest*, ed 5, St Louis, 1985, Mosby.)

Table 11-2 ■ *Selected advances and discoveries facilitating the development of cardiopulmonary bypass*

Advance/discovery	Time period
Blood transfusion	Early 1800s
Antiseptic surgery	1860s
Mechanical oxygenation of blood	1860s
Direct suture of heart	1890s
ABO blood compatibility	1900
Endotracheal thoracic anesthesia	Early 1900s
Blood vessel surgery	Early 1900s
Development of plastics	Early 1900s
Discovery of heparin	1916
Elucidation of acid-base balance	1920s
Discovery of antibiotics	1920s
Elucidation of shock	1930s
Titration of protamine sulfate	1940s
Measurement of intracardiac pressures	1940s
Clinical use of hypothermia	1940s
Understanding of metabolic effects of surgery	Early 1950s
First clinical use of a heart-lung machine	1953
Use of cross-circulation (using parent to act as biologic oxygenator for child)	Early 1950s
Azygos (low-flow) principle: heart and brain can be sustained with reduced blood flow (e.g., when SVC and IVC are occluded and only azygos venous return contributes to preload and cardiac output)	1950s

Modified from Johnson SL: *The history of cardiac surgery 1896-1955*, Baltimore, 1970, Johns Hopkins Press; Shumacker HB: *The evolution of cardiac surgery*, Bloomington, 1992, Indiana University Press; and Brieger GH: The development of surgery. In Sabiston DC, editor: *Textbook of surgery*, ed 14, Philadelphia, 1991, WB Saunders. (See also Chapter 1.)

arch and the descending thoracic aorta is achieved best with a posterolateral incision. Aneurysms of the distal thoracic aorta extending into the abdominal aorta may be approached with the left side of the chest tilted at a 45-degree angle (anterolateral position) and the lower portion of the torso supine. Subxiphoid incisions have been used for pericardial drainage and the insertion of pacemaker electrodes. Nursing considerations related to these incisions are discussed in Chapter 8, and the indications for their use can be found in subsequent chapters.

CARDIOPULMONARY BYPASS

The idea that blood could be infused into organs to maintain their viability had been suggested in the early part of the nineteenth century. But the development of the modern-day heart-lung machine could not have become a reality without the work of researchers whose discoveries provided the theoretic and scientific basis for extracorporeal circulation (Table 11-2). The most notable achievement was Gibbon's (1954) development of the first heart-lung machine to be used in humans.

Gibbon's contribution was to provide a method of perfusing the organs without relying on the heart and the lungs. By diverting venous return to a device that could remove carbon dioxide and add oxygen, and then propel the oxygen-saturated blood back into the body, the use of CPB enabled clinicians to isolate the heart and lungs from the rest of the body. In addition, because oxygenation and ventilation (removal of carbon dioxide) were achieved with a mechanical lung, the patient's own lungs could be deflated and allowed to fall back out of the way of the surgical site.

The heart and the other organs of the body are more tolerant of anoxia than is the brain. With a method to perfuse the brain while the heart was arrested, surgeons were no longer limited to a 6-minute period or less of cerebral anoxia during which they had to complete intracardiac repairs. Gibbon (1954) demonstrated this by using CPB in an 18-year-old girl who underwent a 26-minute period of normothermic cardiac arrest—considerably longer than the 6-minute period tolerated by the ischemic brain—while the operation was performed. Other researchers were able to prolong the period of ischemia safely by combining the already-familiar technique of hypothermia with CPB.

Hypothermia

Prior to the introduction of CPB, topical hypothermia was used to arrest the heart during surgery. Studies by Bigelow, Lindsay, and Greenwood (1950) had shown that, like hibernating animals, humans could lower their metabolic rate and oxygen consumption when their body temperature was reduced. Hypothermia alone, however, proved unreliable because of the attendant risks of ventricular fibrillation and the relatively short period of time during which surgery could be performed without incurring irreversible cerebral anoxia. Sealy, Brown, and Young (1958) were among the first to combine the use of hypothermia with extracorporeal circulation, and their work, along with that of many others, enhanced the safety of CPB and paved the way for the techniques of hypothermic circulatory arrest and myocardial preservation.

Cardiopulmonary Bypass Circuit

Even though there are adverse effects associated with its use, present-day CPB is safer and more efficient than the early heart-lung machines. Components of the CPB system are listed in Table 11-3. Venous blood is drained from the right side of the heart via the superior vena cava (SVC) and the inferior vena cava (IVC), arterialized in the oxygenator, and pumped back into the systemic circulation (Fig. 11-17). To prevent thrombosis within the bypass circuit from exposure of the blood to foreign surfaces, the circulatory system is anticoagulated with heparin.

Table 11-3 ■ *Components of the bypass system*

Component	Purpose/mechanism
Pump	Move fluid throughout extracorporeal circuit
Roller pump	Uses positive displacement with rotating roller head to propel fluid; amount of flow is dependent on degree that tubing is occluded and on number of revolutions per minute; additional roller heads are used for cardiotomy suctions and venting catheters
Centrifugal pump	Transforms potential energy generated by electromagnetic forces into kinetic energy; vortex principle
Pneumatic and electrical pumps	Used primarily as cardiac assistive or replacement devices (see Chapter 17)
Oxygenator	Performs gas exchange functions; provides oxygen, removes carbon dioxide; contains an arterial reservoir
Membrane	Uses a semipermeable membrane through which oxygen diffuses into, and carbon dioxide diffuses out of, desaturated blood; no direct blood-gas interface exists; less trauma to blood than with bubble method; preferred method, especially for long bypass runs
Bubble	Injects oxygen directly through a column of blood; direct blood-gas interface exists, and gas bubbles are formed that must be removed in defoaming section; traumatic to blood elements; contributes to protein denaturation and formation of micro-emboli
Heat exchanger	Used to alter temperature of blood by principle of conduction; may be freestanding or, more commonly, incorporated into oxygenator system
Venous reservoir	Collects venous return and stores excess volume; may be incorporated into oxygenator system
Blood filters	Inserted into arterial line to remove gas and particulate emboli
Cardiotomy suction/venting devices	Suction used to aspirate blood from operative site and return to cardiotomy reservoir; intracardiac vent used to decompress cardiac chamber(s) and to aspirate air and blood that is returned to cardiotomy reservoir; aspirated blood is filtered and returned to venous reservoir and oxygenator
Cardioplegia infusion system	Used to cool and deliver cardioplegia solution; uses a separate roller head; when blood cardioplegia is used, system is connected to arterial blood supply
Ultrafiltration device	Removes excess water from perfusate
Bypass tubing	Made from polyvinylchloride or Silastic; thickness and caliber of tubing vary depending on its use (e.g., arterial or venous lines, suction lines); heparin-coated tubing has advantage of making inner surfaces of bypass circuit more blood compatible and reducing inflammatory responses associated with bypass
Priming solution	Often a balanced salt solution, pH corrected, that will produce hemodilution with a hematocrit of 20% to 25%; extra heparin, albumin, and various other ingredients may be added; whole blood is not used unless patient is small and/or severely anemic
Safety mechanisms	To reduce or prevent complications and injury; include air bubble detectors, filters, arterial and venous oxygen saturation sensors, vents, pressure sensors, shutoff valves

Modified from Bell PE, Diffee GT: Cardiopulmonary bypass, *AORN J* 53(6):1480, 1991; and Stammers AH: Trends in extracorporeal circulation for the 1990's: renewed interest and advancing technologies, *J Cardiothorac Vasc Anesth* 6(2):226, 1992.

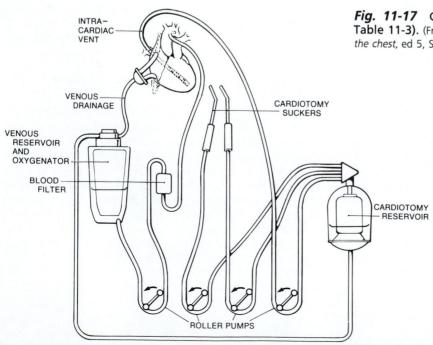

Fig. 11-17 Cardiopulmonary bypass (CPB) circuit (see Table 11-3). (From Walhausen JA, Pierce WS: *Johnson's surgery of the chest*, ed 5, St Louis, 1985, Mosby.)

INTRA-CARDIAC VENT

VENOUS DRAINAGE

CARDIOTOMY SUCKERS

VENOUS RESERVOIR AND OXYGENATOR

BLOOD FILTER

CARDIOTOMY RESERVOIR

ROLLER PUMPS

Heparin and protamine sulfate

Heparin. Heparin, made from bovine lung tissue or porcine intestinal mucosa, prevents the formation of blood clots by producing a conformational change in antithrombin III and converting it to a rapid inhibitor of factor V and factor VIII (Hirsh, 1991). This in turn inhibits the conversion of prothrombin to thrombin and fibrinogen to fibrin (Fig. 11-18).

Heparin prolongs whole-blood clotting time, thrombin time, partial thromboplastin time, and prothrombin time, and has a platelet-inhibiting effect. It is given prior to cannulation for CPB or prior to clamping of blood vessels (e.g., for CPB or during harvesting of the IMA). The initial bolus is approximately 300 units USP/kg (100 units = approximately 1 mg). Thus a patient weighing 70 kg would receive a heparin dose of 21,000 units (or approximately 210 mg). Heparin may be given by the surgeon directly into the right atrium or by the anesthesiologist through a central venous line. Peripheral venous infusion is not recommended, because if CPB must be instituted rapidly, thereby curtailing the time required to measure the blood anticoagulation levels, there is less certainty that the heparin has reached the central circulation (Tinkers and Roberts, 1987).

To determine whether the blood is adequately heparinized, the activating clotting time (ACT) is measured (about 3 minutes) after heparin infusion but before CPB is initiated. A baseline ACT, taken at the start of surgery, is often used for comparison, especially in the presence of coagulation abnormalities. (Because the ACT monitors coagulation but not heparin levels, some clinicians also measure heparin concentration.) Although there is some controversy over the appropriate ACT necessary to initiate CPB safely, a minimum ACT of 400 seconds (four times normal) is generally considered necessary. During bypass, periodic ACTs are measured and additional heparin is given to maintain the ACT well above 400 seconds.

Occasionally it is difficult to achieve adequate anticoagulation with heparin. Some patients on prolonged preoperative heparin regimens demonstrate heparin resistance; the reasons for this are not entirely clear, but increasing the heparin level is usually effective. Inadequate anticoagulation may also be the result of significantly depressed antithrombin III levels; this produces an insufficient amount of the factor for the heparin to affect. Infusion of fresh frozen plasma (FFP) may be necessary to increase the antithrombin III levels (Tinker and Roberts, 1987).

Protamine sulfate. In the absence of heparin, protamine sulfate acts as a mild anticoagulant, but in the presence of heparin, it acts as an antidote to the anticoagulant. Protamine is strongly basic, and it combines with the strongly acidic heparin to form a stable complex. A calculated dosage of 1 to 1.3 times the total heparin dose is usually administered. The ACT is used to guide additional protamine infusion.

Protamine infusion, especially when bolused, is associated with systemic hypotension, thought to be due to arterial vasodilatation and decreased systemic vascular resistance (Kien and others, 1992). In worst cases, a full anaphylactic reaction may occur. Some surgeons may prefer not to remove the arterial cannula before or immediately after the initiation of protamine infusion so that, if necessary, volume may be given to maintain an adequate blood pressure or CPB can be resumed if myocardial function is too depressed (additional heparin may be required to reinstitute bypass). If a serious protamine reaction is going to occur, it is usually apparent shortly after the infusion is started. When minimal or no reaction is evident and the blood pressure is stable, the arterial cannula is removed.

Total and partial cardiopulmonary bypass

Total CPB exists when all of the systemic venous drainage is returned to the oxygenator. This necessitates individual cannulation of the SVC and IVC, with the addition of a tourniquet or caval clamp placed around each of these vessels and tightened against the cannulas within them. This forces all returning systemic venous blood to enter the distal ends of the cannulas. Coronary sinus drainage and bronchial return entering the heart can be removed with an intracardiac venting catheter.

Partial CPB exists when some venous return is allowed to enter the right atrium. This can occur when only one (e.g., two-stage) cannula is placed in the right atrium, or when bicaval cannulas are inserted into the SVC and IVC but tourniquets or caval clamps are not used, allowing some returning blood to drain around the distal ends of the cannulas and into the right atrium.

Pumps and oxygenators

Various types of pumps have been designed to propel blood, but the roller pump (a positive displacement pump) and the centrifugal pump (a constrained vortex pump) are the most widely used (see Fig. 5-19). Unlike the body's normal hemodynamics, nonpulsatile (i.e., no systolic or diastolic phases) flow is usually produced by these pumps. (The roller pump can be modified to provide pulsatile flow.) Although there does not seem to be a significant increase in morbidity from nonpulsatile flow, the potential advantages of pulsatile flow have increased interest in its use. Among these advantages are increased flow in the microcirculation, reduced volume overloading, and improved renal, cerebral, and pancreatic blood flow. Although roller pumps that provide pulsatile flow are available, studies confirming the benefits of pulsatile flow are contradicted by other studies showing no superiority of one method over the other (Stammers, 1992).

Membrane oxygenators have largely replaced bubble oxygenators because of the absence of a direct blood-gas interface. This offers the advantages of less blood cell trauma, reduced incidence of air emboli (especially microemboli), and independent control of oxygenation and ventilation. The absence of a direct blood-gas interface also reduces complement activation.

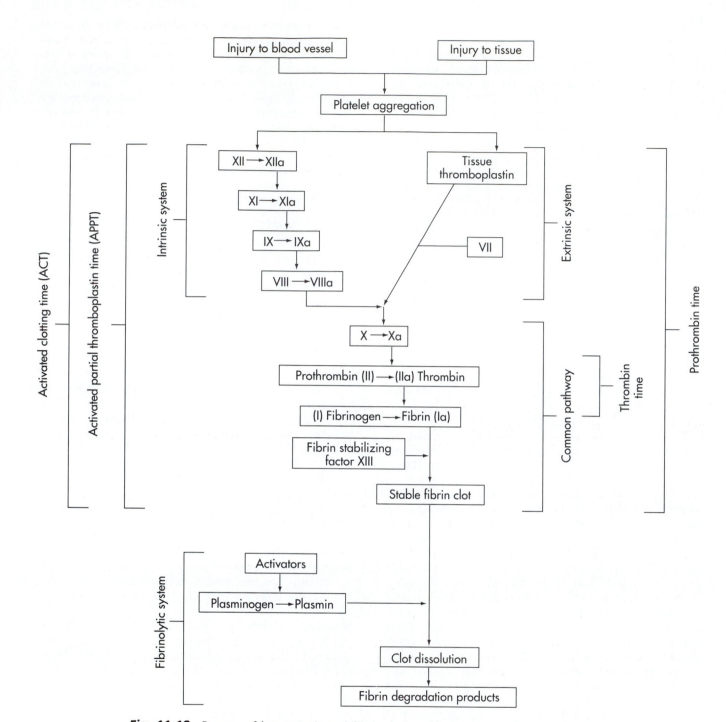

Fig. 11-18 Process of hemostasis and fibrinolysis, with common tests of anticoagulation. Injury to the blood vessel or the tissue activates, respectively, the intrinsic and
extrinsic coagulation pathways, which join to form the common pathway. If the coagulation process is not inhibited, a fibrin clot is formed and then undergoes dissolution
by the fibrinolytic system. The activated clotting time (ACT) is prolonged when factors
of the intrinsic or common pathway are severely decreased. Activated partial thromboplastin time ([a]PPT) is a more sensitive test; it is prolonged when the level of
coagulation factors of the intrinsic and common system decreases to 10% to 40% of
the normal level. Prothrombin time (PT) detects low levels of factors of the extrinsic
or common system. Thrombin time (TT) is prolonged in the presence of abnormally
low fibrinogen. Heparin prolongs the times of all these tests. (Modified from Pagana KD,
Pagana TJ: *Mosby's diagnostic and laboratory test reference,* St Louis, 1992, Mosby; and Tarhan S:
Cardiovascular anesthesia and postoperative care, ed 2, St Louis, 1989, Mosby.)

Suction devices

Aspiration of blood and other fluids is an important component of any surgical procedure, and the ability to reuse shed blood is what makes CPB possible. A variety of suctioning devices is used during cardiac surgery. Indications for their use differ, and a safe and efficient operation is dependent in part on the proper use of these devices (Table 11-4). Some of these are an integral part of the bypass circuit; others that are not are also described in this section.

Cardiotomy suction. One or more cardiotomy suction lines (see Fig. 11-17) aspirate blood directly back to the pump, where it is filtered, oxygenated, and reinfused with the rest of the bypass volume into the arterial circulation. Because blood is returned directly to the pump, the patient must be systemically heparinized before the cardiotomy sucker can be used. Often the perfusionist will "protect" the pump from thrombus formation by not activating the cardiotomy suction until adequate heparinization has been confirmed.

Blood trauma can result from excessive negative pressure and shear forces. The amount of negative pressure can be regulated by perfusionist, and the tip of most cardiotomy suckers has multiple holes (similar to a small Poole tip), which also reduces the negative pressure. The suction should be used to aspirate pools of blood rather than skimming blood away from specific surgical sites (e.g., anastomoses). Another danger occurs when the suction falls off the sterile field and contaminated material is aspirated into the system, increasing the risk of infection. If this happens, the perfusionist should be informed immediately and suction temporarily halted while new tubing is set up.

Cardiotomy suction is used throughout CPB and then terminated once heparin reversal with protamine has been started. Aspiration of irrigating fluids should be avoided, because it can cause excessive hemodilution with a significant drop in the hematocrit of the pump volume. Aspiration of particulate matter should be avoided when possible; even with in-line microfilters, it is safer to minimize the risk of potential emboli entering the circuit. Pleural effusate, pericardial fluid, topical antibiotic solutions, and hemostatic agents should be avoided as well.

Table 11-4 ■ *Safety considerations during cardiopulmonary bypass*

Potential danger	Cause	Safety measures
Embolism Air	Air in arterial line	Constant vigilance Minimum distraction (avoid loud talking or music) Before connecting arterial cannula to arterial line and during connection, check for air (look at highest point) Ensure that tubing clamps are tight; do not use clamps too small for caliber of tubing Notify surgeon and perfusionist immediately of air in arterial line or cannula Test venting catheters before use to ensure they are suctioning (and not infusing) Be aware that perfusion circuit air sensors may trigger shutoff valve if air is detected Be aware that left side of heart should never be opened before aorta is cross-clamped Ensure identification of outflow (e.g., venous and venting lines) and inflow (e.g., arterial and cardioplegia lines) tubing; label if necessary
Thrombus	Inadequate heparinization; old blood clots entering opened arterial line; coagulation agents introduced into circuit	Ensure that proper heparin dose is given before initiating CPB Keep field free of formed blood clots, especially before arterial line is connected to cannula Avoid aspiration of coagulation agents into pump via cardiotomy suction; discontinue use of cardiotomy suction shortly after protamine has been started Monitor ACT (activated clotting time); additional heparin is given as needed If CPB must be reinstituted after heparin reversal with protamine sulfate, ensure that heparin is given before reinitiating CPB Note and notify perfusionist of existing cold antibodies, which promote agglutination of red blood cells at low temperatures (determined by laboratory blood testing)
Particulate debris	Free bone fragments, bone wax, suture pieces, calcium, fat, and so forth	Keep field free of loose debris; monitor lines

Modified from Pae WE and others: Prevention of complications during cardiopulmonary bypass. In Waldhausen JA, Orringer MB: *Complications in cardiothoracic surgery,* St Louis, 1991, Mosby. Data also from O'Connell J, Yorde W: Personal communication, 1991.
CPB, Cardiopulmonary bypass; *CVP,* central venous pressure.

Continued.

Table 11-4 ■ *Safety considerations during cardiopulmonary bypass—cont'd*

Potential danger	Cause	Safety measures
Inadequate venous return	Cannula(s) too small for adequate venous drainage; cannula(s) clogged by caval or atrial tissue; table too low; cannula(s) malpositioned or compressed	Discuss size of cannula(s) with perfusionist/surgeon to ensure sufficient size for adequate drainage Establish good venous return before instituting hypothermia (e.g., adjust cannulas, tighten tourniquets/pursestring sutures, increase CVP, change heart position) Note that right atrium is decompressed (collapsed) and CVP is 0-3 mm Hg when venous return is adequate Anticipate adjusting patient volume if flow is too low Use cardiotomy suction whenever possible to return volume to pump
Interruption of venous return	Tubing kinked or clamped; air lock; tubing/cannulas disrupted or dislodged	If holding heart, avoid compression of right atrial lines Avoid clamping lines (during CPB), or stepping or leaning on lines Avoid large amounts of air in venous line; be able to "chase air" down venous line (raising and lowering line to move air toward pump); refill venous line if necessary During open right-sided heart cases (atrial septal defect, tricuspid valve surgery), be prepared to use double venous cannulation, caval clamps, or tourniquets to avoid sucking air into venous circuit Use caution when walking near lines
Interruption of arterial inflow	Arterial line occluded or kinked (can cause rupture of bypass circuit); tubing/cannula dislodged	Do not occlude arterial line with clamp Avoid kinks in line Refrain from leaning on line Protect line during pleural chest tube insertion
Contamination of circuit	Contaminants introduced into CPB circuit	Monitor location of cardiotomy suction tip; suction must be turned off immediately if tip falls off field Ensure that components of circuit are assembled aseptically Ensure that additives (fluids, drugs, etc.) are administered aseptically Fill venous lines only with appropriate solutions; discuss with perfusionist/surgeon Avoid aspiration of topical antibiotics or other contraindicated fluids Maintain sterility of lines when OR table is raised or lowered
Excessive hemodilution	Excess volume aspirated into circuit	Avoid aspirating excessive amounts of irrigating or topical hypothermic solutions into circuit; use discard suction or autotransfusion
Cellular destruction	Trauma to red blood cells, platelets, and other blood cells	Use cardiotomy suction gently and sparingly Avoid unnecessary connectors in bypass tubing Position bypass lines in gentle curves; avoid tight angles or kinks

Autotransfusion suction. Although not part of the bypass circuit, autotransfusion systems conserve red blood cells (RBCs) by returning them to a reservoir from which they can be processed and reinfused back into the patient. Because of the time required for processing, blood return to the patient cannot be achieved as quickly as it can with the cardiotomy sucker. (Thus it is always preferable to use the cardiotomy suction for large amounts of blood.)

The suction apparatus has greater negative pressure than the cardiotomy suction, allowing it to be used for more selective and precise suctioning. Often a T & A (tonsil and adenoidectomy) tip is used. Significant blood trauma occurs when too high a negative pressure is exerted on the blood.

To prevent clotting within the system, an anticoagulant (i.e., heparin) is added to the circuit. The suction tubing has a double lumen; the smaller-caliber tubing infuses the anticoagulant solution to the tip of

the tubing, where it mixes with aspirated blood and is suctioned back to the reservoir. Because the system has its own method of maintaining anticoagulation, autotransfusion suction can be used throughout the procedure and is not dependent on systemic heparinization. When the patient is systemically heparinized, the autotransfusion anticoagulation flow can be reduced or halted, and restarted when heparin reversal is begun.

Irrigating solutions containing a significant amount of blood can be aspirated back to the reservoir, where processing will remove the excess volume. When the fluid is mostly asanguineous, use of the discard suction is preferable to avoid overloading the autotransfusion reservoir. Other fluids contraindicated for cardiotomy suction (e.g., antibiotic solutions, fibrin "glue") are similarly contraindicated with this system.

The system can also be used in conjunction with the CPB circuit. After termination of CPB, blood remaining within the circuit can be pumped over to the autotransfusion reservoir by connecting the arterial CPB line to the autotransfusion suction tubing.

Discard suction. The standard discard suction system used for many noncardiac procedures is used to rapidly aspirate fluid that cannot or should not be reinfused. This includes crystalloid irrigating solutions, hypothermic lavage fluid, and the fluids and debris contraindicated for cardiotomy aspiration and autotransfusion.

The T & A tip is often used. With the addition of a microsuction tip, the discard suction can be used to aspirate blood from anastomotic sites; the small amount of blood involved (a few milliliters) does not appreciably affect circulating blood volume. Discard suction with an open-ended tip ("debridement" tip) is valuable for aspirating calcium debris during heart valve procedures.

Venting devices and methods to deair the heart

One of the most serious complications associated with cardiac surgery is air embolism, especially to the brain, where it can cause a cerebrovascular accident. Air embolism can occur in a number of ways. The risk is most pronounced when the heart has been opened and trapped air is introduced into the arterial circulation when the aortic occlusion clamp is removed. During CABG, air is introduced into the coronary arteries, and if it is not aspirated, it can cause transient (or permanent) myocardial dysfunction. Patients with intracardiac shunts are also at risk, because air within peripheral or central venous lines can be shunted to the left side of the heart and embolize to the brain.

Because the danger of air embolism is ever-present, the surgical team must be vigilant in preventing entry of air, detecting its presence, and instituting measures to remove it. One of the safest ways to protect the brain is to avoid opening the left side of the heart before the aortic occlusion clamp has been applied. After the heart has been opened, Kirklin and Barratt-Boyes (1993) stress four principles for deairing the heart: (1) the heart is filled with fluid before it is closed to minimize air entrapment; (2) residual air is aspirated from the heart before it is allowed to eject; (3) the lungs are intermittently inflated to remove air from the pulmonary veins and cardiac chambers; and (4) there is continuous suction on a needle vent or catheter in the ascending aorta as the heart begins to eject so that residual air in the heart or pulmonary veins is aspirated.

Venting catheters provide two other benefits: decompression of the ventricles and prevention of rewarming from blood entering the cardiac chambers. Aspiration of blood within the cardiac chambers, especially the left ventricle, decompresses the ventricle and avoids overdistension; and aspiration of returning systemic, bronchial, and coronary venous drainage (which is relatively warmer than myocardial temperature) minimizes temperature gradients within the heart. Rewarming is avoided when possible, because

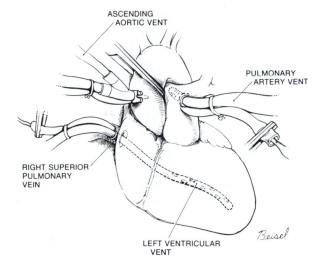

Fig. 11-19 **Types of venting devices.** (From Walhausen JA, Pierce WS: *Johnson's surgery of the chest,* ed 5, St Louis, 1985, Mosby.)

it makes the ventricle, and in particular the subendocardium, less tolerant of ischemia (Hartman, 1992).

Cardiac venting catheters. Cardiac venting catheters are placed within the heart or aorta to remove air. The most common venting device is a needle or catheter placed in the ascending aorta that is connected to suction tubing that aspirates air and blood back to the pump (Fig. 11-19). The same catheter can be used to infuse cardioplegia solution when the inflow line is "Y" connected into the suction line. During infusion the suction line is clamped, and during aspiration the infusion line is clamped. Before the aortic cross-clamp is removed, the vent is turned on slowly to avoid cavitation of the aorta, and then the clamp is opened slowly to allow blood to fill the aortic root.

Additional maneuvers. Additional maneuvers are used to supplement venting devices, because air may be entrapped in the pulmonary veins, the left atrium, the ventricular trabeculations, or other areas of the heart not directly accessible to the venting catheters. Before the aortic cross-clamp is removed, the patient is placed in the steep Trendelenberg position so that air within the aorta will travel preferentially out through the needle vent rather than to the brain; this occurs because air rises and the aortic vent is now in a higher position than the aortic arch vessels.

Another method to dislodge and aspirate air within the cardiac chambers is to pull the heart forward gently and insert a large-bore needle (e.g., 18 gauge) into the left ventricular apex (Fig. 11-20). This may be accompanied by gentle massage of the cardiac chambers. CPB can be slowed temporarily to fill the heart with blood (the venous line is partially clamped to allow some venous return to enter the heart); the anesthesiologist hyperinflates the lungs to allow air in the pulmonary veins to be displaced into the cardiac chambers, where it can be aspirated (Mills and Morris, 1991).

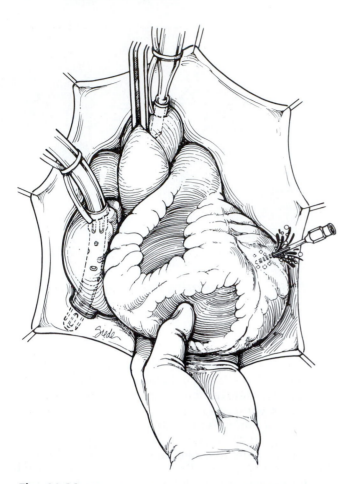

Fig. 11-20 Deairing of the left ventricle. Massage and ballottement of the cardiac chambers with the apex tilted slightly allows air to escape through an apical or aortic vent needle. CPB is slowed to let the heart fill with blood; the anesthesiologist inflates the lungs to dispel remaining air into the heart, and a needle is inserted into the apex of the left ventricle to aspirate air and blood. (From Mills NL, Morris JM: Air embolism associated with cardiopulmonary bypass. In Waldhausen JA, Orringer MB: *Complications in cardiothoracic surgery,* St Louis, 1991, Mosby.)

The heart should not be allowed to eject blood while the presence of air is evident in the aortic vent tubing or air bubbles are seen exiting the left ventricular apical needle. Some surgeons will purposely fibrillate the heart so that it cannot pump potential emboli into the aorta.

When the aorta has been opened, blood and air are allowed to escape through the aortotomy before the incision is completely closed; the aortic vent is not turned on until the aorta has been closed in order to avoid sucking air into the aorta through the aortotomy. During CABG the proximal anastomosis may be allowed to bleed while the suture is being tied, and completed vein grafts may be aspirated with a small-gauge needle (e.g., 27 gauge).

Bypass tubing

Bypass tubing is most often made from polyvinyl-chloride (PVC). At very low temperatures this plastic can become stiff and does not compress well. In the past, when very low temperatures were anticipated, silicone was used in portions of the circuit where flexibility is desired (i.e., in the roller pump head). Recent refinements in the durameter (degree of stiffness or hardness) of PVC tubing have lessened these problems, and silicone inserts are no longer necessary.

Heparin-coated CPB circuits have been evaluated; they are most effective when blood is kept in constant circulation. They reduce the amount of heparin needed but do not supplant it entirely, because areas of stagnant or low flow (within the CPB circuit) require anticoagulation to prevent clot formation (Stammers, 1992). Another advantage may be related to the immune response that accompanies blood exposure to foreign surfaces. The CPB circuit consists of numerous synthetic materials—plastics and metals—and these can also activate platelets, granulocytes, and proteins associated with the coagulation pathways. Research continues to identify bonding techniques applicable to the various components of the CPB circuit and to elucidate blood flow dynamics more fully (Stammers, 1992).

Priming solution

Early bypass systems were primed with whole blood. Current perfusates consist of a balanced electrolyte solution with a near-normal pH and an ionic content similar to that of plasma. Bank blood is now rarely used because of cost considerations, availability, and concern about blood-borne pathogens. Such a policy is usually favorable to patients with religious objections to the use of blood products. Because asanguineous perfusates reduce the hematocrit and hemoglobin (H & H), a unit of packed RBCs may be required occasionally to achieve an adequate, albeit reduced, H & H in patients with relatively small blood volumes compared with the total CPB circuit volume (e.g., small women and children).

Hemodilution is advantageous during hypothermia, which increases blood viscosity. Generally, a hematocrit of 20% to 25% (normal is 40% to 50% in the adult) during moderate hypothermia provides a sufficient number of blood cells for oxygen transport, and it lowers the viscosity and shear rates of blood cells. During rewarming, a higher hematocrit may be needed to meet increased oxyen demands; this can be achieved with ultrafiltration devices, the addition of packed RBCs (Kirlin and Barratt-Boyes, 1993), and/or pharmacologically induced diuresis.

Other additives to the prime may include albumin or hetastarch (to raise the plasma colloidal oncotic pressure), diuretics such as Mannitol and furosemide (to draw fluid from the interstitial space into the vascular space), and vasodilators (to counteract the vasoconstriction produced by catecholamines). Steroids may also be added to improve tissue perfusion and

---

Box 11-2 *Perfusion technology prebypass checklist*

Date: _____   Case No: _____

Nondisposable Equipment

Heart Lung Machine   Ser. No.: Shiley

1. ___ Visually inspect all electrical connections and components. All pumps functional.
2. ___ Emergency power charged and functioning.
3. ___ Clamps, handcranks, and spare fuses available.
4. ___ Gas flow meter and air-oxygen mixer functioning. Emergency oxygen supply available. Regulator and flow meter functional.

Heater—Cooler Unit   Ser. No.: Sarns 1926

5. ___ Visually inspect all electrical connections and components.
6. ___ Heating and cooling modes tested prior to use.
7. ___ Sufficient ice available.

Anticoagulation Monitor   Ser. No.: Hemotec 5003080

8. ___ Visually inspect all electrical connections and components.
9. ___ Monitor self-test completed.
10. ___ Temperature indicator at 37° C (98.6° F).
11. ___ ACT cartridges available.
12. ___ Quality controls completed.

Disposable Equipment

Oxygenator/Venous Reservoir
Cardiotomy Reservoir/Tubing Pack

13. ___ Sterile barrier intact. Outdate noted.
14. ___ Visual check for manufacturing defects.

Assembly

15. ___ Tubing connections secure. Tie band as needed.
16. ___ Cardiotomy vented to atmosphere.
17. ___ Tubing in rollerheads correctly. Checked for kinks and direction of flow.
18. ___ Heat exchanger water to blood leak test performed.
19. ___ Priming and deairing of circuit complete. Oxygen on during priming.
20. ___ Occlusion set on each rollerhead.
21. ___ Blood available. Additional priming solutions, including colloid, available.

Final Checklist

22. ___ Venous saturation meter connected and calibrated.
23. ___ Arterial blood gas monitor operational and calibrated.
24. ___ Cardioplegia pump pressure monitor calibrated and tested. Alarm on.
25. ___ Arterial ultrasonic air detector operational. Alarm on.
26. ___ Arterial line pressure monitored after cannulation.
27. ___ Confirm heparin given. Post-heparin ACT measured prior to bypass.

Comments/corrections:

Perfusionist signature:

1.

2.

Courtesy John O'Connell, CCP.

---

lessen the increases in extracellular water (Kirklin and Barratt-Boyes, 1993).

Safety considerations

Many perfusionists use a written prebypass checklist (Box 11-2) to ensure that the CPB circuit is properly assembled and its integrity tested before CPB is initiated (Pae and others, 1991). Although the conduct of CPB is primarily controlled by the perfusionist in close collaboration with the surgeon and the anesthesiologist, the perioperative nurse also has a vital role in protecting the patient and maintaining a safe operative environment. Among the most important safety considerations (see Table 11-4) are preventing disruption of the bypass circuit, using the various suctioning devices appropriately, and protecting the patient against air or particulate embolism. Perioperative nurses who assist during cardiac procedures may have

additional opportunities to ensure a safe and effective procedure (Box 11-3).

Adverse Effects of Cardiopulmonary Bypass

Although CPB has made possible the repair of congenital and acquired cardiac disorders with relatively low morbidity and mortality, it is not a totally benign intervention. All patients respond physiologically to CPB to one degree or another. Significant adverse reactions can occur—especially in the very young and the very old—producing what is called the "postperfusion syndrome" (Kirklin, 1991). This is evidenced by prolonged pulmonary insufficiency, excessive accumulation of extravascular water, elevated temperature, vasoconstriction, coagulopathy, and variable degrees of renal and other organ dysfunction.

Box 11-3 RN first assistant considerations during cardiopulmonary bypass

Prebypass

If end of arterial line has been cut at the field, do not allow any particulate matter (e.g., bone wax, fat debris) to enter open end of line. Do not unclamp arterial line (may allow entry of air) until necessary.

Ensure that heparin has been given; if you do not either (1) witness surgeon injecting it or (2) hear anesthesia personnel verbalize that it has been (or is being) infused, alert surgeon before any blood vessels are clamped; be especially aware of this when CPB must be reinstituted rapidly and heparin reversal with protamine has been started.

When surgeon attaches arterial cannula to arterial line, look for air—especially at highest point in tubing circuit; if air is noted, ensure immediately that surgeon is aware of it.

Use cardiotomy suction both to retract and to aspirate blood during venous cannulation.

Test intracardiac venting catheters to confirm they are suctioning (and not infusing) before they are inserted into the heart.

Bypass

Do not lean on bypass lines or cause them to kink; be especially alert to perfusionist's warnings that venous return is low or that there is an excessively high pressure in the CPB circuit.

Know purpose and direction of flow of all CPB lines on the field.

Do not clamp any bypass lines except under direct orders from surgeon; never clamp arterial line.

Avoid aspirating significant amounts of irrigating solutions with cardiotomy sucker; avoid aspiration of contraindicated substances (e.g., topical antibiotics, hemostatic agents, surgical debris).

Postbypass

Do not use cardiotomy suction after heparin has been reversed with protamine.

Remove venous cannula quickly (but carefully) to prevent excess blood loss from atriotomy; salvage blood with cardiotomy suction.

Remove arterial cannula with part of your hand covering aortotomy so that blood is not splashed all over the field.

Avoid excess tension when tightening aortic cannula pursestring.

The proposed mechanism for these damaging effects is the exposure of blood to the abnormal surfaces of the CPB circuit, as well as conditions such as hypothermia and altered blood flow, which initiate a systemic inflammatory response. This inflammatory response produces, releases, or alters a host of vasoactive substances that react with specific receptor proteins throughout the body. The resulting vascular smooth muscle and endothelial cell contractions are responsible for many of the morbid complications associated with CPB (Downing and Edmunds, 1992).

Among the numerous substances are endogenous catecholamines; renin, angiotensin, and aldosterone; antidiuretic hormone; atrial natriuretic factor; bradykinin; thyroid hormones; glucagon; platelet-activating factor; vasoactive phospholipids; and complement (Downing and Edmunds, 1992). CPB-induced complement activation is one of the most widely studied reactions.

Complement activation

Complement is a group of circulating glycoproteins that are activated by one of two pathways in response to immunologic injury, infection, or traumatic insult. The classical pathway is usually initiated by an antigen-antibody reaction; protamine infusion at the end of CPB stimulates this pathway. The alternative pathway is activated by exposure of the blood to foreign surfaces, and it is this pathway that seems to be mainly responsible for the activation of the inflammatory response (Kirklin and Barratt-Boyes, 1993).

When the complement proteins are activated, anaphylatoxins, especially C3a, C4a, and C5a, are formed. These toxins increase vascular permeability, release histamine from mast cells, and contract smooth muscle (Chenoweth and others, 1981; Kirklin and others, 1983). C3a has also been shown to cause cardiac dysfunction evidenced by tachycardia, coronary vasoconstriction, and reduced contractility. C3a and C5a concentrations are increased during CPB; plasma C4a appears to be increased immediately after CPB (Downing and Edmunds, 1992).

Modifying the inflammatory response

Attempts to prevent or inhibit the inflammatory response have been directed at modifying the activation of platelets and factor XII, which are the main initiators of the response. Attempts have been made to develop reversible inhibitors of factor XII and platelets, which could attenuate the explosive release of vasoactive materials that is triggered by CPB. Anesthesia, surgery, hemodynamic alterations, heparin, and protamine will still trigger reactions, albeit less dramatically (Downing and Edmunds, 1992).

Cardiopulmonary Bypass Procedures

Cannulation of the aorta for arterial inflow and of the IVC and SVC (or the right atrium) for venous drainage is the most common form of CPB. Other arteries (e.g., the femoral or, rarely, the subclavian) can be cannulated for arterial inflow. The femoral vein can be used to drain venous blood, but venous return may be limited (which then limits arterial flow to the body).

Aortocaval cannulation bypasses both the right and left sides of the heart. Occasionally, left heart bypass or right heart bypass is used to support a failing left or right ventricle, respectively. Left heart bypass does not require an oxygenator, because oxygenated blood is being withdrawn (from the left atrium) and reinfused (into a systemic artery) without its being desaturated. Right heart bypass (e.g., right atrium to

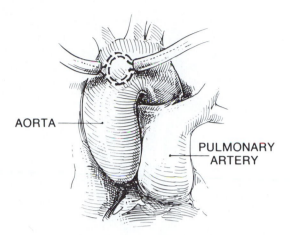

Fig. 11-21   Double pursestring suture with tourniquets in the ascending aorta. (From Walhausen JA, Pierce WS: *Johnson's surgery of the chest*, ed 5, St Louis, 1985, Mosby.)

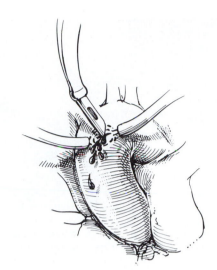

Fig. 11-22   After the stab wound is made in the aorta, the arterial cannula is inserted. (From Walhausen JA, Pierce WS: *Johnson's surgery of the chest*, ed 5, St Louis, 1985, Mosby.)

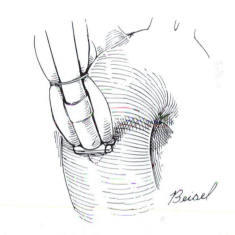

Fig. 11-23   The tourniquets are tightened and tied to the arterial cannula. (From Walhausen JA, Pierce WS: *Johnson's surgery of the chest*, ed 5, St Louis, 1985, Mosby.)

pulmonary artery) does not require an oxygenator either, because the lungs will perform that function. However, whenever desaturated blood is removed from the body, it cannot be infused back into the systemic circulation without prior oxygenation (and ventilation). Doing so would create a shunt and produce hypoxia with cyanosis.

The following procedures are commonly used to achieve CPB.

Operative procedures: arterial cannulation for cardiopulmonary bypass
Cannulation of the aorta

1. After the sternum has been opened, a longitudinal incision is made in the pericardium with scissors and cautery from the pericardial reflection at the aorta to the diaphragmatic portion of the pericardium. The pericardium is often incised laterally at its ends to enhance exposure of the heart. The pericardial edges are sewn to the chest wall. Heparin is given.
2. The aorta is partially dissected from the pulmonary artery.
3. A pursestring double-armed suture is inserted in the ascending aorta just below the great vessels. The needles are removed from the suture, the loose ends of which are threaded with a stylet through a plastic or red rubber catheter. The catheter is clamped with a hemostat so that it does not slide off the suture (but the pursestring is not tightened).
4. A second pursestring suture is placed around the first as described in step 3 (Fig. 11-21).
5. The adventitia inside the pursestring is divided, and a stab wound is made in the aorta (some surgeons use a partial-occlusion clamp on the aorta).
6. The aortic cannula (occluded near the proximal end with a vented cap or a tubing clamp) is inserted into the aorta (Fig. 11-22). The pursestring tourniquets are tightened and held to the cannula with

a heavy tie (Fig. 11-23). If a tubing clamp is used, it is momentarily opened to fill the cannula with blood from the aorta. If there is a cap over the cannula, blood will fill the cannula, displacing any air; the cannula is then clamped, and the cap is removed.
7. While the perfusionist slowly pumps priming solution out of the end of the arterial line (to remove any air), the surgeon connects the proximal end of the aortic cannula to the arterial line, taking care to avoid letting air enter the system (Fig. 11-24). The perfusionist then stops infusing any more solution.

The tubing clamp is removed from the cannula, and the circuit is inspected for air. If any air bubbles are noted, the cannula is reclamped, the connection is opened, priming solution is infused, air

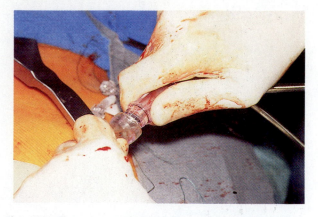

Fig. 11-24 Connecting a cannula to bypass tubing. (Courtesy John R. Garrett, MD; Howard Kaye, photographer.)

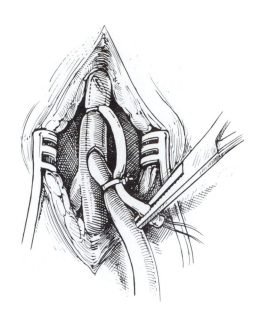

Fig. 11-26 The femoral artery cannula is inserted, and the tourniquet is tightened and tied to the cannula. The femoral vein is adjacent and, when necessary, can be cannulated in a similar manner for venous drainage. (From Walhausen JA, Pierce WS: *Johnson's surgery of the chest*, ed 5, St Louis, 1985, Mosby.)

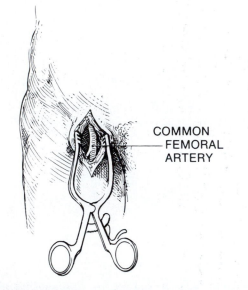

COMMON FEMORAL ARTERY

Fig. 11-25 Exposure of the femoral artery for cannulation. A Weitlaner self-retaining retractor is shown. (From Walhausen JA, Pierce WS: *Johnson's surgery of the chest*, ed 5, St Louis, 1985, Mosby.)

is allowed to escape, and the connection is reestablished. The cannula may also be allowed to fill with blood from the aorta. The arterial line is then attached to the chest with a towel clip or a suture.

Cannulation of the femoral artery

1. A vertical or oblique incision is made in the femoral triangle, and the common femoral artery is exposed (Fig. 11-25).
2. Umbilical tapes are passed around the vessel above and below the planned arteriotomy, and tourniquet catheters are threaded over the tapes. The artery is occluded proximally and distally with femoral artery clamps.
3. An incision is made in the artery and extended with Potts scissors.

4. The arterial catheter (clamped at the proximal end) is inserted into the artery retrogradely as the proximal femoral clamp is removed. The proximal tourniquet is tightened around the cannula in the artery and tied to the cannula (Fig. 11-26).
5. The cannula is attached to the arterial inflow line as described in step 7 and is secured to the drapes. The arterial line should be kept longer to reach the cannula without tension. The distal artery remains occluded with the tourniquet or the femoral artery clamp.

Operative procedure: cannulation for venous return

The two-stage venous cannula is used for most procedures. When entry into the right side of the heart is planned, bicaval cannulation of the IVC and SVC is performed. Occasionally the femoral vein is cannulated when very large thoracic aneurysms obscure the right atrium or pose too great a risk of rupture; the femoral vein is exposed and cannulated in a manner similar to that of femoral artery cannulation. Because femoral venous return drains only the lower body, an SVC cannula is inserted and "Y'd" into the venous line after the aneurysm is controlled.

Cannulation of the right atrium with a two-stage catheter

1. A partial-occlusion clamp is applied to the right atrial appendage.
2. A single pursestring suture is inserted around the appendage, and tourniquets are loosely applied as described in step 3 of the procedure for cannulation of the aorta.

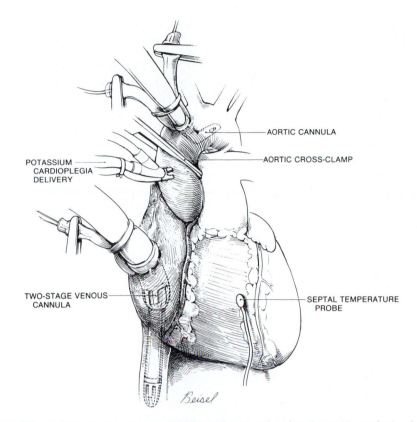

POTASSIUM
CARDIOPLEGIA
DELIVERY

AORTIC CANNULA

AORTIC CROSS-CLAMP

TWO-STAGE VENOUS
CANNULA

SEPTAL TEMPERATURE
PROBE

Beisel

Fig. 11-27 A two-stage venous cannula is shown. The distal openings drain the IVC, and the proximal openings drain venous return from the SVC and the heart via the coronary sinus in the right atrium. The antegrade cardioplegia delivery catheter and the aortic cross-clamp are in place. The temperature probe is placed in the interventricular septum. (From Walhausen JA, Pierce WS: *Johnson's surgery of the chest*, ed 5, St Louis, 1985, Mosby.)

3. The tip of the appendage is excised, and the surgeon and assistant grasp either side of the cut edges. Atrial trabeculations are sharply divided with scissors.

4. With the other hand, the surgeon inserts the venous cannula (with obturator) into the atriotomy and advances the distal fenestrated end into the IVC (Fig. 11-27). The proximal openings of the cannula are positioned in the right atrium. The obturator is removed, and the cannula is allowed to fill with blood. The proximal end is occluded with a tubing clamp.

5. The tourniquet is tightened and attached to the cannula with a tie. The cannula is connected to the venous drainage line. The venous line should be of sufficient length to create a gentle curve on the field.

6. The tubing clamp is removed, and venous drainage is allowed to commence. The perfusionist begins to slowly pump arterial inflow, and CPB is established (Fig. 11-28). Venous return is assessed, and if it is found to be inadequate, the pump is turned off, the tourniquet is loosened, and the venous cannula is repositioned. The tourniquet is retightened and again tied to the cannula.

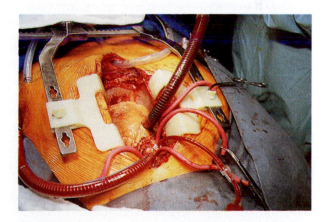

Fig. 11-28 Bypass circuit with an arterial cannula in the ascending aorta and a two-stage venous cannula *(right)* in the right atrium. (Courtesy John R. Garrett, MD; Howard Kaye, photographer.)

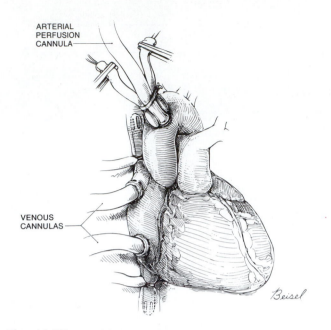

ARTERIAL
PERFUSION
CANNULA

VENOUS
CANNULAS

Beisel

Fig. 11-29 Double venous cannulation of the IVC and SVC. When tourniquets are placed around the cavae and tightened, all systemic venous return is forced into the cannulas, producing total CPB. (From Walhausen JA, Pierce WS: *Johnson's surgery of the chest,* St Louis, 1985, Mosby.)

Bicaval cannulation of the right atrium

Two venous cannulas are used: one to cannulate the SVC and the other to cannulate the IVC (Fig. 11-29). For procedures in the right side of the heart (e.g., tricuspid valve disorders or atrial septal defects) when maximum exposure is required, a right-angle SVC cannula may be used (see Fig. 15-12).

Procedure
1. A partial-occlusion clamp may be placed on the right atrial appendage, and a pursestring suture is placed as described for single venous cannulation. If not already in place, a partial-occlusion clamp is placed on the appendage (outside the pursestring suture). The appendage is excised, and as the assistant opens the clamp, the surgeon inserts the venous cannula; the assistant then tightens the tourniquet. The cannula may be placed in the SVC or the IVC, depending on the surgeon's preference. When the right atrium is to be opened, the cannula is placed in the SVC so that it does not obscure the operative field. The tourniquet is tightened and tied to the cannula. The proximal end of the cannula is occluded with a tubing clamp.
2. A second pursestring suture is similarly placed lower in the right atrium, and the tourniquet is applied. A partial-occlusion clamp may or may not be used; if it is not used, the surgeon makes a stab wound into the atrium and enlarges it with a tonsil hemostat. The cannula is inserted and (usually) threaded to the IVC; the tourniquets are tightened and tied to the cannula.
3. The cannulas are attached to the openings of a Y-connector at the end of the venous line. The tubing clamp is removed, and venous drainage is started.

Discontinuation of cardiopulmonary bypass

After the surgical repair has been completed, the surgeon prepares to discontinue bypass. The patient will have been rewarmed to normothermia (rewarming is started before the cross-clamp is removed), and the heart will be contracting in a regular manner. The anesthesiologist starts to ventilate the lungs, and the surgeon (or perfusionist) gradually occludes the venous line, allowing blood to enter the right atrium. At the same time, the perfusionist reduces the arterial inflow to equal the venous drainage to the pump. As the heart is gradually allowed to accept all the venous return, the surgeon assesses cardiac contractility by monitoring the systemic and pulmonary blood pressures and visually inspecting the heart. When heart action is judged to be sufficient and systemic blood pressures are stable, the venous line is completely clamped, and the heart resumes responsibility for maintaining the circulation. Pump volume remaining in the oxygenator is infused gradually and in increments as necessary to maintain optimal filling pressures (preload) and systemic blood pressure.

Removal of the aortic cannula

After bypass has been discontinued and heparin reversal with protamine sulfate begun, the CPB cannulas are removed. Generally, the venous cannula is removed before the arterial cannula so that blood can continue to be infused if necessary. It is also safer to keep the arterial cannula in place during the beginning of protamine infusion in the event there is a hypotensive reaction to the protamine.

Procedure
1. The towel clip or tie attaching the arterial line to the chest is removed, and the tourniquets are freed from the cannula and loosened.
2. While the surgeon stabilizes the cannula, the assistant removes the tourniquet from one pursestring and makes a throw in the suture, tightening it around the cannula. The assistant holds this stitch taut with one hand and takes the cannula from the surgeon with the other hand.
3. The surgeon then removes the other tourniquet and makes a throw in the stitch. As the assistant removes the cannula, the surgeon tightens the stitch to close the arteriotomy. The assistant hands the cannula to the scrub nurse and then tightens the first pursestring. The surgeon ties his or her pursestring followed by the pursestring held by the assistant.
4. The incision site is inspected for hemostasis, and additional sutures are placed if necessary.

Removal of the femoral artery cannula

1. Tourniquets are detached from the cannula and loosened.
2. As the surgeon slides the cannula out of the arteriotomy, the assistant tightens the tourniquet around the artery. A femoral artery clamp may be

Table 11-5 ■ *Effects of cardiopulmonary bypass*

Effects	Contributing factors	Effects	Contributing factors
Cardiovascular System		**Fluid and Electrolyte Balance**	
Perioperative myocardial infarction	Inadequate myocardial protection and emboli	Interstitial edema	Increased extravascular fluid and organ dysfunction, fluid shifts
Low cardiac output after surgery	Alteration in colloidal osmotic pressure, left ventricular dysfunction, and hypoperfusion injury	Intravascular hypovolemia	Decreased intravascular volume, bleeding, and interstitial edema
Increased afterload	Catecholamine release	Hypokalemia	Dilution, polyuria, intracellular shifts of potassium ions
Hypertension	Elevated renin, angiotensin, and aldosterone levels	Hyperkalemia	Potassium cardioplegia and increased intracellular exchange of glucose and potassium, cellular destruction
Pulmonary System		Hyponatremia, hypocalcemia, and hypomagnesemia	Dilution
Respiratory insufficiency	Alterations in colloidal osmotic pressure, interstitial pulmonary edema, decreased perfusion, and alterations in ventilatory patterns	**Endocrine System**	
		Water and sodium retention	Increase in antidiuretic hormone
Atelectasis	Complement activation, emboli, and alveolar-capillary membrane damage	Hypothyroidism	Increased levels of thyroxine (T_4) and decreased levels of triiodothyronine (T_3) and thyroid-stimulating hormone
Neurologic System		Hyperglycemia	Depressed insulin response
Cerebrovascular accident	Cerebral emboli		
Transient motor deficits	Decreased cerebral blood flow	**Immune System**	
Cerebral hemorrhage	Systemic heparinization	Infection	Exposure to multiple pathogens and decreased immunoglobin levels
Gastrointestinal System			
Gastrointestinal bleeding	Hormonal stress and coagulopathic conditions	Postperfusion syndrome	Release of anaphylactic toxins, complement activation
Intestinal ischemia or infarction	Emboli and decreased perfusion	**Hematologic Factors**	
Acute pancreatitis	Pancreatic vasculature emboli	Bleeding	Blood cell hemolysis, heparin rebound, and reduction in platelet count and coagulation factors
Renal System			
Acute renal failure	Decreased renal blood flow, microemboli, and myohemoglobin release		

Modified from Stewart S: *The physiologic effects and nursing implications of cardiopulmonary bypass,* unpublished master's thesis, Boston, 1985, Boston University. From Kinney MR, Croft MS: The person undergoing cardiac surgery. In Guzzetta CE, Dossey BM: *Cardiovascular nursing: holistic practice,* St Louis, 1992, Mosby.

placed on the artery proximally, and the umbilical tape is removed.

3. The artery is closed with two 4-0 or 5-0 polypropylene sutures; one suture is started on one side and the other on the opposite side of the incision. The stitches are tied at the middle. Tourniquets and clamps are removed, and the incision is checked for hemostasis.

Removal of the venous cannulas

The tourniquet is freed from the cannula and removed from the pursestring. As the assistant removes the cannula, the surgeon tightens the pursestring and then finishes tying the suture. Another pursestring may be placed to achieve hemostasis. If there is a second cannula, it is removed in the same manner.

Postoperative Considerations

Postoperative management of cardiac surgery patients includes assessing not only structural and functional changes associated with the operation and the specific cardiac disease (e.g., coronary artery disease, valvular disorders), but also the clinical sequelae of CPB. Hemodilution, hypothermia, anticoagulation, and the use of the heart-lung machine produce temporary physiologic derangements (Table 11-5) in organ system function (Weiland and Walker, 1986). Whether

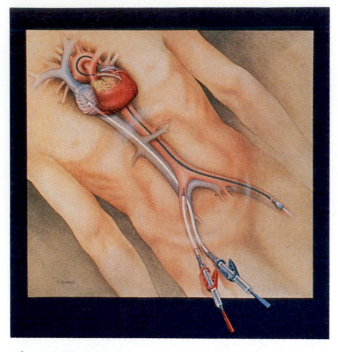

Fig. 11-30   Placement of percutaneous CPB cannulas. (Courtesy Bard Cardiopulmonary Div., Tewksbury, Mass.)

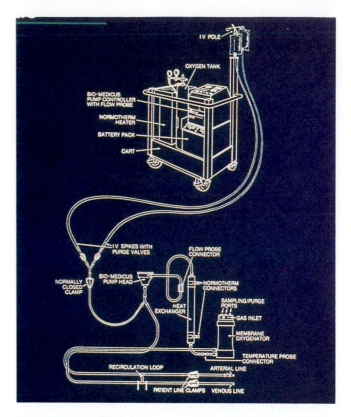

Fig. 11-31   Disposable emergency CPB circuit. (Courtesy Bard Cardiopulmonary Div., Tewksbury, Mass.)

these sequelae resolve spontaneously or require treatment depends in part on effective postoperative management to minimize the deleterious effects of CPB (see Chapter 9 for a discussion of postoperative care).

Emergency Percutaneous Cardiopulmonary Bypass

Portable CPB systems have been used in the past for emergency treatment of sudden death, massive pulmonary embolus, and accidental hypothermia (Cooley, Bell, and Alexander, 1961; Mattox and Beall, 1976). The development of cardiopulmonary support systems using percutaneous femoral vein–femoral artery cannulation techniques has allowed clinicians to expand the use of CPB from the operating room to the emergency department, the critical care unit, the cardiac catheterization laboratory, and other areas where patients may undergo sudden circulatory decompensation (Bruhn and others, 1992; Dillon, Jones, and Shawl, 1992). Patients requiring cardiopulmonary resuscitation and support may benefit from the institution of partial CPB; such patients include those with pulmonary embolus and hypothermia with ventricular fibrillation, as well as those suffering acute myocardial infarction or limb trauma, or those at high risk during coronary angiography and angioplasty (Phillips and others, 1989; Shawl and others, 1990). It is not recommended for multisystem trauma and closed head injuries, primarily because of the large amounts of heparin that must be used (Brown, 1990).

Operative procedure

After the patient has been heparinized, large-bore, thin-walled cannulas are inserted into the femoral artery and one or both femoral veins (Fig. 11-30); some venous catheters are long enough to advance to the IVC–right atrial junction. The cannulas are then connected to the circuit containing an oxygenator and heat exchanger (Fig. 11-31). A centrifugal pump is used to actively drain a sufficient venous return by using negative pressure to suction blood (passive drainage would be inadequate through the cannulas). Blood is then propelled through the membrane oxygenator into the systemic circulation. Flow rates of up to 6 L/min can be established (Phillips and others, 1989; Shawl and others, 1990). Because suction is used to drain the heart, the central venous vascular system is under negative pressure; this can cause intravenous (IV) drip rates to speed up, and there is a risk of air entering the perfusion system via open central venous pressure or IV lines.

Once the system is no longer needed, CPB is terminated and the cannulas are removed. Smaller cannulas (11 French or less) may be withdrawn percutaneously, with pressure applied to the cannulation sites. Larger cannulas often require surgical closure of the femoral vessels. Occasionally bleeding persists or thrombus occludes the femoral artery. Exploration of the artery with thrombectomy can be performed. Additional potential complications are those associated with other forms of CPB; these include air embolism, hemolysis with subsequent renal injury, protamine reaction, and aortic dissection. Because of the special knowledge and experience required to conduct CPB and the risks associated with its use, clinicians using extracorporeal circulation techniques should have appropriate training (Society of Thoracic Surgeons, 1990).

Extracorporeal Membrane Oxygenation

The development of membrane oxygenators and their success in minimizing hemolysis for prolonged periods of time has allowed additional applications of CPB technology. Extracorporeal membrane oxygenation (ECMO), used for pulmonary support, is the most widely recognized technique of prolonged extracorporeal circulation. But the technology has been expanded to support patients with a failing heart, as well as failing lungs, until the affected organ can recover or be replaced with a transplanted organ (Bartlett, 1990). ECMO (using cannulation of a vein and an artery) may be the heart assistive device of choice in infants and children because of the lack of alternative devices of appropriate size. The following discussion focuses mainly on pulmonary support (see Chapter 17 for support of the failing heart).

Commonly, ECMO provides pulmonary support for neonates and adults who have potentially reversible respiratory failure. In neonates acute respiratory failure (ARF) is usually secondary to abnormal pulmonary vasculature, immaturity of the surfactant system, or chemical pneumonitis from meconium aspiration (Levy, O'Rourke, and Crone, 1992; Moront and others, 1989). Adults with ARF from destructive primary lung disease or from adult respiratory distress syndrome causing severe parenchymal injury and fibrosis may derive less benefit from ECMO therapy because the underlying disease is less likely to be reversible (Gersony, 1984).

Types of ECMO

ECMO is achieved by draining venous blood, removing carbon dioxide, adding oxygen, and returning the blood to the circulation via an artery (venoarterial bypass) or a vein (venovenous bypass). In venoarterial bypass (Fig. 11-32, *A*) the function of both the heart and the lungs is replaced by artificial organs. In the neonate the internal jugular vein and the common carotid artery are usually cannulated for venous return and arterial inflow, respectively (Moront and others, 1989).

Venovenous bypass (Fig. 11-32, *B*) is used to support the lungs only; it is not used to support a failing heart. In venovenous ECMO the oxygenated venous blood is returned to the venous circulation, where it raises the oxygen content and lowers the carbon dioxide level of the venous blood. The SVC and IVC or the right atrium and the femoral vein may be cannulated for inflow and outflow. Among the clinical advantages of this method over venoarterial ECMO

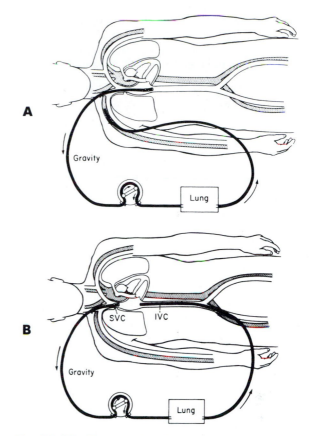

Fig. 11-32 Two modes of long-term extracorporeal circulation. **A,** Venoarterial circuit. Blood is removed from the right atrium, and oxygenated blood is pumped into the subclavian artery. **B,** Venovenous circuit (provides only respiratory support). Blood is removed from the SVC, and oxygenated blood is pumped into the IVC. Other vascular sites can be used. (From Bartlett RH: Extracorporeal life support for cardiopulmonary failure, *Curr Probl Surg* 27[10]:623, 1990.)

is that it is less invasive and as a result can be instituted earlier. Lower flow rates can be used (resulting in less trauma to blood cells), the carotid artery need not be sacrificed, and the potential risk of arterial emboli is avoided (O'Connell, 1993). Subsequently, less aggressive ventilator support (i.e., lower airway pressures and a reduced percentage of oxygen) can be used (Peterson and Brown, 1990). There is, however, some recirculation of blood back into the ECMO circuit, and the patient's lungs may have to augment oxygenation (Levy, O'Rourke, and Crone, 1992).

Systematic heparinization is required; the activated clotting time (ACT) is maintained at approximately 200 seconds. Heparin-coated circuits are under investigation. As with other bypass circuits, complement is activated, but the effect appears to be minimal and subsides within a few hours (Bartlett, 1990). The duration of ECMO is a function of the patient's rate of recovery from the intrinsic disease, improvement in lung compliance, and radiologic evidence of pulmonary improvement (Levy, O'Rourke, and Crone, 1992).

Complications include diffuse bleeding at the cannulation sites; ligation of the internal jugular vein, common carotid artery, or other major blood vessel; and failure of any part of the circuit. The use of topical biologic (fibrin) glue has been used successfully to eliminate bleeding (Moront, O'Connell, and Hoy, 1988). Alternate cannulation sites can sometimes be used, and the risk of component failure may be reduced with adherence to safety guidelines for the use and maintenance of these devices.

Deep Hypothermia with Circulatory Arrest

The technique of deep hypothermia with circulatory arrest is useful for very complex procedures where cerebral flow must be temporarily interrupted and/or where adequate surgical exposure is hampered by the size of the patient or the location of the lesion. In neonates and other very small patients this technique allows removal of both aortic and venous catheters to provide an uncluttered operative field during circulatory arrest; the catheters are reinserted for resumption of CPB and rewarming.

In adults with aneurysms of the transverse arch, application of a cross-clamp on the arch vessels may be difficult or may pose an increased risk of injury to friable aortic tissue (see Chapter 16 on surgery on the thoracic aorta). Moreover, clamping these vessels interrupts cerebral blood flow.

Past experiences with selected cannulation of the arch vessels to perfuse the brain have been disappointing. Current methods to protect the brain use a deeper level of hypothermia (approximately 22° to 24° C [72° to 76° F] or lower) to further reduce cerebral metabolic requirements, as well as circulatory arrest to provide a relatively bloodless field. Although there is some uncertainty about the safe duration of circulatory arrest, it can be inferred from studies that it is inversely proportional to the temperature of the subject (Box 11-4); at 18° C (65° F) the safe period is approximately 45 minutes (Kirklin and Barratt-Boyes, 1993). Others using varying temperatures have noted safe periods of 59 minutes (Griepp and others, 1975) and 104 minutes (Coselli and others, 1988).

Additional cerebral protection is provided with ice bags placed around the patient's head. The ears and nose should be padded to avoid frostbite injury.

Operative procedure

1. CPB is instituted with right atrial venous cannulation, and femoral arterial cannulation for inflow. The patient's body temperature is cooled to 18° to 24° C (65° to 76° F), depending on the surgeon's preference.
2. When the desired temperature is reached, the venous line is occluded and arterial flow discontinued.
3. **Operative repair.** An incision is made (e.g., into the aortic arch; distal and arch anastomoses are completed). Aspiration of blood is limited to that required to visualize the operative site.

Box 11-4 *Comments on cardiopulmonary bypass, profound hypothermia, and circulatory arrest*

A.D. Pacifico, MD
University of Alabama at Birmingham
Birmingham, Alabama

Open heart surgery requires the use of CPB to take over the function of the heart and lungs. In some procedures, profound hypothermia is induced and temporary total circulatory arrest employed to facilitate the technical aspects of the operative procedure. The frequency of the use of total circulatory arrest techniques varies in different medical centers, but they are almost always used for certain specific defects. These would include aortic arch replacement in adults and the repair of total anomalous pulmonary venous connection in infants. In some centers total circulatory arrest techniques are used during the repair of many different congenital heart defects in neonates. There is reasonable evidence that the probability of a "safe" total circulatory arrest period is inversely related to the duration of the arrest. The degree of safety is greater at shorter periods of arrest and at colder temperatures. When the arrest time becomes longer than 45 minutes with the patient at 18° C (65° F) nasopharyngeal, the degree of safety (absence of structural or functional damage) falls precipitously. In addition, there is reasonable evidence that the duration of CPB is related to the probability of postoperative morbidity (cardiac, pulmonary, renal, and coagulation dysfunction). The incidence of morbidity is greater at younger ages than at older ages for the same CPB time. Patient safety, therefore, is improved with shorter CPB times and with shorter periods of hypothermic circulatory arrest.

Considerations regarding the safety of CPB and circulatory arrest techniques demand that the surgical nurse thoroughly understand the surgical procedure. He or she must anticipate the surgeon's needs so as to provide a high level of efficiency to the overall conduct of the operative procedure. This necessitates a thorough understanding of the operative procedure and the need to study the specific steps involved. When this is done properly, the entire operation proceeds as a symphony with each member of the surgical team in harmony culminating in a precise and accurate repair in the shortest period of time with a level and constant momentum and without the need to hurry. Operative procedures that proceed in this manner are thrilling experiences not only for the surgeon and his [or her] surgical assistants, but especially for the surgical nurse. This style of intraoperative personnel cohesiveness clearly enhances the surgical result.

---

4. After sufficient completion of the repair to allow placement of a cross-clamp on the proximal transverse aortic prosthetic graft, arterial perfusion is resumed slowly, and the aorta and arch vessels are filled with blood. Air is allowed to escape from the arch vessels.

5. Arterial perfusion is continued, and rewarming is started at a rate of 3 minutes for each degree Centigrade. The proximal anastomosis is completed during rewarming.

MYOCARDIAL PROTECTION

At one time, early postoperative cardiac failure and death were assumed to be primarily the result of the patient's own disease. It became apparent, however, that diminished left ventricular function and acute cardiac failure might also be due to operative myocardial ischemia or necrosis. Although periods of ischemia and hypoxia are necessary to provide a motionless operative field, ventricular function should not be impaired because protective measures were not taken intraoperatively. Myocardial damage can be minimized by interventions that reduce ischemic time, lower metabolic requirements, conserve energy stores, and maintain an appropriate cellular environment (Foker and others, 1980; Kay and others, 1978).

When the aorta is cross-clamped, blood flow to the myocardium is interrupted, producing hypoxia and ischemia. Deprived of sufficient oxygen, cardiac cells must use alternative methods of energy production if they are to remain viable. These energy demands are determined primarily by myocardial electromechanical work and secondarily by wall tension and temperature (Beuren, Sparks, and Bing, 1958; Gay, 1989). The energy available in high-energy phosphates— adenosine triphosphate (ATP) and creatine phosphate (CP)—must be provided by anaerobic metabolism, which is itself energy dependent and requires the utilization of glucose and oxygen. Anaerobic metabolism is less efficient, however, producing far fewer high-energy phosphates per unit of glucose.

The effects of ischemia are even more deleterious than those of hypoxia, because inadequate coronary blood flow not only impairs oxygen delivery, but also prevents adequate removal of accumulated metabolic waste products (Lell, Huber, and Buttner, 1987). Increased lactate levels lower intracellular pH, which interferes with vital enzyme functions. Glycolysis is eventually inhibited, resulting in energy depletion. Insufficient ATP is available for resumption of excitation-contraction coupling and for energizing the sodium and potassium pumps. Increased levels of intracellular calcium potentiate the utilization of high-energy phosphates, further depleting the energy pool. Without protection, irreversible myocardial damage can occur, the most dramatic being irreversible ischemic contracture, which Cooley, Reul, and Wakasch (1972) termed the "stone heart."

Even when measures are instituted to reduce ischemic time and the accumulation of waste products, ischemia and its adverse consequences cannot be avoided entirely. Some cells will die; others will be damaged slightly or "stunned" (Braunwald and Kloner, 1982). To protect potentially viable cells, corrective measures are necessary to prevent extension of the injury when the cross-clamp is removed and the heart is reperfused. Reperfusion injury includes structural (cellular edema and vascular injury), biochemical (acidosis and decreased ATP production), electrical (increased automaticity and inconsistent activity), and mechanical (impaired systolic and diastolic function) abnormalities (Lell, Huber, and Buttner, 1987).

To minimize the damaging effects of hypoxia and ischemia during cross-clamping, researchers have focused on two factors that have become the basis of myocardial protection and preservation: hypothermia and immediate cardiac arrest. The first reduces the metabolic rate and consequently the workload of the heart (Bigelow, Lindsay, and Greenwood, 1950; Sealy, Brown, and Young, 1958). The second conserves existing energy stores because an arrested heart requires less energy than either a nonworking heart (i.e., one that is not volume loaded, as occurs during CPB) or a fibrillating heart (McKeever, Gregg, and Canney, 1958). The sooner a heart achieves cardiac standstill, the fewer energy resources are used in maintaining the contraction and fibrillation that precedes arrest induced by ischemia and hypothermia alone.

Measures to minimize reperfusion injury focus on structural and functional recovery. Reestablishing homogeneous flow to the coronary vascular bed expedites the delivery of reparative substrates and therapeutic agents (Lell, Huber, and Buttner, 1987).

Hypothermia for Myocardial Protection

Systemic hypothermia is used during CPB to reduce the metabolic rate, and subsequently the energy demands, of the systemic organs. (Shivering, however, must be prevented pharmacologically because it increases the work and energy demands of the heart.) Cooling the myocardium itself achieves the same goals, but additional methods must be used when the heart is separated from the systemic circulation during cross-clamping. Cold solutions can be applied topically, or they can be infused directly into the heart antegradely via the aortic root or retrogradely via the coronary sinus. Because antegrade transmural cooling is especially difficult in the presence of left ventricular hypertrophy and coronary artery disease, which can retard or obstruct an even distribution of the infusate, all three methods—topical, antegrade, and retrograde—may be used in conjunction with prior systemic hypothermia to achieve homogeneous myocardial cooling.

Topical solutions consist of lactated Ringer's solution or normal saline solution that has been chilled in a refrigerator or a device specifically designed for this purpose (see Fig. 5-4). The solution should not be allowed to form large ice particles, because they can injure the phrenic nerves running along the lateral pericardium; some surgeons use an insulating pad between the heart and the pericardium to protect the nerves (Kirklin and Barratt-Boyes, 1993). Other surgeons do not routinely use topical hypothermic irrigation, relying instead on the hypothermic benefits of direct antegrade or retrograde infusion. Topical hypothermia is used adjunctively only when portions of

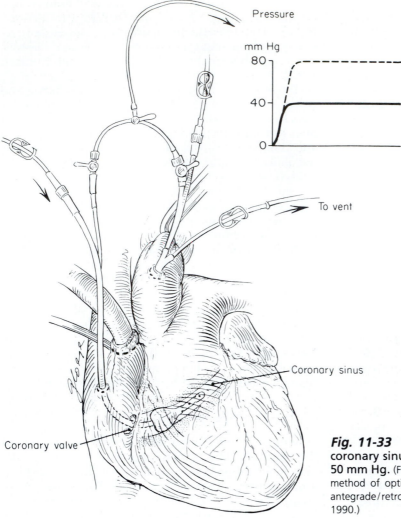

Pressure

mm Hg
80

40

0

To vent

Coronary sinus

Coronary valve

Fig. 11-33 Antegrade/retrograde cardioplegia system. The coronary sinus pressure is monitored; it should remain under 50 mm Hg. (From Drinkwater DC, Laks H, Buckberg GD: A new simplified method of optimizing cardioplegic delivery without right heart isolation: antegrade/retrograde blood cardioplegia, *J Thorac Cardiovasc Surg* 100:56, 1990.)

the heart may not be adequately protected with other methods.

Direct antegrade and retrograde myocardial infusion is accomplished with delivery systems consisting of catheters and tubing incorporated into the bypass circuit (Fig. 11-33). Antegrade infusion is achieved by placing a needle-tipped catheter into the aorta proximal to the aortic CPB cannula and the anticipated site of the aortic cross-clamp. With the aorta clamped, infusion of the solution under sufficient pressure closes the aortic valve, forcing the solution into the right and left coronary ostia and the coronary vascular bed. When aortic valve incompetence is present, antegrade infusions are contraindicated because the solution would enter the left ventricle and distend the ventricular wall. In this situation the surgeon relies on retrograde cardioplegia infusion through a catheter placed in the coronary sinus via the right atrium. Another, less common, method is to open the aorta and infuse the solution directly into each coronary os (see Chapter 14). Selective infusion of coronary bypass grafts can also be performed.

Warm heart surgery

Because there are disadvantages associated with hypothermia, notably adverse effects on enzymatic function, energy generation, and cellular integrity, some researchers have used continuous hyperkalemic infusions of warm blood for cardioplegic arrest during CABG (Lichtenstein and others, 1991). The arrested heart is continuously perfused, thereby obviating the need for hypothermia. With this method of "aerobic arrest," some studies have shown no difference in mortality rates between the warm-blood groups and the cold-blood groups, and myocardial function was improved (e.g., less perioperative myocardial infarction, low-output syndrome, and use of the intraaortic balloon pump) in the warm-blood group. Moreover, the authors propose that this method eliminates reperfusion injury (Kavanagh and others, 1992; Lichtenstein and others, 1991).

One of the disadvantages of this method cited by the authors is that anastomotic sites are obscured by blood, necessitating temporary discontinuation of the infusion of the warm cardioplegia solution. This

Table 11-6 ■ *Objectives of cardioplegia management*

Objective	Potential agents
Immediate arrest to lower energy demands and avoid ATP, glycogen, etc., depletion	K^+, Mg^{++}, lidocaine, hypocalcemia
Temperature reduction and maintenance	Hypothermic cardiopulmonary bypass; topical, intramyocardial hypothermia
Substrate provision for metabolic activity that remains, especially at myocardial temperatures >20° C (68° F)	Infusion and/or topical glucose, oxygen, lactate, Krebs cycle intermediates
Buffering capacity to maintain appropriate myocardial pH	HCO_3, tromethamine, phosphate, blood
Exogenous additives to achieve membrane stabilization	Ca antagonists, steroids, local anesthetics, O_2 radical scavengers
Ideal osmolality with physiologic colloidal oncotic pressure	Albumin, blood

From Thompson AD, Hayden RI, Tyers GFO: Complications related to myocardial preservation in adults. In Waldhausen JA, Orringer MB: *Complications in cardiothoracic surgery*, St Louis, 1991, Mosby. Modified from Buckberg GD: Strategies and logic of cardioplegic delivery to prevent, avoid, and reverse ischemic and reperfusion damage, *Jo Thorac Cardiovasc Surg* 93:127, 1987.
ATP, Adenosine triphosphate; *Ca*, calcium; *K⁺*, potassium; *Mg⁺⁺*, magnesium; *O₂*, oxygen.

makes the technique cumbersome and may produce ischemic injury, especially to the more vulnerable areas of the myocardium. One experimental study (Matsuura and others, 1993) showed no superior myocardial protection with warm continuous retrograde infusion, as compared with antegrade/retrograde, cold-blood cardioplegia. Because this method is relatively new, more sensitive and specific indicators of myocardial damage, in larger numbers of patients, are needed to evaluate it (Lell, 1992).

Cardioplegia

Although hypothermia reduces oxygen consumption, metabolic requirements can be lowered further by reducing, or practically avoiding altogether, the ventricular fibrillation that commonly occurs between the period that the cross-clamp is applied and hypothermic cardiac standstill is achieved. Fibrillation wastes energy resources that could be used when the cross-clamp is removed and the heart must resume beating.

The addition of chemical agents that could quickly arrest the heart with little or no fibrillation had been attempted (Melrose and others, 1955), but results had been poor. Gay and Ebert (1973) demonstrated improved results using components similar to Melrose's but altering the composition of the ingredients of the arresting solution, notably potassium and other ions such as sodium, calcium, and magnesium.

The infusion of hyperkalemic solutions inhibits membrane depolarization and propagation of the action potential. The resulting cardiac paralysis, cardioplegia, produces a reversible diastolic arrest that allows the surgeon to perform delicate procedures on a quiet field. Multidose infusions are needed because the cardioplegia solution eventually washes out and the myocardium rewarms. The solution is reinfused about every 20 minutes (Buckberg, 1989); if cardiac activity is visualized directly or noted on the electrocardiographic (ECG) monitor before 20 minutes has elapsed,

another bolus is given (when the heart is arrested, the ECG is a flat line). Table 11-6 lists the objectives of cardioplegic management.

Cardioplegia solutions may be one of two types: blood or crystalloid. The advantages of blood cardioplegia solutions include providing oxygen to the heart while it is arrested, allowing reoxygenation when the perfusate is replenished, and providing a buffering effect from the plasma. Repeat infusions of blood cardioplegia solution help to maintain hypothermic arrest, remove accumulated acid wastes, treat evolving edema, and provide additional substrate. The cardioplegia solution consists of oxygenated blood from the arterial line of the bypass pump, which is separately cooled to 3° to 4° C (38° to 40° F). Potassium (K^+) is the most common arresting agent, but others such as magnesium (Mg^{++}) may also be used. The solution is adjusted for pH and osmotic pressure (Bell and Diffee, 1991). The ratio of the components is 4 parts blood to 1 part cardioplegia solution (Buckberg, 1989).

Crystalloid cardioplegia solution, once widely used, also contains K^+ and some of the components contained in sanguineous cardioplegia solution (i.e., sodium chloride, sodium bicarbonate). Because of the advantages associated with blood cardioplegia solutions, many surgeons limit the use of crystalloid solutions to special situations. One of these occurs when a patient has a significantly elevated level of cold antibodies that can stimulate RBC agglutination in vital organs during hypothermia. Measures to protect the patient, in addition to the use of crystalloid cardioplegia solution, include maintaining temperatures above the critical point and infusing the heart with warm crystalloid solution before allowing blood to reenter the coronary circulation (Anderson, Stephenson, and Edmunds, 1991).

Reperfusion management

Reperfusion injury can be reduced by measures taken before, during, and after the heart is arrested. Initial infusion of a warm hyperkalemic bolus of cardioplegia solution with substrate-enriched blood is considered advantageous in hearts that are already energy depleted and have reduced ejection fractions (less than 40%) preoperatively. The warm blood enhances global distribution of the cardioplegia solution, especially to the subendocardium (Kirklin and Barratt-Boyes, 1993). Subsequent boluses are cooled to take advantage of the beneficial effects of hypothermia. Hearts that have adequate preoperative ejection fractions (greater than 40%) may receive cold cardioplegia solution initially (Buckberg, 1989).

To lower cardiac energy demands, a warm bolus of cardioplegia solution with reduced levels of K$^+$ is infused antegradely and retrogradely for a few minutes before the cross-clamp is removed to add substrates, buffer acidosis, and limit the calcium load. This bolus is followed by warm, noncardioplegic blood to wash out the cardioplegia solution. When the cross-clamp is removed (or even before), the heart often resumes contraction. If asystole continues, the surgeon may initiate contraction by gently tapping the heart with the finger; temporary pacing may be helpful when asystole is more persistent. If ventricular fibrillation is noted, the heart is defibrillated immediately, because fibrillation interferes with adequate distribution of coronary blood flow (Buckberg, 1989). Warm cardioplegic reperfusion may be prolonged in hearts with evolving myocardial infarction to enhance functional recovery (Allen and others, 1986).

Antegrade/retrograde blood cardioplegia infusion

The blood cardioplegia solution is cooled to the desired temperature via the heat exchanger incorporated into the cardioplegia delivery system (see Fig. 5-14). Antegrade infusion is performed first, followed by retrograde infusion. The doses are never given simultaneously by the two routes (Drinkwater, Laks, and Buckberg, 1990) because this would produce excessive distension of the ventricular wall. The initial bolus contains a higher concentration of K$^+$ than later doses, so that prompt cardiac arrest can be achieved. Later infusions have a lower K$^+$ level.

Retrograde infusion alone may be used in the presence of significant aortic insufficiency. When only retrograde cardioplegia is used, right ventricular protection is less predictable than left ventricular protection. Pericardial lavage with hypothermic solutions can be used to provide additional protection to the right ventricle (Buckberg, 1989). (See Box 11-5 for RNFA considerations.)

Operative procedure: insertion of the antegrade/retrograde cardioplegia infusion catheter *(Buckberg, 1989; Drinkwater, Laks, and Buckberg, 1990)*
Antegrade cannulation

1. After the aortic cannula has been inserted and connected to the arterial CPB line, a double-armed pursestring suture is placed in the aorta proximal

---

Box 11-5　RN first assistant considerations related to myocardial protection

Be sure cardioplegia infusion line is clamped before it is attached to antegrade (aortic) cardioplegia catheter (to prevent introduction of air into systemic circulation).

Use cardiotomy suction both to retract and to aspirate blood during retrograde cardioplegia catheter insertion.

Alert surgeon to presence of air in cardioplegia line before cardioplegia infusion is initiated; when saphenous vein grafts are selectively infused, flush cardioplegia line before attaching it to bypass graft.

When retrograde cardioplegia is being infused, verify that aortic vent is turned on (a momentary delay is acceptable); monitor coronary sinus pressure to determine whether it is too high (greater than 50 mm Hg).

If retrograde cardioplegia catheter requires manual inflation and deflation, ensure that balloon is inflated during infusion and deflated during antegrade infusion (occasionally surgeon will maintain balloon inflation during initial stages of antegrade infusion to enhance myocardial distribution of solution, but balloon must be deflated shortly thereafter); do not overinflate balloon (which can injure coronary sinus).

If topical hypothermic solutions are used, remove large ice particles to prevent phrenic nerve injury.

Monitor electrocardiogram and observe heart directly for cardiac activity to anticipate reinfusion of cardioplegia solution.

Use discard sucker to aspirate cardioplegia solution that may have collected in pericardial well.

---

to the aortic cannula, leaving enough space between the two catheters for future placement of the aortic cross-clamp. The pursestring may be pledgeted to buttress the suture.

2. The needles are removed, and a tourniquet is threaded over the free ends of the suture. A hemostat is placed on the free ends of the suture (or over the tourniquet around the suture).

3. The cardioplegia catheter containing a needle obturator is inserted into the aorta, and the obturator is then removed. The surgeon places a finger over the opened end of the catheter to prevent excessive blood loss from the catheter. The tourniquet is tightened by the assistant.

4. The cardioplegia tubing is handed to the surgeon, who connects the tubing to the cardioplegia catheter. The tubing must be clamped so that air in the cardioplegia system is not drawn into the aorta.

5. With the clamp still occluding the tubing where it is attached to the cardioplegia catheter, the cardioplegia circuit is deaired by circulating cardioplegia solution into the infusion tubing and out the vent (suction) tubing integrated into the circuit (Fig. 11-33).

6. After the circuit is deaired, the cardioplegia inflow

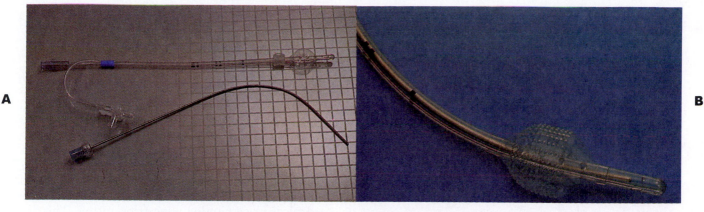
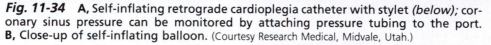

Fig. 11-34 **A,** Self-inflating retrograde cardioplegia catheter with stylet *(below);* coronary sinus pressure can be monitored by attaching pressure tubing to the port. **B,** Close-up of self-inflating balloon. (Courtesy Research Medical, Midvale, Utah.)

line is clamped. The suction line is kept open so that when the clamp between the cardioplegia catheter and the rest of the circuit is removed, remaining air is aspirated back to the pump.

7. The suction line is then clamped, and the cardioplegia line is opened to infuse the cardioplegia. The aortic cross-clamp is placed on the aorta between the aortic cannula and the cardioplegia catheter. The initial bolus of cardioplegia is 300 to 350 ml/min at an aortic pressure ranging from 60 to 80 mm Hg. This is infused over a 2-minute period (Drinkwater, Laks, and Buckberg, 1990). Coronary venous drainage exiting through the coronary sinus combines with systemic venous return going back to the pump.

8. Cardiac arrest should be achieved within 1 minute. Failure to obtain arrest within this time may be due to (1) an inadequate rate of flow (increase flow up to 500 ml per minute), (2) subtotal occlusion of the aorta (the surgeon can readjust the clamp or replace it with another), (3) aortic insufficiency (switch to retrograde infusion), (4) inadequate venous drainage (readjust the venous cannula), or (5) there is no K^+ in the cardioplegia solution or an inadequate amount of K^+ in the solution (add K^+) (Buckberg, 1989).

Retrograde cannulation

1. After venous cannulation (but before CPB is initiated), a double-armed pursestring suture is placed in the lower right atrium. The needles are removed, and a tourniquet is applied as described in step 2 of the procedure for antegrade cannulation. (A full right atrium facilitates insertion of the cannula.)

2. A stab wound is made within the right atrial pursestring, and the opening is enlarged with a tonsil hemostat.

3. The retroplegia catheter with a stylet in place is inserted through the atrial incision, and the tip of the catheter is advanced to the coronary sinus. The

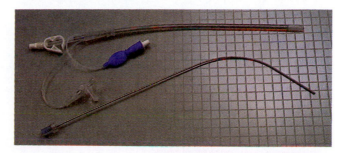

Fig. 11-35 Retrograde cardioplegia catheter with stylet *(below);* the balloon is manually inflated via the attached port. The second port is for pressure tubing to monitor coronary sinus pressure. (Courtesy Research Medical, Midvale, Utah.)

stylet is removed, and blood is aspirated from the cannula to displace air. Correct placement is confirmed by palpating the undersurface of the heart. The tourniquet is tightened and tied to the catheter with a heavy silk tie.

4. The proximal end of the catheter is attached to the cardioplegia infusion tubing.

5. The pressure port of the catheter is connected to a pressure-monitoring line (often passed off the surgical field to a transducer maintained by anesthesia personnel or cardiopulmonary technologists). The coronary sinus pressure is measured.

The catheter may be self-inflating (Fig. 11-34), in which case the infusion of cardioplegia solution will automatically inflate the balloon surrounding the distal opening of the catheter and wedge it into the entrance of the coronary sinus; when cardioplegia infusion is stopped, coronary venous drainage deflates the balloon. If the catheter requires manual inflation and deflation (Fig. 11-35), a small (3-ml) syringe is attached to an inflation port; once the infusion is stopped, the balloon should be deflated to reduce the possibility of injury to the coronary sinus.

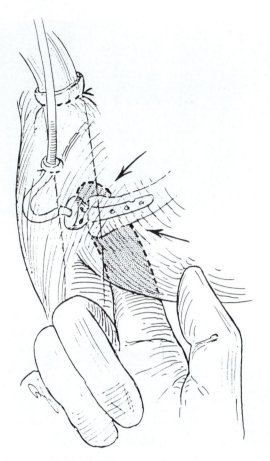

Fig. 11-36 Method of compression of the coronary sinus–right atrial junction to maintain pressure during retroperfusion when the retrograde cannula recoils partially into the right atrium. (From Drinkwater DC, Laks H, Buckberg GD: A new simplified method of optimizing cardioplegic delivery without right heart isolation: antegrade/retrograde blood cardioplegia, *J Thorac Cardiovasc Surg* 100:56, 1990.)

6. Back-bleeding from the coronary sinus is allowed to fill the cardioplegia line back to its connection to the main cardioplegia circuit (see Fig. 11-24), or blood is aspirated. Once the air is displaced, the retroplegia line is clamped.
7. Infusion of the cardioplegia solution is initiated at a rate of 200 to 250 ml/min; coronary sinus pressure should remain between 30 and 50 mm Hg. If the coronary sinus pressure is below 20 mm Hg, the coronary sinus balloon may not be inflated sufficiently to occlude the sinus. When the self-inflating balloon is used, the surgeon may compress the coronary sinus–right atrial junction to increase the pressure (Fig. 11-36).
8. The aortic vent is turned on to aspirate blood exiting via the coronary ostia so that the ventricle is not distended by the retroplegia solution. Blood exits via the aortic cardioplegia catheter and vent tubing connected to it. The aortic (antegrade) cardioplegia infusion line should be clamped.

Removal of cardioplegia catheters

1. The antegrade catheter tourniquet is removed, and one throw is placed in the pursestring. The surgeon holds the stitch taut with one hand and removes the catheter with the other; as this is done, the assistant places a finger over the aortotomy to prevent excessive blood loss. After the surgeon makes a second throw in the suture, the assistant removes the finger, and the surgeon completes the tie. Another stitch can be placed if necessary to achieve hemostasis.
2. After the tourniquet is removed, the retrograde catheter is withdrawn (the balloon should be deflated before removal of the catheter) and one throw is placed in the pursestring suture. The surgeon finishes tying the stitch, the wound is assessed for hemostasis, and another stitch is inserted if necessary.

REFERENCES

Allen BS and others: Studies of controlled reperfusion after ischemia. XVI. Consistent early recovery of regional wall motion following surgical revascularization after eight hours of acute coronary occlusion, *J Thorac Cardiovasc Surg* 92(suppl 3):636, 1986.

Anderson DR, Stephenson LW, Edmunds LH: Management of complications of cardiopulmonary bypass: complications of organ systems. In Waldhausen JA, Orringer MB: *Complications in cardiothoracic surgery*, St Louis, 1991, Mosby.

Baisden CE, Greenwald LV, Symbas PN: Occult rib fractures and brachial plexus injury following median sternotomy for open heart operations, *Ann Thorac Surg* 38:192, 1984.

Bartlett RH: Extracorporeal life support for cardiopulmonary failure. In Wells SA, editor: *Curr Probl Surg* 27(10):623, 1990.

Bell PE, Diffee GT: Cardiopulmonary bypass: principles, nursing implications, *AORN J* 53(6):1480, 1991.

Beuren A, Sparks C, Bing RJ: Metabolic studies on arrested and fibrillating perfused heart, *Am J Cardiol* 1:103, 1958.

Bigelow WG, Lindsay WK, Greenwood WF: Hypothermia: its possible role in cardiac surgery: an investigation of factors governing survival in dogs at low body temperatures, *Ann Surg* 132:849, 1950.

Braunwald E, Kloner RA: The stunned myocardium: prolonged, postischemic ventricular dysfunction, *Circulation* 66:1146, 1982.

Brown CV: Portable extracorporeal circulation: a new standard in myocardial infarction care? *J Emerg Nurs* 16(3):226, 1990.

Bruhn PS and others: A team approach to emergency portable cardiopulmonary support, *Crit Care Nurs Q* 15(1):33, 1992.

Buckberg GD: A proposed "solution" to the cardioplegic controversy, *J Thorac Cardiovasc Surg* 77:803, 1979.

Buckberg GD: Antegrade/retrograde blood cardioplegia to ensure cardioplegic distribution: operative techniques and objectives, *J Cardiac Surg* 4(3):216, 1989.

Chenoweth DE and others: Complement activation during cardiopulmonary bypass: evidence for generation of C3a and C5a anaphylatoxins, *N Engl J Med* 304(9):497, 1981.

Conti VR and others: Cold cardioplegia vs. hypothermia for myocardial preservation: randomized clinical study, *J Thorac Cardiovasc Surg* 76:577, 1978.

Cooley DA: *Techniques in cardiac surgery*, ed 2, Philadelphia, 1984, WB Saunders.

Cooley DA, Beall AL, Alexander JK: Acute massive pulmonary embolism successful surgical treatment using temporary cardiopulmonary bypass, *JAMA* 177:283, 1961.

Cooley DA, Reul GJ, Wakasch DC: Ischemic contracture of the heart: "stone heart," *Am J Cardiol* 29:575, 1972.

Coselli JS and others: Determination of brain temperatures for safe circulatory arrest during cardiovascular operation, *Ann Thorac Surg* 45:638, 1988.

Craver JM and others: Management of postcardiotomy mediastinitis. In Waldhausen JA, Orringer MB: *Complications in cardiothoracic surgery*, St Louis, 1991, Mosby.

Crawford FA, Kratz JM: Thoracic incisions. In Sabiston DC, Spencer FC: *Surgery of the chest*, ed 5, vol 1, Philadelphia, 1990, WB Saunders.

Culliford AT and others: Sternal and costochondral infections following open heart surgery: review of 2,594 cases, *J Thorac Cardiovasc Surg* 72:714, 1976.

Dillon ML, Jones RG, Shawl F: A nursing guide for patient care after percutaneous cardiopulmonary support, *Heart Lung* 21(3):228, 1992.

Downing SW, Edmunds LH: Release of vasoactive substances during cardiopulmonary bypass, *Ann Thorac Surg* 54:1236, 1992.

Drinkwater DC, Laks H, Buckberg GD: A new simplified method of optimizing cardioplegic delivery without right heart isolation: antegrade/retrograde blood cardioplegia, *J Thorac Cardiovasc Surg* 100:56, 1990.

Edmunds LH, Norwood WI, Low DW: *Atlas of cardiothoracic surgery*, Philadelphia, 1990, Lea & Febiger.

Foker JE and others: Adenosine metabolism and myocardial preservation: consequences of adenosine catabolism on myocardial high energy compounds and tissue blood flow, *J Thorac Cardiovasc Surg* 80:506, 1980.

Garrett HE, Matthews J: Reoperative median sternotomy, *Ann Thorac Surg* 48:305, 1989.

Gay WA: Potassium-induced cardioplegia: evolution and present status, *Ann Thorac Surg* 48:441, 1989.

Gay WA: *Atlas of adult cardiac surgery*, New York, 1990, Churchill Livingstone.

Gay WA, Ebert PA: Functional, metabolic, and morphologic effects of potassium-induced cardioplegia, *Surgery* 74:284, 1973.

Gersony WM: Neonatal pulmonary hypertension: pathophysiology, classification and etiology, *Clin Perinatol* 11:517, 1984.

Gibbon JH Jr: Application of a mechanical heart and lung apparatus to cardiac surgery, *Minn Med* 37:171, 1954.

Griepp RB and others: Prosthetic replacement of the aortic arch, *J Thorac Cardiovasc Surg* 70:1051, 1975.

Harlan BJ, Starr A, Harwin FM: *Manual of cardiac surgery*, vol 1, New York, 1980, Springer-Verlag.

Hartman AR: Myocardial preservation techniques. In Vlay SC, editor: *Medical care of the cardiac surgical patient*, Boston, 1992, Blackwell Scientific Publications.

Hirsh J: Heparin, *N Engl J Med* 324(22):1565, 1991.

Kavanagh BP and others: Effect of warm heart surgery on perioperative management of patients undergoing urgent cardiac surgery, *J Cardiothorac Vasc Anesth* 6(2):127, 1992.

Kay HR and others: Effects of cross clamp time, temperature and cardioplegic agents on myocardial function after induced arrest, *J Thorac Cardiovasc Surg* 76:590, 1978.

Kien N and others: Mechanism of hypotension following rapid infusion of protamine sulfate in anesthetized dogs, *J Cardiothorac Vasc Anesth* 6(2):143, 1992.

Kirklin JK: Prospects for understanding and eliminating the deleterious effects of cardiopulmonary bypass, *Ann Thorac Surg* 51:529, 1991.

Kirklin JW, Barratt-Boyes: *Cardiac surgery*, ed 2, vol 1, New York, 1993, Churchill Livingstone.

Kirklin JW and others: Complement and the damaging effects of cardiopulmonary bypass, *J Thorac Cardiovasc surg* 86(6):845, 1983.

Lell WA: Hot or cold, continuous or intermittent? What goes around comes around, *J Cardiothorac Vasc Anesth* 6(2):125, 1992, (editorial).

Lell WA, Huber S, Buttner EE: Myocardial protection during cardiopulmonary bypass, In Kaplan JA: *Cardiac anesthesia*, ed 2, vol 2, Philadelphia, 1987, WB Saunders.

Levy FH, O'Rourke PP, Crone RK: Extracorporeal membrane oxygenation, *Anesth Analg* 75:1053, 1992.

Lichtenstein SV and others: Warm heart surgery, *J Thorac Cardiovasc Surg* 101:269, 1991.

Loop FD and others: Trends in selection and results of coronary reoperations, *Ann Thorac Surg* 36(4):380, 1983.

Macmanus Q and others: Surgical considerations in patients undergoing repeat median sternotomy, *J Thorac Cardiovasc Surg* 69(1):138, 1975.

Matsuura H and others: Warm versus cold blood cardioplegia—is there a difference? *J Thorac Cardiovasc Surg* 105:45, 1993.

Mattox KC, Beall AC: Resuscitation of the moribund patient using portable cardiopulmonary bypass, *Ann Thorac Surg* 22:436, 1976.

McKeever WP, Gregg DE, Canney PC: Oxygen uptake of the nonworking ventricle, *Circ Res* 6:612, 1958.

McLaughlin JS: Positional and incisional complications of thoracic surgery. In Waldhausen JA, Orringer MB: *Complications in cardiothoracic surgery*, St Louis, 1991, Mosby.

Melrose DG and others: Elective cardiac arrest: preliminary communication, *Lancet* 2:21, 1955.

Mills NL, Morris JM: Air embolism associated with cardiopulmonary bypass. In Waldhausen JA, Orringer MB: *Complications in cardiothoracic surgery*, St Louis, 1991, Mosby.

Moront MG and others: The use of fibrin glue in neonatal ECMO cannulation sites, *Surg Gynecol Obstet* 166:358, 1988.

Moront JG and others: Extracorporeal membrane oxygenation for neonatal respiratory failure: a report of 50 cases, *J Thorac Cardiovasc Surg* 97(5):706, 1989.

O'Connell J: Personal communication, 1993.

Ottino G and others: Major sternal wound infection after open-heart surgery: a multivariate analysis of risk factors in 2,579 consecutive operative procedures, *Ann Thorac Surg* 44:173, 1987.

Pae WE and others: Prevention of complications during cardiopulmonary bypass. In Waldhausen JA, Orringer MB: *Complications in cardiothoracic surgery*, St Louis, 1991, Mosby.

Pairolero PC, Arnold PG, Harris JB: Long-term results of pectoralis major muscle transposition for infected sternotomy wounds, *Ann Surg* 213:583, 1991.

Peterson KJ, Brown MM: Extracorporeal membrane oxygenation in adults: a nursing challenge, *Focus Crit Care* 17(1):40, 1990.

Phillips SJ and others: Percutaneous cardiopulmonary bypass: application and indication for use, *Ann Thorac Surg* 47:121, 1989.

Robicsek F, Daugherty HK, Cook JW: The prevention and treatment of sternum separation following open heart surgery, *J Thorac Cardiovasc Surg* 73:267, 1977.

Robicsek F and others: The embolization of bone wax from sternotomy incision, *Ann Thorac Surg* 31:357, 1981.

Sealy WC, Brown IW, Young WG: A report on the use of both extracorporeal circulation and hypothermia for open heart surgery, *Ann Surg* 147:603, 1958.

Shawl FA and others: Percutaneous cardiopulmonary bypass support in the catheterization laboratory: technique and complications, *Am Heart J* 120(1):195, 1990.

Society of Thoracic Surgeons: Report: the use of extracorporeal circulation (ECC) for circulatory support during PTCA, *Ann Thorac Surg* 49:514, 1990.

Stammers AH: Trends in extracorporeal circulation for the 1990's: renewed interest and advancing technologies, *J Cardiothorac Vasc Anesth* 6(2):226, 1992.

Sutherland RD, Martinez HE, Guynes WA: A rapid, secure method of sternal closure, *Cardiovasc Dis* 8:54, 1981.

Tinker JH, Roberts SL: Management of cardiopulmonary bypass. In Kaplan JA: *Cardiac anesthesia*, ed 2, vol 2, Philadelphia, 1987, WB Saunders.

Waldhausen JA, Pierce WS: *Johnson's surgery of the chest*, ed 5, St Louis, 1985, Mosby.

Weiland AP, Walker WE: Physiologic principles and clinical sequelae of cardiopulmonary bypass, *Heart Lung* 15(1):34, 1986.

12

Surgery for Coronary Artery Disease

In certain cases of angina pectoris, when the mouth of the coronary arteries is calcified, it would be useful to establish a complementary circulation for the lower parts of the arteries.

Alexis Carrel, MD, 1910

Surgical therapy for ischemic heart disease was proposed in the late nineteenth century by Francois-Franck, a French physiologist, whose suggestion to divide the cardiac sympathetic pain fibers was based on the theory that the patient would be unable to perceive angina pectoris. Thoracic sympathectomy did relieve angina in many patients, but it did not alter the underlying disease or ameliorate its adverse effects. More direct efforts to treat ischemia by increasing the myocardial blood supply, suggested by Carrel in 1910, were attempted by Claude Beck in the 1930s. Beck's belief that the heart could be perfused by surrounding tissue led him to devise various techniques whereby pectoral muscle, pericardial tissue, or omentum was grafted to the denuded epicardium of patients. Eventually these procedures were abandoned, but they did set the stage for Vineberg's implantation in 1948 of the bleeding end of an internal mammary artery into the myocardium of a patient. This indirect method of revascularizing the myocardium remained popular until Favaloro's large-scale success with direct revascularization using aortocoronary bypass grafts (and extracorporeal circulation) superseded previous techniques for the surgical treatment of coronary artery disease (Rankin and Sabiston, 1991).

CORONARY ARTERY DISEASE

Coronary artery disease (CAD) is the result of chronic and progressive atherosclerosis of the coronary arteries. It is the leading cause of morbidity and mortality in the United States, affecting more than 5 million Americans (American Heart Association, 1989). Commonly hypothesized to develop in response to endothelial injury (Ross, 1992), atherogenesis is characterized by endothelial accumulations of fatty and fibrous tissue that produce atheromas (particularly in the epicardial portions of the coronary arteries), which grad-

ually decrease the cross-sectional area of the affected coronary artery (Fig. 12-1). This is a multifactorial process involving the proliferation of smooth muscle cells within the arterial intima. Large amounts of connective tissue are formed by these proliferating cells, in combination with an accumulation of lipid within the cells and the surrounding connective tissue. The process demonstrates great variability, with some lesions of atherosclerosis being dense and fibrous whereas others may be more lipid and necrotic (Ross, 1992).

As the atherosclerotic process continues, perfusion is reduced to the coronary bed distal to the stenosis. When the eventual reduction in myocardial blood flow becomes inadequate to meet the heart's oxygen demand (determined by heart rate, contractility, preload, and afterload) and hinders the adequate removal of metabolic waste products, myocardial ischemia results (Box 12-1). This may be well tolerated at rest when the myocardial oxygen supply is sufficient to meet the demands of the heart (and collateral circulation provides alternate routes for blood flow), but during periods of physical exertion or emotional stress, the blood supply to the myocardium (and in particular the innermost layer of the myocardium: the subendocardium) becomes insufficient to meet cellular oxygen demands. The imbalance that is created between myocardial oxygen supply and myocardial oxygen demand (MVo_2), requires therapy to restore the balance by either decreasing the demand for, or increasing the supply of, oxygen and nutrients.

Decreasing the myocardial oxygen demand by reducing the workload of the heart forms the basis for most medical therapy in treating ischemia. Treatment includes rest, risk factor modification, and pharmacologic therapy. Among the medications used are beta-blocking agents (which decrease heart rate and contractility), calcium channel blocking agents (which

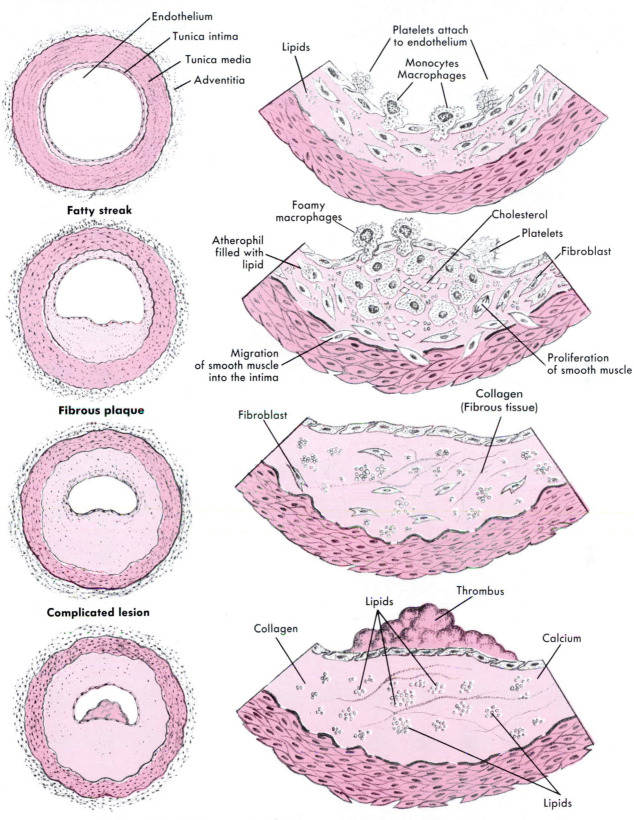

Fig. 12-1 Progression of atherosclerotic coronary artery disease according to the response-to-injury hypothesis (see text). (From McCance KL, Huether SE: *Pathophysiology: the biological basis for disease in adults and children*, St Louis, 1990, Mosby.)

Box 12-1   Types of oxygen deprivation in the heart

Hypoxia/hypoxemia Reduced oxygen supply to myocardial tissues despite adequate perfusion (example: anemia, congenital cyanotic lesions, right-to-left shunts).

Anoxia Absence of oxygen supply despite adequate perfusion (e.g., carbon monoxide poisoning).

Ischemia Oxygen deprivation and inadequate removal of metabolic products as a result of reduced perfusion; leads to lactic acid accumulation and decrease in intracellular pH (e.g., obstructive coronary artery disease, myocardial infarction).

Modified from Braunwald E, Sobel BE: Coronary blood flow and myocardial ischemia. In Braunwald E: *Heart disease*, ed 3, Philadelphia, 1988, WB Saunders.

reduce wall tension and heart rate), antihypertensive medications (which decrease afterload), antidysrhythmic drugs (to treat conduction disturbances), and nitrates (which alter preload and afterload). In general, medications are used to reduce MVo_2 and are less effective at increeaasing myocardial oxygen supply. Coronary vasodilating drugs (e.g., nitrogylcerin) are useful to increase blood flow, but in severe forms of the disease the fixed atherosclerotic obstructions can restrict the usefulness of these drugs.

Increasing the myocardial oxygen supply can be achieved with interventions such as coronary artery bypass grafting (CABG), percutaneous transluminal coronary angioplasty (PTCA), and atherectomy.

These procedures increase the blood supply to the myocardium by creating conduits to bypass the obstructions (CABG) or compressing (PTCA) or excising (atherectomy) the intraluminal plaque and thereby enlarging the artery. Without these interventions, increasing the myocardial oxygen supply is difficult, because the heart already removes about 65% of the oxygen from the blood it receives at rest and 80% during strenuous exercise (Wolff and Nugent, 1988).

Ischemia and Angina Pectoris

Patients with CAD often complain of angina pectoris, the precordial chest discomfort associated with myocardial ischemia. Patients whose presenting symptom is angina will undergo a history and physical examination (H & P) and have an electrocardiogram (ECG) performed. An exercise stress test and other diagnostic studies are used to evaluate the extent and severity of the disease. Cardiac catheterization may be ordered to identify the affected arteries and myocardial tissue at risk (Table 12-1) and to assess wall motion abnormalities and other signs of left ventricular malfunction (Box 12-2).

Anginal syndromes can be classified as stable or unstable. The symptoms of stable angina are predictable and recurrent, and they tend to be consistent in pattern and severity. The patient complains of tightness or pressure in the chest that may radiate to the jaw and the left arm. Symptoms usually subside within 15 minutes and often disappear with rest (which reduces MVo_2) and the administration of nitroglycerin.

Unstable angina refers to pain that increases in frequency, intensity, and duration, and that often occurs

Table 12-1 ■ *Cardiac structures and their coronary arterial supply*

Structure	Coronary artery
Sinus node	Sinus node artery from right coronary artery (RCA): 55%* Sinus node artery from left circumflex artery: 45%
Right atrium	Sinus node artery from RCA: 55% Sinus node artery from left circumflex artery: 45%
Atrioventricular (AV) node	RCA: 90%; left circumflex artery: 10%
Bundle of His	RCA: 90%; left circumflex artery: 10%
Right ventricle	
Anterior	Major supply from RCA; minor supply from left anterior descending (LAD) coronary artery
Posterior	Major supply from RCA and posterior descending branch of RCA; minor supply from distal LAD
Left atrium	Major supply from left circumflex artery
Left ventricle	
Anterior	Left coronary artery (LCA), left circumflex, and LAD
Posterior (diaphragmatic)	Major supply from posterior descending branch of RCA (90%) or left circumflex artery (10%); minor supply from distal LAD
Apex	Major supply from LAD
Left ventricular papillary muscles	
Anterior	Diagonal branch of LAD; other branches of LAD and left circumflex artery
Posterior	RCA and left circumflex artery
Interventricular septum	Major supply from septal perforating branches of LAD; minor supply from posterior descending branch of RCA and AV nodal branch of RCA

Modified from Halpenny CJ, Bond EF: Cardiac anatomy. In Underhill SL and others: *Cardiac nursing*, ed 2, Philadelphia, 1989, JB Lippincott.
*Percentages refer to frequency of occurrence found on postmortem examination.

Box 12-2 Types of impaired ventricular wall motion

Hypokinesia Part of the ventricular wall has weak or poor contraction; motion is diminished but not absent.
Akinesia Part of the ventricular wall has no motion; contraction is absent.
Dyskinesia Paradoxical motion of part of the ventricular wall during systole; abnormal bulging during contraction (e.g., left ventricular aneurysm).

Modified from Kern MJ, editor: *The cardiac catheterization handbook,* St Louis, 1991, Mosby.

Table 12-2 ■ Risk factors for coronary artery disease

Type	Factor
Major: nonmodifiable	Inherited traits
	Male sex
	Increasing age
Major: modifiable	Cigarette smoking
	High blood pressure
	Elevated blood cholesterol
Contributing	Diabetes mellitus
	Obesity
	Physical inactivity
	Emotional stress

Modified from the American Heart Association: *1990 heart and stroke facts,* Dallas, Tex, 1989, The Association.

at rest. This syndrome has been given various names, such as preinfarction angina, accelerated angina, intermediate anginal syndrome, and acute coronary insufficiency (Gazes, 1988a, 1988b). More aggressive treatment (e.g., CABG, PTCA) may be required for this form of angina.

In some patients with ischemic heart disease, anginal symptoms are not always present. This condition, known as "silent ischemia," places patients at increased risk because they do not have pain—one of the important warning signals that would prompt them to seek medical attention. Ambulatory ECG (Holter) monitoring has been used to identify ischemic episodes in this population, but the difficulty remains of determining which patients should receive continuous monitoring (Wolff and Nugent, 1988). The presence of known risk factors (Table 12-2) can alert the clinician to the possibility of ischemic heart disease.

In some cases, fatal or nonfatal myocardial infarction (MI) may be the first manifestation of CAD.

In addition to angina, myocardial ischemia can lead to depressed ventricular function, decreased ventricular compliance, tachydysrhythmias and other conduction disturbances, and systemic embolization from thrombi originating within the left ventricular cavity. In severe cases MI with irreversible cellular injury occurs (Fig. 12-2). In survivors of MI, the mechanical sequelae are related to the location of the blockage and the area of the heart perfused by the blocked artery. Sequelae include left ventricular aneurysm, ventricular septal perforation, left ventricular rupture, and acute mitral valvular insufficiency due to rupture of chordae tendineae or a papillary muscle.

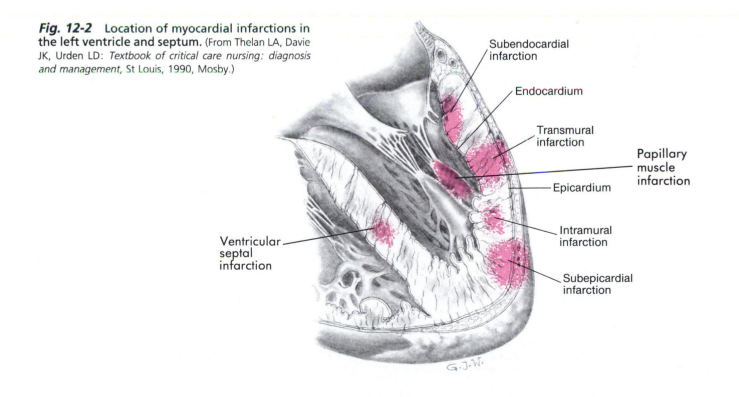

Fig. 12-2 Location of myocardial infarctions in the left ventricle and septum. (From Thelan LA, Davie JK, Urden LD: *Textbook of critical care nursing: diagnosis and management,* St Louis, 1990, Mosby.)

The prognosis is poor for patients in whom these mechanical lesions have acutely and severely compromised ventricular function, and emergency surgical repair is often indicated.

Death from MI is usually attributed to dysrhythmias or low cardiac output from left ventricular failure. Patients who sustain an acute MI and die in cardiogenic shock may have destruction of over 40% of the left ventricular muscle (Magilligan and Ullyot, 1991).

THROMBOLYTIC THERAPY

Patients presenting emergently with symptoms of acute coronary thrombosis (intense, unrelieved chest pain, overwhelming weakness, diaphoresis, nausea and vomiting), may be candidates for thrombolytic therapy. The benefit appears to be greatest when therapy is initiated less than 6 hours after the onset of pain (Pasternak, Braunwald and Sobel, 1992). Among the most commonly used lytic agents, infused intravenously or directly into the coronary artery under fluoroscopy, are streptokinase and recombinant tissue-type plasminogen activator (rt-PA). Because there is a danger of bleeding, invasive procedures such as CABG and PTCA are avoided unless thrombolysis fails to improve coronary blood flow. If surgery is required, bleeding problems will be influenced by the type of lytic agent used. For instance, the longer half-life of streptokinase as compared with that of rt-PA, is likely to create more bleeding problems during the perioperative period (Niemyski and Hellstedt, 1989). Interventional procedures performed in the cardiac catheterization laboratory are associated with persistent bleeding from the catheter insertion site (usually in the groin). Measures to minimize bleeding include direct pressure to arterial and venous puncture sites, application of pressure dressings, and administration of volume or blood products.

PERCUTANEOUS TRANSLUMINAL CORONARY ANGIOPLASTY

Fibrinolytic therapy, PTCA, and surgery are common methods of increasing myocardial oxygen supply. Among the interventional procedures performed in the cardiac catheterization laboratory, PTCA is the most frequently performed, although other revascularization procedures are available, including lasers that vaporize atherosclerotic plaques (Dougherty and others, 1991), atherectomy cutting devices to excise the atheroma (Good and Gentzler, 1991), and intracoronary stents (Fig. 12-3) that prevent occlusion or restenosis of arteries following PTCA (Muller and others, 1990).

The concept of PTCA was first described by Dotter, Rosch, and Judkins (1968), when they suggested the use of mechanical force to dilate atherosclerotic vascular obstructions by inserting progressively larger catheters through a stenosed coronary artery. In 1977 Gruentzig (Gruentzig, Senning, and Siegenthaler,

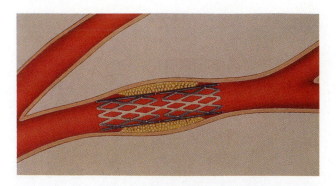

Fig. 12-3 Intracoronary stent in place at the site of the lesion. The long-term consequences of these devices is still unknown. Newer stents are bioabsorbable, and research is underway to incorporate atheroma-inhibiting drugs into the stents. (Courtesy Johnson & Johnson Interventional Systems Co.)

1979) refined the process by developing a small catheter with an inflatable balloon at the tip, which he used to perform the first transluminal coronary angioplasty (Kent, 1987). The number of PTCAs has increased dramatically and in the United States now exceeds the number of coronary artery bypass operations (Massie and Sokolow, 1991).

Much of the popularity of angioplasty is attributed to an acceptable level of success, greater procedure-related comfort for the patient (as compared with CABG), a shorter hospital stay, and less initial cost than CABG (Hlatky and others, 1990; Hochberg and others, 1989). However, restenosis of the repaired coronary arteries is approximately 30% within 6 months (Vlietstra and Holmes, 1988), and the need for repeat cardiac catheterization and additional PTCAs make the difference in cost (compared with surgery) less pronounced. Repeat interventions occur significantly more often in patients undergoing PTCA versus surgery, and there is greater evidence of residual or recurrent ischemia (Vacek and others, 1992). The long-term outcome may be another significant difference, because more complete revascularization can be achieved with surgery versus PTCA in patients with multivessel disease.

The technique consists of positioning the inflatable balloon across a stenosed segment of coronary artery and inflating the balloon, thereby compressing the atheroma and enlarging the lumen (Fig. 12-4). This enhances perfusion of the distal coronary vascular bed. During this process, the atherosclerotic plaque is ruptured and the intraluminal debris is subsequently reabsorbed during the healing process.

PTCA is considered successful when the lumen size is increased at least 20% and the systolic pressure gradient between the proximal and distal portion of the affected artery is abolished or significantly reduced. Restenosis of the repaired arteries may require CABG if repeat PTCA is not feasible.

PTCA is performed in the cardiac catheterization laboratory with the patient under local anesthesia. It

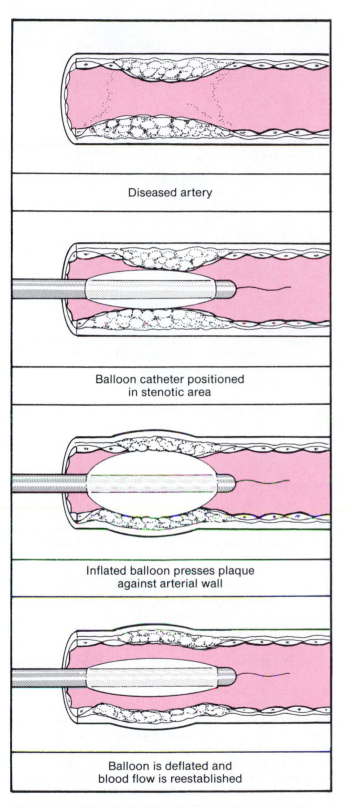

Diseased artery

Balloon catheter positioned
in stenotic area

Inflated balloon presses plaque
against arterial wall

Balloon is deflated and
blood flow is reestablished

Fig. 12-4 Coronary balloon angioplasty procedure. (From Canobbio MM: *Cardiovascular disorders, St Louis, 1990, Mosby.*)

may be coincident with a diagnostic catheterization, or it may be performed at a later date. Surgical standby for PTCA is required in most institutions because of the possibility of dissection of the artery and subsequent acute coronary occlusion. In these cases immediate bypass surgery can prevent or minimize MI and is required in 3% to 5% of PTCA procedures (Kirklin and others, 1991).

In the past, indications for PTCA were limited to selected patients with single-vessel disease and proximal, discrete lesions. At present, the indications have been expanded considerably with improved catheter systems and experienced clinicians. PTCA is performed in patients with multivessel disease and numerous lesions, as well as in patients with stenosed bypass grafts. It can also be used adjunctively with thrombolytic therapy in the emergency treatment of patients with acute MI, although some recommend delaying angioplasty when it is possible to do so in order to reduce the possibility of bleeding complications at the catheterization site (Sherry, 1990).

PERCUTANEOUS TRANSLUMINAL CORONARY ANGIOPLASTY VERSUS CORONARY ARTERY BYPASS GRAFTING

Debate continues over the comparative advantages of angioplasty and CABG, but available data suggest that, within subsets of patients, there are differences in survival and recurrence of angina. With respect to survival, CABG provides greater benefit to patients with left main and three-vessel coronary disease, although some patients with two-vessel disease receive considerable comparative benefit. Some studies have shown that few patients with single-vessel disease receive comparative benefit from CABG, but follow-up data are still incomplete. Most of these patients are more likely to undergo PTCA (Massie and Sokolow, 1991). Recurring angina is less after initial CABG as compared with initial PTCA. The occurrences of MI after CABG and after PTCA have been found to be similar, although there are studies that demonstrate an advantage of the bypass operation (Kirklin and others, 1991).

Another area of study has been the number of patients who did require bypass surgery after angioplasty; this is commonly reported at 1-, 3-, and 5-year intervals. Data indicate that for all patients undergoing PTCA, 10% to 15% require CABG within 1 year, 19% within 3 years, and 10% to 25% within 5 years (Kirklin and others, 1991). Thus the number of patients who "cross over" from PTCA to surgery tend to increase yearly. Rather than severely limiting the number of coronary bypass procedures performed, PTCA has in fact contributed to an increase in the surgical population by expanding the number of patients with documented CAD who, after undergoing one or more angioplasty procedures, often receive surgical revascularization.

SURGERY FOR CORONARY ARTERY DISEASE

Pioneered in 1969 by Favaloro (Box 12-3) and his respective colleagues, CABG using saphenous vein conduits has become one of the most widely performed operations in the United States, and one of the most thoroughly studied (Kirklin and others, 1991). Although there has been debate in the past about the indications for surgical revascularization, there is now general agreement that surgery is appropriate for patients with significant (1) left main coronary artery stenosis, (2) triple-vessel disease (left anterior descending, circumflex, and right coronary systems), (3) severe double-vessel disease involving the proximal left anterior descending and dominant right coronary arteries), and (4) persistent and unacceptable symptoms after maximal medical therapy or after failure of medical therapy. Surgery is also considered in patients with impaired left ventricular function. Usually major arteries and secondary branches 1 mm in size and with 50% or greater stenoses are anastomosed. The arteries should have relatively good distal blood flow (Society of Thoracic Surgeons, 1992).

Use of the internal mammary artery (IMA) has increased dramatically since the publication of results (Cosgrove, Loop, and Sheldon, 1982; Lytle and others, 1983) demonstrating improved long-term patency and minimal atherosclerosis as compared with vein grafts. At least 90% of IMA grafts are patent 10 years postoperatively, compared with 50% of saphenous vein grafts. Because early graft closure of vein grafts is commonly due to thrombosis, patients may be placed on antiplatelet regimens (e.g., aspirin, dipyridamole) to retard this process. Surgical technique in the preparation of bypass conduits and their anastomosis to the coronary arteries is critical to surgical outcome, as is adequate blood flow through the newly constructed graft (Quist, Haudenschild, and LoGerfo, 1992; Roberts, 1991). Extremes in temperature and distension pressure should be avoided during dissection and preparation of the saphenous vein (Fuchs, 1986).

Late closure of grafts is attributed to the progressive atherosclerosis (Lytle and others, 1992). Dietary adjustments, pharmacologic treatment for hypercholesterolemia and hypertension, and cardiovascular risk factor modification (see Table 12-2) are aimed at decelerating the atherosclerotic process.

Other procedures developed to reverse the mechanical sequelae of coronary ischemia include coronary endarterectomy, repair of left ventricular aneurysms, repair of postinfarction ventricular septal defects, and surgery for ischemia-related mitral valve regurgitation (see Chapter 13). Operations to treat electrical disturbances include insertion of pacemakers, resection or ablation of dysrhythmogenic tissue, and antitachycardia devices (see Chapter 19).

In otherwise healthy patients with good left ventricular function, the mortality associated with CABG is between 1% and 3%. The impact on mortality from

---

Box 12-3   Comments on coronary artery bypass grafting

Rene G. Favaloro, MD
Instituto de Cardiologia y
Cirugia Toracica y
Cardiovascular
Buenos Aires, Argentina

I believe that for this delicate type of surgery, even more precise since the application of the internal mammary–coronary anastomosis, the nurse is of paramount significance in our work. If the nurse is not acquainted with every single step and is not ready to help us, especially in difficult situations, our work will be impossible to accomplish.

Even though the extracorporeal circulation has improved very much, I always say that when the patient is connected to the pump, really the patient is dying, because extracorporeal circulation is far from being close to our normal circulation. As a consequence, we have to organize the operation; simplification and standardization are the most important steps to be able to perform the operation with dexterity using the least possible time. In this respect the work of the nurses is really significant. Without their help in an organized manner it would be impossible to carry out the complicated myocardial revascularization combination that we are doing at present.

---

the increase in the number of high-risk and older patients with complex multivessel lesions receiving CABG has yet to be determined precisely (Kirklin and others, 1991).

Women and Coronary Artery Disease

A number of reports have described differences in the use of diagnostic and therapeutic procedures for women and men with coronary artery disease. Ayanian and Epstein (1991) found that angiography and operations for revascularization were significantly higher for men than for women; as a result of these findings, more aggressive management has been pursued in women with coronary artery disease (Steingart and others, 1991).

Surgical outcomes and hospital mortality tend to be higher in women as compared with men. However, some studies that closely matched women and men according to age, anginal status, ejection fraction, number of bypasses, and year of operation, showed no significant differences in mortality. Women did tend to have more frequent postoperative chest pain than men (Jeffrey and others, 1986).

Anatomic differences may account for some of the technical difficulties associated with CABG in women. Hearts and coronary arteries in women are generally smaller than those in men, and this can affect anastomotic techniques. Graft patency is lower in women; smaller vessels, thin-walled saphenous veins, and more diabetes and hypertension have been cited as possible reasons. Another factor may be that women are referred for surgery later in the course of the disease, after left ventricular function has been impaired (Penckofer and Holm, 1990). Bickell and co-workers (1992) found that among patients with a low risk for cardiac death, women have been less likely than men to be referred for CABG. In recent years, women with more severe CAD are at least as likely as men to be referred for CABG.

Preoperative Evaluation

Minimum requirements for preoperative evaluation of patients with ischemic heart disease established by the Society of Thoracic Surgeons (1992) include:

- History and physical examination
- Chest roentgenogram
- Urinalysis
- Electrocardiogram
- Blood typing and crossmatching for homologous transfusion, or autologous donation
- Blood analysis for complete blood count, platelet count, chemistries, and bleeding times
- Blood gas analysis
- Assessment of nutritional status
- Medical consultation as indicated

Prior to surgery, the surgeon again reviews the cardiac catheterization data to assess the patient's coronary anatomy and to determine the severity and location of coronary lesions. Coronary angiography also identifies whether circulation to the posterior aspect of the left ventricle is supplied by the right coronary artery (right dominant), by the circumflex branch of the left coronary artery (left dominant), or by both the right and the left arteries (balanced system). This knowledge is used by the surgeon to select the anastomotic sites (Cooley, 1984). The surgeon will also want to evaluate the function of the left ventricle and the mitral apparatus, especially in patients who have sustained an MI and whose ventricular wall motion may be impaired.

Coronary Artery Bypass Grafting with the Saphenous Vein and Internal Mammary Artery

CABG is the attachment of conduits, most commonly the autogenous greater saphenous vein and/or the IMA, directly to the coronary artery at a point distal to the narrowed artery. Mammary arteries may be as small as 1 mm, and surgeons and their assistants must be able to perform the delicate anastomoses with dexterity and in the least possible time (Favaloro, 1991).

Patient teaching considerations

Teaching considerations focus on the nature of the disease, the surgical intervention, expected perioperative events, and postoperative activities designed to enhance the recuperative process (Table 12-3). Many of these considerations are applicable to all cardiac procedures, but the nurse can specify certain aspects, such as the care of the leg incision, the pro-

gressive nature of the atherosclerotic process, and the modification of coronary risk factors. (Kinney and Craft, 1992).

When alternative conduits are to be used, additional considerations are included in the teaching plan. For example, use of the gastroepiploic artery (described later) is associated with increased pain and gastrointestinal discomfort postoperatively. This information is useful both to the patient and to the postoperative caregivers. Likewise, use of one or both cephalic or basilic arm veins affects postoperative arm movement, and potential self-care deficits should be incorporated into patient care planning.

In emergency situations (e.g., for failed PTCA) when patients are unstable, the surgeon may elect to use only the saphenous vein as a conduit because an assistant can dissect and prepare the leg vein while the surgeon is opening the sternum and cannulating for cardiopulmonary bypass. Dissecting the IMA would delay cannulation for bypass. If the patient is relatively stable, however, the IMA is often used.

Procedural considerations

Perioperative management focuses on preventing myocardial ischemia by maintaining the oxygen supply while reducing the oxygen demand. ECG leads II and V_5 are commonly used to detect signs of ischemia in the left ventricle. Tachycardia and hypotension also alert the clinician to suspect ischemia, but these hemodynamic alterations may not always be present during ischemic episodes.

Nitroglycerin acts as a coronary vasodilator, and patients may come to the operating room with nitroglycerine tablets or dermal patches. When skin patches are present, nurses should wear gloves to remove these patches so that the medication does not contact the nurse's skin (and possibly cause a hypotensive episode). The patches can be removed after consulting with the anesthesiologist and before the skin preparation.

Coronary artery instruments (Box 12-4) are added to the basic setup for cardiac surgery; these include delicate blades to incise the coronary artery, fine forward- and backward-cutting Potts scissors to extend the incision, and forceps and needle holders for the anastomoses. Additional supplies may include one or more cannulas that are inserted into the distal (ankle) end of the saphenous vein, syringes to distend the vein, and blunt-tipped needles for dilating the IMA (and gastroepiploic artery if used) and infusing it with papaverine to reduce spasm. If coronary endarterectomy is to be performed, dissectors and endarterectomy loops may be required (Fig. 12-5). Cotton gloves help the assistant to grasp the heart securely for circumflex marginal and posterior descending coronary artery anastomoses.

Patient care standards for myocardial revascularization (Table 12-3) include the shave preparation along the center of the anterior chest, the groin, and the inner aspect of both legs (along the path of the greater saphenous vein). A more extensive shave

Table 12-3 ■ *Standards of nursing care for myocardial revascularization*

Nursing diagnosis	Patient outcome	Nursing actions
Anxiety/fear of death, changes in life-style or quality of life, ability to modify risks factors	Patient verbalizes concerns/fears and demonstrates a reduction in level of apprehension	Describe perioperative routine that patient will encounter while awake: transport to operating room (OR), insertion of intravascular lines, description of OR (size, color, temperature, number of people and their roles, etc.) Provide comfort measures (warm blankets, etc.) Answer questions to patient's (and family's) level of understanding; respect coping mechanisms (such as denial) if they do not interfere with ability to cooperate with therapeutic regimen Allow patient to verbalize any concern; if necessary, refer to appropriate person
Knowledge deficit related to inadequate knowledge of planned surgery and perioperative events	Patient demonstrates knowledge of physiologic and psychologic responses to myocardial revascularization	Determine patient's understanding of chronic and progressive nature of coronary artery disease (CAD) Determine patient's understanding of surgical procedure; describe (briefly) immediate preoperative events (that will take place while patient is awake); reinforce or clarify what patient (and family) has been told by surgeon; reconcile conflicting time frames given to family (make family aware of preparation and transport time) Assess patient's understanding of planned conduits for bypass grafts (e.g., greater saphenous vein, internal mammary artery, alternative conduits); answer questions or refer as needed If saphenous vein is to be used, inform patient of leg incision(s), leg discomfort, and adequacy of venous drainage even with removal of saphenous vein If additional myocardial revascularization procedures are to be performed (resection or repair of left ventricular aneurysm, coronary endarterectomy, closure of post–myocardial infarction ventricular septal defect), assess patient's understanding and clarify as necessary Determine where family will be waiting during and immediately after surgery; inform them of patient's appearance postoperatively (chest and leg dressings in addition to drains and invasive lines; pallor, cool skin)
High risk for infection related to surgery	Patient is free of infection related to aseptic technique	Shave anterior chest, groin, and inner aspect of both legs Perform circumferential skin preparation of legs and feet Confine and contain instruments and supplies used to excise saphenous vein Change gown and gloves before moving from groin/leg to chest and if contaminated Wrap dressing around leg from ankle to groin to avoid venous stasis and seroma formation If table height is adjusted for exposure of mammary artery, protect sterility of drapes and bypass lines; use additional drapes if necessary
High risk for injury related to positioning, use of mammary retractor	Patient is free of injury related to surgical positioning or use of retraction devices	Place internal mammary artery (IMA) retractor so as to avoid injury to brachial plexus; do not overextend; have all table parts available If IMA retractor post(s) impinges on arm, remove after completion of dissection; pad arms Use caution when elevating legs to perform circumferential skin preparation; raise and lower legs simultaneously; have additional personnel if required If arm veins are to be used, place arms on boards without overextending (to avoid injury to brachial plexus) If lesser saphenous vein is to be used, expose posterior aspect of leg using caution to avoid injury to leg or contamination of field

Modified from Seifert PC: Cardiac surgery. In Rothrock JC: *Perioperative nursing care planning*, St Louis, 1990, Mosby.   *Continued.*

Table 12-3 ■ *Standards of nursing care for myocardial revascularization—cont'd*

Nursing diagnosis	Patient outcome	Nursing actions
High risk for injury related to:	Patient is free of injury related to:	
Retained foreign objects	Retained foreign objects	Account for bulldog clamps, IMA infusion needles, coronary artery knives or blades, saphenous vein cannulas, coronary dilators, epicardial retractors; remove coronary plaque from field to reduce possibility of becoming emboli
Chemical hazards	Chemical hazards	Label syringes containing papaverine, heparinized saline, or other solutions; use only physiologically compatible solutions to distend vein
Physical hazards	Physical hazards	If left ventricular aneurysm (LVA) is to be resected, have felt strips and pledgets, suture, patch material, and vents available as needed
		If coronary endarterectomy is to be performed, have dilators, spatulas, and clamps as needed
		If postinfarction ventricular septal defect (VSD) is to be performed, have felt strips and pledgets, suture, and patch material available
		If reoperation is to be performed, have lateral and posteroanterior chest x-ray films taken to determine location of mediastinal structures relative to sternum and to count number of chest wires; be prepared to cannulate femoral artery for cardiopulmonary bypass if necessary
Electrical hazards	Electrical hazards	Place unused cautery pencil where it cannot be inadvertently discharged; test defibrillator paddles prior to start of procedure; if using long cautery tip during IMA dissection, insulate all but distal end to avoid injury to retrosternal structures
Thermal injury	Thermal injury	Avoid pouring ice chips on IMA; test warm solutions prior to application
High risk for decreased cardiac output/decreased tissue perfusion related to coronary artery disease	Patient's fluid and electrolyte balance is maintained	If reoperation, anticipate need for additional blood/blood products; on all cases monitor blood loss
		If patient has had bypass surgery with IMA, have bulldog clamp available to clamp IMA when cardioplegia infusion is initiated (persistent IMA flow will prevent cardioplegic arrest)
		Insert urinary drainage catheter to monitor urinary drainage, renal perfusion (cardiac output)

Box 12-4 *Myocardial revascularization: procedural considerations*

Instrumentation
Internal mammary artery (IMA) retractor and table parts
Epicardial retractor
Vein, IMA excision instruments (dissecting instruments)
Coronary anastomosis instruments (needle holders, forceps, scissors)
Endarterectomy instruments (spatulas, dilators, clamps)
Coronary, IMA dilators

Supplies
Coronary anastomotic suture (5-0, 6-0, 7-0, 8-0 size)
Micro bulldog clamps
Vein cannulas
Blunt-tipped needles
Syringes to irrigate vein
25-, 27-gauge needle to deair vein grafts
Cotton glove(s) for assistant to retract heart
If resection/repair of left ventricular aneurysm (LVA) or repair of postinfarction ventricular septal defect (VSD)

*Label syringes and containers of solutions, medications.

to be performed, have felt strips and pledgets, heavy suture, and graft material available
Topical hemostatic agents

Medications*
Papaverine
Heparin, heparinized saline solution
Topical antibiotic irrigating solution

Positioning
Supine, legs slightly everted
Leg holder for skin preparation; legs raised and lowered simultaneously
Pillows or positioning pad for legs
If arm veins are used, arms placed on boards without overextending to avoid injury to brachial plexus; arms tucked after dissection is completed
If lesser saphenous vein is used, leg positioned to expose posterior aspect of calf (may need to suspend leg)

Continued.

Box 12-4 *Myocardial revascularization: procedural considerations—cont'd*

Skin Preparation

Midline of chest, inner aspect of both legs shaved

Legs and feet washed circumferentially

Arms and hands washed circumferentially (if arm vein used)

Draping

Anterior chest exposed

Legs exposed from groin to ankle

Feet wrapped

Arm veins exposed from shoulder to wrist; hand(s) wrapped

Special Infection Control Measures

Confine and contain groin and leg instruments

Change gown and gloves before moving from groin to chest

Change gown and gloves if contaminated (e.g., by team member's back during retraction of heart)

Apply dressing to leg incision(s), then wrap elastic bandage around leg from ankle to groin to avoid venous stasis and seroma formation

If table height is adjusted for exposure of IMA, protect sterility of drapes and bypass lines; add additional drapes if necessary

Insulate all but distal tip of long cautery pencil

Place IMA retractor so as to avoid injury to arms; if retractor impinges on arm, remove immediately after IMA dissection (pad arm)

Prevent topical cold solutions from contacting IMA

Avoid use of ice chips (can injure phrenic nerve)

Account for all bulldog clamps, IMA infusion needles, vein cannulas, blades, dilators, epicardial retractors

Remove coronary atheromatous material from field to reduce possibility of emboli

Prepare for selective infusion of cardioplegia solution into coronary grafts; have appropriate tubing, connectors, etc.

Observe for ECG signs of ischemia (ST segment changes) denoting possible incomplete revascularization; if noted, prepare for revision of graft(s) or additional grafts

Monitor presence of ventricular failure and possible need for mechanical ventricular support (intraaortic balloon or ventricular assist device)

Documentation/Report to Cardiac Surgical Intensive Care Unit*

Procedure; bypass grafts: number, type, location

Chest tubes: number, location (mediastinal and pleural)

Monitoring lines: type, location

Epicardial pacemaker lead placement (single, dual), and if being paced

Patient problems, concerns related to coronary heart disease, surgery

Preoperative left ventricular function (e.g., ejection fraction)

*In addition to standard documentation/postoperative report; see Chapter 9.

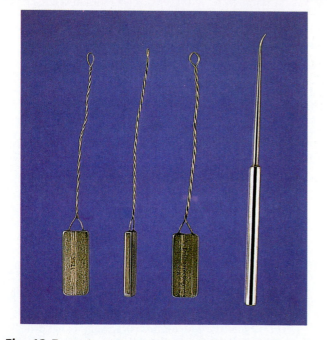

Fig. 12-5 Endarterectomy loops *(left)* and Penfield dissector *(far right)* used for coronary endarterectomy procedures. (From Brooks-Tighe SM: *Instrumentation for the operating room: a photographic manual,* ed 3, St Louis, 1989, Mosby.)

preparation may be requested by some surgeons. The patient is placed in the supine position, and standard precautions, outlined in Chapter 9, are taken to avoid nerve/pressure injury. The legs and feet are washed circumferentially.

Draping is accomplished to expose the chest, the groin, and the legs; the feet are covered with towels, stockinette, or other material. The legs are everted slightly with folded sterile towels or drapes, or they are placed onto a special positioning device (Fig. 12-6) that has been covered with sterile sheets. RN first assistant (RNFA) considerations are listed in Box 12-5.

In some patients requiring grafts to the right coronary artery or the left anterior descending (LAD) coronary artery (in particular, patients with heavily calcified aortas where there is an increased risk of dissection, rupture, or embolization), CABG has been performed without cardiopulmonary bypass (Pfister and others, 1992). The heart is not arrested, and hypothermia is not used. Bleeding from the arteriotomy can be controlled with small clamps, tourniquets, or direct pressure with the blunt end of an instrument. Exposure is achieved with gentle traction and moist, warm laparotomy pads placed under the heart. Monitoring the ECG for ischemia and maintaining ade-

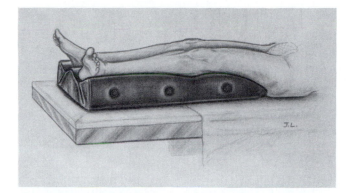

Fig. 12-6 Padded support that elevates and externally rotates the legs to improve exposure of the saphenous vein. (Courtesy Tony Rodono, Leatherette Specialty, Cleveland Heights, Ohio.)

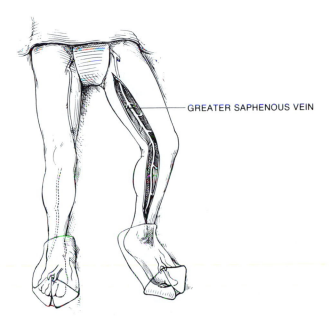

GREATER SAPHENOUS VEIN

Fig. 12-7 Dissection of the greater saphenous vein, which runs along the medial aspect of the leg. A cannula is inserted into the distal (ankle) end, and the vein is gently dilated with physiologic solution. Tributaries are ligated. (From Waldhausen JA, Pierce WS: *Johnson's surgery of the chest*, ed 5, St Louis, 1985, Mosby.)

Box 12-5 *RN first assistant considerations during myocardial revascularization*

Dissection of Saphenous Vein

Clamp tributaries on vein side, leaving a pedicle, or "neck," to tie without causing adventitial constriction of vein lumen.

Clip tributaries on leg side close to leg to avoid impinging on vein.

Avoid excessive distension of vein with irrigating solution.

Dissection of Internal Mammary Artery (IMA)

Suction away cautery plume during IMA dissection.

Avoid touching orifice of IMA (may cause arterial spasm).

Retract lung with ribbon or other retractor.

If pericardium is to be incised to provide "window" for IMA, note location of, and avoid injury to, phrenic nerve.

In emergency situations with unstable patient, there may be insufficient time to dissect IMA; saphenous vein only may be used.

Coronary Anastomoses

Anticipate and avoid suture snagging on instrument handles, pericardial stitch or cannulation suture knots, sternal edges, fingers, etc.

Cover protruding items with damp laparotomy sponge or towels.

Keep fingers moist to allow suture to slip easily.

If retracting heart and it begins to slip, notify surgeon before heart slips from your grasp.

Suction coronary artery with caution; avoid contact with endothelium.

Prevent twisting of bypass graft.

Repair of Left Ventricular Aneurysm

Stabilize and maintain alignment of tissue and prosthetic material with forceps.

When following suture to close infarctectomy, maintain sufficient tension to prevent leaking from suture line.

Repair of Ventricular Septal Defect (VSD)

If retracting heart for closure of posterior VSD, use a cotton glove to maintain a secure grasp of ventricle (repair may be lengthy).

Assist surgeon in maintaining alignment of felt pledgets and felt strips.

Keep interrupted stitches in order.

---

quate volume status are essential. If the heart becomes ischemic, the team should be prepared to institute cardiopulmonary bypass.

Operative procedure

1. A median sternotomy is performed.
2. Vein preparation:
   a. The necessary length of the greater saphenous vein is harvested from the medial aspect of one or both legs (Fig. 12-7). The initial skin incision can be made proximally at the saphenous bulb in the groin or distally at the medial malleolus. The incision is then extended as far as necessary to expose a sufficient length of vein. Tributaries are identified and ligated with 3-0 silk ties and vascular clips on the vein and the leg sides, respectively.

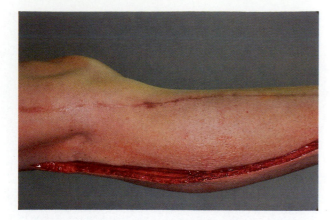

Fig. 12-8 Dissection of the lesser saphenous vein. The incision is made posterior to the lateral malleolus and extended up over the calf. Note the incisional scar where the greater saphenous vein had been excised. (Courtesy Edward A. Lefrak, MD.)

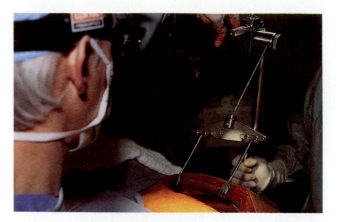

Fig. 12-9 IMA retractor positioned to elevate the left chest wall. (Courtesy John R. Garrett, MD; Howard Kaye, photographer.)

The distal (ankle) end of the vein is identified and cannulated with a blunt-tipped needle to which is attached a syringe of flush solution. The vein is flushed with heparinized (10,000 U/L) physiologic solution to distend it and inspect it for leaks. Tears in the vein may be repaired with a figure-eight suture (usually 6-0 or 7-0 polypropylene). The vein should be kept moist.

Caution is taken to reverse the vein so that the semilunar valves do not interfere with the flow of blood: the proximal (groin) end of the vein will be attached to the coronary artery to become the distal anastomosis, and the distal (ankle) end of the vein will become the proximal (aortic) anastomosis. (The vein is not turned inside out.)

b. The lesser saphenous vein (also known as the short saphenous vein) may be used to augment available venous conduits. The vein runs along the posterior aspect of the lower leg, which can make exposure difficult. The patient may be placed in the prone position to expose the vein (requiring the patient to be rolled over and a new sterile field created); or the leg may be elevated (Fig. 12-8) by an assistant or suspended in a sling. A sterile IMA retractor can be used to hold the sling. The vein is removed and prepared in a manner similar to that of the greater saphenous vein, although the lessor saphenous vein tends to have more tributaries than the greater saphenous vein. Caution is taken during dissection to avoid injury to the sural nerve and the posterior cutaneous nerve.

3. When the IMA is used, the left and/or the right IMA is dissected free after the sternal incision is made. A special retractor (Fig. 12-9) can be used to expose the IMA within its pedicle in the retrosternal bed, and cautery and/or scissors can be used to dissect out a sufficient length of the vessel (Fig. 12-10). Small vascular ligating clips are used on the arterial branches. Before the artery is divided, the patient is heparinized to prevent thrombosis of the artery. The IMA is then divided distally, and the blood flow is assessed. A bulldog clamp is placed across the artery to control blood flow. The distal artery remaining in the lower chest wall is ligated with a heavy tie.

A small (1 mm) dilator may be inserted into the end of the artery to dilate the opening, after which a solution of papaverine may be injected into the IMA to distend it and to reduce arterial spasm (the assistant momentarily opens the bulldog while this is done). The pedicle may be sprayed with the solution as well. Connective tissue surrounding the distal end of the artery is removed. The pedicle is placed in the ipsilateral pleural cavity until needed; the pedicle may or may not be wrapped in a sponge moistened with papaverine.

4. Cardiopulmonary bypass is instituted as previously described. Usually, mild to moderate hypothermia (28° to 32° C [82.4° to 89.6°F]) is used; cooling may be initiated either before or after the cross-clamp is applied. The aorta is cross-clamped, and cardioplegia solution is infused antegradely and/or retrogradely (through the aortic root and/or the coronary sinus, respectively). Both distal (coronary) and proximal (aortic) anastomoses may be performed during a single cross-clamping (with the heart arrested); or all distals are performed with the cross-clamp, the heart is defibrillated, and proximal anastomoses are performed with a partial occlusion clamp (and a beating heart). Some surgeons prefer to perform the proximal anastomoses first.

5. Coronary anastomosis:

a. The surgeon assesses the heart and identifies the arteries to be bypassed, comparing anatomic findings with the cineangiograms taken during cardiac catheterization (and usually reviewed

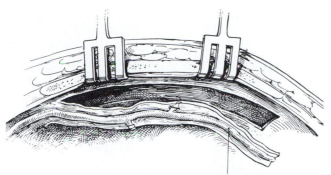

INTERNAL MAMMARY
ARTERY

Fig. 12-10 Dissection of the left internal mammary artery from the retrosternal bed. The artery is dissected proximally from the subclavian artery and distally to the costal margin. The artery and accompanying vein are dissected out together within the pedicle; the vein (and its tributaries) and the arterial branches are ligated with clips. (From Walhausen JA, Pierce WS: *Johnson's surgery of the chest,* ed 5, St Louis, 1985, Mosby.)

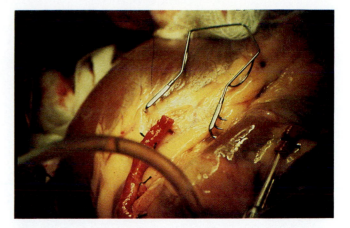

Fig. 12-11 A coronary epicardial retractor improves exposure of the left anterior descending coronary artery embedded in adipose tissue. Note the silk ties on tributaries of the vein graft. (Courtesy Edward A. Lefrak, MD; Doug Yarnold, CRNA, photographer.)

just before surgery). Cardioplegia infusion allows the surgeon to visualize the artery and note a suitable incision site.

Left anterior descending, diagonal coronary arteries: Cold laparotomy pads are placed under the left side of the heart; additional retraction may be provided by the assistant. If there is a great deal of epicardial fat obstructing the coronary artery, an epicardial retractor may be used to improve exposure (Fig. 12-11).

Circumflex obtuse marginal coronary arteries: Cold laparotomy pads may be used to elevate the heart; more commonly, the assistant holds the heart (Fig. 12-12). Wearing a cotton glove provides greater traction and allows the heart to be held securely; a special sling may be used.

Right coronary artery: The proximal or mid–right coronary artery may be exposed with a suture around the artery and tagged to the

Fig. 12-12 Retraction of the heart to expose the obtuse marginal arteries of the circumflex system; a completed anastomosis is shown. (From Waldhausen JA, Pierce WS: *Johnson's surgery of the chest,* ed 5, St Louis, 1985, Mosby.)

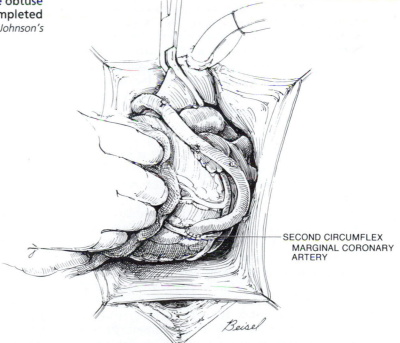

SECOND CIRCUMFLEX
MARGINAL CORONARY
ARTERY

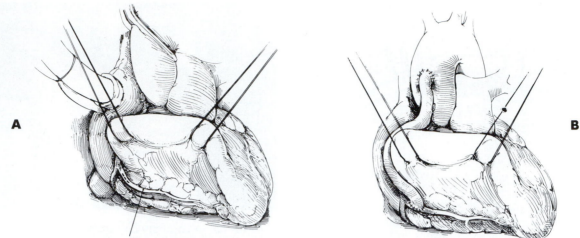

POSTERIOR DESCENDING CORONARY ARTERY

Fig. 12-13 **A,** Use of retention sutures to expose the posterior descending coronary artery. **B,** Completed anastomosis. (From Waldhausen JA, Pierce WS: *Johnson's surgery of the chest,* ed 5, St Louis, 1985, Mosby.)

drapes to elevate the heart. An assistant may provide additional retraction.

Posterior descending coronary arteries: The assistant holds the heart (with a cotton glove [Fig. 12-12]), or a retention suture is used (Fig. 12-13) to expose the artery.

b. The coronary artery is incised with a fine blade; the cardioplegia infusion is turned off, and suction is turned on. The incision is extended forward and backward with delicate angled scissors, and a probe is inserted to measure and dilate the arterial lumen. External pressure with small bulldog clamps or a pill sponge may be applied proximally and/or distally to the arteriotomy to prevent bleeding during the anastomosis, although suctioning through the aortic venting needle usually provides a sufficiently dry field. Placement of the coronary suction tip within the artery should be done carefully (if at all) to avoid injury to the vascular intima.

c. The distal end of the vein is beveled with scissors to approximate the coronary incision for the end-to-side anastomosis, which can be performed with a continuous stitch technique (Fig. 12-14) or with interrupted stitches.

   If a side-to-side sequential graft is to be performed, a venotomy is made with a blade (or small punch) and extended with scissors (Fig. 12-15).

d. The anastomosis is made with fine cardiovascular suture. With the continuous stitch technique a 6-0 or 7-0 monofilament is commonly used; an interrupted stitch technique is performed by some surgeons with fine silk stitches.

   Before the distal anastomosis is completed, the coronary artery may be probed to ensure patency. The stitch is tied carefully to avoid compromising the size of the lumen. Physiologic solution may be injected into the vein

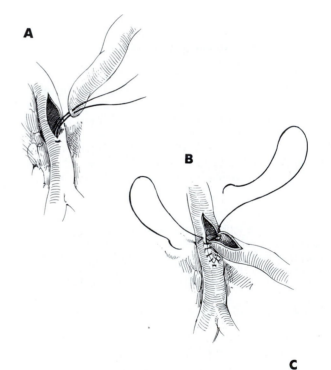

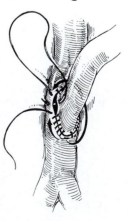

Fig. 12-14 **A,** A continuous end-to-side anastomosis begins distally at the "toe" and, **B,** continues along the edge of the arteriotomy toward the "heel." **C,** The anastomosis almost completed. After the knot is tied, cardioplegia solution can be infused through the graft to test for leaks and assess distal flow, and is delivered to the myocardium distal to the coronary blockage. (From Waldhausen JA, Pierce WS: *Johnson's surgery of the chest,* ed 5, St Louis, 1985, Mosby.)

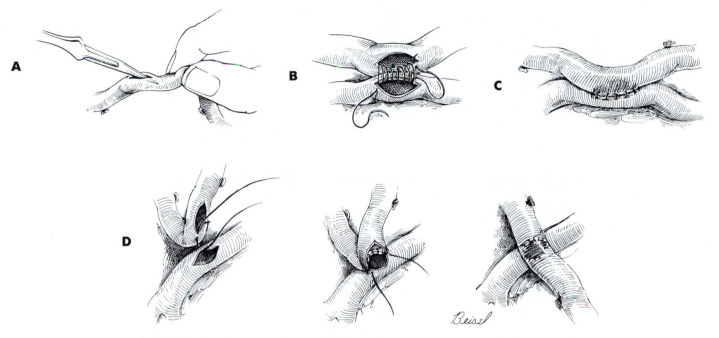

Fig. 12-15   Continuous side-to-side anastomosis for sequential grafts. **A,** Longitudinal incision of the vein. **B,** The anastomosis is started at the distal end. **C,** Completed anastomosis, **D,** Diamond anastomosis. (From Waldhausen JA, Pierce WS: *Johnson's surgery of the chest,* ed 5, St Louis, 1985, Mosby.)

grafts to detect any leaks, to assess distal flow into the coronary bed, and to unravel a twisted graft. Cardioplegia solution may be selectively infused into the completed graft to protect the myocardium beyond the stenosis.

e. A small bulldog clamp may be placed on the proximal portion of the vein to prevent air from entering the coronary artery. The proximal anastomosis may be performed at this time, or after all of the distal anastomoses are completed.

f. Steps a through e are repeated for each subsequent vein graft anastomosis. Grafts to the LAD artery and its branches require little manipulation of the heart and are usually performed last to minimize disruption of previously placed grafts (Gay, 1990). When the IMA is used on the LAD, it is the last distal anastomosis performed so that tension on that critical graft is avoided.

6. The distal IMA anastomosis to the coronary artery is performed as described for the anastomosis of the saphenous vein to the coronary artery. The IMA pedicle is brought out of the pleura with the bulldog clamp in place (to prevent blood flow from obscuring the field and rewarming the heart). No aortic proximal anastomosis is required, because the IMA remains attached to its takeoff from the subclavian artery (Fig. 12-16).

Occasionally, IMA free grafts are used, with the

IMA proximal anastomosis made on the aorta (Tector, Schmahl, and Canino, 1986). Sequential side-to-side anastomoses also may be performed; these are accomplished in a manner similar to that used for vein grafts.

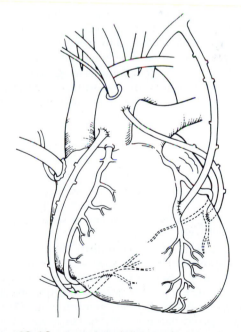

Fig. 12-16   Completed internal mammary artery and vein graft anastomoses.

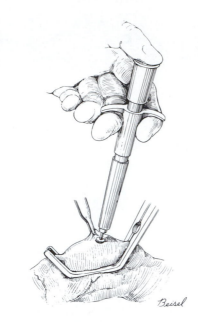

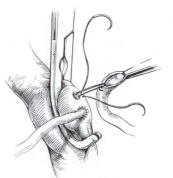

Fig. 12-17 **A,** A partial occlusion clamp is placed on the anterior aorta (away from areas of calcification) for the proximal anastomosis. A small incision is made in the aorta with a knife, and the aortic punch is then used to create the aortotomy (4.5 mm). **B,** Anastomosis of the vein graft is performed with 5-0 polypropylene. (From Waldhausen JA, Pierce WS: *Johnson's surgery of the chest,* ed 5, St Louis, 1985, Mosby.)

After completion of the anastomosis, the pedicle is tacked to the epicardium with a fine suture. The pericardium may be incised at the point where the IMA crosses it to allow sufficient room for the IMA graft once the lungs are reinflated; caution is taken to avoid injuring the phrenic nerve running along the lateral borders of the pericardium.

If concomitant mitral valve repair or replacement is performed, the coronary anastomoses are performed first, followed by the valve surgery. The procedure is done in this order so that cardioplegia solution can be infused into the grafts to protect the distal myocardium and so that during manipulation of the heart for anastomoses, injury does not occur to the atrioventricular groove from the valve prosthesis.

7. Aortic anastomoses. The proximal vein graft anastomoses may be performed while the aorta is still cross-clamped and the heart arrested, or with the clamp removed and the heart beating. In the latter case, an angled, partial-occlusion clamp, such as a Beck clamp, is used to isolate a segment of aorta (Fig. 12-17).

   a. A segment of aorta slightly smaller than the diameter of the vein graft is resected. A knife blade (e.g., No. 11 or 15) is used to incise the aorta, and a punch is inserted into the aortotomy to create an oval opening (Fig. 12-17, *A*).

   b. The proximal end of the saphenous vein is anastomosed to the side of the aorta with 5-0 vascular suture (Fig. 12-17, *B*, and 12-18). The

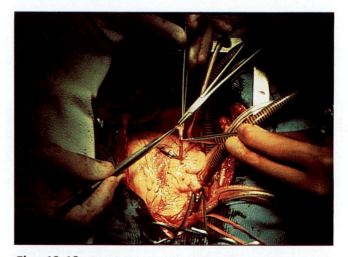

Fig. 12-18 Proximal anastomosis. The assistant holds apart the edges of the proximal vein graft while the surgeon places stitches into the vein and then into the aortotomy. The vein will be seated onto the aorta, and the anastomosis will be completed. (Courtesy Edward A. Lefrak, MD; Doug Yarnold, CRNA, photographer.)

site may be marked with a radiopaque ring or clip for future identification of the graft.

   c. The partial-occlusion clamp, or the cross-clamp, is removed, and the suture lines are checked. Air is removed from the vein graft using a fine (25- or 27-gauge) hypodermic nee-

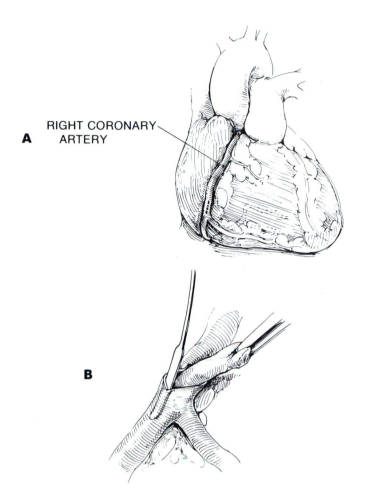

A RIGHT CORONARY ARTERY

B

Fig. 12-19 Endarterectomy of the right coronary artery. An endarterectomy spatula is used to bluntly dissect the atheromatous inner core. (From Waldhausen JA, Pierce WS: *Johnson's surgery of the chest,* ed 5, St Louis, 1985, Mosby.)

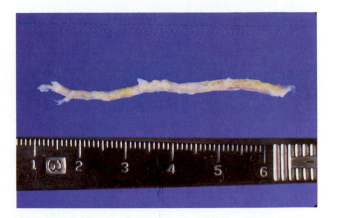

Fig. 12-20 Native coronary atheroma. (Courtesy Alan M. Speir, MD; Kip Seymour, photographer.)

dle and the bulldog clamp or clamps are removed. The IMA bulldog clamp is also removed at this time. An angled chest tube is inserted to drain one or both pleural cavities that may have been opened during the IMA dissection. (Or, the distal end of the straight mediastinal drainage tube can be inserted into the pleural cavity.)

Coronary Endarterectomy

Coronary endarterectomy is usually reserved for removal of plaque from the right coronary artery system in situations where the right coronary artery is occluded and no distal branches are available for anastomosis. Endarterectomy of the left coronary artery system is performed less often and remains controversial (Cooley, 1984).

Operative procedure

1. An arteriotomy is made above the plaque, commonly near the bifurcation of the right coronary artery and the posterior descending coronary artery.

2. An endarterectomy spatula is used to bluntly dissect the atheromatous intimal core from the inner wall of the artery (Fig. 12-19).
3. The atheroma (Fig. 12-20) is freed circumferentially as far as possible from each separate branch of the artery and removed by gentle traction with a small clamp. The distal ends should have feathered ends, indicating complete removal of the plaque (Cooley, 1984).
4. A probe can be inserted distally to ensure patency.
5. The arteriotomy site is then used for anastomosing a bypass graft.

Other Coronary Artery Bypass Conduits

Although the saphenous vein and the IMA are the vessels of choice, there are situations that preclude their use. These include patients with previous bilateral vein stripping, extensive varicosities, or previous bypass surgery using these conduits, or the presence of vessels that are too small, too short, or too fragile. Alternative autologous venous and arterial conduits that have been used include the cephalic vein and the basilic vein, and the right GEA, radial artery, splenic artery, and inferior epigastric artery (Fig. 12-21). The cephalic or basilic vein is often used if the saphenous vein and the IMA are insufficient or unavailable. There are drawbacks that limit their use: there is a higher failure rate than with the saphenous vein or the IMA (Prieto, Basile, and Abdulnour, 1984; Stoney and others, 1984); positioning for access to the vein is cumbersome and difficult, and the skin incision is uncomfortable and disfiguring.

Among the allografts that have been used are the umbilical vein and the greater saphenous vein. Synthetic grafts made of Dacron or polytetrafluoroethylene (PTFE) have been used on occasion as well (Edmunds, Norwood, and Low, 1990).

Many of the investigational studies of alternative conduits have consisted of small sample sizes, thus their conclusions may not be generalizable. However,

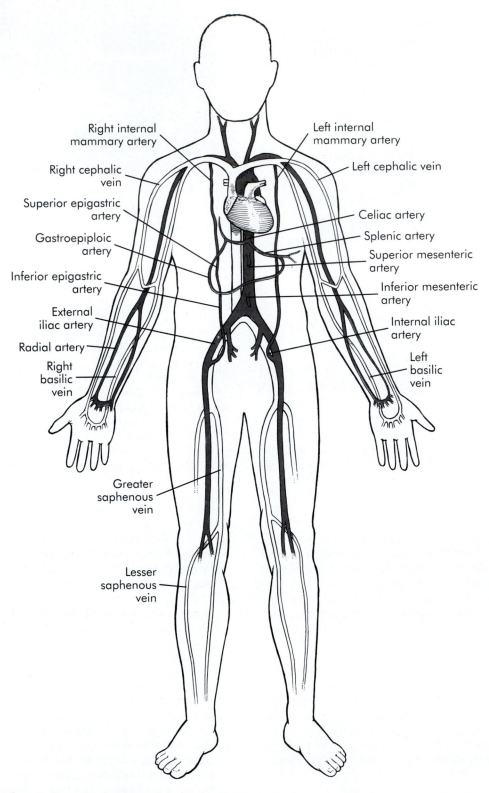

Fig. 12-21 Alternative autologous arterial and venous conduits for coronary bypass grafting. (Drawing by Peter Stone.)

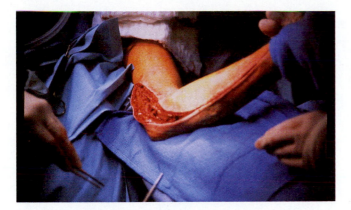

Fig. 12-22 Incision site for (basilic) arm vein. (Courtesy John R. Garrett, MD.)

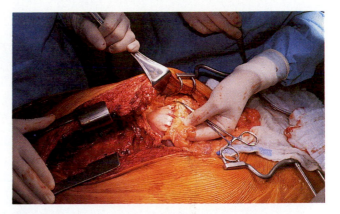

Fig. 12-23 Dissection of the right gastroepiploic artery (GEA). The surgeon is holding the GEA pedicle; the clamp is placed on the distal portion of the right GEA. Branches of the GEA can be seen penetrating the stomach wall (pale smooth area). A Balfour retractor is in the abdomen; a Cooley sternotomy retractor is in the chest. (Courtesy John R. Garrett, MD.)

there are encouraging data about the patency rates of the GEA (Glick, Liddicoat and Karp, 1990; Lytle and others, 1989) and the inferior epigastric artery (Buche and others, 1992; Milgalter and others, 1992). Alternative conduits described here include arm veins and the GEA.

Operative procedure: arm veins (cephalic or basilic)

1. One or both arms are placed on armboards and prepared from the shoulder to the hands. The hands are wrapped with towels or sterile stockinette. (Intravascular lines in the wrist are avoided when possible, but if necessary, they are covered with sterile drapes.) The necessary length of vein is excised: the **cephalic vein** from the radial aspect of the wrist to the inner aspect of the antecubital space up to the deltopectoral groove and the **basilic vein** from the ulnar aspect of the wrist to the elbow and upper arm, where it courses toward the axilla. Variations in the venous patterns are common and numerous (Fig. 12-22).
2. Tributaries are ligated with 3-0 silk ties and vascular clips on the vein and arm sides, respectively. The distal (hand) end is cannulated with a blunt-tipped needle. The vein is prepared in a manner similar to that for the saphenous vein, but because the arm vein has thinner walls, it may be more difficult to handle (Edmunds, Norwood, and Low, 1990). Subcutaneous tissue and skin are closed with absorbable suture; staples may be used on the skin. Dressings are applied to the arm(s).
3. If the abducted position of the arms interferes with the surgeon's or the assistant's access to the chest, the arms may be tucked along the patient's side after the dressings are applied. Additional drapes may be placed along the lateral borders to maintain the sterility of the field.
4. Arm vein graft anastomoses are similar to those using saphenous vein.

Operative procedure: gastroepiploic artery

1. The median sternotomy incision is extended along the midline abdominal fascia to a point just above the umbilicus. An abdominal retractor, such as a Balfour, may be inserted (Fig. 12-23).
2. The peritoneal cavity is entered, and the right GEA is identified along the greater curvature of the stomach. Branches to the omentum are ligated with silk ties or clipped with staples (Fig. 12-24, *A*) branches to the stomach are ligated with silk ties (Fig. 12-24, *B*). The GEA is isolated from the greater curvature of the stomach (to a point where the artery becomes less than 1 mm in diameter) back to the level of the pylorus, just distal to its takeoff from the gastroduodenal artery. The patient is heparinized before the GEA is divided (Lytle and others, 1989). Papaverine can be injected into the distal (cut) end of the GEA to reduce arterial spasm.
3. If the GEA is to be used in situ, the vessel is divided distally and brought through an opening made into the diaphragm to the site of the coronary anastomosis. In situ grafts are commonly performed on the main right coronary artery and its posterolateral branches and the posterolateral branches of the circumflex coronary artery (Fig. 12-24, *C*). They can also be attached to the LAD if there is sufficient length to reach the planned anastomotic site.
4. Free GEA grafts may be used. They allow greater versatility, but early results are not as good as they are for in situ grafts. Anastomotic techniques are similar to those for the IMA free graft. When used as a free graft, the GEA is divided at both the distal and proximal ends and remaining portions of the artery tied off with heavy ties.
5. The abdominal incision is closed in layers.

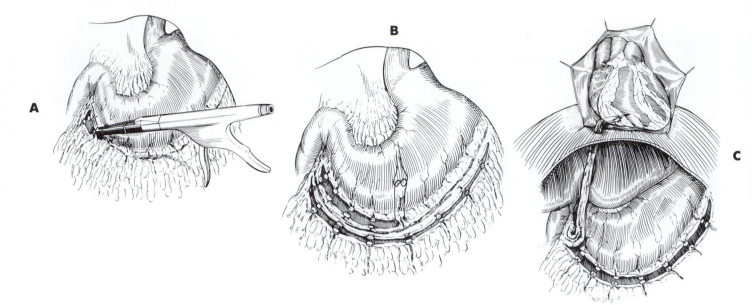

Fig. 12-24 Use of the right GEA for coronary artery bypass grafting. **A,** A staple gun is used to divide omental branches of the GEA. **B,** Branches to the stomach are ligated with silk ties. **C,** The right GEA is brought through the diaphragm and anastomosed to the right coronary artery. (From Lytle BW and others: Coronary artery bypass grafting with the right gastroepiploic artery, *J Thorac Cardiovasc Surg* 97[6]:826, 1989.)

Repair of a Left Ventricular Aneurysm

A left ventricular aneurysm is one of the complications of acute myocardial infarction, with anterolateral and anteroseptal aneurysms seen more frequently than diaphragmatic or posterior aneurysms. It is thought to occur in muscular areas where the artery has been occluded and where there is an absence of significant collateral circulation. Without treatment, patients generally succumb to congestive heart failure or recurring dysrhythmias and are at risk for embolization and/or rupture of the ventricle.

The aneurysmal tissue, often clearly delineated from the surrounding myocardium, appears as a thinned-out transmural scar devoid of trabeculations normally seen in the ventricular endocardium. Chest x-ray films show enlargement of the left ventricle, and cardiac cineangiography, echocardiography, or radionuclide imaging techniques may reveal akinesis or dyskinesis (paradoxical motion with bulging of the affected area) during systole (Box 12-2).

Operative mortality ranges from 3% to 30% depending on the patient's age, general status, associated disease, and extent of myocardial involvement (Society of Thoracic Surgeons, 1992).

The goal of surgical repair is to remove the dysfunctional tissue while retaining the geometry of the left ventricle as much as possible in order to optimize left ventricular function. With early reparative techniques, there was distortion of the cardiac anatomy because the repair produced a linear, rather than a circular or elliptic, suture line (Fig. 12-25). Patients

often required early postoperative support with an intraaortic balloon pump (Cooley, 1989).

The technique of ventricular endoaneurysmorrhaphy described by Jatene (1985) and refined by Cooley (1989) was developed to preserve the surface anatomy and restore the internal contour of the ventricle. Endoaneurysmorrhaphy, as well as the conventional repair that involves resecting and plicating ventricular tissue, are described here.

Procedural considerations

Teflon felt strips, patch material (woven Dacron, PTFE, or pericardium), and additional sutures (1, 0, 2-0, or 3-0) of polypropylene or polyester with large needles are needed in addition to instruments and supplies for coronary artery bypassing. The left side of the heart is vented with a catheter placed in the ventricle via the right superior pulmonary vein or the ventriculotomy. The superior and inferior vena cavae are cannulated for venous return.

Operative procedure: apical ventricular endoaneurysmorrhaphy (Cooley, 1989)

1. A median sternotomy is performed, and cardiopulmonary bypass is instituted as previously described. Moderate hypothermia (28° to 30° C [82.4° to 86° F]) is used. The aorta is cross-clamped, and the heart is arrested with cardioplegia. To reduce the possibility of dislodging a mural thrombis, the aneurysm is generally not palpated until the cross-clamp has been applied and the heart arrested.

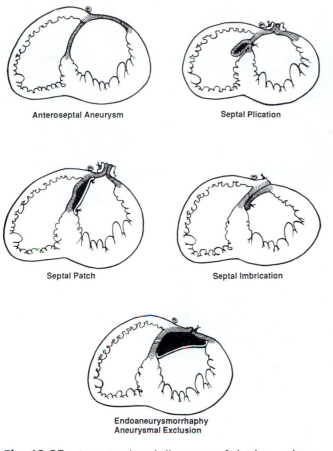

Anteroseptal Aneurysm

Septal Plication

Septal Patch

Septal Imbrication

Endoaneurysmorrhaphy
Aneurysmal Exclusion

Fig. 12-25   Cross-sectional diagrams of the heart showing the methods of repair for anteroseptal ventricular aneurysm and a comparison with the technique of endoaneurysmorrhaphy. (From Cooley DA: Ventricular endoaneurysmorrhaphy, *Tex Heart Inst J* 16[2]:72, 1989.)

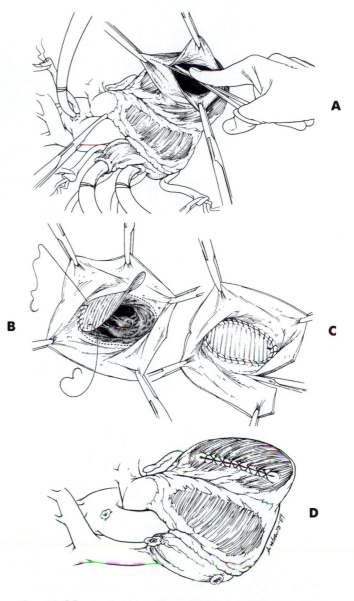

Fig. 12-26   Technique of ventricular endoaneurysmorrhaphy. **A,** The apex is incised lateral and parallel to the interventricular groove, and any thrombus is removed. The mitral apparatus is inspected. **B,** and **C,** A patch of woven Dacron is fashioned to replace the diseased area of the ventricular cavity and secured with 3-0 polypropylene. **D,** The ventriculotomy is repaired directly or with buttressing felt strips. (From Cooley DA: Ventricular endoaneurysmorrhaphy, *Tex Heart Inst J* 16[2]:72, 1989.)

Adhesions between the left ventricular apex and the pericardium are sharply divided.

2. The aneurysm is identified and inspected, and a longitudinal incision is made in the aneurysmal tissue over the apex lateral and parallel to the interventricular groove.

3. The aneurysmal endocardium is inspected, and any thrombus is removed. The boundary between viable myocardium and fibrotic scar is noted. The mitral apparatus is inspected.

4. An oval patch of low-porosity woven Dacron (patch graft or a section of the tube graft) is cut to duplicate the infarcted area in the ventricular cavity (Fig. 12-26). It is secured with continuous sutures of 3-0 polypropylene placed in the fibrotic tissue that forms the boundary between infarcted and healthy myocardium. Care is taken not to damage the mitral papillary muscles.

5. The ventriculotomy edges are then reapproximated over the patch by direct suture or buttressed with felt strips using heavy suture. Care is taken not to suture the left anterior descending coronary artery.

6. If coronary artery bypass surgery is planned, it is often performed after the aneurysm is repaired.

Operative procedure: conventional repair of a left ventricular aneurysm *(Waldausen and Pierce, 1985)*

1. Median sternotomy, cardiopulmonary bypass, and hypothermic cardioplegic arrest are instituted. Adhesions are dissected free.

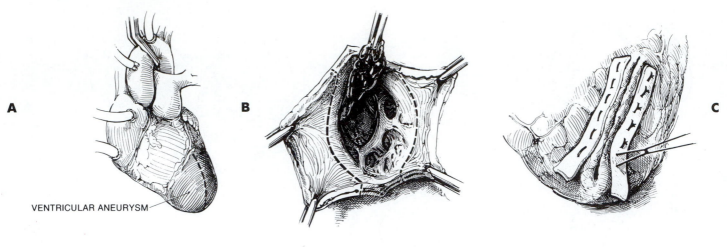

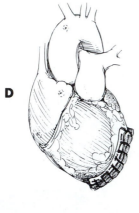

Fig. 12-27 Conventional repair of a left ventricular aneurysm. **A,** The apex is incised. **B,** Thrombus is removed. The mitral valvular apparatus is then inspected. **C,** The ventriculotomy edges are plicated with buttressing felt strips using an interrupted suture technique, followed by, **D,** oversewing with a continuous suture. (From Waldhausen JA, Pierce WS: *Johnson's surgery of the chest,* ed 5, St Louis, 1985, Mosby.)

2. The central portion of the aneurysm is incised, and existing clot is removed. Boundaries of viable myocardium are identified, and the endocardium and mitral apparatus are inspected.
3. Clamps (such as straight Kocher clamps) are placed along the edges of the aneurysm, and the thinned-out scar tissue is excised, leaving a rim of fibrous tissue to close the aneurysm. Normal tissue should not be compromised in the repair.
4. Two strips of Teflon felt (approximately 2 cm by 15 cm) are fashioned and placed along each side of the incision (one strip along each edge). The needle of a double-armed heavy (No. 1, 0, 2-0) suture is passed through the edge of one felt strip, through the edge of the fibrous tissue below the felt, across to the other edge of the tissue, and up through the opposing felt strip. The needles are cut off, and the suture ends are tagged. A series of these interrupted stitches is made along the length of the ventriculotomy (Fig. 12-27).
5. A venting catheter may be placed at the apex of the incision.
6. The interrupted stitches are tied.
7. A secondary, continuous suture of polyester or polypropylene is run down and back the length of the incision to oversew the repair. An additional felt strip may be placed over the middle of the incision to prevent leakage of the fibrous walls

(Cooley, 1984). Additional pledgeted sutures may be placed as necessary to achieve hemostasis.
8. Air is removed from the left ventricle, the vent is removed, and the vent site is closed with a previously placed suture.

Repair of a Postinfarction Ventricular Septal Defect

Rupture of the ventricular free wall or the interventricular septum is an additional complication of myocardial infarction originating in the zone of necrotic myocardium. Free wall ruptures with immediate cardiac tamponade and cardiovascular collapse are almost uniformly fatal because there is insufficient time to close the left ventricle.

Ventricular septal ruptures also represent a surgical emergency and are commonly located in the anterior septum near the apex of the heart. Defects may also appear in the posterior septum and the midseptum. Postinfarction ventricular septal defects (VSDs) usually occur within 2 weeks of the infarction (Heitmiller, Jacobs, and Daggett, 1986).

Incidence and pathophysiology

Septal ruptures are rare (1% to 2% incidence), but they are often lethal, with a 24% mortality in the first 24 hours. Clinical manifestations include pulmonary artery hypertension, pulmonary edema, and, frequently, cardiogenic shock (e.g., systolic blood pressure less than 80 mm Hg, oliguria or anuria, elevated creatinine level, and cool, clammy skin [Komeda, Fremes, and David, 1990]).

There is an increase ("step-up") in the oxygen content of the blood in the right ventricle and pulmonary artery after septal rupture because of the left-to-right shunting of oxygenated blood from the left ventricle through the defect into the right ventricle. Pulmonary flow may be twice that of systemic flow. Blood returning to the right atrium may reflect a lower than normal oxygen saturation because of the body's extraction of more oxygen in the presence of a lowered cardiac output. A loud holosystolic murmur can be heard at the lower left sternal border (Fecteau, 1986).

Preoperative care

Patients often undergo echocardiography and/or cardiac catheterization and cineangiography to visualize the left-to-right shunt, the coronary arteries, and cardiac valve function, especially signs of mitral valve incompetence. Unstable patients may be supported with an intraaortic balloon pump during these studies, after which they are transported directly to the operating room. Because of the critical nature of this complication, patients and their families are extremely frightened and anxious. This fear and anxiety may be aggravated by the lack of preanesthetic medication in patients too unstable to tolerate the depressive effects of the drugs. Although detailed teaching or instruction is unrealistic, it is possible (and important) to reduce some of the fear and anxiety through a calm and caring manner that is at the same time efficient and quick. The family can be directed to the waiting area and kept informed of the patient's progress by a designated person such as a case manager, a patient representative, or a unit-based nurse.

Perioperative nursing considerations

Once the patient enters the operating room, intravascular lines and a urinary drainage catheter are inserted if they are not already in place. Skin preparation and draping are done as soon as possible; the sternum is incised, and the patient is placed on bypass. The aim of surgery is to excise infarcted tissue and close the defect with a patch of prosthetic material or pericardium (bovine or autologous). Concomitant valve repair and/or coronary artery bypassing of documented coronary obstructions is performed as indicated. Saphenous vein grafts are used most often, because in most instances there is insufficient time to dissect out the IMA.

The mortality from ventricular septal rupture is due largely to multisystem failure resulting from hypoperfusion of peripheral organs rather than from cardiac failure per se (Daggett, 1991). Thus one of the main considerations is to avoid delay in operating on the patient. Cardiopulmonary bypass (with bicaval cannulation and systemic cooling to 20° to 24° C [68°

to 75° F]) should be instituted expeditiously, and meticulous attention should be given to myocardial protection. Surgical mortality may range from 10% to 60% depending on the preoperative status (Society of Thoracic Surgeons, 1992).

Implications for the perioperative nurse include having necessary instruments and supplies immediately available, including basic sternotomy and coronary instruments, heavy suture such as that used for left ventricular aneurysms (0 to 2-0 polyester, double-armed), felt strips, felt pledgets (1 cm by 1 cm, or smaller) patch material, and woven graft material. There should be sufficient cold topical solutions for pericardial lavage.

Freshly infarcted myocardial tissue tends to be very friable and does not hold sutures securely. For this reason, suture lines are often buttressed with felt strips and/or felt pledgets to prevent disruption of the repair and to distribute stresses more evenly along the suture line. Strips of felt and individual pledgets may be cut from prepackaged felt squares (6 inches by 6 inches). Some repairs use 4 or more strips and 25 or more individual pledgets. Multiple pledgeted sutures are used for many repairs; if the suture with the size pledget desired by the surgeon is not prepackaged, a scrub nurse may need to pledget 20 to 30 stitches. (It is very helpful if another scrub nurse is available to do this.)

Operative procedure: repair of a postinfarction ventricular septal defect

Cooley and associates (1957) were the first to report a successful repair of a postinfarction VSD. Since then, a number of techniques have evolved. Notable has been the work of Daggett and colleagues (1977, 1982; see also Box 12-6), who are credited with developing a number of reparative techniques for this complication. Among the refinements that have improved survival are (1) using Teflon felt to buttress suture lines of friable myocardium, (2) repairing larger defects with prosthetic patch material and thereby reducing tension on the tissue edges, (3) incising the ventricle through infarcted rather than normal tissue (thereby sparing functional myocardium), and (4) instituting intraaortic counterpulsation to support the heart (Heitmiller, Jacobs, and Daggett, 1986). Because bleeding from the suture lines occasionally can be a problem, some authors (Komeda, Fremes, and David, 1990) have described the use of (more pliable) bovine pericardium rather than Dacron material to repair defects.

Each defect is anatomically unique, with the condition of the tissue uncertain. Therefore the surgeon may not be certain of the precise technique needed. After the institution of cardiopulmonary bypass and the aorta is cross-clamped, the nurse should anticipate a period of inspection of the anatomy before the final surgical plan is formulated. Repair of anterior, apical, and posteroinferior defects are described here and reflect the principles enumerated by Daggett.

Box 12-6 *Comments on the repair of postinfarction ventricular septal defects*

Willard M. Daggett, MD
Massachusetts General Hospital
Boston, Massachusetts

Increasingly we view the patient with a postinfarction ventricular septal rupture as a surgical emergency, not dissimilar to the patient with a leaking abdominal aortic aneurysm. We tend to operate on patients with postinfarction septal rupture as they present. Operations in these patients will occur at odd hours and, of course, on weekends as well. This has a lot of meaning for cardiac surgical nursing, as this type of operation is complex in its planning and execution and, paradoxically, relatively infrequent in its occurrence. This means that experience with this type of procedure needs to be concentrated in the hands of highly trained cardiac surgical nurses who will be on call for this type of emergent procedure nights and weekends.

It is our distinct impression that each of these defects is in some way anatomically unique; therefore the repair to be instituted in a given patient may in itself be unique, requiring flexibility in the conduct of the operation both for the surgeon and the cardiac perioperative nurse. A wide variety of suture material may be used in these repairs, again requiring some flexibility. The first priority to achieve success for these patients is complete closure of the defect itself, this repair being accomplished without tension on the adjacent muscle to prevent recurrence of the defect or free wall left ventricular rupture.

Each of these operations is a little like "weaving a rug" in that different locations of the defect, the extent of muscle loss, and the extent of coronary artery disease require flexibility in both the planning and the execution of the operation.

This is the type of procedure wherein operative outcome will depend a great deal on the specific knowledge, experience, and planning of the operating room team. Reading appropriate articles and discussion with all of the surgical staff will aid greatly in making sure that all possible contingencies have been covered and thought out in advance.

Procedure

1. Bicaval cardiopulmonary bypass is established, and the heart is arrested with cold cardioplegia.
2. An incision is made through the infarcted left ventricular wall.
3. Infarcted left ventricular tissue is trimmed to viable myocardium (rarely is there fibrotic tissue between viable and nonviable muscle because there has been insufficient time for healing and scar formation).
4. The mitral apparatus is inspected. If there is a ruptured papillary muscle, valve replacement is performed through a conventional left atrial approach. This avoids tearing of friable myocardium that could occur with ventricular exposure of the valve.
5. Repair (Heitmiller, Jacobs, and Daggett, 1986):
   Anterior defects:
   The heart is elevated with cold laparotomy pads to expose the left anterior coronary artery.
   a. Small defects beneath anterior infarcts can be closed without a patch by approximating the septal margin of the defect to the right ventricular free wall. Horizontal mattress sutures with felt pledgets are all placed and then tied.
   b. Larger anterior defects (Fig. 12-28) require a patch to reduce tension on the suture line; tension can cause delayed rupture postoperatively.

   Interrupted felt pledgeted sutures are placed through the edge of the defect and then into the VSD patch. When all the sutures are placed, the patch is seated against the left ventricular side of the VSD, and an additional pledget is attached to each suture. The needles are cut, and all the stitches are tied.

   The ventriculotomy is closed by patching or by approximation of the edges with felt buttressed sutures.

   Apical defects:
   The principles of closing anterior VSDs are also applied to apical defects (Fig. 12-28).
   a. The apex is elevated with cold laparotomy pads.
   b. The infarcted left ventricular apex is incised, and necrotic myocardium is debrided.
   c. Closure of the remaining apical portion of the left and right ventricular free wall and the apical septum is accomplished with felt strips and pledgets sandwiched between these layers.
   d. Interrupted mattress sutures are placed through felt pledgets into the ventricular septum and the edge of the right ventricular anterior wall. The sutures are placed into the edges of a patch (Dacron, PTFE, autologous or bovine pericardium) that is placed against the septum and the right ventricular free wall. The needles are cut, and the stitches are tied. The ventriculotomy is closed with a woven patch that may be buttressed with a felt strip or pledgets.

   Inferoposterior septal defects:
   a. The surgeon may identify the margins of the infarct before clamping the aorta and note whether the infarct involves the diaphragmatic aspect of the left ventricle or both ventricles.
   b. The heart is arrested and retracted to expose the posterior descending coronary artery.
   c. The septal defect is exposed through a left ventricular infarctectomy. (The surgeon may stand on the patient's left side for better visualization of the defect.)
   d. The mitral valve is inspected and replaced if indicated.
   e. Infarcted left ventricular tissue is debrided. Right ventricular muscle is conservatively trimmed as necessary to identify the margins of the defect.

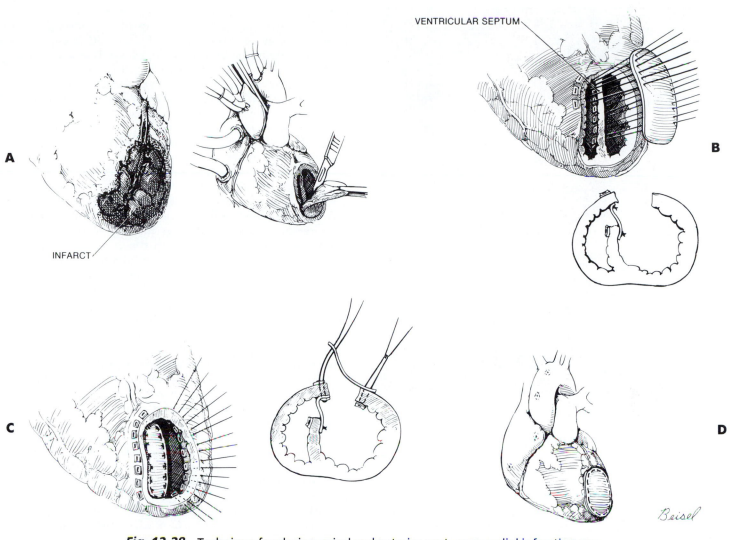

VENTRICULAR SEPTUM

INFARCT

Beisel

Fig. 12-28 Technique for closing apical and anterior post–myocardial infarction ventricular septal defects. **A,** The apex is incised, and necrotic tissue is excised. The mitral apparatus is then inspected, with special attention focused on the papillary muscles. **B,** Pledgeted mattress sutures are placed in the right ventricular septum and the right ventricular wall. The stitches are inserted into the edges of a patch that is placed against the left ventricular side of the septum and the endocardial side of the right ventricular free wall. **C,** The ventriculotomy is closed with another felt-buttressed patch. **D,** Completed repair. (From Walhausen JA, Pierce WS: *Johnson's surgery of the chest*, ed 5, St Louis, 1985, Mosby.)

f. If the defect is small, it may be closed by approximating the edge of the septum to the right ventricular free wall with mattress sutures buttressed with felt strips. Larger defects require a patch inserted with individually pledgeted mattress sutures. Additional free pledgets are attached to all sutures. The patch is seated against the septum, and the sutures are tied.

g. The ventricular wall is closed using another patch (to avoid excessive tension and subsequent hemorrhage from the suture line). The

epicardial technique, developed by Daggett (1982), is used. Pledgeted mattress sutures are inserted on the endocardial surface and brought out through the epicardial surface around the circumference of the ventriculotomy. In the region of the septal repair, the sutures are passed through the edge of the septal patch and exit on the epicardial surface of the right ventricle.

h. A woven Dacron patch is cut to overlap the perimeter of the ventriculotomy. The previously placed sutures (step g) are passed through the

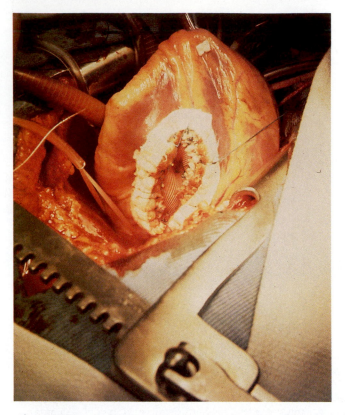

Fig. 12-29 Completed repair of a posterior ventricular septal defect. The ventricular free wall has been closed with an elliptic patch of low-porosity graft material and buttressed with a strip of felt. The left ventricular apex is elevated to expose the posterior wall. (Courtesy Edward A. Lefrak, MD.)

edges of the patch and then through individual pledgets. The patch and overlying pledgets are seated, and the stitches are tied (Fig. 12-29).

6. Coronary artery grafting to major coronary arteries with significant proximal lesions may be performed at this time.

7. Air is removed from the heart, and the cross-clamp is removed. The surgeon confirms that the shunt is closed.

COMPLETION OF PROCEDURES

After the surgical repair is completed and a stable rhythm resumes, the surgeon assesses the anastomoses and the bypass grafts, and other repairs for hemostasis. Small clips may be used on saphenous or internal mammary vein tributaries, or IMA branches. Occasionally a stitch may be required on the conduit or at the anastomosis for hemostasis. The proximal anastomoses can be marked with radiopaque rings or metal clips for future reference.

If a vein graft is too long, a number of options are available. Topical collagen hemostatic agents can be used to tack the graft to the heart; or a fine suture can be used to attach the adventitia of the vein to the

epicardium of the heart. Usually the graft is attached in at least two places so that it lies in a gentle curve rather than at an acute angle, which could cause occlusion of the graft. Another method is to resect excess tissue. This can be accomplished with a small curved partial-occlusion clamp placed over the graft and the excess tissue pulled into the jaws. While an assistant steadies the clamp, the surgeon excises the excess vein and reanastomoses the cut ends. Air is removed from the graft, and the clamp is removed. Usually this can be performed on a beating heart.

Temporary epicardial pacing wires are attached. If the patient is bradycardic, the pacing wires can be attached to a temporary external generator and the heart paced at 90 to 100 beats per minute. Maintaining an adequate blood pressure is especially critical for maintaining blood flow through the conduits. Transient hypotension due to decreased contractility may be treated with inotropic medications. Treatment for volume-related hypotension depends on the cause of the problem. Interventions include fluid replacement if volume is low, infusion of clotting factors to correct deficiencies, and/or repair of surgical bleeding sites.

The patient is weaned from cardiopulmonary bypass. Chest tubes are inserted into the pericardial cavity and into the pleural cavity that was opened during IMA dissection. Hemostasis is achieved, incisions are closed, and dressings are applied. The leg incision is dressed, and the leg is wrapped from ankle to thigh with an elastic pressure dressing (taking care not to apply excessive pressure). The perioperative nurse can assess the pedal pulse and the capillary refill of the toes to determine perfusion of the affected leg.

Before the patient is transferred to the bed for transport to the post–cardiac surgery intensive care unit (SICU), the patient's hemodynamic stability is reconfirmed, and chest tube drainage reassessed (from both mediastinal and pleural drainage tubes). Pleural tubes on the side of an IMA dissection should be evaluated for bleeding from the IMA pedicle. Early drainage of 200 to 400 ml/hr is almost always "surgical" and requires exploration (Waldhausen and Orringer, 1991). Because of the possibility of having to reopen the chest, instruments, back tables, and defibrillator paddles should be kept sterile until the patient has at least left the operating room.

After the patient has been transferred to the postoperative bed, hemodynamic stability is again reconfirmed. The patient's ECG and blood pressure are monitored during transport, and a portable defibrillator accompanies the patient.

POSTOPERATIVE CONSIDERATIONS AND COMPLICATIONS

The goals of postoperative care are to maintain hemodynamic stability and avoid complications (Table 12-4). For the patient who has undergone myocardial revascularization, major considerations (in addition to those outlined in Chapter 9) include monitoring the ECG for dysrhythmias and signs of ischemia or peri-

Table 12-4 ■ *Postoperative complications of myocardial revascularization*

Complication	Interventions
Bleeding	Monitor chest tube drainage, inspect wounds for bleeding Report excessive bleeding (greater than 200-400 ml/hr) Report sudden cessation of chest tube drainage Monitor laboratory values: PT, PTT, platelet count, H & H, DIC screen, ACT Administer blood, blood products, fluids as indicated Reinfuse shed blood with autotransfusion Infuse DDAVP as ordered Monitor VS and hemodynamics for hypotension, tachycardia, hypovolemia, tamponade Promote normothermia with warming blankets, warmed solutions If cardiac tamonade occurs, be prepared to open chest to evacuate hematoma and relieve compression, if heart has arrested, be prepared to perform open cardiac massage; anticipate return to OR (see Box 5-3 for emergency)
Respiratory complications	Monitor for fluid shifts and left ventricular dysfunction during transition from mechanical to spontaneous ventilation Evaluate gas exchange and respiratory parameters: respiratory rate, vital capacity, tidal volume Monitor skin color, ABGs, restlessness, decreased LOC Promote expansion of atelectasis by deep breathing and coughing, incentive spirometry, suctioning, mobilizing patient Monitor for phrenic nerve injury reducing strength of respiratory efforts Monitor for signs and symptoms of pneumothorax, pneumonia, hemothorax, mediastinal shift
Neurologic complications	Assess for signs and symptoms: peripheral neuropathy, stroke, coma Avoid air in intravascular lines Assess for postoperative delirium: agitation, disorientation, hallucinations, paranoia Initiate interventions to maintain mental stability and foster orientation to environment Use alternative communication techniques with intubated patients Relieve discomfort/agitation due to pain, hypoxia, full bladder, fear, anxiety

Cardiac complications
Myocardial failure
	Monitor peripheral pulses, foot and toe temperature, urinary output, arterial blood pressure, central venous pressure, pulmonary artery pressure, and thermodilution CO measurements
	Report MAP below 65 mm Hg, especially in presence of IMA graft
	Manipulate determinants of CO to optimize perfusion:
	    Increase preload—institute volume replacement
	    Decrease afterload—administer vasodilators
	    Augment contractility—administer inotropic drugs
	    Heart rate—institute cardiac pacing
	Augment ventricular function with mechanical assistance (IABP, LVAD)

Myocardial infarction	Assess ECG changes, significant increase in cardiac enzymes (creatine kinase MB fraction greater than 8%)
Dysrhythmia	Institute cardiac pacing for bradycardia, supraventricular dysrhythmias Administer antidysrhythmic drugs Monitor potassium levels Cardiovert ventricular tachycardia or fibrillation If cardiac arrest occurs, be prepared to open chest and perform internal chest massage; anticipate return to OR
Infection and wound disruption	Monitor temperature, report if above 38° C (100.4° F) Inspect incisions for evidence of swelling, redness, exudate, and tenderness Administer antibiotics as prescribed Wash hands often, and before and after contact with patient May require return to OR for sternal debridement Mediastinitis may require repair with pectoralis major muscle or omental flap
Renal complications	Assess urinary output, BUN, creatinine, and urine specific gravity Measure weight daily Assess CO, central venous pressure, electrolyte levels, acid-base balance Maintain adequate volume, reduce afterload Promote adequate renal blood flow (dopamine) and fluid management (diuretics)
Gastrointestinal complications	Assess NG tube drainage and stool, bowel sounds, gastric pH, signs of abdominal distension Assess for signs and symptoms of gastroduodenal ulcer, cholecystitis, pancreatitis, intestinal ischemia, perforation, or bleeding In patients with gastroepiploic grafts, anticipate increased pain, abdominal discomfort, prolonged ileus Administer vasopressors judiciously; avoid aspirin

Modified from Kinney MR, Craft MS: The person undergoing cardiac surgery. In Guzzetta CE, Dossey BM: *Cardiovascular nursing: holistic practice*, St Louis, 1992, Mosby; and Mahfood SS, Higgins TL, Loop FD: Management of complications related to coronary artery bypass surgery. In Waldhausen JA, Orringer MB: *Complications in cardiothoracic surgery*, St Louis, 1991, Mosby.

ABG, Arterial blood gasses; *ACT,* activated clotting time; *BUN,* blood urea nitrogen; *CO,* cardiac output; *DDAVP,* desmopressin acetate; *DIC,* disseminated intravascular coagulopathy; *ECG,* electrocardiogram; *H & H,* hemoglobin and hematocrit; *IABP,* intraaortic balloon pump; *IMA,* internal mammary artery; *LOC,* level of consciousness; *LVAD,* left ventricular assist device; *MAP,* mean arterial pressure; *MB,* myocardial band; *NG,* nasogastric tube; *OR,* operating room; *PT,* prothrombin time; *PTT,* partial thromboplastin time; *VS,* vital signs.

operative infarction; maintaining adequate blood pressure to ensure sufficient blood flow through vein grafts and especially the IMA; preventing bradycardia, which can decrease cardiac output and tissue perfusion; and monitoring for tamponade resulting from excessive bleeding into the pericardium without adequate drainage.

If the patient tamponades or has a cardiac arrest from some other cause, the sternum is opened in the SICU and manual cardiac compressions are performed. Chapter 5 lists supplies and other items that should be kept in the SICU in the event that emergency sternotomy is required. After being stabilized, the patient is transported back to the operating room for closure of the chest once the hemodynamic status is stable. For further information about postoperative care, the reader is referred to Guzzetta and Dossey (1992).

Long-term Outcome and Quality of Life

Several preoperative variables are important predictors of long-term outcome. These include the presence of congestive heart failure, extensive regional ventricular wall motion abnormalities (indicating poor left ventricular function), and associated medical diseases. In patients with three-vessel CAD, complete revascularization (defined as grafts to the three vessels involved and major branches) appears to be most beneficial to patients with severe angina and left ventricular dysfunction. Bypassing three or more vessels versus one or two vessels in these patients has been associated with improved survival and a reduced incidence of fatal MI, especially when bypass was performed to a diseased LAD coronary artery. After 5 years, patients also tended to be more likely to be asymptomatic or to have less severe recurring angina pectoris (Lytle and Casgrove, 1992).

The effect of increasing age on functional recovery and the quality of life after myocardial revascularization has received increased attention. Older patients undergoing elective CABG have reported functional benefits related to activities of daily living and social and emotional functioning similar to those reported by younger patients (Guadagnoli, Ayanian, and Cleary, 1992).

A number of studies comparing surgically treated patients with medically treated counterparts have demonstrated that although survival is similar, quality of life is improved in patients who have undergone surgery; they have greater relief of symptoms, fewer activity limitations, less requirement for medications, and improved functional capacity (Rogers and others, 1990). Subsets of older patients have shown similar results, confirming the efficacy of bypass in this patient population (Carey, 1992).

REOPERATION FOR CORONARY ARTERY DISEASE

As more patients undergo myocardial revascularization, an increasing number of these patients require a second or third operation for their disease because of the failure of vein grafts to stay patent. The most common cause of late graft failure is atherosclerotic changes in the saphenous vein grafts, producing stenosis and impaired myocardial blood flow.

In particular, late stenoses of 50% to 99% in saphenous vein grafts to the LAD coronary artery are associated with a significantly worse survival than that in patients having a similar degree of stenosis who have not had a graft to a native LAD (Lytle and others, 1992). This is thought to be related to the differences between native vessel lesions and graft lesions.

Native atherosclerotic lesions of the coronary arteries tend to be focal, eccentric, and proximal, with encapsulated plaques. In contrast, saphenous vein atherosclerotic lesions are more diffuse and concentric and do not have a fibrous cap; intimal debris from these lesions may embolize. Studies have demonstrated that venous tissue surpasses arterial tissue in its uptake of serum lipids (Fuchs, 1986). It is not surprising, then, that these friable and fragile lesions are more prone to embolization and should be manipulated with extreme caution during reoperation (Lytle and others, 1992).

Although the patency of IMA grafts is significantly greater than vein graft patency (Lytle and others, 1985), many patients undergoing reoperation do not have IMA grafts, because the initial surgery was performed at a time when IMA use was not widespread. In addition, vein grafts are needed to supplement the conduits needed for complete revascularization. Until more suitable conduits are available, saphenous vein grafts will continue to be used for bypass procedures.

When reoperation is indicated, previous chest wires are exposed and removed. In many institutions, the sternum is divided with an oscillating saw (see Chapter 11 for a discussion of repeat sternotomy). Care is taken to avoid lacerating previously placed IMA or saphenous vein grafts that may be lying under the sternum. At reoperation, when possible, the initial aortic cannulation site is used for aortic inflow. Venous return is achieved with a two-stage cannula in the right atrium.

Conduits

At reoperation, when one or both IMAs are available, they can be used as conduits as an alternative to the greater saphenous vein. The lesser saphenous vein or other conduits described previously (see Fig. 12-21) are used as necessary. The presence of a preexisting IMA graft may make exposure of the marginal arteries in the left lateral wall difficult. Also, an already-present IMA graft may require temporary occlusion with a small bulldog clamp so that blood flow through the IMA does not rewarm the heart and prevent cardioplegic arrest during the period of cross-clamping. Retroplegia may be used for achieving cardioplegic arrest (Owen and others, 1990).

Overall operative mortality for reoperation is 3% to 4% (Lytle and others, 1992) and is related to abnormal left ventricular function, advanced age, and hypertension (Lytle and others, 1987).

REFERENCES

American Heart Association: *1990 heart and stroke facts*, 1989, Dallas, The Association.

Ayanian JZ, Epstein AM: Differences in the use of procedures between women and men hospitalized for coronary heart disease, *N Engl J Med* 325(4):221, 1991.

Bickell NA and others: Referral patterns for coronary artery disease treatment: gender bias or good clinical judgment? *Ann Int Med* 116(10):791, 1992.

Buche M and others: Use of the inferior epigastric artery for coronary bypass, *J Thorac Cardiovasc Surg* 103(4):665, 1992.

Carey JS, Cukingnan RA, Singer LK: Quality of life after myocardial revascularization: effect of increasing age, *J Thorac Cardiovasc Surg* 103(1):108, 1992.

Carrel A: On the experimental surgery of the thoracic aorta and the heart, *Ann Surg* 52:83, 1910.

Cooley DA: *Techniques in cardiac surgery*, ed 2, Philadelphia, 1984, WB Saunders.

Cooley DA: Ventricular endoaneurysmorrhaphy: results of improved method of repair, *Tex Heart Inst J* 16(2):72, 1989.

Cooley DA and others: Surgical repair of ruptured intraventricular septum following acute myocardial infarction, *Surgery* 41:930, 1957.

Cosgrove DM, Loop FD, Sheldon WC: Results of myocardial revascularization (an 11 year experience), *Circulation* 65 (suppl 2):37, 1982.

Daggett WM: Surgical technique for early repair of posterior ventricular septal rupture, *J Thorac Cardiovasc Surg* 84:306, 1982.

Daggett WM. Personal communication, 1991.

Daggett WM and others: Surgery for post-myocardial infarct ventricular septal defect, *Ann Surg* 186:260, 1977.

Dotter CT, Rosch J, Judkins MP: Transluminal dilatation of atherosclerotic stenosis, *Surg Gynecol Obstet* 127:794, 1968.

Dougherty KG and others: Laser ablation of coronary arteries, *AORN J* 54(2):244, 1991.

Edmunds LH, Norwood WI, Low DW: *Atlas of cardiothoracic surgery*, Philadelphia, 1990, Lea & Febiger.

Favaloro RG.: Personal communication, 1991.

Fecteau DL: Nursing care in rupture of the interventricular septum following MI, *Cardiothorac Nurse* 4(2):1, 1986.

Fuchs JC: Pathologic changes occurring in venous autografts. In Sabiston DC, editor: *Textbook of surgery*, ed 13, Philadelphia, 1986, WB Saunders.

Gay WA: *Atlas of adult cardiac surgery*, New York, 1990, Churchill Livingstone.

Gazes PC: Angina pectoris: classification and diagnosis, part 1, *Mod Concepts Cardiovasc Dis* 57(4):19, 1988a.

Gazes PC: Angina pectoris: classification and diagnosis, part 2, *Mod Concepts Cardiovasc Dis* 57(5):25, 1988b.

Glick DB, Liddicoat JR, Karp RB: Alternative conduits for coronary artery bypass grafting: *Advances in cardiac surgery*, vol 2, St Louis, 1990, Mosby.

Good LP, Gentzler RD: Coronary atherectomy, *AORN* 53(1):32, 1991.

Gruentzig AR, Senning A, Siegenthaler WE: Non-operative dilatation of coronary artery stenosis—percutaneous transluminal coronary angioplasty, *N Engl J Med* 301:61, 1979.

Guadagnoli E, Ayanian JZ, Cleary PD: Comparison of patient-reported outcomes after elective coronary artery bypass grafting in patients aged ≥ and < 65 years, *Am J Cardiol* 70(1):60, 1992.

Guzzetta CE, Dossey BM: *Cardiovascular nursing: holistic practice*, St Louis, 1992, Mosby.

Heitmiller R, Jacobs ML, Daggett WM: Surgical management of postinfarction ventricular septal rupture, *Ann Thorac Surg* 41:683, 1986.

Hlatky MA and others: Resource use and cost of initial coronary revascularization: coronary angioplasty versus coronary bypass surgery, *Circulation* 82 (suppl 4):4-208, 1990.

Hochberg MS and others: Coronary angioplasty versus coronary bypass: three-year follow-up of a matched series of 250 patients, *J Thorac Cardiovasc Surg* 97(4):496, 1989.

Jatene AD: Left ventricular aneurysmectomy: resection or reconstruction, *J Thorac and Cardiovasc Surg* 89(3):321, 1985.

Jeffrey DL and others: Results of coronary bypass surgery in elderly women, *Ann Thorac Surg* 42:550, 1986.

Kent KM: Coronary angioplasty: a decade of experience, *N Engl J Med* 316(18):1148, 1987.

Kinney MR, Craft MS: The person undergoing cardiac surgery. In Guzzetta CE, Dossey BM: *Cardiovascular nursing: holistic practice*, St Louis, 1992, Mosby.

Kirklin JW and others: Guidelines and indications for coronary artery bypass graft surgery, *J Am Coll Cardiol* 17(3):543, 1991.

Komeda M, Fremes SE, David TE: Surgical repair of postinfarction ventricular septal defect, *Circulation* 82(5) (suppl 4):4-244, 1990.

Lytle BW, Cosgrove DM: Coronary artery bypass surgery, *Curr Probl Surg* 29(10):737; 1992.

Lytle BW and others: Multivessel coronary revascularization without saphenous vein: long-term results of bilateral internal mammary artery grafting, *Ann Thorac Surg* 36:540, 1983.

Lytle BW and others: Long-term (5 to 12 years) serial studies of internal mammary artery and saphenous vein coronary bypass grafts, *J Thorac Cardiovasc Surg* 89(2):248, 1985.

Lytle BW and others: Fifteen hundred coronary reoperations: results and determinants of early and late survival, *J Thorac Cardiovasc Surg* 93:847, 1987.

Lytle BW and others: Coronary artery bypass grafting with the right gastroepiploic artery, *J Thorac Cardiovasc Surg* 97(6):826, 1989.

Lytle BW and others: Vein graft disease: the clinical impact of stenoses in saphenous vein bypass grafts to coronary arteries, *J Thorac Cardiovasc Surg* 103(5):831, 1992.

Magilligan DJ, Ullyot DJ: The heart. I. Acquired diseases. In Way LW: *Current surgical diagnosis and treatment*, ed 9, Norwalk, Conn, 1991, Appleton & Lange.

Massie BM, Sokolow M: Heart and great vessels. In Schroeder SA and others, editors: *Current medical diagnosis and treatment 1991*, Norwalk, Conn, 1991, Appleton & Lange.

Milgalter E and others: The inferior epigastric arteries as coronary bypass conduits: size, preoperative duplex scan assessment of suitability, and early clinical experience, *J Thorac Cardiovasc Surg* 103(3):463, 1992.

Muller DW and others: Quantitative angiographic comparison of the immediate success of coronary angioplasty, coronary atherectomy and endoluminal stenting, *Am J Cardiol* 66:938, 1990.

Niemyski P, Hellstedt LF: Patient selection and management in thrombolytic therapy: nursing implications, *Crit Care Nurs Q* 12(2):8, 1989.

Owen EW and others: The third time coronary artery bypass graft: is the risk justified? *J Thorac Cardiovasc Surg* 100(1):31, 1990.

Pasternak PC, Braunwald E, Sobel BE: Acute myocardial infarction. In Braunwald E: *Heart disease*, ed 4, Philadelphia, 1992, WB Saunders.

Penckofer SM, Holm K: Women undergoing coronary artery bypass surgery: physiological and psychosocial perspectives, *Cardiovasc Nurs* 26(3):13, 1990.

Pfister AJ and others: Coronary artery bypass without cardiopulmonary bypass, *Ann Thorac Surg* 54:1085, 1992.

Prieto I, Basile F, Abdulnour E: Upper extremity vein graft for aortocoronary bypass, *Ann Thorac Surg* 37(3):218, 1984.

Quist WC, Haudenschild CC, LoGerfo FW: Qualitative microscopy of implanted vein grafts: effects of graft integrity on morphologic fate, *J Thorac Cardiovasc Surg* 103(4):671, 1992.

Rankin JS, Sabiston DC: The coronary circulation. In Sabiston DC, editor: *Textbook of surgery*, ed 14, Philadelphia, 1991, WB Saunders.

Roberts WC: Changes in venous autografts used as aortocoronary conduits. In Sabiston DC, editor: *Textbook of surgery*, ed 14, Philadelphia, 1991, WB Saunders.

Rogers WJ and others: Ten-year follow-up of quality of life in patients randomized to receive medical therapy or coronary artery bypass graft surgery: the Coronary Artery Surgery Study (CASS) registry, *Circulation* 82:1647, 1990.

Ross R: The pathogenesis of atherosclerosis. In Braunwald E: *Heart disease*, ed 4, Philadelphia, 1992, WB Saunders.

Sherry S: Bleeding complications in thrombolytic therapy, *Hosp Pract* 25(suppl 5):1, Nov 1990.

Society of Thoracic Surgeons: Practice guidelines in cardiothoracic surgery: ischemic heart disease, parts I-III, *Ann Thorac Surg* 53:930, 1992.

Steingart RM and others: Sex differences in the management of coronary artery disease, *N Engl J Med* 325(4):226, 1991.

Stoney WS and others: The fate of arm veins used for aorta-coronary bypass grafts, *J Thorac Cardiovasc Surg* 88(4):522, 1984.

Tector AJ, Schmahl TM, Canino VR: Expanding the use of the internal mammary artery to improve patency in coronary artery bypass grafting, *J Thorac Cardiovasc Surg* 91(1):9, 1986.

Vacek JL and others: Comparison of percutaneous transluminal coronary angioplasty versus coronary artery bypass grafting for multivessel coronary artery disease, *Am J Cardiol* 69:592, 1992.

Vlietstra RE, Holmes DR: Percutaneous transluminal coronary angioplasty, *J Cardiovasc Surg* 3:53, 1988.

Waldhausen JA, Orringer MB: *Complications in cardiothoracic surgery*, St Louis, 1991, Mosby.

Waldhausen JA, Pierce WS: *Johnson's surgery of the chest*, ed 5, St Louis, 1985, Mosby.

Wolff PR, Nugent M: Mechanisms of myocardial ischemia and infarction, *Anesthesiol Clin North Am* 6(3):461, 1988.

13

Mitral Valve Surgery

I anticipate that with the progress of cardiac surgery some of the severest cases of mitral stenosis will be relieved by slightly notching the mitral valve.

D.W. Samways, MD, 1898

A quarter of a century after Samways' prediction, Cutler and Levine (1923) performed the first effective operative procedure in the treatment of valvular heart disease with a closed mitral commissurotomy on an 11-year-old girl suffering severe mitral stenosis. Although this initial experience was successful, subsequent attempts by Cutler and others were failures, largely because of the mitral insufficiency created by resecting portions of the valve. The resulting controversy diminished enthusiasm for direct valvular surgery, which was not reintroduced until after World War II (Johnson, 1970; Lefrak and Starr, 1979). The next era of valvular surgery was stimulated by the efforts of Harken and others (1948) and Bailey (1949), who promoted greater understanding of the underlying pathophysiology and the importance of mobilizing the leaflets without creating mitral insufficiency during commissurotomy (Cosgrove and Stewart, 1989). The introduction of cardiopulmonary bypass and the development of biologically compatable prosthetic materials enabled further advances in technology and operative technique, which culminated in the first mitral valve replacement in 1960 by Starr (1961).

ATRIOVENTRICULAR VALVES

Heart valves enable efficient cardiac function by providing unimpeded forward blood flow and preventing backflow into the originating chamber. Unlike the more simple aortic and pulmonary semilunar valves, the atrioventricular mitral and tricuspid valves reflect a complex interplay between the valve leaflets, annulus fibrosis, chordae tendineae, papillary muscles, and the intraventricular wall (see Chapter 5). Structurally and functionally, the mitral valve (Fig. 13-1) is similar to the tricuspid valve, the atrioventricular valve found in the right side of the heart, except that the mitral valve is slightly smaller and is composed of two leaflets or cusps and the tricuspid valve is composed of three, as the names would imply.

MITRAL VALVE APPARATUS

The larger anterior (septal, or aortic) mitral leaflet is roughly triangular in shape, inserting into approximately one third of the annulus. It is in fibrous continuity with the aortic valve and forms one boundary of the left ventricular outflow tract. The posterior (mural, or ventricular) leaflet is narrower and has a scalloped appearance; it inserts into about two thirds of the annulus (Kirklin and Barratt-Boyes, 1993).

Valvular opening and closing is related to pressure changes between the atria and ventricles. Opening of the valve leaflets occurs during ventricular diastole after the left atrium has filled with blood and the pressure in the atrium exceeds the pressure in the left ventricle. The valve leaflets then are forced open. Near the completion of ventricular filling, the atrium contracts, providing an additional 20% to 30% to the left ventricular end-diastolic volume.

At the beginning of ventricular systole, the papillary muscles contract. As the inner ventricular pressure rises, these muscles and the attached chordac tendineae, which insert into the valve leaflets, prevent the leaflets from everting into the atrium. Each leaflet receives chordae from both the anterolateral and the posteromedial papillary muscles. The chordae, which tether the leaflets to the papillary muscles, are divided into three categories: primary chordae insert into the leaflet edges, secondary chordae insert into the leaflet undersurface, and tertiary chordae (arising from trabeculations within the posterior left ventricular wall) are prominent in the ventricular aspect of the posterior leaflet (Harlan, Starr, and Harwin, 1980). The free edges of the valve leaflets coapt firmly along their atrial surface, with the remainder of each leaflet bulging somewhat toward the atrium like a parachute. The annulus decreases in size and becomes more elliptic, thereby reducing the area the leaflets must cover. Abnormalities in any of these components (Table 13-1)

241

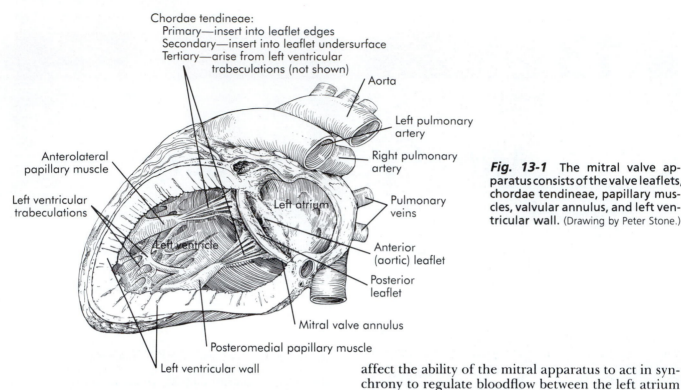

Chordae tendineae:
  Primary—insert into leaflet edges
  Secondary—insert into leaflet undersurface
  Tertiary—arise from left ventricular
    trabeculations (not shown)

Aorta

Left pulmonary artery

Right pulmonary artery

Anterolateral papillary muscle

Left ventricular trabeculations

Left atrium

Pulmonary veins

Left ventricle

Anterior (aortic) leaflet

Posterior leaflet

Mitral valve annulus

Posteromedial papillary muscle

Left ventricular wall

Fig. 13-1 The mitral valve apparatus consists of the valve leaflets, chordae tendineae, papillary muscles, valvular annulus, and left ventricular wall. (Drawing by Peter Stone.)

Table 13-1 ■ *Abnormalities of the mitral apparatus producing stenosis and regurgitation*

Stenosis	Regurgitation
Valve Leaflets	
Fibrosis	Retraction of cusps
Calcification (preventing leaflet opening)	Calcification (preventing leaflet closure)
Thickening	Perforation, tearing
Rigidity	Myxomatous degeneration
Commissural fusion	Congenital deformity (cleft leaflet)
Annulus	
Fibrosis	Dilatation
Calcification (impinging on orifice)	Calcification (preventing annular contraction)
Chordae Tendineae	
Shortened	Elongated
Fused	Ruptured
	Shortened
	Fused
Papillary Muscle	
Thickened	Ruptured (head or body)
	Dysfunctional (ischemic or infarcted)
	Congenitally malformed
Inner Ventricular Wall	
(Usually not a factor)	Dilated left ventricle
	Hypokinetic left ventricle
	Cardiomyopathy

Modified from Braunwald E: Valvular heart disease. In Braunwald E: *Heart disease*, ed 4, Philadelphia, 1992, WB Saunders.

affect the ability of the mitral apparatus to act in synchrony to regulate bloodflow between the left atrium and the left ventricle.

MITRAL VALVE DISEASE

Most often mitral valve disease is a disorder of the valve and not, as was first thought, primarily a disorder of the myocardium (Brieger, 1991). (An important exception is mitral valve incompetence due to ischemic coronary artery disease.) The two most common functional anomalies affecting the opening and closing motions of the valve are increased leaflet motion and restricted or diminished leaflet motion (Carpentier, 1983). Not infrequently, the two conditions coexist because the diminished leaflet opening (producing obstructed flow) is often accompanied by incomplete leaflet closing (resulting in regurgitation). Occasionally there is impaired blood flow even in the presence of normal leaflet motion, such as occurs with leaflet perforation or cleft mitral valve.

Impedance to flow from the left atrium to the left ventricle is caused by mitral **stenosis,** a narrowing of the valve orifice (normally 4 to 6 cm²). This process usually occurs gradually. Mitral valve **regurgitation** (or **incompetence,** or **insufficiency**) occurs when the valve leaflets do not coapt properly and thus are unable to prevent backflow into the left atrium during ventricular systole. This process may be gradual or may occur suddenly when the chordae or the papillary muscles supporting the valve leaflets rupture suddenly. Either of these conditions, stenosis or regurgitation, creates hemodynamic alterations that impose a progressively greater myocardial workload to maintain a sufficient cardiac output. The aim of surgery is to correct existing mechanical derangements in order to restore valve function as close to normal as possible (Carpentier, 1983).

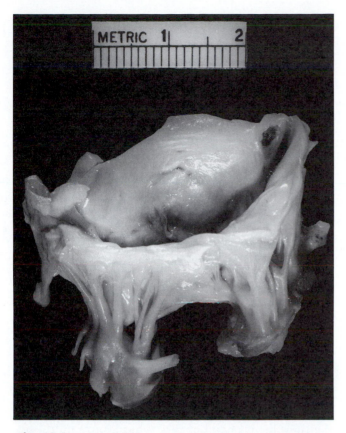

Fig. 13-2 Stenotic, rheumatic mitral valve. Note the typical, smooth thickened leaflets, the shortened and fused chordae tendineae arising from the tips of the papillary muscles. (Courtesy William C. Roberts, MD; Michael Spencer, photographer.)

Mitral valve disease in adulthood is often attributable to rheumatic fever in childhood, although it can also result from coronary artery disease, infection, degenerative changes, trauma, tumors, congenital anomalies, or failure of a previously implanted prosthesis. It is thought that the initial injury to the valve is further aggravated by the higher pressures in the left side of the heart and greater mechanical trauma to the valve, particularly when it is closed, as compared with the valves in the right side of the heart.

An awareness of the etiology is helpful to perioperative nurses because they can anticipate and prepare for adjunctive procedures and interventions. These may include culturing infected valve tissue, debriding calcified leaflets, repairing a septal defect created by excision of an atrial tumor causing stenosis or regurgitation, performing a valve replacement if it becomes apparent that valve repair cannot be achieved, or planning for concomitant coronary artery bypass grafting in patients with ischemic coronary heart disease.

Mitral Stenosis

Mitral stenosis occurs when deformities of the valve leaflets or other components of the apparatus produce narrowing of the mitral valve orifice and create an

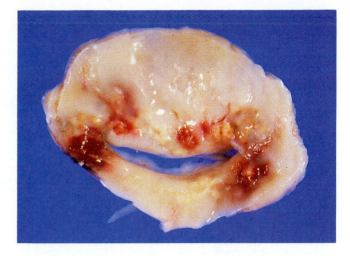

Fig. 13-3 Stenotic mitral valve demonstrating a "fish mouth" appearance. Note the calcium deposits in the area of the commissures. (Courtesy Edward A. Lefrak, MD.)

impedance to blood flow across the valve. These deformities produce turbulent blood flow, which can result in further injury to the valve itself (e.g., calcification) or promote the formation of thrombus. The most common causes of mitral stenosis include rheumatic fever, bacterial vegetations, and tumors.

Rheumatic fever

The most common etiologic factor of mitral stenosis remains rheumatic fever. Although it has become less common in the United States, new outbreaks continue to occur (Rahimtoola, 1989b). As one of the sequelae of beta-hemolytic streptococcal infection, rheumatic fever is a systemic immune process that can be self-limiting but may lead to progressive valvular deformity. Rheumatic fever may be associated with pericarditis and congestive heart failure; presenting signs include cardiomegaly and mitral or aortic murmurs.

The isolated mitral valve is affected in the majority of cases; aortic valve lesions are seen less commonly, and tricuspid valve involvement is usually seen only in association with mitral or aortic valve disease. The pulmonary valve is rarely affected (Stollerman, 1988).

When rheumatic carditis affects the mitral valve, the valve cusps become rigid and deformed, and this is often accompanied by varying amounts of calcium. The commissures fuse, and the chordae tendineae thicken and shorten (Fig. 13-2). The fixed stenotic orifice is often described as having a "fish mouth" appearance (Fig. 13-3). Mobilization of the valve leaflets by commissurotomy is often effective during the earlier stages of the rheumatic process when there is some leaflet pliability and heavy calcification is absent.

Over years or decades, the turbulence in blood flow produced by the fibrosis and calcification of the valve tissue causes further thickening of the leaflets and chordae tendineae. Leaflet motion is restricted, and the valve orifice narrows, in severe cases to less than

1 cm². Valve replacement is usually necessary at this stage, particularly when the valve is heavily calcified (Deloche and others, 1990).

Bacterial endocarditis

The infectious process of bacterial endocarditis attacks the valve leaflets and may extend to the perivalvular tissue (annulus, chordae tendineae, and papillary muscles). Often there are vegetations composed of bacterial colonies, fibrin, white blood cells, and red blood cells. When the destruction of the valve and adjacent tissue is severe, surgery is performed to remove infected tissue and to reconstruct the annulus so that a prosthetic valve can be securely anchored. Mitral insufficiency accompanies stenosis when endocarditis causes perforation of the leaflet(s).

Other causes

Left atrial thrombus or tumor, such as atrial myxoma, may obstruct left ventricular inflow. Degenerative processes may cause calcification of the leaflets and annulus.

Pathophysiology of Mitral Stenosis

The various physiologic derangements of mitral stenosis have similar clinical manifestations. The most significant effects are seen in the left atrium and the pulmonary vasculature. In severe cases the right ventricle may be affected (Fig. 13-4).

As the mitral and subvalvular orifices narrow, left atrial pressure increases to maintain normal flow across the valve, and a pressure gradient is created between the left atrium and ventricle throughout diastole. As increased left atrial pressure becomes sustained as a result of impedance to forward flow, the pulmonary vessels become congested, producing pulmonary edema. The patient may complain of dyspnea, especially when in the supine position or when the legs are elevated. Chronic pulmonary congestion leads to an increased volume and pressure load on the right side of the heart, which compensates by increasing the heart rate. The problem is exacerbated with exercise, which increases venous return to the right side of the heart in addition to the tachycardia, which shortens the time period for diastolic filling. This results in a reduced cardiac output and insufficient peripheral perfusion, which in turn produces fatigue.

With longstanding pulmonary venous hypertension, medial thickening and fibrosis of the pulmonary arterioles occurs, and pulmonary artery pressures are increased, often to systemic levels. Because the right side of the heart must now work against nearly systemic pressures, the right ventricle hypertrophies, then dilates, and eventually fails.

The majority of patients also develop transient or chronic atrial fibrillation as the left atrium dilates and hypertrophies in response to chronic atrial overloading. Because atrial fibrillation is not as effective as normal sinus rhythm in providing an adequate left

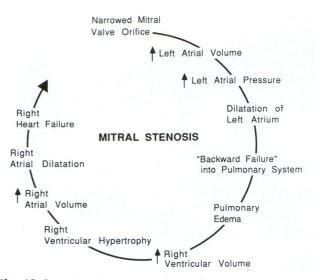

Fig. 13-4 Pathophysiology of mitral stenosis. (From Kinney MR and others: *Comprehensive cardiac care*, ed 7, St Louis, 1991, Mosby.)

ventricular preload, cardiac output will be reduced. Another problem associated with atrial fibrillation is venous stasis, which increases the risk of thrombus formation and embolization (Rankin, 1991).

Although pathologic changes in the left atrium and the right heart chambers are typical, pure mitral stenosis (unlike mitral regurgitation) does not stress the left ventricle itself. Thus the left ventricle is often normal in configuration and does not demonstrate hypertrophy or dilatation. Because left ventricular function has not been impaired by chronic hemodynamic stresses, patients who undergo surgery often show remarkable improvement with a significant decrease or disappearance of pulmonary hypertension (Spencer, 1989).

Mitral Regurgitation

When valvular regurgitation exists, the heart must eject the regurgitant fraction of blood, as well as its normal volume. Valvular and subvalvular abnormalities of the mitral apparatus (see Table 13-1) producing mitral regurgitation may have inflammatory, degenerative, infective, structural, or congenital causes (Braunwald, 1992).

Rheumatic fever remains a significant but less frequent etiology. More common are mitral valve prolapse, fibroelastic degeneration, infective endocarditis, dilatation of the annulus or the left ventricle, trauma, and coronary heart disease. Valve leaflets that are thickened, noncompliant, and retracted as a result of the inflammatory process of rheumatic carditis may fail to coapt. These valves commonly display symptoms of both stenosis and regurgitation.

Mitral valve prolapse

Mitral valve prolapse is an increasingly recognized clinical syndrome known by various names: Barlow's

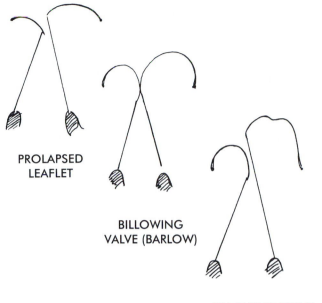

PROLAPSED
LEAFLET

BILLOWING
VALVE (BARLOW)

BILLOWING VALVE
+ PROLAPSED LEAFLET

Fig. 13-5 Surgical classification of prolapsed valve *(left),* billowing valve (Barlow's valve), and prolapsed billowing valve *(right).* (From Carpentier A: Cardiac valve surgery: the "French correction," *J Thorac Cardiovasc Surg* 86[3]:323, 1983).

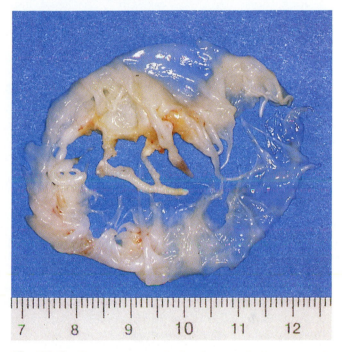

Box 13-1 *Terms associated with mitral valve prolapse*

Billowing mitral valve Ballooning or protruding of leaflet tissue into the left atrium; the valve edges coapt and regurgitation does not occur unless complicated by prolapse.
Floppy mitral valve Exaggerated billowing.
Prolapse of the mitral valve Billowing without leaflet coaptation; produces regurgitation.
Flail mitral valve Produced when chordae (or papillary muscle) rupture and the untethered leaflet is flung into the left atrium; produces acute regurgitation.

Data from Cosgrove and Stewart (1989), Carpentier (1983), and Barlow (1992).

Fig. 13-6 Myxomatous mitral valve producing regurgitation. The degenerative process causes the leaflets to become thinned out and elongated. (Courtesy Edward A. Lefrak, MD.)

syndrome, floppy valve syndrome, billowing mitral valve syndrome, and systolic click/murmur syndrome. It is common in women and in its milder form may not cause mitral regurgitation.

The multiple names given to the syndrome, the diverse etiologies, the nonspecific findings, and the lack of consistent definitions in the terminology occasionally create difficulty in describing the syndrome and planning treatment. For surgeons, for instance, the term "prolapse" (Fig. 13-5; Box 13-1) refers to valve leaflets that do not coapt and by definition are incompetent (Barlow, 1992; Carpentier, 1983; Cosgrove and Stewart, 1989; Shah, 1992). Barlow (1992) himself prefers the term "billowing mitral valve" to describe the condition bearing his name. "Billowing" or "floppy" valves are incompetent (dysfunctional) when they prolapse into the left atrium. Prolapsed leaflets require repair (or replacement) to regain functional valve performance.

Changes in the fibroelastic components of the valvular tissue, such as myxomatous proliferation (Fig. 13-6), produce thinning, elongation, and redundancy of valve leaflet tissue, which prolapses into the atrium during systole. Numerous mechanisms are thought to produce the syndrome, including hereditary disorders, thoracic deformities, coronary heart disease, and, most commonly, abnormal collagen metabolism and other connective tissue disorders that produce degenerative changes. Severe hemodynamic disturbances result from extensive calcification, elongation of the chordae, and asymmetric dilatation of the annulus (Anderson, 1987; Braunwald, 1992).

Other leaflet disorders

Valve leaflets may become perforated or chordae may rupture as a result of infective endocarditis or trauma and produce sudden regurgitation, requiring emergency surgery. Rarely, congenital clefts, organized thrombus, or tumors prevent secure leaflet closure. Previously implanted bioprostheses may degenerate, causing tears or perforations of the leaflets, producing regurgitation (Fig. 13-7).

Annular dilatation

The most common abnormality of the mitral valve annulus is primary dilatation of the annulus. Annular

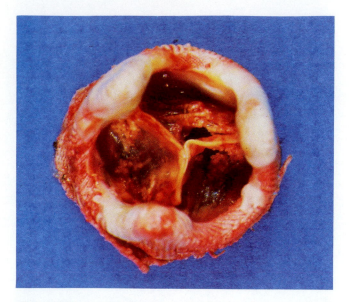

Fig. 13-7 Explanted porcine mitral valve prosthesis; note the tears and calcification of the leaflet tissue. (Courtesy Edward A. Lefrak, MD.)

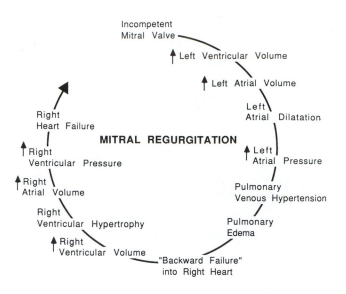

Fig. 13-8 Pathophysiology of mitral regurgitation. (From Kinney MR and others: *Comprehensive cardiac care*, ed 7, St Louis, 1991, Mosby.)

dilatation may also be produced secondary to the dilatation of the left ventricle surrounding the annulus, which normally constricts during left ventricular contraction. Severe idiopathic calcification of the annulus in the elderly may be a common cause of regurgitation and may be accelerated by systemic hypertension, aortic stenosis, diabetes, chronic renal failure, and fibrous skeletal disease (Braunwald, 1992).

Chordal dysfunction

Chordae tendineae affected by rheumatic disease restrict leaflet closure when they are shortened and fused. When attacked by bacterial endocarditis, they may rupture, resulting in sudden prolapse of the untethered leaflet. Chordal rupture may also result from trauma or acute ventricular dilatation.

Papillary muscle dysfunction

Papillary muscle dysfunction secondary to coronary artery disease is an increasingly common cause of mitral regurgitation. Papillary muscles are especially vulnerable to ischemia because of their terminal position in the coronary vascular bed. In severe cases papillary muscle necrosis and rupture create acute, severe regurgitation. Trauma to the muscles is a less common but important cause of regurgitation.

Left ventricular aneurysm and left ventricular dilatation occuring with increased volume loads or cardiomyopathy alter the ventricular geometry. Stretching of the chordae and the papillary muscles prevents leaflet coaptation.

Pathophysiology of Mitral Regurgitation

An incompetent valve is incapable of preventing the backflow of blood into the left atrium during ventric-

ular systole. Left atrial pressure rises from the additional regurgitant volume, and the left atrial chamber dilates and may then hypertrophy to overcome the additional volume (Fig. 13-8). Enlargement of the left atrium is not necessarily proportional to the degree of regurgitation, however, and only a slight increase in size may be seen in patients with significant disease, whereas a giant left atrium may be present in others with less severe disease (Spencer, 1989). Pulmonary vascular changes appear later in the course of the disease process as compared with the changes seen in mitral stenosis, depending on the ability of the atrium to dilate and adjust to gradual increases in volume over time (Hurst, 1990). When mitral regurgitation occurs suddenly (e.g., rupture of a papillary muscle), the heart is unable to compensate for the acutely increased volume load presented to it, and heart failure ensues rapidly. Acute regurgitation requires immediate surgical treatment.

When the ventricle contracts, more than 50% of its volume can be preferentially ejected into the left atrium, thereby significantly reducing the amount of blood entering the aorta (Carabello, 1988). As the amount of regurgitation increases and the volume overload becomes progressively greater, the left ventricle attempts to maintain an adequate cardiac output through the compensatory mechanisms of an increased heart rate, hypertrophy, and dilatation (Schakenbach, 1987).

DIAGNOSTIC EVALUATION OF MITRAL VALVE DISEASE

Chronic valvular stenosis and/or regurgitation develop gradually but are frequently first detectable by a murmur after about 10 years (Table 13-2). The electrocardiogram commonly shows abnormalities of the

Table 13-2 ■ *Signs, symptoms, and findings of mitral valve disease*

Mitral stenosis	Mitral regurgitation
Signs	
Atrial fibrillation	*Chronic*
Low-pitched, rumbling diastolic murmur	Atrial fibrillation
Opening snap (unless leaflets are immobile)	High-pitched, blowing systolic murmur
Hepatomegaly, ascites	Atrial pulsation at third left intercostal space
Jugular venous distension	Jugular venous distension
Peripheral edema	Hepatomegaly
	Point of maximal impulse downward and to left
	Acute
	Signs of infective endocarditis
	Sinus tachycardia
	High-pitched, blowing systolic murmur at apex
Symptoms	
Dyspnea	*Chronic*
Orthopnea	Fatigue, exhaustion
Paroxysmal nocturnal dyspnea	Palpitations
Hemoptysis	Atypical chest pain
Hoarseness	Dysphagia
	Acute
	Pulmonary edema
Chest X-Ray Film	
Large LA indenting esophagus	Enlarged LA and LV
Large RV and PA with pulmonary hypertension	
Calcification occasionally seen	
Echocardiography	
Restricted valve movement	Prolapsed, flail leaflet
Thickened, immobile annulus, leaflets	Enlarged LV
LA enlargement	Vegetations on leaflets
Subvalvular fibrosis	Regurgitant flow mapped (color Doppler)
Prolonged flow across valve	
Cardiac Catheterization	
Confirms valve lesion	Confirms valve lesion
Assesses LV function	Assesses degree of regurgitation, LV function, PA pressures
Detects coronary artery disease	Detects coronary artery disease
Measures valve orifice, pressure gradient	

Modified from Schakenbach LH: Physiologic dynamics of acquired valvular heart disease, *J Cardiovasc Nurs* 1(3):1, 1987.
LA, Left atrium; *LV*, left ventricle; *PA*, pulmonary artery; *RV*, right ventricle.

left atrium, including atrial fibrillation. The chest roentgenogram often demonstrates an enlarged left atrium and, in advanced states, pulmonary artery and right ventricular enlargement; occasionally calcium is seen on the mitral valve.

Preoperative diagnostic ultrasound methods with two-dimensional echocardiography, Doppler echocardiography, and color flow imaging provide detailed anatomic and functional information about the cardiac valves. Chest wall deformities or marked obesity may impede the penetration of ultrasound waves, necessitating cardiac catheterization and angiography. Transesophageal echocardiography (TEE) and Doppler color flow imaging are used widely during the intraoperative period to provide immediate structural and functional assessment of the valve after repair or replacement (Figs. 13-9 and 13-10).

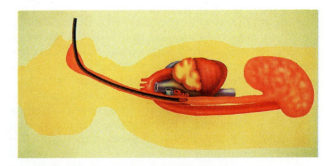

Fig. 13-9 Diagram of the transesophageal echocardiography (TEE) probe in position, demonstrating the orientation of the TEE probe, esophagus, heart, lungs, diaphragm, and stomach. The close proximity between the probe tip and the structures of the heart facilitates intraoperative assessment of cardiac function. (Courtesy Hewlett-Packard Co.)

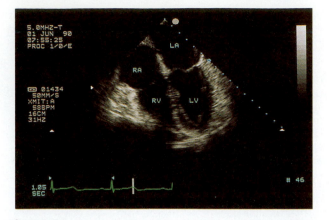

Fig. 13-10 Echocardiographic four-chamber view of the heart. In addition to evaluating ventricular and valvular function, TEE is also useful to detect air in the chambers and within the trabeculations of the ventricles. Air bubbles appear as tiny, light specks. (Courtesy Hewlett-Packard Co.)

In patients with concomitant coronary artery disease requiring myocardial revascularization, selective coronary arteriography remains the most accurate method for delineating the coronary arterial anatomy and the location of obstructive lesions. Coronary angiography also may be done to evaluate pulmonary hypertension, mitral insufficiency, aortic valve disease, and left ventricular function (Spencer, 1990). Computed tomography (CT) scanning and magnetic resonance imaging (MRI) are not yet standard diagnostic methods, but they are becoming increasingly useful for evaluating mitral valve disease.

SURGERY FOR MITRAL VALVE DISEASE

Surgical options, particularly for mitral regurgitation, have increased dramatically since the 1960s, when only commissurotomy and prosthetic replacement were technically feasible. Perioperative nurses, including RN-first assistants (RNFA's) (Box 13-2) can actively participate in the development and implementation of these procedures.

Carpentier and colleagues (1971, 1983; see also Box 13-3) are credited with many of the technical advancements associated with mitral valve repair and bioprosthetic replacement. Their description and categorization of the anatomic changes that occur with mitral (and tricuspid) insufficiency and the clinical application of their research findings have led to a number of improvements. These include the creation of the annuloplasty ring to correct annular dilatation (see Chapter 5) and the development of a wide array of procedures to repair not only the annulus, but also the leaflets, the chordae tendineae, and the papillary muscles. Carpentier and colleagues also introduced the glutaraldehyde-treated porcine heterograft in 1969, thereby expanding the number and type of valvular prostheses.

Box 13-2 *RN first assistant considerations during mitral valve surgery*

Keep sutures from tangling: use suture holder or tag with small clamps and arrange in orderly fashion around operative site, or tag and hold each stitch.

Keep running count of stitches in each leaflet (or annular segment), as well as a total count.

Be alert to calcium particles, thrombus, pieces of resected chordae, or other debris that could be retained and subsequently embolize; notify surgeon and remove from field.

Use open tip suction to remove calcium pieces and other debris; suction after each particle removed.

Keep bioprostheses moist with frequent saline irrigation (with bulb syringe); prevent drying out.

Monitor instruments and wipe clean of debris with moist sponge (sterile nurse may not be able to see).

Assist in keeping suture pledgets from twisting.

Hold prosthesis (annuloplasty ring or valve) securely with handle (or manually); do not twist prosthetic rings.

Avoid excess pressure on tissue when using hand-held retractor(s).

Avoid aggressive manipulation of rigid suction tip or venting catheter (may tear endocardial ventricular wall).

If heart must be elevated to inspect suture lines and anastomoses, do so cautiously to avoid puncturing ventricle with prosthetic struts.

Occasionally surgeons need to tilt their head over the field to see the operative site; avoid having prosthesis handle or other long instruments touch surgeon's head.

Avoid damage to prosthetic valves from instruments and other sharp objects.

At present, patients can benefit from a variety of possible interventions. Decisions regarding the timing and the selection of the procedure (repair or replacement) are determined on an individual basis and are influenced by the lesion and associated cardiac anatomy, the age of the patient, the past medical history, symptoms, and the patient's life-style (Weiland, 1983). Heavily calcified and deformed valves may not be amenable to repair; bulky valves may obstruct blood flow in a small ventricle. Ideally, a prosthetic valve should last the expected lifetime of the patient without degeneration or significant complications.

The past medical history provides information about the status of the left ventricle (functional class), previous surgery, thromboembolic episodes, atrial fibrillation, and disease processes (such as hepatic disease, gastric ulcers, and coagulopathies, which could contraindicate the use of valve prostheses requiring continuous anticoagulation). Aspects of the patient's life-style influencing the selection of a prosthesis include the ability and/or desire to comply with prescribed medication regimens. In addition, the prosthetic orifice should be large enough to accommodate

Box 13-3 *Comments on mitral valve repair: the "French correction"*

Alain Carpentier, MD
Hospital Broussais
Paris, France

Surgeons are not basically concerned with lesions. We care more about function. Therefore one may define the aim of a valve reconstruction as restoring normal function rather than normal valve anatomy.

There are only two functional anomalies [of valve motion]: The opening and closing motions of each leaflet are either increased as with *leaflet prolapse* or diminished as with *restricted leaflet motion*.

New surgical tools impose new surgical goals. It is not enough to save patients' lives; we must also take into consideration the quality of life given to the patient and the socioeconomic impact of our surgical actions.

Excerpted from Carpentier A: Cardiac valve surgery: the "French Correction," *J Thorac Cardiovasc Surg* 86(3):323, 1983.

a stroke volume commensurate with the activity level and size of the patient (Weiland, 1983).

Increasingly, patients are considered for surgery before symptoms become severe and permanent myocardial damage develops. Surgery for patients with symptomatic mitral insufficiency is often indicated earlier after the onset of symptoms as compared with that for patients with mitral stenosis because of the greater risk to left ventricular function seen in insufficiency (Cosgrove and Stewart, 1989). Surgery becomes necessary when left ventricular function deteriorates to a point that activities of daily living are curtailed.

Mitral Valve Repair

Reparative procedures that preserve the native valve are popular because the complications associated with prosthetic replacement and anticoagulation can be avoided. The availability of reparative techniques, their lower rate of complications as compared with valve replacement, and the improved results seen with preservation of the native valve have made mitral valve repair especially attractive in children. These advantages have also prompted surgical intervention for adults earlier in the course of their disease.

It may be premature to state unequivocally that repair is better than replacement, but there is increasing evidence that functional improvement and survival are greater with repair (David, 1990). Good results are also related to institutional factors such as familiarity with reparative techniques, appropriate patient selection, and an adequate case volume to maintain proficiency (Rahimtoola, 1989a). As repair techniques become more complex and widespread, however, new potential complications may arise (Grossi and others, 1992).

Procedures to reconstruct incompetent valves may not always be curative (Kirklin, Blackstone, Kirklin, 1988). Reoperation may be required in patients who have undergone initial commissurotomy at a younger age if commissural fusion recurs over time. Biologic or synthetic material used in the repair of the valve may degenerate, and patients should be informed of this possibility when their informed consent for surgery is granted. In addition, reparative procedures often require more time (and additional training) than a standard valve replacement. These considerations also necessitate excellent myocardial protection (MacNeil, Balasundaram, and Duran, 1991).

Patient teaching considerations

Patient teaching considerations focus on the patient's ability to adapt physiologically and psychologically. Including the family in the teaching process reinforces patient learning, enhances compliance with prescribed therapy postoperatively, and provides a supportive social structure. Patient teaching is directed at the disease, its etiology, anticipated treatment, associated complications, and information about the postoperative course. The patient should be aware of the possibility of valve replacement and be prepared accordingly.

The use of reparative techniques generally obviates the need for long-term anticoagulation (unless the patient has a history of chronic atrial fibrillation). This is significant in children, women of childbearing age, and patients with bleeding tendencies for whom anticoagulation poses an increased risk of hemorrhagic complications. Patients who do receive anticoagulant medications postoperatively need to be aware of reportable signs and symptoms of bleeding, such as pink urine, black stools, excessive nosebleeds, unusual vaginal or anal bleeding, purple or red skin discoloration, or bleeding gums (Canobbio, 1990).

Prevention of infective endocarditis is another important teaching area. Patients benefit from understanding the importance of antibiotic prophylaxis and the need to inform dentists and physicians about their history of valve disease and its treatment.

Procedural considerations

The terms **annuloplasty** and **valvuloplasty** are often used to categorize the type of repair. The former designates procedures performed on the valve annulus; valvuloplasty is a broad category that refers to reconstruction of the leaflets, chordae, and/or papillary muscles. Very selective repairs such as chordal transfer fall under this category.

Because the technique must be tailored to the unique pathophysiologic findings, a careful evaluation of the leaflets and the subvalvular mechanism is performed before the technique is selected. If damage to the valve is more extensive than anticipated, valve replacement may become necessary. Consequently, the nurse should be ready with instruments, prostheses, and related supplies to excise the valve and implant a mechanical or biologic prosthesis.

Box 13-4 *Mitral valve surgery: procedural considerations*

Instrumentation

Self-retaining mitral valve retractor with changeable blades

Hand-held mitral valve retractors

Small dental mirror (to assess subvalvular structures)

Mitral valve hook

Longer scissors, forceps, needle holders, and other instruments

Long, angled Babcock clamp to grasp valve leaflets for retraction

Valve Prostheses and Accessories

Annuloplasty rings

Mechanical heart valves

Bioprostheses (porcine)

Sizers (obturators), range of sizes, specific to prosthesis

Sizer (obturator) handles

Prosthetic valve holders and handles (some prostheses are packaged with an attached holder); sterile nurse applies handle into holder

Supplies

Valve suture, single and multipack (multicolored)
  Pledgeted
  Nonpledgeted

Suture organizer (if used)

French-eye needles (to adjust suture if needle has been removed)

Free pledgets, precut or cut to size

18- or 19-gauge needle to deair ventricle

Long (spinal) 18-gauge needle for transseptal deairing of ventricle

Additional basins for bioprosthetic saline rinse (three), antibiotic solutions, or glutaraldehyde preparation of autologous pericardium

Culture tubes (for valve tissue, suture, rinse solutions)

Venting lines for deairing left ventricle

Separate venous cannulas for inferior and superior venae cavae

Umbilical tapes and tourniquets (or caval clamps) to isolate cavae

ECG cables for cardioversion (patients with atrial fibrillation)

Positioning

Supine

If coronary bypass grafts to be performed, patient positioned as for removal of leg vein (see Chapter 12)

Skin Preparation

Midline of chest, inner aspect of both legs shaved

Legs washed at least to knees

Draping

Anterior chest exposed

Legs exposed from groin to knees (can be covered with a towel if access is not required)

Anesthesia screen placed over lower legs to keep drapes off feet

Special Infection Control Measures

Confine and contain tissue and instruments from infected tissue

Culture valve tissue, rinse solutions, and other items as requested by surgeon

Place mechanical prostheses in antibiotic solution prior to insertion as requested by surgeon

Keep instruments free of debris

Document lot and serial numbers of all implants

Special Safety Measures

Label syringes and containers of solutions, medications:
  Antibiotic solution
  Heparinized saline
  Glutaraldehyde

Account for all sizers, handles, and holders used to size and insert a prosthesis, as well as pledget material, suture needles, hypodermic needles, retractor parts

Monitor for presence of ventricular failure and possible need for mechanical ventricular support (intraaortic balloon pump or ventricular assist device)

Keep prostheses stored in a cool, dry, contamination-free location

Have at least two of each size valve available (may need to borrow from another hospital)

Follow institutional policy/procedure for complying with Safe Medical Devices Act

Documentation/Report to Cardiac Surgical Intensive Care Unit*

Procedure: repair or replacement, type of prosthesis

Serial and lot numbers of prostheses

Preoperative diagnosis (stenosis, regurgitation, or both; onset)

Epicardial pacemaker lead placement (single, dual) and if being paced

History of atrial fibrillation (chronic or recent onset)

Patient problems, concerns related to valvular heart disease, surgery

Preoperative left ventricular function (e.g., ejection fraction)

Completion of valve implant card (and card sent to manufacturer)

*In addition to standard documentation/postoperative report; see Chapter 9.

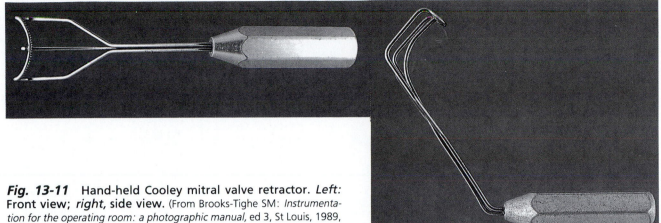

Fig. 13-11 Hand-held Cooley mitral valve retractor. *Left:* Front view; *right,* side view. (From Brooks-Tighe SM: *Instrumentation for the operating room: a photographic manual,* ed 3, St Louis, 1989, Mosby.)

In preparation for surgery, mitral valve instruments (Box 13-4) are added to the basic setup. Special retractors designed for exposure of the mitral valve may be used (Fig. 13-11; also see Chapter 5). Because the decision as to the most appropriate reparative technique is made only after careful inspection, nurses should have available (but not necessarily opened) a variety of sutures and prosthetic materials. Some surgeons may use autologous pericardium treated with glutaraldehyde solution to patch-repair leaflets. Discussing possible surgical options with the surgeon preoperatively guides the nurse and helps to avoid delay once a definitive repair is selected.

Patient care standards for mitral valve surgery (Table 13-3) include skin preparation on the supine patient from chin to knees. Access to the femoral artery should be retained in the event that arterial pressure monitoring lines or an intraaortic balloon pump

Table 13-3 ■ *Standards of nursing care for mitral valve surgery*

Nursing diagnosis	Patient outcome	Nursing actions
Anxiety related to disease, surgery, and postoperative events	Patient demonstrates acceptable level of anxiety and is able to cooperate with therapeutic regimen	Elicit questions and concerns about disease and proposed treatment Identify and reinforce effective coping mechanisms; respect some denial Provide comfort measures; identify perceived needs and expectations
Knowledge deficit related to inadequate knowledge of planned surgery and perioperative events	Patient demonstrates knowledge of physiologic and psychologic responses to mitral valve surgery	Determine patient's understanding of mitral valve disease; possible surgical interventions (annuloplasty, valvuloplasty, commissurotomy, valve replacement); types, benefits, and risks of prostheses; and preferences if any Determine patient's understanding of surgical procedure; describe (briefly) immediate preoperative events (while patient is awake); reinforce or clarify what patient (and family) has been told by surgeon; elicit expected outcome of surgery Assess patient's life-style (exercise limits, geographic location, proximity to laboratory facilities, community resources, support groups); note age and, if female, ability or desire to have children If additional myocardial revascularization procedures are to be performed (coronary artery bypass grafts), assess patient's understanding and clarify as necessary Assess patient's ability to comply with possible anticoagulation regimen Assess family support mechanism
High risk for infection related to surgery	Patient is free of infection related to aseptic technique	Culture excised valve and suture as requested Confine and contain instruments and supplies used to excise infected valve tissue Place mechanical prosthesis in antibiotic solution prior to implantation as requested by surgeon Keep instruments free of debris Document lot and serial numbers of implants

Modified from Seifert PC: Cardiac surgery. In Rothrock JC: *Perioperative nursing care planning,* St Louis, 1990, Mosby.

Continued.

Table 13-3 ■ *Standards of nursing care for mitral valve surgery—cont'd*

Nursing diagnosis	Patient outcome	Nursing actions
High risk for altered skin integrity	Patient's skin integrity is maintained	In severely thin and malnourished patients (cardiac cachexia), use additional padding to protect skin, joints, and bony prominences
High risk for injury related to use of valve retractor	Patient is free of injury from use of retraction devices	Use hand-held valve retractors with caution to avoid injury to perivalvular tissue (e.g., conduction tissue)
High risk for injury related to: Retained foreign objects	Patient is free of injury related to: Retained foreign objects	Account for valve sizers, holders, and handles, and other items Keep instruments free of tissue, suture, and calcium debris
Chemical hazards	Chemical hazards	Label syringes containing antibiotic solutions, heparinized saline, or other solutions; use only physiologically compatible solutions to rinse bioprosthetic valve; do not place bioprosthesis in antibiotic solution; follow protocol for removing glutaraldehyde from bioprostheses (rinsing in three baths of saline for at least 2 minutes each); keep bioprostheses moist with saline during implantation
Physical hazards	Physical hazards	Have available type and sizes of valvular prostheses desired by surgeon; store valves in cool, dry location; have appropriate accessories to size and insert valve; have necessary suture available (pledgeted, nonpledgeted, multicolored); be prepared with needles and venting catheters to deair left ventricle
Electrical hazards	Electrical hazards	Have appropriate ECG cables and confirm defibrillator setting with surgeon if cardioversion is planned for patients with atrial fibrillation
Thermal injury	Thermal injury	Avoid pouring ice chips directly on phrenic nerve (in lateral pericardium)
High risk for self-care deficit related to inadequate knowledge of rehabilitation period	Patient demonstrates knowledge of rehabilitation period as it relates to self-care abilities	Assess patient's knowledge of signs/symptoms of valve failure Assess patient's understanding of medications prescribed; signs/symptoms of anticoagulation-related hemorrhage, thrombosis, emboli; need for antibiotic prophylaxis prior to invasive procedures; need for follow-up laboratory work (prothrombin time). Identify signs/symptoms of anticoagulation-related hemorrhage (notify physician): Nosebleeds, bleeding gums Red or brown urine Red or black bowel movements Bleeding from cuts that cannot be stopped, bruises that get larger Severe and persistent headaches Abdominal pain Faintness, dizziness, or unusual weakness Excessive menstrual flow Identify signs/symptoms of suboptimal anticoagulation (notify physician): Stroke, transient ischemic attacks Closing sound of prosthesis no longer audible; absent "click" Sudden-onset congestive heart failure List precautions for patients on anticoagulants: Use a soft-bristled toothbrush Use electric shavers rather than razors Wear gloves when gardening Do not go barefoot Trim nails with a soft emery board instead of scissors or clippers Avoid sports in which skin may be broken or internal injuries may occur Provide patient with name of person to contact if questions/problems arise Wear medical alert bracelet

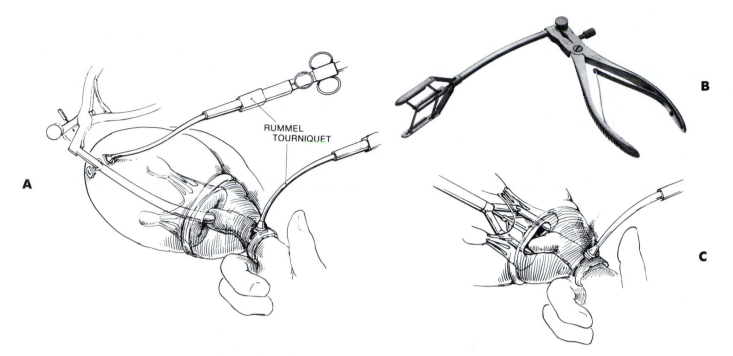

Fig. 13-12 Closed mitral commissurotomy. **A,** A tourniquet is applied to the atrial pursestring, and the surgeon's finger is inserted through the atriotomy. A Rummel tourniquet is applied over a heavy polyester suture, buttressed with felt pledgets, and placed near the left ventricular apex. **B,** A Tubbs dilator is inserted through the ventriculotomy and advanced into the mitral valve orifice. **C,** The dilator is opened by squeezing the handle; a tip guard can be adjusted to limit the opening of the dilator blades. (**A** and **C** from Waldhausen JA, Pierce WS: *Johnson's surgery of the chest,* ed 5, 1985, Mosby. **B** courtesy Baxter Healthcare Corp., V. Mueller Div.)

must be inserted or if a segment of saphenous vein is needed for revascularization.

Patients receiving oral warfarin anticoagulation medications (Coumadin) preoperatively will have them discontinued. Patients then are often switched to heparin prior to surgery because heparin can be given intravenously, acts more rapidly, and has a shorter half-life than warfarin (Christopherson and Froelicher, 1990). Heparin is the anticoagulant of choice during cardiopulmonary bypass because it can be reversed quickly with its antagonist, protamine sulfate.

Operative procedure: mitral commissurotomy for mitral stenosis

Closed mitral commissurotomy was the first effective surgical technique in treating valvular heart disease. The operation is now less commonly performed because of the drawbacks associated with the procedure, primarily lack of direct visualization and inadequate access to all cardiac structures. For example, in patients with severe mitral valve disease, the tricuspid valve may be affected. Adequate repair of the tricuspid valve is difficult with a closed mitral commissurotomy (Spencer, 1989).

Although there are disadvantages to the closed technique, it is of value in less technologically advanced countries where open procedures may not be feasible. Closed commissurotomy generally is performed with a Tubbs dilator, which mechanically dilates the commissures and enlarges the valve orifice (Fig. 13-12).

Open mitral commissurotomy, first performed in 1956 by Lillehei (1958), is the separation of fused, adherent leaflets (Fig. 13-13) under direct vision. It is effective in patients without serious mitral regurgitation, left atrial thrombis, calcification, or severe chordal fusion and shortening. Operative results are best if the procedure is performed before the onset of chronic atrial fibrillation or heart failure (Braunwald, 1992). The operative risk is usually less than 1% (Spencer, 1990).

Procedural considerations. The patient is placed in a supine position for a median sternotomy. TEE (with color flow Doppler) may be performed to establish a baseline for later comparison. A left or right thoracotomy approach may be used, but there are disadvantages related to exposure of the mediastinal structures, ease of cannulation, venting of air, and incisional pain (Starr, Grunkemeier, Fessler, 1988). Mitral valve instruments are added to the basic sternotomy setup and should include instruments and supplies not only for valve repair, but also for valve replacement should this be necessary (see Box 13-4).

Procedure

1. A median sternotomy is performed. The surgeon

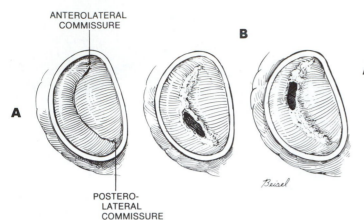

ANTEROLATERAL
COMMISSURE

B

A

POSTERO-
LATERAL
COMMISSURE

Beisel

Fig. 13-13 **A,** Normal mitral valve. **B,** Stenotic mitral valve with thickened, fused, and calcified leaflets. The orifice is narrowed and irregular. (From Waldhausen JA, Pierce WS: *Johnson's surgery of the chest,* ed 5, St Louis, 1985, Mosby.)

may place a finger through the right atriotomy prior to cannulation for bypass to determine whether functional tricuspid valve insufficiency is present.

Double venous cannulation is performed to reduce the amount of venous return to the right atrium and to enhance exposure of the left atrium. Antegrade and/or retrograde cardioplegia catheters are inserted. Cardiopulmonary bypass is instituted, and the heart is arrested.

2. The left atrium is incised, and a self-retaining or hand-held retractor is inserted. A wet laparotomy pad may be placed under the left ventricular apex to facilitate exposure of the valve.

3. The valve is grasped with forceps and inspected. Retraction sutures may be placed.

4A. The fused leaflets are separated at the commissures with scissors and/or a knife, and a long clamp such as a tonsil (Fig. 13-14). The mitral valve dilator (see Fig. 13-12, *B*) may be used to spread apart the leaflets and to measure the orifice.

4B. Chordal splitting: Obstruction in the subvalvular apparatus must be relieved as well. To improve flow in the presence of fused chordae, the chordae inserting into the leaflets may be divided at the commissural level, with the longitudinal incision extending to the head of the papillary muscles (Antunes, 1989). Rewarming is started.

5. The valve is tested for competency. Fluid is injected through the orifice into the left ventricle with a bulb syringe, and the presence of residual insufficiency is noted. If there is an unacceptable amount of regurgitation, annular plication may be performed.

6. The left atrium is closed with a continuous cardiovascular suture technique. Usually two sutures are used; one suture is started at one end of the atrial incision, and the second suture is started at the other end. The sutures are tied where they join.

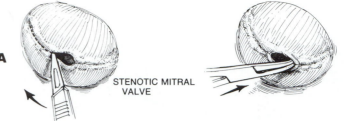

A

STENOTIC MITRAL
VALVE

B

Fig. 13-14 Open mitral commissurostomy. **A,** A knife is used to incise the fused commissures. **B,** The commissurotomy is extended with a tonsil clamp. (From Waldhausen JA, Pierce WS: *Johnson's surgery of the chest,* ed 5, St Louis, 1985, Mosby.)

7. The heart returns to a regular rhythm spontaneously or with defibrillation, and the patient is weaned from cardiopulmonary bypass. TEE is used to evaluate residual insufficiency and to confirm the effectiveness of the valve repair.

Operative procedure: mitral annuloplasty for mitral regurgitation

Mitral annuloplasty is the reduction in size of a dilated annulus through the use of a suturing technique or, more commonly, through application of a prosthetic ring. Placement of the annuloplasty ring is performed to correct dilation of the mitral annulus, to increase leaflet coaptation by reforming the deformed annulus, to reinforce the annular sutures when part of the valve leaflet has been resected; and to prevent further dilatation of the annulus (Chachques and others, 1990).

Procedural considerations. Annuloplasty rings may be semirigid (Carpentier, 1983) or flexible (Duran, 1980). Proponents of the preshaped, rigid ring (Fig. 13-10) stress the importance of restoring the shape, as well as the size of the dilated orifice. Flexible rings (see Chapter 5) offer the advantage of not compromising the ability of the annulus to change size and shape throughout the cardiac cycle. Both types of rings reduce the annular circumference by gathering excess posterior leaflet tissue and redistributing it toward the larger anterior leaflet to produce a competent valve. The size of the ring is determined by measuring the anterior leaflet with special sizing obturators. Carpentier (even-numbered) ring sizers have angled metal holders (see Chapter 5) that fit firmly into a slot in the middle of the sizer. Duran (odd-numbered) ring sizers do not have their own holder and must be grasped through a central opening with a tonsil or Kelly clamp from the nurse's basic instrument set. The side of the obturator displaying the letter "M" (mitral) should be facing the operator (the reverse side with "T" is used for tricuspid sizing).

Carpentier ring sizes of 28, 30, and 32 mm are appropriate for most female patients, and sizes 30, 32, and 34 mm are common for male patients. Duran ring sizes are similar except that the obturators and rings come in odd-numbered sizes (e.g., 27, 29, and 31 mm, and 29, 31, and 33 mm, respectively).

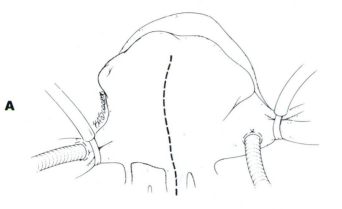

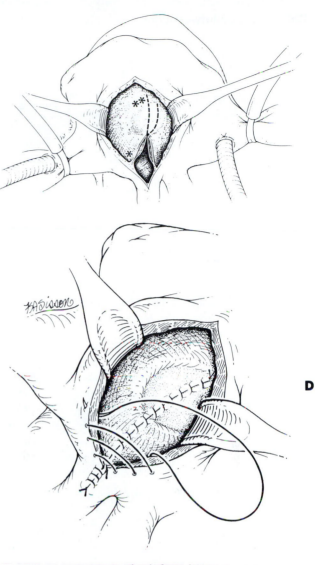

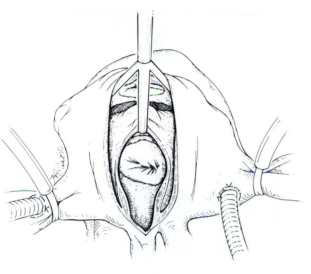

Fig. 13-15 Oblique right atriotomy and right septotomy to expose the left atrium. **A,** An oblique incision is made through the right atrium. **B,** The atrial septum is divided from the junction of the pulmonary vein *(asterisk)* and the muscular septum through the fossa ovalis. The incision is never made caudal to the limbus *(double asterisk)* or the fossa ovalis, so that injury to the coronary sinus and conduction system can be avoided. **C,** A self-retaining retractor beneath the septum exposes the mitral valve and retracts the tricuspid valve anteriorly. **D,** The septum is closed with one suture. The pulmonary vein and right atriotomy are closed with separate sutures. (From Hartz RS and others: Oblique transseptal left atriotomy for optimal mitral exposure, *J Thorac Cardiovasc Surg* 103[2]:282, 1992.)

Prostheses may be hand-held (Carpentier) or attached to a holder with a handle (Duran) for insertion of the stitches. The flexibility of the Duran ring requires that it be grasped firmly (even though it is attached to the ring holder) during insertion of stitches into the prosthesis. The method of insertion is similar for both kinds of rings.

Children are generally poor candidates for ring annuloplasty because of the risk of evolving valvular stenosis as growth occurs. Suture techniques have been successfully used in younger age groups and in women wishing to become pregnant (Reed, Pooley, and Maggio, 1980). Experimental work on an absorbable (biodegradable) prosthetic ring made from polydioxanone may help obviate problems with secondary stenosis and enable surgeons to perform annuloplasty techniques in younger patients (Chachques and others, 1990).

A median sternotomy approach is generally preferred, although a right or left thoracotomy can be used in special cases. Patients with chronic mitral insufficiency often have large atria, facilitating exposure of the mitral apparatus. When insufficiency is of acute onset, the atrium has not had time to dilate, and exposure may be difficult. This may also be a problem in the presence of dense adhesions from previous surgery, calcification, thrombosis, or chest deformities. In these situations, exposure can be enhanced by incising the right atrium and the atrial septum to expose the mitral valve as first described by Dubost and others (1966) and later modified by Hartz and others (1992) and Smith (1992) (Fig. 13-15).

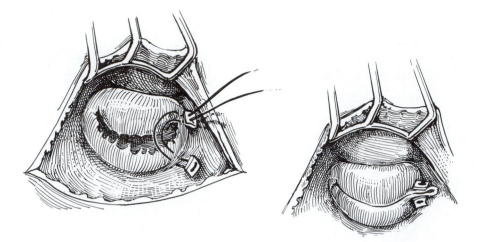

Fig. 13-16 Mitral annuloplasty by commissural plication with pledgeted suture. (From Waldhausen JA, Pierce WS: *Johnson's surgery of the chest,* ed 5, St Louis, 1985, Mosby.)

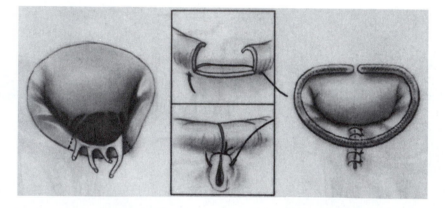

Fig. 13-17 Repair of mural leaflet prolapse by rectangular resection; the corresponding annulus is plicated, and an annuloplasty ring is inserted to remodel the annulus. (From Carpentier A: Cardiac valve surgery: the "French correction," *J Thorac Cardiovasc Surg* 86:[3]323, 1983.)

Procedure

1. A median sternotomy is performed, cardiopulmonary bypass with double venous cannulation is instituted, and the heart is arrested. Right or left thoracotomy may be performed for patients undergoing reoperation.

2. The left atrium is incised from the superior vena cava to the inferior vena cava posterior and parallel to the interatrial groove. In small left atria, right atriotomy and right septotomy may be required for adequate exposure (Fig. 13-15).

   Cardiotomy suction tips are inserted into the atrium. Special hand-held or self-retaining atrial retractors may be inserted to expose the valve. Additional exposure may be provided by placing cold laparotomy tapes under the left ventricle anteriorly, laterally, and inferiorly (Oury and others, 1986).

3. The valve annulus, leaflets, and related structures are identified and inspected. Annular dilatation is evaluated.

4A. **Plication:** Segmental disease of the posterior leaflet can be repaired with the use of a nonabsorbable mattress suture to plicate the commissure adjacent to the leaflet. The suture is buttressed with a felt pledget (Fig. 13-16). An alternative is to plicate both commissures (Reed and others, 1980).

4B. **Suture technique:** A suture technique may be used: a double-armed suture is placed around most of the circumference of the annulus and tied, thereby pursestringing the annulus to the desired size. The technique is more commonly used for tricuspid valve insufficiency and is described in more comprehensive detail in Chapter 15.

4C. **Resection and plication:** Redundant posterior leaflet tissue may be resected and the cut edges sewn together; the corresponding annular segment is plicated. An annuloplasty ring is inserted to reinforce the repair and correct the annular dilatation (Fig. 13-17).

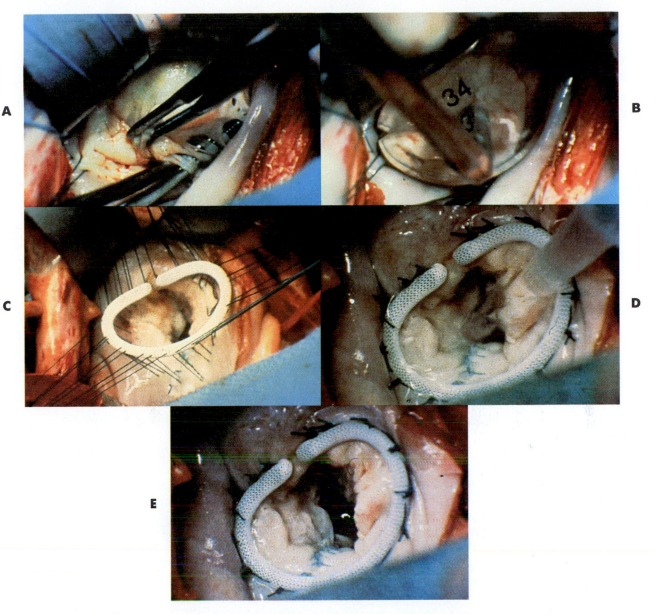

Fig. 13-18 Annuloplasty ring. **A,** The valve and subannular structures are assessed. **B,** The sizing obturator is used to measure the anterior leaflet. **C,** Interrupted sutures are placed in the annulus and the prosthetic sewing ring. **D,** Completed repair. **E,** A bulb syringe is used to test the competency of the valve. (Courtesy Baxter Healthcare Corp., Edwards CVS Div., Santa Ana, Calif.)

4D. **Ring annuloplasty:** Annular dilatation of the posterior (mural) leaflet is most commonly seen; annuloplasty with a semirigid or flexible ring is performed. A sizing obturator is used to measure the area of the anterior leaflet (Fig. 13-18, *A* and *B*), and the comparable annuloplasty ring is delivered to the field.

5. In the Carpentier (1983) technique interrupted sutures are placed around the circumference of the annulus and then into the ring (Fig. 13-18, *C*). Because the anterior leaflet is less dilated than the posterior leaflet, spacing of the sutures is done so that when the stitches are tied, the excessive posterior leaflet tissue is evenly drawn up against the prosthesis and the anterior leaflet retains its original shape and size (Fig. 13-18, *D*).

6. Competency of the repair is tested as described in step 5 of the operative procedure for mitral commissurotomy (Fig. 13-18, *E*).

7. The Duran annuloplasty techniue is similar (Fig. 13-19).

8. The left atrial appendage may be excised and oversewn (or stapled) to reduce the risk of thrombus formation and subsequent embolization.

Fig. 13-19 Duran annuloplasty technique with a flexible ring. (Courtesy Medtronic, Inc., Minneapolis, Minn.)

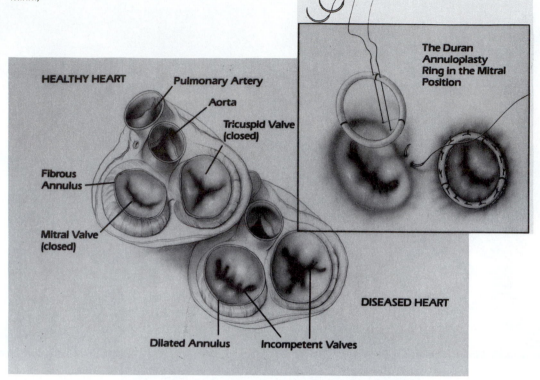

9. The atrial incision is partially closed (and the lungs are inflated) to allow air to exit the left ventricle. The heart is allowed to resume beating. TEE may be used before and after the discontinuation of cardiopulmonary bypass to evaluate ventricular function and valve performance.

Operative procedure: mitral valvuloplasty for mitral regurgitation

Procedural considerations. Valvuloplasty represents an array of techniques to repair the valve leaflets and related structures. Not infrequently, there are abnormalities in one or more components of the apparatus, such as a dilated annulus with elongated chordae.

Procedure

1. After the left atrium is opened and the valve exposed, a thorough evaluation of the valvular and subvalvular structures is made.

2A. **Patch repair:** Perforations of the anterior or posterior leaflets may be patched with autologous pericardium (Fig. 13-20) that has been treated by immersion in glutaraldehyde solution (available from pharmaceutical companies). Resection of the torn portion of the leaflet and annular plication with annuloplasty (see Fig. 13-17) may be used to repair the posterior leaflet. This technique is not generally used for the anterior leaflet, which does not tolerate much loss of its free edge (Antunes, 1989).

2B. **Debridement:** Leaflets with discrete areas of

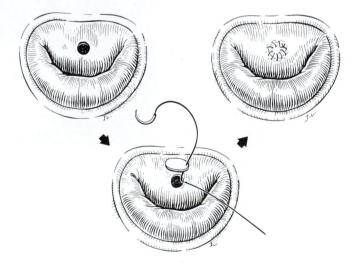

Fig. 13-20 Perforations of the leaflet may be patched with autologous pericardium. (From Cosgrove DM, Stewart WJ: Mitral valvuloplasty, *Curr Prob Cardiol* 14[7]:353, 1989.)

calcification may be debrided. If the calcium extends through the leaflet, the remaining defect in the leaflet after excision of the calcium may be patched with pericardium (Fig. 13-20) as described in step 2A. In some situations extensive calcification can be removed by debridement (Fig. 13-21).

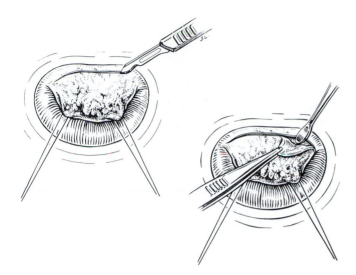

Fig. 13-21 Extensive fibrosis and calcification removed by debridement. (From Cosgrove DM, Stewart WJ: Mitral valvuloplasty, *Curr Probl Cardiol* 14[7]:353, 1989.)

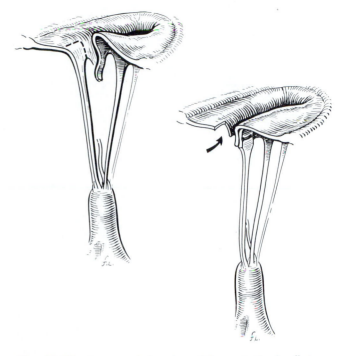

Fig. 13-23 Ruptured chordae of the anterior leaflet are corrected by chordal transfer from the posterior to the anterior leaflet and repair of the posterior leaflet. (From Cosgrove DM, Stewart WJ: Mitral valvuloplasty, *Curr Probl Cardiol* 14[7]:353, 1989.)

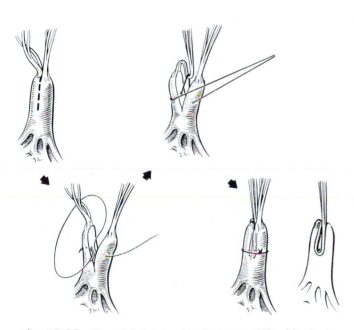

Fig. 13-22 Chordal shortening is accomplished by incising the papillary muscle and burying the chordae in it. (From Cosgrove DM, Stewart WJ: Mitral valvuloplasty, *Curr Prob Cardiol* 14[7]:353, 1989.)

2C. **Mobilization:** Shortened, fused chordae tendineae can be mobilized and lengthened by their division into secondary chordae or by incising the tip of the papillary muscle.

2D. **Chordal shortening:** Redundant tissue of elongated chordae may be implanted into the incised papillary muscle head (Fig. 13-22) or folded over itself and secured with a suture.

2E. **Chordal transfer:** Ruptured chordae of the anterior leaflet may be corrected by transfer of chordae from a portion of the posterior leaflet to the unsupported segment of the anterior leaflet (Fig. 13-23). The transferred chordae are sutured to the free edge of the anterior leaflet. An alternative method is to transfer a healthy secondary chorda to the free edge of the anterior leaflet, and have the transferred chorda thereby take on the function of a primary chorda (Cosgrove and Stewart, 1989).

2F. **Papillary muscle repair:** One head of a ruptured papillary muscle can be sutured to an immediately adjacent papillary muscle (Fig. 13-24).

Mitral Valve Replacement

Mitral valve replacement is the excision of one or both mitral valve leaflets, as well as supporting chordae and papillary muscle tips, and replacement with a mechanical or biologic prosthesis. There is increasing evidence that preserving the posterior (mural) leaflet and associated chordae minimizes impaired postoperative left ventricular function by maintaining the normal geometry and mechanics of the left ventricle (David, 1990).

Replacement is indicated for patients in whom extensive valvular damage precludes repair. Patients may be moderately or severely symptomatic (func-

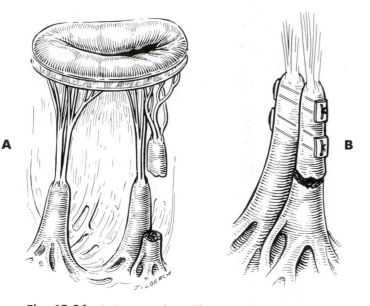

Fig. 13-24 **A,** Ruptured papillary muscle sutured to, **B,** adjacent papillary muscle with pledgeted sutures. (From Cosgrove DM, Stewart WJ: Mitral valvuloplasty, *Curr Probl Cardiol* 14[7]:353, 1989.)

Box 13-5 *Patient-related factors and risks associated with mitral valve surgery*

Left ventricular function (e.g., functional class, coronary artery disease, congestive heart failure)
Age
Sex
Residence
Preoperative endocarditis
History of atrial fibrillation
Connective tissue disorders (e.g., Marfan's syndrome)
Congenital anomalies (e.g., cleft mitral valve)
Enlarged left atrium
Left atrial thrombus
History of transient ischemic attacks
Anticoagulation compliance
Preexisting health problems (e.g., diabetes mellitus, pulmonary or systemic hypertension, hepatic or renal disease)
Valve lesion
Previous cardiac surgery

Modified from Mitchell RS and others: Significant patient-related determinants of prosthetic valve performance, *J Thorac Cardiovasc Surg* 91:807, 1986.

---

tional class 3 or 4). Impaired ventricular function may be documented by diagnostic evaluation with echocardiography, ventriculography, or nuclear studies.

Patient teaching considerations

In addition to patient-related factors (Box 13-5), prosthetic valve–related factors (Box 13-6) must be con-

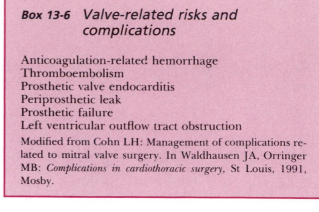

Box 13-6 *Valve-related risks and complications*

Anticoagulation-related hemorrhage
Thromboembolism
Prosthetic valve endocarditis
Periprosthetic leak
Prosthetic failure
Left ventricular outflow tract obstruction

Modified from Cohn LH: Management of complications related to mitral valve surgery. In Waldhausen JA, Orringer MB: *Complications in cardiothoracic surgery*, St Louis, 1991, Mosby.

---

sidered when replacement is performed. This includes not only anticoagulation-related hemorrhage and endocarditis, but also other complications related to prosthetic performance (Finkelmeier, Hartz, and Michaelis, 1989).

Signs of prosthetic failure vary according to the prosthesis inserted. A thrombosed disk valve will no longer be audible if the opening and closing mechanism is impaired. A perforated bioprosthetic leaflet (Fig. 13-6) may produce sudden regurgitation, as can a valve that has a dehisced sewing ring. Periprosthetic leaks resulting from detachment of part of the sewing ring from the annulus are suggested by the presence of new murmurs, varying degrees of regurgitation, and signs of hemolysis secondary to blood trauma from being squeezed between the prosthesis and the annulus.

Thromboembolism is a risk with all prostheses, but there is a higher incidence in patients with mechanical valves whose bleeding times are not sufficiently prolonged with anticoagulants. The risk increases significantly in patients with a history of chronic atrial fibrillation. Warfarin therapy is used to maintain the prothrombin time (PT) to at least 1.5 times normal. Regular laboratory follow-up of PTs is necessary to adjust and maintain warfarin levels in a range that causes neither excessive bleeding nor increased risk of thrombus formation.

Plans for patient teaching during the perioperative, recuperative, and rehabilitative periods will incorporate information related to risks and complications, as well as diet, life-style, and habitat (Whitman and Guzzetta, 1992).

The decision as to which prosthesis to use should be a joint effort between the surgeon, the cardiologist, and the patient. The perioperative nurse can assist the patient by clarifying the reasons for the selection of a particular prosthesis and providing information about the possible effects such a choice will have on the patient's future life-style.

Procedural considerations

Choice of a prosthesis. Since the introduction of a prosthetic valve in the 1960s, many prostheses have been developed with a variety of configurations and

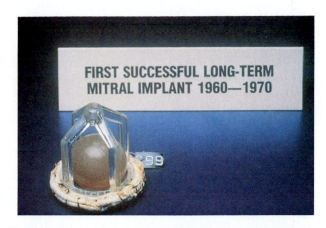

Fig. 13-25 Original Starr-Edwards ball-and-cage valve (explanted 10 years after implantation when the patient died from an accident). (Courtesy Baxter Healthcare Corp., Edwards CVS Div., Santa Ana, Calif.)

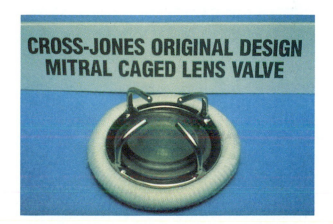

Fig. 13-26 The Cross-Jones valve had a low-profile cage with a lens-shaped, free floating disk. (Courtesy Baxter Healthcare Corp., Edwards CVS Div., Santa Ana, Calif.)

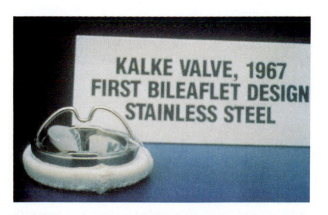

Fig. 13-27 The Kalke double-leaflet valve was a forerunner of the modern-day bileaflet prostheses. (Courtesy Baxter Healthcare Corp., Edwards CVS Div., Santa Ana, Calif.)

Box 13-7 Cardiac valve prostheses developed since the 1960s

A variety of prosthetic valves have been designed and developed. The opening and closing mechanism of synthetic valves is usually one of two configurations: the ball and cage, or the single or double tilting disk. The prostheses below are listed under their respective headings; they are no longer available for implantation in the United States.

Ball and Cage
Braunwald-Cutter
Braunwald-Morrow
Cooley-Bloodwell-Liotta-Cromie
DeBakey-Surgitool
Harken ball and cage (see Fig. 14-1)
Hufnagel (see Fig. 14-2)
Magovern-Cromie
Smeloff-Cutter
Smeloff-Cutter-Davey-Kaufman
Starr-Edwards (other than 1260, 6120)(see Fig. 13-25)

Tilting Disk
Bjork-Shiley
Hufnagel trileaflet
Lillehei-Kastor
Wada-Cutter

Caged Disk
Barnard-Goosen
Beall-Surgitool
Cooley-Bloodwell-Cutter
Cooley-Cutter
Cross-Jones (see Fig. 13-26)
Hufnagel-Brunswick
Kay-Shiley
Kay-Suzuki
Starr-Edwards disk

Bileaflet Disk
Edwards-Duromedics
Gott-Daggett
Kalke (see Fig. 13-29)

Modified from Akins CW: Mechanical cardiac valvular prostheses, *Ann Thorac Surg* 52:161, 1991; and Lefrak EA, Starr A: *Cardiac valve prostheses*, Norwalk, Conn, 1979, Appleton-Century-Crofts.

closing mechanisms (Figs. 13-25 through 13-27). Box 13-7 lists those implanted at one time but no longer approved by the U.S. Food and Drug Administration (FDA). Patients who present for reoperation may have one of these valves, and knowledge of their design may be helpful for radiologic identification and surgical excision.

FDA-approved mechanical and bioprosthetic valves are listed in Table 13-4 with considerations for use, advantages, and disadvantages.

The choice of a mechanical or biologic prosthesis is complicated by the fact that each type of prosthesis has drawbacks. Increased risk of thromboembolism is associated with mechanical valves, and durability can be a problem with biologic valves (Table 13-4). In addition, all prosthetic heart valves are inherently stenotic because attachment of the sewing ring to the annulus takes up a portion of the native orifice. Starr, Grunkemeier, and Fessler (1988) stress the importance of proper selection to achieve optimal results for a particular patient. They recommend selection criteria that include the patient's age and the safety of anticoagulation.

Age is a factor because biologic valves deteriorate. In children and young adults degenerative calcification occurs at an accelerated rate and is thought to be related to the active calcium metabolism within this age group. In adults the reasons for the calcific stenosis are less clear but are thought to be associated with altered metabolism of calcium and other substances. (This may also be a factor in patients with

renal disease who also demonstrate accelerated bioprosthetic failure.)

Enhanced durability is seen in elderly patient groups where the failure rate has decreased. According to Jamieson and colleagues (1988), 83% of patients 60 years of age and older are free of significant leaflet degeneration at 10 years. At 15 years only 25% of patients are free of significant leaflet degeneration (Starr, Grunkemeier, and Fessler, 1988).

The durability of mechanical valves is an important factor, especially in patients who may have to face reoperation because their life expectancy is longer than that of a bioprosthesis. Another consideration is that when chronic anticoagulation therapy has already been instituted in patients with a history of atrial fibrillation, it is logical to select the more durable, mechanical valve.

Hemodynamic function is comparable for most mitral prostheses, especially in the larger sizes. There

Table 13-4 ■ *Commonly used mechanical and biologic valve prostheses*

	Mechanical	
Ball and cage	**Tilting disk**	
Starr-Edwards	**Medtronic-Hall, Omniscience**	**St. Jude Medical**
Model/Description		
6120 Mitral 1260 Aortic	Spherical single tilting disk	Bileaflet tilting disk
Advantages		
Long-term durability Good hemodynamics Inaudible Least risk of sudden thrombosis	Long-term durability Good hemodynamics in all sizes Low profile	Long-term durability Good hemodynamics in all sizes Low TE rate for a mechanical valve Low profile
Disadvantages		
Anticoagulation required Higher incidence of TE than with disk valves Suboptimal hemodynamics in small aortic sizes (less than 23 mm) High profile not optimal in small LV or aortic root Higher risk of TE in mitral position	Anticoagulation required Sudden thrombosis Noisy Higher risk of TE in mitral position If warfarin must be discontinued, there is increased risk of catastrophic thrombosis	Anticoagulation strongly recommended Sudden thrombosis Some noise Higher risk of TE in mitral position If warfarin must be discontinued, there is increased risk of catastrophic thrombosis
Special Considerations		
Sizers and handles specific to prosthesis; must be sterilized Poppet of aortic valve removable to facilitate tying sutures; replaced before aorta closed; mitral poppet not removable Aortic model has three struts; mitral has four	Sizers and handles specific to prosthesis; must be sterilized	Sizers and handles specific to prosthesis; must be sterilized Frequently used in children needing prosthetic valve
Resterilization*		
Yes; steam preferred over EO gas	Yes; steam preferred over EO gas	Yes; steam preferred over EO gas

Modified from Jones EL and others: Complications from cardiac prostheses. I. Infection, thrombosis, and emboli associated with intracardiac prostheses; and Salzman EW, Ware JA: Complications from cardiac prostheses. II. Thromboembolic complications of cardiac and vascular prostheses. In Sabiston DC, Spencer FC: *Surgery of the chest*, ed 5, vols 1 and 2, New York, 1990, WB Saunders.
TE, Thromboembolism; *LV,* left ventricle; *EO,* ethylene oxide; *AVR,* aortic valve replacement.
*Follow manufacturer's instructions. All prostheses should be stored in a cool, dry, contamination-free area.

may be some differences in patients with a small native mitral valve annulus (less than 29 mm), but the small valve orifice is more often a problem in aortic valve surgery (see Chapter 14). Thrombosis can occur with all prosthetic valves, although the biologic valves may have a somewhat lower rate (Morgan, Davis, and Fraker, 1985).

Perioperative considerations. A complete range of prosthesis with sizers should be available, as well as pledgeted and nonpledgeted suture (see Fig. 5-34). Obturators can be arranged in order of size on the back table (with the size written on the table cover next to each obturator). Individual obturator and

prosthetic valve holders may appear similar; the nurse can identify these with labels or by writing the name of the corresponding prosthesis next to each one.

Three basins capable of holding at least 500 ml of normal saline for rinsing glutaraldehyde-stored bioprostheses should be arranged on the back table or on a separate sterile field. Forceps, suture scissors, one to three syringes (10 ml), and one to four culture tubes are added. Biologic valves require rinsing for at least 2 minutes in each of the three basins. They should be kept moist with frequent saline irrigation during implantation but should not be moistened with topical antibiotic solution.

Table 13-4 ■ *Commonly used mechanical and biologic valve prostheses—continued*

Biologic		Homograft
Heterograft		
Carpentier-Edwards; Hancock	**Carpentier-Edwards pericardial valve**	**Homograft**
Model/Description		
Porcine heterograft (from excised pig aortic valves)	2700 Aortic Bovine pericardium (cut and shaped into a trileaflet valve)	Aortic or pulmonary valve allograft (cadaver, organ donor, excised from cardiomyopathic heart removed from transplant recipient)
Advantages		
Incidence of TE very low; anticoagulation rare, especially after AVR No hemolysis Good hemodynamics Central flow Gradual failure allows elective reoperation	Incidence of TE very low; anticoagulation rare, especially after AVR No hemolysis Good hemodynamics in all sizes Central flow Gradual failure allows elective reoperation Residual gradient minimal	Incidence of TE very low; anticoagulation rare (used mainly for AVR) No hemolysis Excellent hemodynamics, (especially with stentless technique) Central flow Gradual failure allows elective reoperation No residual gradient
Disadvantages		
Durability usually less than 10-15 years Accelerated fibrocalcific degeneration in children, patients with hypertension or on chronic renal dialysis Suboptimal hemodynamics and residual gradient in smaller sizes (less than 23 mm aorta or 29 mm mitral) May be contraindicated in small, hypertrophied LV	Durability not yet established Available only for AVR Accelerated calcification may be a problem in children, renal patients, or those with hypertension	Limited durability Limited availability
Special Considerations		
Sizers and handles specific to prosthesis; must be sterilized Prior to insertion, must be rinsed in saline to remove glutaraldehyde storage solution Frequent irrigation recommended to prevent drying Diets low in calcium recommended for children, renal patients	Sizers and handles specific to prosthesis; must be sterilized Prior to insertion, must be rinsed in saline to remove glutaraldehyde storage solution Frequent irrigation recommended to prevent drying Diets low in calcium recommended for children, renal patients Approved for aortic position only	No specific sizers; may use sizers for heterografts (e.g., biologic prostheses) Cryopreserved homograft must be thawed per protocol Used for aortic valve replacement; stent attached for use in mitral and tricuspid position; pulmonary allograft may be used for pediatric reconstruction
Resterilization*		
Not recommended	Not recommended	Not recommended

Additional basinware may be needed for heparinized saline and other solutions.

Operative procedure

1. Cardiopulmonary bypass with double venous cannulation is instituted. Caval clamps or umbilical tapes with tourniquets may be placed around the inferior and superior venae cavae to isolate the heart from any venous return.
2. The left atrium is incised, blood is suctioned away, and the incision is enlarged to expose the mitral valve (Fig. 13-28, *A* and *B*). The atrium is inspected, and any thrombotic material is removed.
3. Retraction stitches may be placed in the anterior leaflet for exposure and mobilization, and the valvular apparatus is inspected. Stitches may be placed in each commissure.
4. The valve leaflets with their respective chordae tendineae and tips of the papillary muscle heads are excised with a blade and scissors, leaving a fibrous margin of the valve annulus to insert fixation sutures to the valve prosthesis (Fig. 13-28, *C*). Caution is taken not to transect too much of the papillary muscle, since this can weaken the ventricular wall and lead to rupture (Harlan, Starr, and Harwin, 1980). The valvular tissue may be sent to the laboratory for bacterial examination and culturing, even if the patient has not had an episode of endocarditis.

   Increasingly, only the anterior leaflet and subvalvular structures are removed; the posterior leaflet and attached chordae are left intact as support structures for the left ventricle.

   Rongeurs may be used to debride calcium particles; the rongeur tips should be rinsed in saline and wiped clean with a wet sponge. The atrium and ventricle are inspected, and all loose debris is removed.
5. The valve annulus is sized with obturators corresponding to the specific prosthesis desired, and the appropriate-size valve is selected, verified by the circulating nurse and the sterile nurse, and delivered to the field.
   a. **Mechanical valve:** The sterile nurse attaches the appropriate handle, cuts the identification label, wraps the prosthesis in a sponge soaked with heparinized saline or antibiotic solution, and places the prosthesis in a protected area of the field until it is needed.
   b. **Biologic valve:** The sterile nurse attaches the appropriate handle and removes any packing material from the prosthesis. The identification tag is cut and removed before the rinsing procedure is begun (agitation of the prosthesis with the tag attached could lacerate the prosthetic leaflets).

   The bioprosthesis is then rinsed for at least 2 minutes in each of three basins of normal saline (total minimum time: 6 minutes). Rinse solution from the third basin (5 to 10 ml) is placed in a tube and sent for culture; cultures may be taken from all three of the basins if requested. The bioprosthesis is wrapped in a saline-moistened sponge and placed in a protected area of the field until needed. It should not be allowed to dry or come into contact with antibiotic solutions (which can damage the tissue).
6. Nonabsorbable, alternately colored individual cardiovascular sutures (about 20) are placed in the retained fibrous annular margin (avoiding the muscular wall, which could tear when the sutures are tied) and then into the prosthetic sewing ring (Fig. 13-28, *D*). The needles are then removed.

   Some surgeons prefer to insert stitches into the prosthetic sewing ring only after all the annular stitches are in place.
7. The sutures are held taut as the prosthesis is guided into position. Sprinkling normal saline on the sutures makes them slide more easily through the sewing ring. (The surgeon may also want to keep his or her fingers moist to facilitate tying each stitch.) The sutures are tied and cut, and the surgeon confirms that no stitches are entangled in the prosthetic struts. A small dental mirror (prewarmed in saline to prevent fogging) can be used to assess the subvalvular placement of stitches in bioprostheses.
8. Occasionally a catheter may be placed through the orifice of a mechanical valve to keep the valve incompetent, thereby allowing air to escape from the left ventricle (Fig. 13-28, *E*).
9. In patients with an enlarged left atrium or history of embolic episodes, the atrial appendage is often ligated or stapled to prevent the subsequent formation and embolization of thrombus.
10. The atriotomy is partially closed with nonabsorbable sutures (Fig. 13-28, *F*). The patient is placed in the Trendelenburg position so that residual air in the left ventricle will exit preferentially through the venting needle placed in the anterior ascending aorta (rather than travel to the brain and cause an air embolus). The lungs are inflated to expel intracardiac air.

    Air is also aspirated from the left ventricle with a hand-held hypodermic needle (or less frequently, an apical venting catheter). Caution is taken to avoid excessive elevation of the ventricle, which could produce a ventricular wall tear or rupture. In reoperations where ventricular apical adhesions remain, a spinal needle can be placed transseptally from the right ventricle to the left ventricle to remove air. If bleeding from the needle holes persists, a stick tie may be used for repair.
11. Additional venting measures may be used (moving the table from side to side, gently jiggling the heart. The cross-clamp is removed, and the heart is allowed to fibrillate. The ventricle is not allowed to eject blood until the surgeon is assured that sufficient air is evacuated. After adequate venting, the heart is defibrillated. The transvalvular cath-

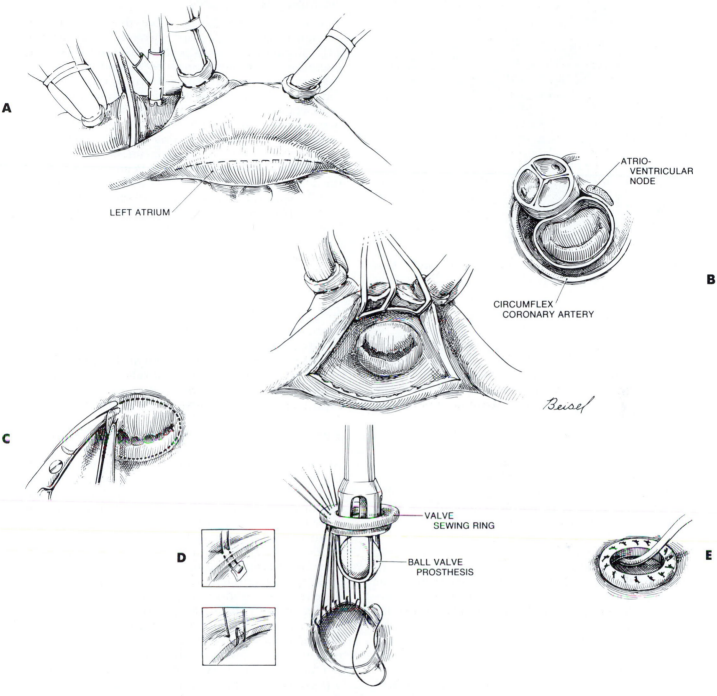

Fig. 13-28 Mitral valve replacement. **A,** Line of incision along the posterior interatrial groove. **B,** Cooley atrial retractor in the left atrium, exposing the mitral valve. **C,** Valve excision. The posterior leaflet and chordae may be retained. **D,** Insertion of interrupted stitches into the annulus and prosthetic sewing ring. Two suture techniques are shown in the boxes: a figure-eight without a pledget may be used when there is a firm fibrous annular margin; felt-pledgeted suture helps reduce the risk of perivalvular leaks when there is a fragile or calcified annulus. The pledget may be positioned in the subannular position (shown) or in the supraannular position. **E,** Catheter inserted through the valve orifice to maintain incompetence of the prosthesis, allowing air to escape from the left ventricle. (This technique is no longer commonly used.) **F,** Closure of the left atrial incision. (From Walhausen JA, Pierce WS: *Johnson's surgery of the chest,* ed 5, St Louis, 1985, Mosby.)

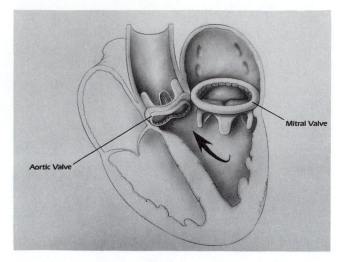

Fig. 13-29 Double valve replacement with bioprostheses in the mitral and aortic positions. (Courtesy Medtronic, Inc., Minneapolis, Minn.)

eter (if used) is removed, and the atrial closure is completed.

12. Rewarming is completed, and the patient is weaned from cardiopulmonary bypass. TEE may be used to assess ventricular function (and detect the presence of residual air).

Additional Procedures

Reoperation for mitral valve disease

Patients with a prior commissurotomy may require reoperation for recurring mitral stenosis. If the initial approach was via thoracotomy, few if any sternal adhesions will be present. If repeat sternotomy is planned, additional dissecting time and increased bleeding can be anticipated. Some surgeons may elect to use a right or left thoracotomy approach for repeat valve replacement in patients who had an initial sternotomy. Exposure is critical, and the surgeon will use the approach that allows optimal visualization of the operative site (David, 1990). Operative risk is increased with repeat valve replacement (Kirklin and Barratt-Boyes, 1993).

The nurse can anticipate some difficulty in removing the prosthetic valve. Reconstruction of the annulus with autologous or bovine pericardium may be necessary.

Infective endocarditis

Infective endocarditis of the native valve or a prosthetic valve is an indication for surgery when there is heart failure, septic emboli, conduction disturbances, prosthetic valve dysfunction, or persistent signs of infection (Hendren and others, 1992). Repair may be feasible in some native valves, but replacement is necessary with infected prostheses or with valves that are severely damaged.

Multiple valve surgery

When concomitant aortic valve disease is serious enough to warrant surgical correction (see Chapter 14), valve replacement is performed during the same operation. Both valves may be excised first. Mitral valve replacement is then performed, with the prosthesis seated and the sutures tied, followed by aortic valve replacement (Fig. 13-29). Performing the surgery in this order avoids injury to aortic structures from a rigid prosthesis during manipulation of the mitral valve. Closure of the atrial incision can be completed after the aortic valve has been implanted and the aorta closed.

Tricuspid valve surgery is performed after mitral valve replacement. Generally, suture or ring annuloplasty is performed for tricuspid regurgitation, and commissurotomy is performed for stenotic lesions. Valve replacement is uncommon (see Chapter 15). Multiple-valve surgery poses an increased risk to the patient.

Coronary artery disease

Distal coronary artery bypass grafts are performed first, followed by valve replacement and then proximal anastomoses. If resection of an apical left ventricular aneurysm is planned, the mitral valve can be replaced through the ventriculotomy, after which the aneurysm is resected and the ventricle closed.

COMPLETION OF THE PROCEDURE

At the completion of the repair, the surgeon inspects the suture line(s) for hemostasis. In patients with recent onset of atrial fibrillation, the heart may return to normal sinus rhythm; cardioversion may be attempted if atrial fibrillation is present. In patients with chronic atrial fibrillation (or mechanical prostheses), warfarin therapy is begun a few days postoperatively, after the danger of surgical bleeding has passed.

Surgical manipulation and local edema may produce transient conduction disturbances, so temporary ventricular and atrial pacing wires are attached prophylactically. (Atrial pacing is ineffective in converting fibrillation to sinus rhythm; ventricular wires may be necessary to maintain an adequate heart rate.)

One or two mediastinal drainage catheters are inserted; pleural drainage tubes are unnecessary unless the pleura has been opened. Occasionally the superior portion of the pericardium is closed to prevent extensive adhesions from developing. This is helpful in patients for whom there is a high probability of reoperation at a later time. Although the pericardium generally is left open (to preclude the risk of tamponade when mediastinal blood cannot drain properly), it may be partially closed over the base of the heart and the great vessels so that fewer adhesions form after surgery. This may be considered in patients who are expected to require reoperation, such as young patients or recipients of bioprostheses with a greater than 10- to 15-year life expectancy.

Table 13-5 ■ *Postoperative complications of mitral valve surgery*

Complication	Interventions
Rupture of left ventricular free wall or atrioventricular groove	If chest is still open, reinstitute cardiopulmonary bypass to decompress heart, and control hemorrhage with fingers; if prosthesis is implicated in rupture, replace with different valve; repair perforation with heavy suture in manner similar to repair of left ventricular aneurysm
	If chest is closed, sudden massive chest tube drainage will be noted; perform immediate sternotomy and proceed as above
	Repair may compromise circumflex coronary artery, producing ischemic changes or infarction; coronary artery bypass grafting should be anticipated
Prosthetic failure; thrombosed occluder (disk or ball), or degeneration of bioprosthesis	Cessation of valve noise alerts patient or clinician; sternotomy, assessment of valve, and possible replacement required
	If bioprosthesis is damaged, a new murmur will appear with elevated pulmonary pressures; replacement is indicated
Prosthetic dehiscence; perivalvular leak	A new murmur with elevated pulmonary pressures alerts clinician; surgical exploration may necessitate insertion of additional stitches or prosthetic replacement; hemolysis producing a decreased hematocrit may be apparent
Prosthetic valve endocarditis	Elevated temperature and positive blood cultures alert clinician; valve replacement is indicated
Anticoagulation-related hemorrhage	Readjust warfarin dosage; recommend more frequent laboratory studies until prothrombin time is within acceptable range
	Refer for additional teaching and family support
Thromboembolism, embolism related to surgical intervention	Anticoagulation dosage adjusted to prolong prothrombin time; neurologic deficits should be reported; meticulous intraoperative cleaning of instruments and removal of particulate debris can reduce risk of surgical emboli
Residual regurgitation after valve repair	Echocardiographic assessment, new murmurs, or congestive heart failure may indicate suboptimal repair; surgical exploration required to revise, repair or perform valve replacement

Modified from Cohn LH: Management of complications related to mitral valve surgery. In Waldhausen JA, Orringer MB: *Complications in cardiothoracic surgery*, St Louis, 1991, Mosby.

POSTOPERATIVE COMPLICATIONS

Complications of mitral valve surgery are related to the valve repair or replacement, the insertion and function of the particular prosthesis, and the patient factors that affect the outcome of surgery. Patients with longstanding mitral valve disease preoperatively, for example, may be at increased risk for multiorgan dysfunction postoperatively as a result of their chronic low cardiac output. These patients tend to be sicker and may not make as rapid a recovery as the patient with acute-onset valvular dysfunction (Cohn, 1991).

Table 13-15 lists complications associated with mitral valve surgery. One of the most serious, albeit infrequent, complications is rupture of the left ventricle (Bjork, Henze, and Rodriquez, 1977). Whether occurring intraoperatively (usually after the termination of cardiopulmonary bypass when the heart resumes its pressure-volume work) or in the immediate postoperative period, this complication is associated with a high mortality (Karlson, Ashraf, and Berger, 1988). A number of causes have been suggested. It may result from anatomic factors that predispose the ventricle to injury (e.g., ischemic or weakened myocardium), or it may be related to the technique of valve excision and insertion of a prosthesis (Seifert and Speir, 1990). Other factors may include excessive tilting of the ventricle during venting (which pushes the valve struts into the ventricular endocardial wall) and aggressive manipulation of rigid suction or venting catheters. When the complication is detected (by the appearance of sudden, massive hemorrhage), the location of the rupture will guide the type of repair used (Figs. 13-30 and 13-31).

In the postoperative period clinicians should be aware that external chest compressions during cardiac resuscitation may produce injury as a result of the prosthesis pushing against the ventricle and causing it to rupture. Immediate sternotomy is performed to repair the ventricle.

Complications related to prostheses such as anticoagulation-related hemorrhage and endocarditis may be modified by the patient's and family's ability to anticipate problems and seek help when signs and symptoms arise (Table 13-3). Patient teaching is critical in avoiding many of these risks.

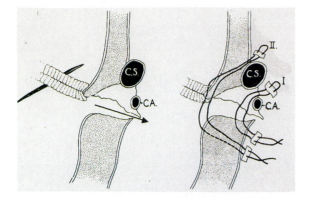

Fig. 13-30 Type I rupture of the left ventricle occurs at the atrioventricular junction. The repair is performed with a double layer of buttressed sutures penetrating the left atrial wall on each side of the coronary sinus (*cs*) and left ventricular myocardium. The circumflex coronary artery (*ca*) is avoided; sutures are passed through the prosthetic sewing ring. Occasionally the prosthesis must be replaced with another that is smaller or of a different configuration. (From Bjork VO, Henze A, Rodriquez L: Left ventricular rupture as a complication of mitral valve replacement, *J Thorac Cardiovasc Surg* 73:14, 1977.)

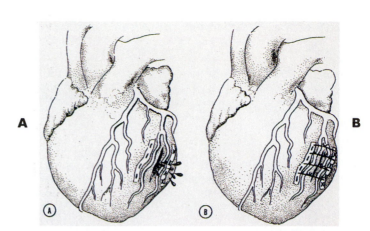

Fig. 13-31 Type II rupture of the left ventricle occurs in the ventricular wall near the location of an excised papillary muscle. The repair consists of, **A**, a first layer of isolated mattress sutures buttressed with felt strips. These may not be able to hold friable myocardium, **B**. A second, reinforcing layer of isolated over-and-over sutures may be required to achieve hemostasis. Note the similarity to conventional repair of a left ventricular aneurysm (see Chapter 12). (From Bjork VO, Henze A, Rodriquez L: Left ventricular rupture as a complication of mitral valve replacement, *J Thorac Cardiovas Surg* 73:14, 1977.)

REFERENCES

Akins C: Mechanical cardiac valvular prostheses, *Ann Thorac Surg* 52:161, 1991.

Anderson UK: Mitral valve prolapse: a diagnosis for primary nursing intervention, *J Cardiovasc Nurs* 1(3):41, 1987.

Antunes MJ: *Mitral valve repair*, Federal Republic of Germany, 1989, RS Schulz.

Bailey CP: The surgical treatment of mitral stenosis (mitral commissurotomy), *Dis Chest* 15:377, 1949.

Barlow JB: Idiopathic (degenerative) and rheumatic mitral valve prolapse: historical aspects and an overview, *J Heart Valve Dis* 1(2):163, 1992.

Bjork VO, Henze A, Rodriquez L: Left ventricular rupture as a complication of mitral valve replacement, *J Thorac Cardiovasc Surg* 73:14, 1977.

Braunwald E: Valvular heart disease. In Braunwald E: *Heart disease*, ed 4, Philadelphia, 1992, WB Saunders.

Brieger GH: The development of surgery. In Sabiston DC: *Textbook of surgery*, ed 14, New York, 1991, WB Saunders.

Canobbio MM: *Cardiovascular disorders*, St Louis, 1990, Mosby.

Carabello BA: Mitral regurgitation. 2. Proper timing of mitral valve replacement, *Mod Concepts Cardiovasc Dis* 57(11):59, 1988.

Carpentier A: Cardiac valve surgery: the "French Correction," *J Thorac Cardiovasc Surg* 86(3):323, 1983.

Carpentier A and others: Biological factors affecting long-term results of valvular heterografts, *J Thorac Cardiovasc Surg* 58:467, 1969.

Carpentier A and others: A new reconstructive operation for correction of mitral and tricuspid insufficiency, *J Thorac Cardiovasc Surg* 61:1, 1971.

Chachques JC and others: Absorbable rings for pediatric valvuloplasty: a preliminary study, *Circulation* 82(suppl IV, No 5):IV-82, 1990.

Christopherson DJ, Froelicher ES: Anticoagulant, antithrombotic, and platelet-modifying drugs. In Underhill SL and others: *Cardiovascular medications for cardiac nursing*, Philadelphia, 1990, JB Lippincott.

Cohn LH: Management of complications related to mitral valve surgery. In Walhausen JA, Orringer MB: *Complications in cardiothoracic surgery*, St Louis, 1991, Mosby.

Cosgrove DM, Stewart WJ: Mitral valvuloplasty, *Curr Probl Cardiol* 14(7):359, 1989.

Cutler EC, Levine SA: Cardiotomy and valvulotomy for mitral stenosis: experimental observations and clinical notes concerning an operated case with recovery, *Boston Med Surg J* 188:1023, 1923.

David TE: A rational approach to the surgical treatment of mitral valve disease. In Karp RB, Laks H, Wechsler AS, editors: *Advances in cardiac surgery*, vol 2, St Louis, 1990, Mosby.

Deloche A and others: Valve repair with Carpentier techniques: the second decade, *J Thorac Cardiovasc Surg* 99(6):990, 1990.

Dubost C and others: Nouvelle technique d'ouverture de l'oreillette gauche en chirurgie a coeur ouvert: l'abord bi-auriculaire transseptal, *Tech Chir* 30:1607, 1966.

Duran CG and others: Conservative operation for mitral insufficiency: critical analysis supported by postoperative hemodynamic studies in 72 patients, *J Thorac Cardiovasc Surg* 79:326, 1980.

Finkelmeier BA, Hartz RS, Michaelis LL: Implications of prosthetic valve implantation: an 8-year follow-up of patients with porcine bioprostheses, *Heart Lung* 18(6):565, 1989.

Grossi EA and others: Experience with twenty-eight cases of systolic anterior motion after mitral valve reconstruction by the Carpentier technique, *J Thorac Cardiovasc Surg* 103(3):466, 1992.

Harken DE and others: The surgical treatment of mitral stenosis: valvuloplasty, *N Engl J Med* 239:801, 1948.

Harlan BJ, Starr A, Harwin FM: *Manual of cardiac surgery*, vol 1, New York, 1980, Springer-Verlag.

Hartz RS and others: Oblique transseptal left atriotomy for optimal mitral exposure, *J Thorac Cardiovasc Surg* 103(2):282, 1992.

Hendren WG and others: Mitral valve repair for bacterial endocarditis, *J Thorac Cardiovasc Surg* 103(1):124, 1992.

Hurst JW: *The heart*, ed 7, vols 1 and 2, New York, 1990, McGraw-Hill.

Jamieson WRE and others: Carpentier Edwards standard porcine bioprosthesis: primary tissue failure (structural valve deterioration) by age groups, *Ann Thorac Surg* 46:155, 1988.

Johnson SL: *The history of cardiac surgery 1896-1955*, Baltimore, 1970, Johns Hopkins Press.

Karlson KJ, Ashraf MM, Berger RL: Rupture of left ventricle following mitral valve replacement, *Ann Thorac Surg* 46:590, 1988.

Kirklin JW, Barratt-Boyes BG: *Cardiac surgery*, ed 2, New York, 1993, Churchill Livingstone.

Kirklin JW, Blackstone EH, Kirklin JK: Cardiac surgery. In Braunwald E: *Heart disease*, ed 3, Philadelphia, 1988, WB Saunders.

Lefrak EA, Starr A: *Cardiac valve prostheses*, Norwalk, Conn, 1979, Appelton-Century-Crofts.

Lillehei CW and others: The surgical treatment of stenotic or regurgitant lesion of the mitral and aortic valves by direct vision utilizing a pump oxygenator, *J Thorac Surg* 35:154, Feb 1958.

MacNeil C, Balasundaram S, Duran C: Cardiac valve repair: experiences in Saudi Arabia, *AORN J* 53(4):976, 1991.

Morgan RJ, Davis JT, Fraker TD: Current status of valve prostheses, *Surg Clin North Am* 65(3):699, 1985.

Oury JH and others: Mitral valve reconstruction for mitral regurgitation, *J Cardiac Surg* 1(3):217, 1986.

Rahimtoola SH: Comments on Cosgrove DM, Stewart WJ: Mitral valvuloplasty, *Curr Probl Cardiol* 14(7):359, 1989a.

Rahimtoola SH: Perspective on valvular heart disease: an update, *J Am Coll Cardiol* 14(1):1, 1989b.

Rankin JS: Mitral and tricuspid valve disease: In Sabiston DC: *Textbook of surgery*, ed 14, New York, 1991, WB Saunders.

Reed GE, Pooley R, Moggio R: Durability of measured mitral annuloplasty: seventeen-year study, *J Thorac Cardiovasc Surg* 79(3):321, 1980.

Samways, DW: Cardiac peristalsis: its nature and effects, *Lancet* 1:927, 1898. From Lefrak EA, Starr A: *Cardiac valve prostheses*, 1979, New York, Appleton-Century-Crofts, p 3.

Schakenbach LH: Physiologic dynamics of acquired valvular heart disease, *J Cardiovasc Nurs* 1(3):12, 1987.

Seifert PC, Speir AM: Left ventricular rupture: a collaborative approach to emergency management, *AORN J* 51(3):714, 1990.

Shah P: Mitral valve prolapse: the elusive definitions and differing criteria of diagnosis, *J Heart Valve Dis* 1(2):160, 1992 (editorial).

Smith CR: Septal superior exposure of the mitral valve, *J Thorac Cardiovasc Surg* 103(4):623, 1992.

Spencer FC: Acquired heart disease. In Schwartz SI: *Principles of surgery*, ed 5, New York, 1989, McGraw-Hill.

Spencer FC: Acquired disease of the mitral valve. In Sabiston DC, Spencer FC: *Surgery of the chest*, ed 5, vols 1 and 2, New York, 1990, WB Saunders.

Starr A, Edwards ML: Mitral replacement: clinical experience with a ball-valve prosthesis, *Ann Surg* 154:726, Oct 1961.

Starr A, Grunkemeier GL, Fessler CL: Tissue and mechanical valves: mutually advantageous interplay, *J Cardiac Surg* 3(3):437, 1988.

Stollerman GH: Rheumatic fever and other rheumatic diseases of the heart. In Braunwald E: *Heart disease*, ed 4, Philadelphia, 1992, WB Saunders.

Weiland AP: A review of cardiac valve prostheses and their selection, *Heart Lung* 12(5):498, 1983.

Whitman GR, Guzzetta CE: Cardiac surgery. In Dossey BM, Guzzetta CE, Kenner CV, editors: *Critical care nursing: body-mind-spirit*, Philadelphia, 1992, JB Lippincott.

14

Aortic Valve Surgery

Diseases of the aortic valve present many anatomic and clinical syndromes. Aortic insufficiency with a dilated left ventricle in failure has been totally refractory to surgical intervention. Because of the clear diagnosis and grave prognosis of these patients, we are not only eager to intervene but have an obligation to undertake whatever we may regard as the most reasonable therapy. It is to this group that we address ourselves here.

Dwight E. Harken, MD, and associates, 1960 (p. 744)

With the above introductory paragraph, Harken and his co-workers proceeded to describe the first successful aortic valve replacement with a ball valve prosthesis (Fig. 14-1) implanted in the normal subcoronary anatomic position. Technologic advances during the previous decade had helped to make Harken's achievement a reality.

In the year before Gibbon (1954) introduced the first successful clinical application of a mechanical heart-lung machine, Hufnagel (Hufnagel and Harvey, 1953) had inserted a prosthetic ball valve (Fig. 14-2) into the descending aorta of a patient with aortic regurgitation. Although it provided only partial hemodynamic relief, this accomplishment stimulated further research into the development of valvular prostheses, which led to Harken's subcoronary aortic valve replacement.

Ironically, Harken and Starr (Starr and Edwards, 1961) independently developed the ball valve at the same time, and each used his own prosthesis to perform the first aortic valve replacement and the first mitral valve replacement, respectively.

ANATOMY AND PHYSIOLOGY OF THE AORTIC VALVE

The aortic valve (see Figs. 4-7 and 4-12), normally tricuspid morphologically, is located at the junction of the left ventricle and the origin of the ascending aorta (the aortic root). The valve is composed of fibrous leaflets that insert into a fibrous annular skeleton, and the sinuses of Valsalva, which are slightly dilated pouches between the valve cusps and the aortic wall. The valve annulus and attached leaflets are located below the openings to the right and left coronary arteries. The area between adjacent cusps is called a commissure. The sinuses of Valsalva and correspond-

ing valve cusps are respectively named after the right and left coronary arteries that originate within the sinuses. The third cusp, containing no coronary os, is named the noncoronary cusp (see Chapter 4).

The aortic valve lies in an oblique plane with the left coronary cusp slightly superior to the right coronary cusp. This explains why during surgery prosthetic valves appear slightly tilted when they are implanted into the aortic root.

Opening of the valve occurs when left ventricular pressure exceeds aortic pressure. The construction of the valve leaflets is such that the free edge of each cusp approaches the aortic wall, thereby allowing maximum opening of the orifice. This is enhanced by an increase in the diameter of the aortic root during systole. The pressure difference between the ventricle and the aorta disappears by midsystole, and forward blood flow is maintained by the effect of mass acceleration. On reversal of the flow, the cusps fall back and their edges contact each other to close the valve and prevent backflow (Nolan and Muller, 1986; Titus and Edwards, 1991).

The skeleton of the aortic valve is in fibrous continuity with the anterior leaflet of the mitral valve (which forms part of the ventricular outflow tract) and with the membranous septum. Conduction tissue lies below the right coronary cusp. It is essential that surgeons and perioperative nurses exercise great caution during operations performed on either valve so that they can avoid injury to the conduction pathways and to the structural components of the adjacent valve.

AORTIC VALVE DISEASE
Etiology and Pathology

Aortic valve stenosis and/or regurgitation may be the result of a number of conditions that affect the valve

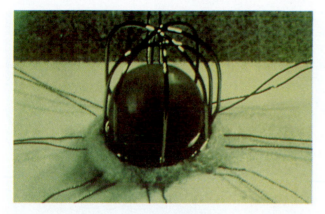

Fig. 14-1 Original Harkin caged-ball valve. The sewing ring could be trimmed to facilitate its insertion into the aortic root. (Courtesy Baxter Healthcare Corp., Edwards CVS Div., Santa Ana, Calif.)

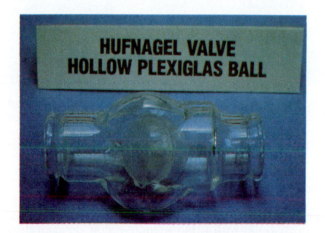

Fig. 14-2 Hufnagel valve. Although this valve was placed in the descending aorta and did not "replace" the aortic valve, it did show that foreign material could be implanted in the bloodstream without disastrous effects. (Courtesy Baxter Healthcare Corp., Edwards CVS Div., Santa Ana, Calif.)

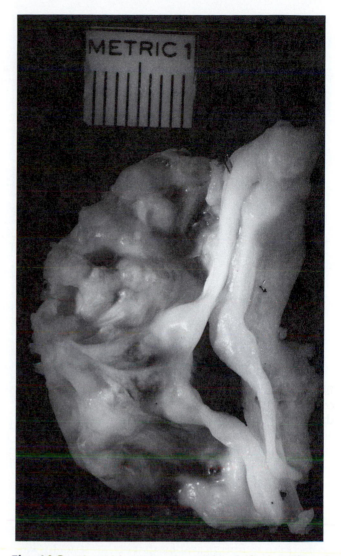

Fig. 14-3 Bicuspid aortic valve with calcified, stiffened leaflets producing stenosis. Note the greatly reduced orifice area. (Courtesy William C. Roberts, MD; Michael Spencer, photographer.)

leaflets and/or the annulus. Stenotic lesions obstruct left ventricular outflow and may be located at the valve level, below the valve (subvalvular), or above the valve (supravalvular).

Congenital malformations

Congenital malformations are a common cause of aortic stenosis, with the bicuspid aortic valve (Fig. 14-3) being the most common cause of aortic stenosis (Roberts, 1970). Bicuspid valves are rarely symptomatic at birth, but the turbulent flow across the leaflets produces fibrosis, stiffening, and calcification, which leads to symptomatic stenosis generally in the sixth decade (Subramanian, Olson, and Edwards, 1984). Aortic regurgitation may be associated with a bicuspid valve, but this is less common.

Unicuspid and dome-shaped valves are rare in the adult. Occasionally a patient may have a unicuspid

valve that goes undetected until calcification and fibrotic degeneration produce symptoms (Fig. 14-4). Severe forms usually cause immediate stenotic symptoms in early life; valvotomy is performed to enlarge the orifice.

Rheumatic fever

Rheumatic fever continues to be a significant etiologic factor in aortic valve disease. Inflammatory changes affect the aortic valve in a manner similar to that of the mitral valve, although it occurs less frequently. Granulation tissue and scarring produce contracted leaflets with rolled edges (Fig. 14-5). These changes make the valve more susceptible to degeneration from atherosclerosis and calcium deposition. Eventually there is stiffening of the cusps and fusion of the commissures, producing a stenotic orifice. The rheumatic process may also destroy fibrous tissue within the an-

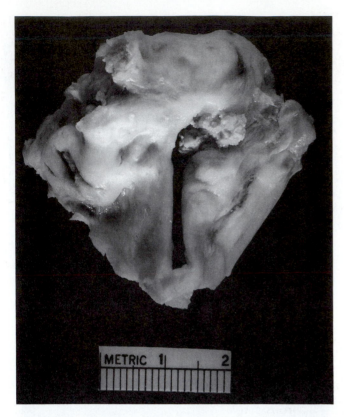

Fig. 14-4 Stenotic unicuspid aortic valve with fibrosed leaflets. Note the calcium particles. (Courtesy William C. Roberts, MD; Michael Spencer, photographer.)

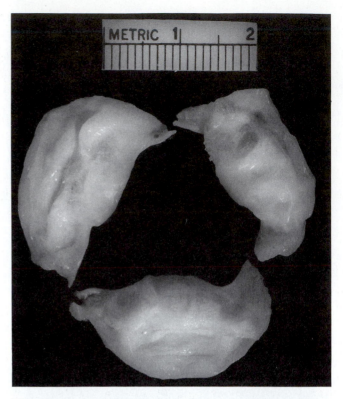

Fig. 14-5 Rheumatic trileaflet (e.g., morphologically normal) aortic valve. The thickened, glistening, and smooth leaflets are typical of rheumatic changes. (Courtesy William C. Roberts, MD; Michael Spencer, photographer.)

nulus, which can lead to annular dilatation and regurgitation through the incompetent valve. Mixed lesions occur in fibrotic leaflets that both restrict forward flow and fail to prevent backward flow.

Senile calcific aortic stenosis

With the decline of acute rheumatic fever in the United States and a growing geriatric population, the predominant cause of aortic stenosis has shifted from inflammatory lesions to degenerative lesions associated with aging (Lombardy and Selzer, 1987). These valves are heavily calcified but normally have a tricuspid configuration (Fig. 14-6).

Bacterial endocarditis

Bacterial endocarditis is an increasingly important etiologic factor in the development of aortic valve disease. It may occur on a structurally normal valve but more often affects rheumatically scarred or congenitally malformed aortic valves (Jacobs and Austen, 1990). Staphylococcus aureus is the most common organism. Vegetations and thrombus developing on the leaflets may break off and embolize to the heart, brain, or other organs; and they may cause valvular obstruction. However, the infectious process more often produces valvular incompetence from destruction of the valve and supporting structures. If there is erosion or perforation of the leaflets (Fig. 14-7), acute regurgitation occurs with rapid hemodynamic deterioration. Especially virulent cases of endocarditis are seen among intravenous drug users who use unsterile needles (Byrd and Cheitlin, 1987).

Marfan's syndrome

Chronic or acute regurgitation in an aortic valve with apparently normal leaflets occurs with annular dilatation associated with Marfan's syndrome. This is a generalized connective tissue disorder that weakens the wall of the aorta, producing dilatation and aneurysmal formation of the annulus, the sinuses of Valsalva, and/or the ascending aorta (see Chapter 16). Acute intimal tearing and dissection of the aorta stretches the supporting structures of the valve in such a way that the leaflets are unable to coapt.

Similar degenerative changes appear in some patients who do not have Marfan's syndrome. This is termed a "forme fruste" of the syndrome.

Other conditions

Trauma. Aortic insufficiency may be caused by blunt trauma or extreme muscular exertion, which can rupture or perforate the leaflet(s). Frequently this occurs in a previously diseased valve (Nolan and Muller, 1986).

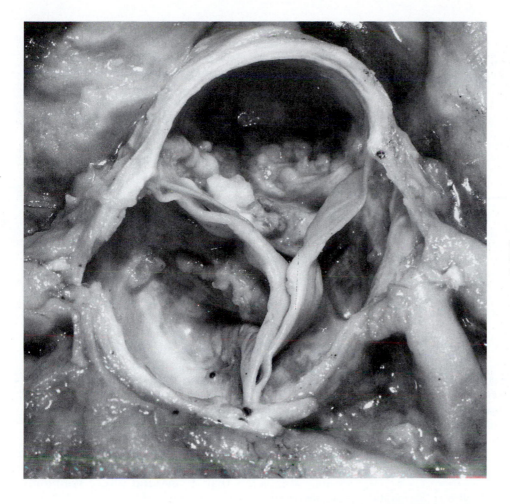

Fig. 14-6 Degenerative calcific stenosis of a trileaflet aortic valve. (Courtesy William C. Roberts, MD; Michael Spencer, photographer.)

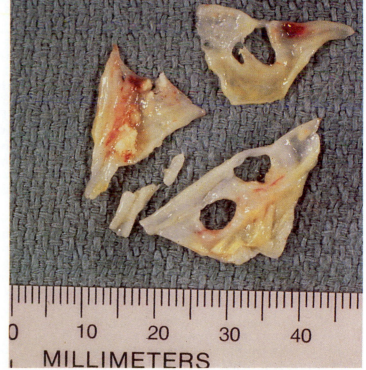

Fig. 14-7 Perforated aortic valve leaflets resulting from bacterial endocarditis. The patient had acute aortic insufficiency. (Courtesy Edward A. Lefrak, MD.)

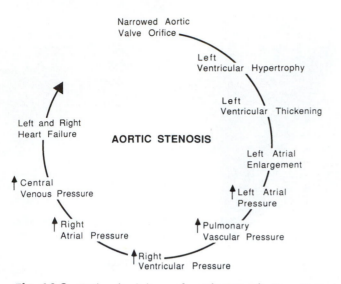

AORTIC STENOSIS

Narrowed Aortic Valve Orifice

Left Ventricular Hypertrophy

Left Ventricular Thickening

Left Atrial Enlargement

↑ Left Atrial Pressure

↑ Pulmonary Vascular Pressure

↑ Right Ventricular Pressure

↑ Right Atrial Pressure

↑ Central Venous Pressure

Left and Right Heart Failure

Fig. 14-8 Pathophysiology of aortic stenosis. (From Kinney MR and others: *Comprehensive cardiac care,* ed 7, St Louis, 1991, Mosby.)

Tertiary syphilis. Syphilitic aortitis, once a major cause of aortic root and annular dilatation, has declined significantly since the introduction of antimicrobial therapy (Pedersen and Goldenberg, 1991).

Pathophysiology

Aortic stenosis

Gradual, chronic obstruction to left ventricular outflow resulting from congenital or acquired aortic stenosis creates an increasing pressure load on the left ventricle (Fig. 14-8). The ventricle must work harder to generate a pressure higher than the aortic pressure in order to propel blood through the narrowed orifice (afterload) into the systemic circulation. Ventricular muscle is able to maintain a relatively normal cardiac output by the compensatory mechanism of concentric hypertrophy.

Hypertrophy develops as a result of the increased energy expenditure demanded of each cardiac cell. Pressure overloading stimulates the myocyte to produce new contractile proteins so that these energy demands can be met. Individual cells enlarge, but the overall number of cells, as well as the capillary network that replenishes their energy resources, remain constant. Although the capillary-to-myocyte ratio is the same, the distances between them is increased in proportion to the degree of cellular hypertrophy. This is most evident in the deeper myocardial layers of the subendocardium and papillary muscles, which are particularly vulnerable to ischemia. Even pharmacologic coronary vasodilatation fails to perfuse the subendocardium adequately, further jeopardizing these cells. The situation is aggravated by increased wall stress (a determinant of myocardial oxygen consumption) in the severely hypertrophied heart. Compounding the problem is the reduced diastolic compliance

associated with the thickened ventricle. Thus when the ventricle becomes stiff, diastolic filling (preload) is impaired (Jorgensen, 1991; Selzer, 1987).

The ventricle cannot compensate indefinitely. Eventually the reduction in energy-producing mitochondria within the cells and the increased distance between capillaries and the interior of the myocyte produce an adverse metabolic environment.

Although cardiac output can be maintained for a considerable period of time in aortic stenosis, derangements in afterload, preload, and contractility will eventually produce heart failure. Left ventricular dilatation occurs, which predisposes the heart to left-sided failure and left atrial enlargement. Right-sided heart failure eventually develops as backward volume creates increased pulmonary pressure, which cannot be accommodated by the low-pressure right heart circuit. Contractility of both ventricles decreases, and myocardial cell death can occur without treatment (Morton, 1987).

The cardinal symptoms of aortic stenosis are syncope, angina pectoris, and dyspnea (Table 14-1). These are related respectively to insufficient blood flow to the brain and the heart, and to impaired left ventricular function. Concomitant coronary artery disease exacerbates anginal episodes. Ventricular decompensation results in pulmonary congestion and dyspnea. Exercise-induced fatigability is associated with the reduction in cardiac output. Nonspecific symptoms include dizziness, palpitations, and fatigue. Symptoms usually become apparent when the valve orifice area is less than 1 cm^2, and severe symptoms are seen with an orifice area of less than 0.5 cm^2 (Spencer, 1989). The time interval between the discovery of a systolic murmur and the appearance of symptoms can vary from 1 month to 10 years (Lombardy and Selzer, 1987).

The appearance of symptoms, particularly dyspnea, is an ominous sign and warrants surgical intervention. The mean time of survival in patients presenting with angina is 4.7 years; with syncope it is less than 3 years, and with dyspnea and congestive heart failure it is 1 to 2 years (Whitman and Harken, 1991). The urgent need for surgery in patients with symptoms of failure is underscored by the fact that there is a significant incidence of sudden death in patients with aortic stenosis (Walker, 1988). The mechanism is unclear, but is thought to be related to syncopal attacks or ischemically induced ventricular fibrillation.

Irreversible left ventricular dysfunction can develop before symptoms become apparent. Given the importance of preoperative left ventricular function on the surgical outcome, surgery for aortic stenosis, unlike operations for most other valvular disorders, may be indicated even before the appearance of any functional disability.

Other forms of left ventricular outflow tract obstruction

Subvalvular impedance to outflow may also be caused by asymmetric hypertrophy of the ventricular septum,

Table 14-1 ■ *Signs, symptoms, and findings of aortic valve disease*

Aortic stenosis	Aortic regurgitation (insufficiency)
Signs Powerful, heaving PMI to left and below MCL Systolic thrill over aortic area, sternal notch Slowly rising carotid pulse BP normal or systolic BP normal with high diastolic reading Harsh, midsystolic murmur over sternum or apex	*Chronic* Hyperdynamic PMI to left and below MCL Forceful apical impulse displaced to left and down Prominent, and rapidly rising and collapsing carotid pulse Wide pulse pressure with diastolic BP less than 60 mm Hg Faint diastolic murmur along left sternal border *Acute* Weakness Congestive failure Pulmonary edema Tachycardia Short diastolic murmur Hypotension
Symptoms Syncope Angina pectoris Exertional dyspnea Fatigue Paroxysmal nocturnal dyspnea Dizziness Palpitations Sudden death	*Chronic* Orthopnea Atypical chest pain Exertional dyspnea Palpitations Paroxysmal nocturnal dyspnea Nocturnal angina with diaphoresis *Acute* Dyspnea
Chest X-Ray Film Prominent ascending aorta (poststenotic dilatation) Calcification on valve Concentric LV hypertrophy Pulmonary congestion	LV enlargement Pulmonary congestion
Electrocardiogram LV hypertrophy Ventricular tachycardia Sinus bradycardia	LV hypertrophy
Echocardiography Persistent echoes from obstructed flow Poor leaflet movement LV hypertrophy Poststenotic dilatation of aorta Increased velocity through valve Pressure gradient between LV and aorta	Diastolic vibrations of anterior leaflet of MV and septum Vegetations on leaflets Regurgitant flow mapped (color Doppler)
Cardiac Catheterization Confirms valve lesion Assesses LV function Detects coronary artery disease, MV problems Measures valve orifice, pressure gradient	Assesses degree of regurgitation, LV and MV function, PA pressures Detects coronary artery disease (less common with AI)

Modified from Braunwald E: *Heart disease*, ed 4, Philadelphia, 1992, WB Saunders.
AI, Aortic insufficiency; *BP*, blood pressure; *LA*, left atrium; *LV*, left ventricle; *MCL*, midclavicular line; *MV*, mitral valve; *PA*, pulmonary artery; *PMI*, point of maximal impulse.

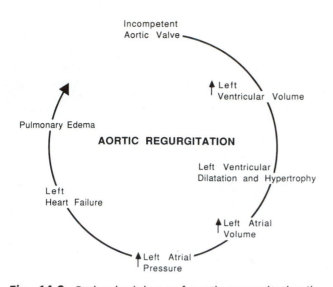

Fig. 14-9 Pathophysiology of aortic regurgitation/insufficiency. (From Kinney MR and others: *Comprehensive cardiac care,* ed 7, St Louis, 1991, Mosby.)

which protrudes into the left ventricular outflow tract (LVOT). The condition, often referred to as idiopathic hypertrophic subaortic stenosis (IHSS), is now more commonly known as hypertrophic cardiomyopathy (HCM). It is probably an inherited disorder, but it does occur in patients without a family history. Medical therapy initially consists of beta-adrenergic blocking medications to lower ventricular contractility and pharmacologic control of frequently associated dysrhythmias. Surgery is indicated when there is a significant left ventricular-aortic gradient, and symptoms persist despite medical treatment (Hazinski, 1992).

Septal hypertrophy is often associated with systolic anterior motion (SAM) of the aortic leaflet of the mitral valve; the leaflet protrudes toward the septal bulge, further obstructing flow (Kirklin and Barratt-Boyes, 1993). Surgery for this problem is included in this chapter.

Aortic insufficiency

From a mechanical viewpoint, aortic insufficiency is the result of a primary valve disorder or aortic root disease (Pedersen and Goldenberg, 1991). The volume overload associated with mild, chronic aortic insufficiency in a majority of cases can be tolerated for almost two decades before the patient becomes symptomatic, because the heart gradually dilates to compensate for the additional burden placed on it (Fig. 14-9). Regurgitant aortic volume is added to blood coming from the left atrium during diastole. As end-diastolic volume increases (preload), the left ventricle contracts more forcefully to expel the blood volume. This chronic overload state stimulates the eventual development of left ventricular hypertrophy.

Left ventricular decompensation will occur, and increased chamber pressure is reflected backward to the left atrium, the pulmonary vasculature, and the right side of the heart (Abramczyk and Brown, 1991). Without timely surgical intervention, failure becomes irreversible. Patients with a severely compromised left ventricle preoperatively have a less favorable outcome.

In contrast to chronic aortic insufficiency, acute aortic insufficiency is poorly tolerated for several reasons. The normal-size left ventricle is incapable of accommodating the increased, regurgitant volume and ejecting it with each heartbeat (and increasing the cardiac output). The lowered diastolic pressure that results from volume regurgitating into the ventricle impairs coronary filling by lowering perfusion pressure. Heart failure ensues rapidly.

DIAGNOSTIC EVALUATION OF AORTIC VALVE DISEASE

Evaluation of the patient with aortic valve disease begins with the history and physical examination. Diagnosis is often made using only routine tests such as the standard electrocardiogram and the chest x-ray film, although invasive and noninvasive imaging techniques (see Table 14-1) may provide additional detail useful to clinical decision making.

Aortic Stenosis

Cardiomegaly is not seen commonly in patients undergoing radiologic and electrocardiographic examinations unless severe valvular stenosis producing dilatation is present. Cardiac size may appear normal, although valvular calcification and left ventricular hypertrophy are often apparent on chest x-ray films.

Echocardiography can identify the level of left ventricular outflow tract obstruction: supravalvular, valvular, or subvalvular. Supravalvular and subvalvular lesions are generally congenital in origin; most acquired lesions are at the valvular level. When obstruction is caused by asymmetric hypertrophy of the left ventricular septum, bulging septal tissue can be observed.

In elderly and hypertensive patients, a systolic ejection murmur may be the result of aortic sclerosis rather than significant aortic stenosis. Echocardiography can distinguish between the thickened, but mobile leaflets of sclerosis and the relatively immobile cusps of the stenotic valve. Often the structure of the valve (e.g., bicuspid) can be determined, as well as left ventricular chamber and aortic root size, ventricular wall thickness, and other abnormalities. Regional and global left ventricular wall motion can be assessed with two-dimensional imaging.

The addition of color flow Doppler imaging allows quantification of the obstruction and measurement of the gradient, although cardiac catheterization-derived gradients may be more precise (Assey, Usher, and Hendrix, 1989). The aortic valve area can be calculated with reasonable accuracy.

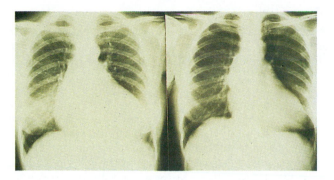

Fig. 14-10   Aortic insufficiency. *Left:* Preoperative chest x-ray film shows dilated left ventricle. *Right:* Postoperatively, the ventricle has returned to a more normal size and contour. (Courtesy Edward A. Lefrak, MD.)

Cardiac catheterization is not necessary for the diagnosis of aortic stenosis but is mandatory for evaluating the presence and significance of coronary artery disease. There is a high incidence of coronary artery disease in adults, and the need for myocardial revascularization should be considered prior to valve replacement.

Cardiac catheterization may also be performed to assess left ventricular function and to measure the pressure gradient across the valve. Occasionally a severely obstructed aortic valve orifice will not allow retrograde passage of a catheter into the left ventricle for injection of dye (to visualize ventricular contractility) or measurement of systolic intraventricular pressure. In severe stenosis, pressure gradients may be 50 mm Hg or more between the left ventricle and the ascending aorta. To attain an aortic pressure of 100 mm Hg beyond the valvular obstruction, the ventricle must generate a pressure of 150 mm Hg. Absence of a significant gradient may not be benign, however; it can reflect a weakened left ventricle incapable of generating sufficient pressure.

Aortic Insufficiency

Left ventricular enlargement (Fig. 14-10) with the apex displaced downward and to the left is commonly seen on the x-ray film. An enlarged ascending aorta may also be seen. Serial chest x-ray films are examined for increasing cardiac enlargement as an indication of the progression of the disease. The electrocardiogram will show signs of left ventricular hypertrophy. If atrial fibrillation is present (and not related to another disorder), it is usually a sign of elevated left ventricular end-diastolic pressure referred back to the left atrium and an indication of advanced disease (Hurst, 1990).

Echocardiography is used to determine the size of the ventricle, assess left ventricular function, and estimate regurgitant flow. It is particularly valuable as a noninvasive method of serially following the patient's progress.

Cardiac catheterization is used to visualize the degree of reflux and associated pathologic conditions of the aortic root, other valves, and coronary arteries. Elevated pulmonary and ventricular pressures are important prognostic indicators and provide information about optimal timing of surgery (Jacobs and Austen, 1990). Unfortunately, deciding when to operate is less precise for aortic insufficiency than it is for aortic stenosis. The problem is compounded in the asymptomatic patient with severe aortic regurgitation, because the degree of left ventricular impairment (an important predictor of survival) may be difficult to determine. However, surgery is rarely contraindicated, because death is virtually a certainty without it. To a great extent, timing of surgery for insufficiency still depends on clinical intuition as well as quantitative data (Spotnitz and Antunes, 1990).

SURGERY FOR AORTIC VALVE DISEASE
Reparative techniques

Techniques to repair the stenotic aortic valve have been less successful than those for the mitral valve and are less commonly performed. This is due in part to the more precise closing mechanism of the aortic valve. There is little overlap of the leaflets when the aortic valve is closed, as compared with the mitral leaflets when the mitral valve is closed. Thus imprecise repairs can produce regurgitation that is not well tolerated by the ventricle. Some patients, however, are unable to take anticoagulants or undergo reoperation for bioprosthetic failure or other valve-related complications. These patients may receive temporary benefit from balloon valvuloplasty (performed by the cardiologist in the cardiac catheterization laboratory) or surgical debridement under direct visualization. Allograft valve replacement may be an alternative.

Percutaneous aortic balloon valvuloplasty

Balloon valvuloplasty is increasingly being preferred to surgical valvulotomy in children and adolescents with noncalcific congenital aortic stenosis, although its value appears limited in adults with acquired calcific aortic stenosis. However, it is performed occasionally as an alternative to surgical replacement in patients who are very elderly and debilitated, disabled, and considered high-risk or unsuitable candidates (Braunwald, 1992). Age alone is not a contraindication to surgery.

One or two balloon catheters are passed through the aortic orifice and are inflated to "crack" the calcium that is restricting leaflet motion. The procedure generally enlarges the valve area by only 50% and is associated with a 3% to 10% mortality (Block and Palacios, 1988; Safian and others, 1988). If massive aortic insufficiency develops as a complication of balloon valvuloplasty, emergency surgical repair is performed (Seifert and Auer, 1988). Balloon valvuloplasty techniques for both mitral valve stenosis and aortic stenosis have limited applications.

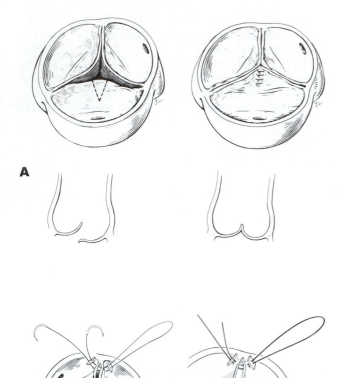

Fig. 14-11 A, Triangular resection of the free edge of the prolapsing cusp results in normal leaflet size and coaptation. **B,** Annuloplasty performed by placement of horizontal mattress sutures buttressed with felt at each commissure. The suture goes through the annulus (but not the leaflet) into the outflow tract and back through the annulus. (From Cosgrove DM and others: Valvuloplasty for aortic insufficiency, *J Thorac Cardiovasc Surg* 102[4]:571, 1991.)

Surgical valvuloplasty

Attempting to improve on the results of closed balloon techniques and to avoid prosthetic replacement, surgeons have devised a number of reparative procedures. King and others (1991); Mindich, Guarino, and Goldman (1986); and McBride and others (1990) have used ultrasonic high-speed drills to debride calcified stenotic leaflets. The best results have been seen in valves that are tricuspid and without commissural fusion or insufficiency. Valvuloplasty for aortic regurgitation has been described by Cosgrove and others (1991), who have attempted to repair prolapsed aortic leaflets. With these techniques, excess cusp tissue is resected or plicated; annular dilatation is repaired by reducing the annular circumference with pledgeted mattress sutures placed through the valve commissures (Fig. 14-11).

Aortic valvotomy

Valvotomy is performed under direct visualization in infants and children with congenital aortic stenosis. The fused leaflets are sharply divided with a knife.

Aortic Valve Replacement

Because reconstruction and repair of acquired lesions of the aortic valve have met with limited success, valve replacement is still considered the treatment of choice for aortic valve disease. Because of the risks associated with prosthetic valves, surgery may be delayed until symptoms warrant intervention but is performed before irreversible failure has developed.

Timing of surgery and results

In aortic stenosis, the presence of symptoms usually prompts the timing for valve replacement. Left ventricular hypertrophy often resolves following surgery, but left ventricular dilatation may not (Whitman and Harken, 1991). Operative mortality in patients with good left ventricular function is 2% to 8% (Kirklin and Barratt-Boyes, 1993). Operative mortality for patients in congestive heart failure can reach 24% (Sethig and others, 1987).

In aortic insufficiency, the optimum timing of surgery is less easily determined because the severity of the lesion is more difficult to quantitate as compared with aortic stenosis. The point of irreversible failure is hard to establish because the effects of volume overloading are less predictable than those associated with pressure overloading. Operative and late mortality tend to be higher in patients with aortic insufficiency because of the presence of more severe left ventricular dysfunction preoperatively. Long-term survival is approximately 85% to 90% at 5 years (Marshall and Kouchoukos, 1989).

Other considerations affect the timing and subsequent success of surgery. A thorough dental assessment is performed, and abscessed or carious teeth are repaired or removed prior to surgery so that they are not an entry site for bacteria. Infections in other parts of the body are a strict contraindication to surgery and must be resolved before valve surgery is performed. Antiplatelet medications such as aspirin and dipyridamole, and anticoagulants such as warfarin (Coumadin) (e.g., for patients with chronic atrial fibrillation) are discontinued preoperatively to reduce the incidence of excessive perioperative bleeding.

Prostheses and their selection

Aortic valve prostheses tend to have a less bulky sewing ring than their mitral prosthetic valve counterparts. They are constructed in this way to reduce as much as possible the amount of material that would take up space within the valve orifice. This provides greater flow through the opening of the prosthesis. Some porcine aortic valve manufacturers (who produce the modified orifice Hancock valve, for example) further modify the valve by removing the leaflet con-

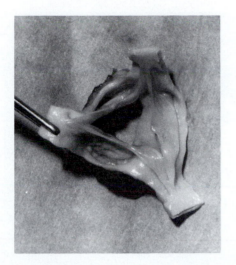

Fig. 14-12 Unstented aortic valve allograft (homograft). The attached aorta and subvalvular tissue have been removed by the surgeon. "Stented" allografts are mounted on a frame. (Courtesy CryoLife, Inc., Marietta, Ga.)

Box 14-1   Allografts (homografts): clinical considerations

No emboli, turbulence, or hemolysis
Deterioration occurs gradually
Degeneration manifested at about 7 years
Incidence of degeneration uncertain
Slow process of degeneration; valve-related deaths rare
Patient survival better than with prosthetic valves
Satisfactory valve for children
Quality of life is excellent
May be immunologically active

Modified from Ross D: Application of homografts in clinical surgery, *J Cardiac Surg* 1(3, suppl):175, 1987.

---

taining a muscle shelf (found in all pig aortic valves) and replacing it with a leaflet from another pig valve that does not have this restrictive leaflet. Thus two pig valves are necessary to produce these bioprostheses.

Unfortunately, all prosthetic valves have inherent disadvantages (see Box 13-6 and Table 13-4). The hemodynamic performance of a prosthesis is critical in aortic valve surgery, and the residual transvalvular gradients associated with prosthetic aortic valves can make selection of a suitable replacement prosthesis difficult. For example, an active life-style requires an increased cardiac output during exercise. This is hemodynamically significant, especially in patients with small aortic roots having annular diameters of 19 to 21 mm or less. Although a 19 mm prosthesis generally provides acceptable transvalvular blood flow, in large or very active persons the orifice of a 19 mm prosthesis may not allow a sufficient stroke volume and cardiac output to meet tissue demands. (One could expect to see postoperative tachydysrhythmias as a compensatory mechanism for the decreased cardiac output.) With the further narrowing of the orifice from the presence of the prosthetic sewing ring, increasing the cardiac output requires greater ventricular work to overcome the pressure load. In these cases a significant residual pressure gradient restricts the potential effectiveness of valve replacement.

When the annulus is smaller than 19 mm, the surgeon may consider enlargement procedures so that a 19 mm or larger prosthetic valve can be implanted. A mechanical valve is usually selected in order to avoid reoperation, which is more likely with a bioprosthesis that can deteriorate over time.

In general, hemodynamic performance is acceptable for most currently available prostheses with an annular diameter of 25 mm or more (Morgan, Davis, and Fraker, 1985). In the smaller annulus (23 mm or less) the excellent flow characteristics of the St. Jude Medical valve make it a popular prosthesis (Arom and others, 1989) in many patients who can tolerate lifelong anticoagulation. In patients unable to take anticoagulants, a biologic valve is often the prosthesis of choice (Frater and others, 1992). An unstented allograft (homograft) is also an option, and it may be preferable in the small aortic root because there is no sewing ring to reduce the size of the orifice. ("Allograft" is now the correct term for tissue from one person's body placed in another person. The term is used preferentially by the Food and Drug Administration to regulate these grafts, which were commonly known as "homografts.")

Aortic valve allograft (homograft)

Patients requiring valve replacement but who are considered unsuitable candidates for insertion of a mechanical or biologic prosthesis may benefit from an aortic valve allograft (homograft) (Fig. 14-12; Box 14-1). Unstented aortic valve allografts are advantageous in small aortic roots because there is no sewing ring to decrease the size of the orifice. In addition, allografts do not require anticoagulation.

Ross (1962; see also Box 14-2), Barratt-Boyes (1964), and O'Brien, McGriffin, and Stafford (1989), who laid the groundwork for the use of allografts, stress the excellent long-term results and advocate the use of these grafts in all patients with pathologic conditions of the aortic valve and root. One of the few exceptions is the elderly patient in whom a bioprosthesis would give a comparable result.

Pulmonary allografts (Fig. 14-13), another graft source, may also be used. Both aortic and pulmonary allografts are procured from cadavers without a history of communicable disease, disseminated malignancy, diabetes, hypertension, hyperlipidemia, or previous sternotomy (Lange and Hopkins, 1989). The grafts are obtained from cadaver hearts under sterile conditions in an operating room, subjected to micro-

When retracting aorta, be especially cautious to avoid lacerating aortic wall, coronary ostia, and adjacent structures.

If hand-held coronary ostial cannulas are used for cardioplegia, ensure that no air is present in tubing before infusion; prepare cannulas for infusion (e.g., flush) when ECG activity is noted or surgeon requests it; left coronary ostial cannula is usually shaped like an L, and right coronary ostial cannula is usually shaped like a J.

When retroplegia cardioplegia is used, anticipate back bleeding from the coronary ostia and the need to suction more frequently (unless there is a pause in suturing while cardioplegia solution is given).

Adjust position of aortic root retractors as stitches are placed into each commissure.

Assist in keeping valve suture pledgets aligned.

Keep sutures from tangling with use of suture holder, suture tags, or other method per protocol.

Keep running count of stitches in each leaflet (or annular segment), as well as total count.

Use moist sponges to clean instruments, suction tips, etc., of loose calcium particles or other debris.

Use open-tip suction to remove calcium pieces and other debris; suction frequently and whenever loose material is noted in operative field; alert surgeon to presence of material.

Keep bioprostheses moist with frequent saline irrigation (with bulb syringe); prevent drying out.

Watch for calcium particles in crevices of aorta or aortic root (especially where surgeon's view may be obscured) and on tips of instruments and suction catheters. Do not hesitate to wipe tips of instruments used by team members when debris is present (and before instruments are inserted into surgical site).

If heart must be elevated to inspect coronary anastomosis suture lines, do so cautiously to avoid puncturing ventricle with prosthetic struts.

If patch enlargement is performed, maintain alignment of material while surgeon cuts and shapes patch and during insertion into aortic root.

If eye cautery (battery powered) is used to create an opening in prosthetic graft for anastomosis, remove all pieces of excised graft material.

When implanting a Starr-Edwards 1260 aortic ball-and-cage prosthesis, ball poppet can be removed to facilitate insertion of stitches; ball should be stored in safe place until needed; it is easily reinserted into cage after stitches are tied and cut.

When surgeon is tying annular stitches, use Freer or similar instrument to separate sutures.

After the heart resumes beating, monitor the ECG for signs of ischema, which may be an indication of coronary ostial obstruction by the prosthesis.

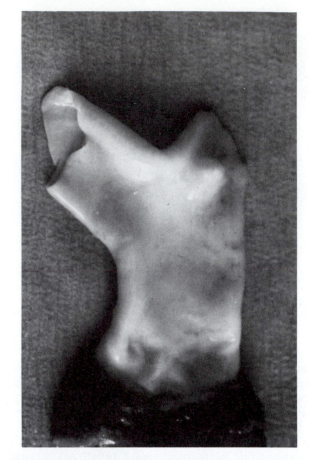

Fig. 14-13 Pulmonary allograft (homograft) containing the pulmonary valve, main pulmonary artery, and proximal portion of the bifurcation of the right and left pulmonary arteries. (Courtesy CryoLife, Inc., Marietta, Ga.)

bial testing, treated with nutrient media and antibiotics, and cryopreserved in a special freezer (Stelzer and Elkins, 1989). Prior to freezing, the leaflets of the valve are assessed for proper function, and the diameter of the annulus is measured. The allograft is sealed in a plastic bag and frozen in liquid nitrogen. Long-term storage is maintained at approximately minus 196° C (O'Brien, McGriffin, and Stafford, 1989). When needed for surgery, an array of grafts in different sizes is transported in a portable freezer. Once the appropriate graft is selected, it is thawed and implanted.

Pulmonary autografts are also being used more often. The patient's pulmonary valve may be used to replace the aortic valve, and a pulmonary allograft is inserted to replace the autograft.

Advantages of the allograft include excellent hemodynamics, nonthrombogenicity, and a lower incidence of infection postoperatively. They are especially attractive in young women and children and may be advantageous for patients with recurrent endocarditis, in whom it is preferable to avoid synthetic foreign material (Miller and Shumway, 1987). A disadvantage may be long-term durability, but Matsuki and colleagues (1988) describe excellent results 20 years after surgery. Although primary tissue failure does occur, the onset is not sudden, and it does not progress rapidly, as compared with some other bioprosthetic valves.

Patient teaching considerations

Teaching considerations for patients undergoing aortic valve surgery are based on the particular lesion, the type of surgery performed, and the impact that the disease and the treatment have on the patient (Table 14-2). As in all patients with valvular heart disease, the perioperative nurse will want to elicit the patient's understanding of the anticipated procedure and answer questions of the patient and family.

Nurses explain that the procedure will be tailored to the patient's needs, with anatomic considerations often playing a decisive role. Assessing the patient's life-style and activity level is important because an active 80-year-old, for example, may require a more hemodynamically satisfactory prosthesis than a seden-

Table 14-2 ■ *Standards of nursing care for aortic valve surgery*

Nursing diagnosis	Patient outcome	Nursing actions
Anxiety related to disease, surgery, and postoperative events	Patient demonstrates reduced levels of anxiety that promote therapeutic regimen	Elicit questions and concerns about disease and proposed treatment Identify and reinforce effective coping mechanisms; respect some denial Provide comfort measures; identify perceived needs and expectations
Knowledge deficit related to inadequate knowledge of planned surgery and perioperative events	Patient demonstrates knowledge of physiologic and psychologic responses to aortic valve surgery	Determine patient's understanding of aortic valve disease; possible surgical interventions (aortic valve or root enlargement, valve replacement); types, benefits, and risks of prostheses; and preferences if any Determine patient's understanding of surgical procedure; describe (briefly) immediate preoperative events (that will occur while patient is awake); reinforce or clarify what patient (and family) has been told by surgeon; elicit expected outcome of surgery Assess patient's life-style (exercise limits, geographic location, proximity to laboratory facilities, community resources, support groups); note age and, if female, ability or desire to have children, possible need for anticoagulation If additional myocardial revascularization procedures are to be performed (coronary artery bypass grafts), assess patient's understanding and clarify as necessary Assess patient's ability to cooperate with possible anticoagulation regimen; assess family support mechanism
High risk for infection related to surgery	Patient is free of infection related to aseptic technique	Culture excised valve and suture as requested Confine and contain instruments and supplies used to excise infected valve tissue Place mechanical prosthesis in antibiotic solution prior to implantation as requested by surgeon Keep instruments free of debris Document lot and serial numbers of implants
High risk for altered skin integrity	Patient's skin integrity is maintained	In severely thin and malnourished patients (cardiac cachexia), use additional padding to protect skin, joints, and bony prominences
High risk for injury related to use of valve retractor	Patient is free of injury from use of retraction devices	Use hand-held valve retractors with caution to avoid injury to aortic wall, coronary ostia
High risk for injury related to: Retained foreign objects	Patient is free of injury related to: Retained foreign objects	Account for valve sizers, holders, handles, and other items Keep instruments free of tissue, suture, and calcium debris Confirm that Starr-Edwards ball poppet is securely replaced in cage (model 1260 prosthesis)
Chemical hazards	Chemical hazards	Label syringes containing antibiotic solutions, heparinized saline, or other solutions; use only physiologically compatible solutions to rinse bioprosthetic valve; do not place bioprosthesis in antibiotic solution (injures valve); follow protocol for removing glutaraldehyde from bioprostheses (rinsing in three baths of saline for at least 2 minutes each); keep bioprostheses moist with saline during implantation

Modified from Seifert PC: Cardiac surgery. In Rothrock JC: *Perioperative nursing care planning,* St Louis, 1990, Mosby.

Continued.

Table 14-2 ■ *Standards of nursing care for aortic valve surgery—cont'd*

Nursing diagnosis	Patient outcome	Nursing actions
Physical hazards	Physical hazards	Have available type and sizes of valvular prostheses desired by surgeon; store valves in cool, dry location; have appropriate accessories to size and insert valve; have necessary suture available (pledgeted, nonpledgeted, multicolored) Cardioplegia solution may be infused directly into coronary ostia; have hand-held cannulas available (L-shaped tip for left coronary os; J-shaped tip for right coronary os); have appropriate tubing for retrograde cardioplegia infusion; determine if initial bolus of cardioplegia solution will be given via aortic root (patients with aortic stenosis and minimal or no insufficiency) and have tubing, connectors, and others items as needed If aortic enlargement is planned, have patch material and suture per surgeon's request Be prepared with needles and venting catheters to deair left ventricle (superior right pulmonary venous catheter is often inserted); test vents to ensure they are suctioning
Thermal injury	Thermal injury	If aortic valve allograft is used, avoid contact with graft in frozen condition; follow manufacturer's instructions for thawing graft in warm water baths; use insulated gloves when handling cryopreserved valve; if allografts are stored on premises, monitor temperature of storage tank to protect viability of allograft; replace coolant as necessary In patients with left ventricular hypertrophy, anticipate need for additional topical cold solutions and more frequent infusion of cardioplegia solution to provide transmural cooling/cardioplegic arrest
High risk for self-care deficit related to inadequate knowledge of rehabilitation period	Patient demonstrates knowledge of rehabilitation period as it relates to self-care abilities.	Assess patient's knowledge of signs/symptoms of valve failure Assess patient's understanding of medications prescribed; signs/symptoms of anticoagulation-related hemorrhage, thrombosis, emboli; need for antibiotic prophylaxis prior to invasive procedures; need for follow-up laboratory tests (prothrombin time) Identify signs/symptoms of anticoagulation-related hemorrhage (notify physician): 　Nosebleeds, bleeding gums 　Red or brown urine 　Red or black bowel movements 　Bleeding from cuts that cannot be stopped, bruises that get larger 　Severe and persistent headaches 　Abdominal pain 　Faintness, dizziness, or unusual weakness 　Excessive menstrual flow Identify signs/symptoms of suboptimal anticoagulation (notify physician): 　Stroke, transient ischemic attacks 　Closing sound of prosthesis no longer audible; absent "click" 　Sudden onset of congestive heart failure List precautions for patients receiving anticoagulants: 　Use a soft-bristled toothbrush 　Use electric shavers rather than razors 　Wear gloves when gardening 　Do not go barefoot 　Trim nails with a soft emery board instead of scissors or clippers 　Avoid sports in which skin may be broken or internal injuries may occur Provide patient with name of person to contact if questions/problems arise Provide information for obtaining and using medical alert bracelet

Box 14-3 Aortic valve surgery: procedural considerations

Instrumentation
Hand-held aortic valve retractors

Valve Prostheses and Accessories
Mechanical heart valves
Bioprostheses (porcine or bovine pericardium)
Sizers (obturators), range of sizes, specific to prosthesis
Sizer (obturator) handles
Prosthetic valve holders and handles (some prostheses are packaged with an attached holder); sterile nurse applies handle into holder

Supplies
Valve suture, single and multipack (multicolored):
    Pledgeted
    Nonpledgeted
Suture organizer (if used)
Preferred patch material (for enlarging aortic root)
Free pledgets, precut or cut to size
18- or 19-gauge needle to deair ventricle
Long (spinal) 18-gauge needle for transseptal deairing of ventricle
Additional basins for bioprosthetic saline rinse, antibiotic solutions, allograft thawing/preparation, or glutaraldehyde preparation of autologous pericardium
Culture tubes (for valve tissue, suture, rinse solutions)
Venting lines for deairing left ventricle
Left superior pulmonary venting catheter (apical vent rare)
Two-stage venous cannula commonly used

Positioning
Supine
If coronary bypass grafts to be performed, patient positioned as for removal of leg vein (see Chapter 12)

Skin Preparation
Midline of chest, inner aspect of both legs shaved
Legs washed at least to knees

Draping
Anterior chest exposed
Legs exposed from groin to knees (can be covered with a towel if access is not required)
Anesthesia screen placed over lower legs to keep drapes off feet

Special Infection Control Measures
Confine and contain tissue and instruments from infected tissue
Culture valve tissue, rinse solutions, and other items as requested by surgeon
Place mechanical prostheses in antibiotic solution prior to insertion as requested by surgeon
Keep instruments free of debris
Document lot and serial numbers of all implants

Special Safety Measures
Label syringes and containers of solutions, medications:
    Antibiotic solution
    Heparinized saline
    Glutaraldehyde
Account for all sizers, handles, and holders used to size and insert a prosthesis, as well as pledget material, suture needles, hypodermic needles
Monitor presence of ventricular failure and possible need for mechanical ventricular support (intraaortic balloon or ventricular assist device)
Keep prostheses stored in a cool, dry, contamination-free location
If using Starr-Edwards ball-and-cage valve, keep poppet in safe place while suturing valve ring

Documentation/Report to Cardiac Surgical Intensive Care Unit*
Procedure, type of replacement prosthesis
Lot and serial numbers of prosthesis
Preoperative diagnosis (stenosis, regurgitation, or both; congestive heart failure; syncope; angina pectoris; onset)
Epicardial pacemaker lead placement (single, dual), and if being paced
Patient problems, concerns related to valvular heart disease, surgery
Preoperative left ventricular function (e.g., ejection fraction)
Completion of valve implant card (and sent to manufacturer)

*In addition to standard documentation/postoperative report; see Chapter 9.

---

tary 60-year-old. Various options and reasons provided by the surgeon for the selection of one prosthesis over another can be clarified for the patient.

As with patients undergoing mitral valve replacement, the ability and desire to follow recommended therapeutic regimens must be evaluated. Anticoagulation-related hemorrhage and endocarditis should be discussed and safety measures identified (Whitman and Guzzetta, 1992). Bioprosthetic failure, thrombosis of the disk occluder, and dehiscence can also occur. Laboratory follow-up is required to adjust warfarin levels and maintain prothrombin times within an acceptable range.

Procedural considerations
Aortic valve instruments are added to the basic cardiac setup (Box 14-3). Longer knife handles, needle holders, scissors, and forceps may be required, particularly in patients with a deep chest cavity. One or two hand-held aortic valve leaflet retractors (Fig. 14-14) are used for exposure (see Box 14-2 for RN first assistant considerations).

Because of the presence of extensive calcification on many native valves, some surgeons prefer to use a taper cutting needle (rather than a plain taper needle) for easier insertion of the stitches into the calcified

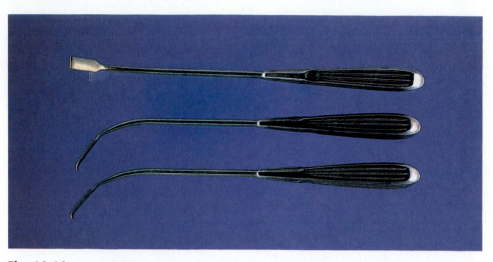

Fig. 14-14 **Aortic valve leaflet retractors.** (From Brooks-Tighe SM: *Instrumentation for the operating room: a photographic manual,* ed 3, St Louis, 1989, Mosby.)

annulus. Alternately colored stitches are used (as they are for mitral valve replacement).

Prosthetic valves and accessories for sizing and implanting the prosthesis should be immediately available and distinguishable from each other. The nurse should be able to quickly select the appropriate type and size obturator requested. Even if the surgeon plans to use a specific type of prosthesis (e.g., a mechanical or biologic valve), obturators for both should be on the field because anatomic conditions noted during assessment of the native valve may require a change in plan. It is helpful to arrange and label the obturators according to size and type, especially when multiple valve replacement is planned. Prosthesis handles also differ depending on the manufacturer and should be differentiated as well.

The surgeon may elect to enlarge a small aortic root. Preferred graft material should be available to perform this procedure.

If an aortic (or pulmonary) valve allograft (Box 14-4) is used, additional basins for thawing and reconstitution of the graft are needed, along with scissors, and clamps or forceps for preparation. Insulated gloves are required to protect the hands of the person retrieving the frozen allograft from the portable freezer. Additional scissors and forceps will be needed when the surgeon trims the graft at the field.

Basins are also necessary for rinsing glutaraldehyde-preserved biologic valves; the valve should be rinsed for at least 2 minutes in each of three basins (total time: 6 minutes) containing normal saline. An additional sterile nurse is helpful for procedures that require preparation (thawing, rinsing) of implants. When tissue implants are used, cultures are often taken of the rinse solution, a small piece of the discarded excess allograft, and/or the needles used for suturing.

Myocardial protection is achieved with retrograde cardioplegia infusion. This method is reliable and easier than the antegrade method, and it reduces the

---

Box 14-4 **Comments on aortic valve homografts (allografts)**

Donald Ross
Fellow, Royal College of Surgeons
National Heart Hospital, London

Aortic valve homografts are centrally flowing and are consequently nonobstructive and give rise to neither emboli nor turbulence. They do, however, undergo a slow process of degeneration, giving plenty of time for an elective low-risk second operation. An additional advantage is that they can be used in children.

The quality of life of the homograft patient, who is removed from the dangers of embolism and anticoagulant hemorrhage, the ingestion of pills, regular hematologic checks, restrictions on pregnancy, and the danger of sudden death, is considerably better than that of the mechanical valve patient and very close to normal living.

This quality of life as opposed to quantity is not something that can be evaluated statistically. From the patient's point of view, however, it is a very important feature and is reflected in the fact that most patients ask for a homograft for their second operation.

Long-term results indicate that the unmounted homograft (in contrast to one attached to a stent) in the aortic area gives better results than currently used bioprostheses, and in the right ventricular outflow tract there is no comparable valve.

Since 1982 homografts have remained our preferred method of replacement of the aortic valve, irrespective of age, sex, and the severity of the lesion.

Modified and excerpted from Ross D: Application of homografts in clinical surgery, *J Cardiac Surg* 1(3, suppl):175, 1987.

potential injury to the coronary ostia associated with the use of hand-held antegrade infusion cannulas. Standard retrograde cardioplegia systems need no special additional preparation for aortic valve surgery.

Occasionally coronary ostial cardioplegia catheters are needed for antegrade cardioplegia infusion if retroplegia cannot be used. The disposable or nondisposable infusion tips are preshaped to facilitate insertion into the left or right coronary os. Generally, the left coronary cannula is L-shaped, and the right coronary cannula is J-shaped.

In patients with coronary artery disease (and aortic stenosis with minimal or no insufficiency), both antegrade and retrograde cardioplegia infusion is used, with the initial bolus of cardioplegia solution infused antegradely through the aortic root before the aorta is opened. This is unfeasible in the presence of aortic insufficiency because the incompetent valve leaflets will allow the cardioplegia solution to flow preferentially through the valve orifice into the left ventricle rather than into the coronary ostia. This produces ventricular distension and a delay in achieving car-

dioplegic arrest. If this occurs, the surgeon uses retrograde cardioplegia infusion; bypass grafts are selectively infused antegradely with cardioplegia solution through tubing connected to the retroplegia system.

Operative procedure: aortic valve replacement

Aortic valve replacement is the excision of the diseased aortic valve and replacement with a biologic or mechanical prosthesis or an aortic valve homograft. Before the procedure begins, the sterile nurse prepares a sterile field on a small table. On this is placed three small round basins, suture scissors, and a pair of forceps. Prosthesis handles specific to the types of prostheses available can be arranged nearby. Culture tubes and syringes are added if a bioprosthesis is selected.

Procedure

1. A median sternotomy is performed, cardiopulmonary bypass is instituted using a two-stage cannula for venous drainage, and the patient is cooled to approximately 22° C (72° F) (Fig. 14-15, *A*). A

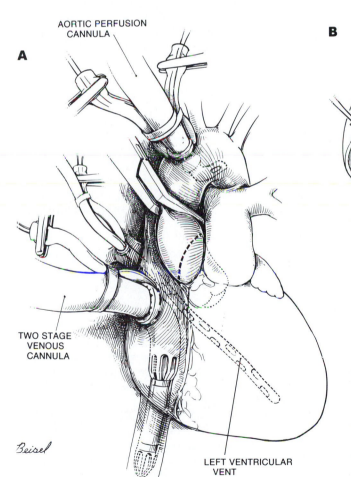
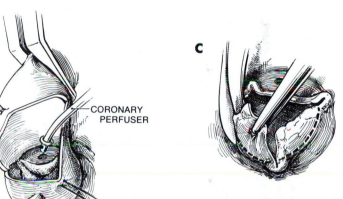

Fig. 14-15 Aortic valve replacement. **A,** Arterial inflow is established with an aortic perfusion cannula in the ascending aorta distal to the cross-clamp. The two-stage venous cannula is inserted into the right atrium; the distal openings receive blood from the inferior vena cava, and the proximal openings (in the atrium) drain blood returning from the superior vena cava and the coronary sinus. A catheter is inserted through the right superior pulmonary vein and passed into the left ventricle to suction away blood during the valve replacement and to vent air after the valve is implanted and before the cross-clamp is removed. A retrograde cardioplegia infusion catheter (not shown) can be inserted into the coronary sinus via the right atrium. **B,** The aortotomy is made above the aortic valve, and two retraction sutures are placed in the aorta. If retroplegic arrest cannot be used, hand-held coronary ostial perfusers are inserted into the coronary ostia. Shown is the left cannula tip which is often L-shaped for ease of insertion. The right coronary ostium is below and under the aortic incision; a perfuser with a J-shaped tip makes insertion into the right ostium easier. **C,** Valve leaflets are resected. *Continued.*

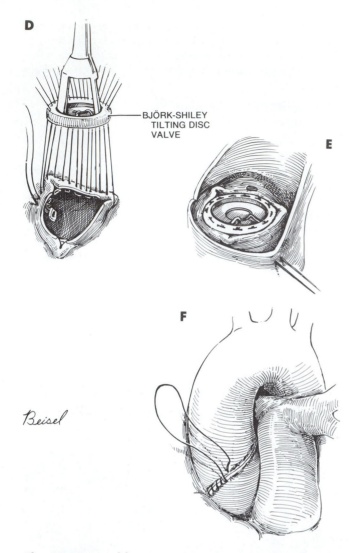

D

BJÖRK-SHILEY
TILTING DISC
VALVE

E

F

Beisel

Fig. 14-15, cont'd. **D,** Stitches with pledgets in the subannular position are placed in the annulus and then into the sewing ring of a low-profile prosthesis. **E,** Prosthesis in position with the stitches tied and cut. (Note that the prosthesis shown—the Bjork-Shiley—is no longer available in the United States.) **F,** The aorta is closed with a running suture. (For clarity, the cross-clamp is not shown) (From Waldhausen JA, Pierce WS: *Johnson's surgery of the chest,* ed 5, St Louis, 1985, Mosby.)

venting catheter is passed through the right superior pulmonary vein, past the mitral valve, and into the left ventricle, where it will suction blood and vent air after the valve is implanted.

The aorta is clamped. Cardioplegia solution is given antegradely through the root or retrogradely through a catheter in the coronary sinus. Direct ostial infusion is accomplished with hand-held catheters (Fig. 14-15, *B*). A cooling pad may be wrapped around the ventricle to enhance cooling.

The valve is exposed through a transverse aortotomy above the coronary ostia (Fig. 14-16).
2. The aortic valve leaflets are excised with a knife or scissors, leaving a rim of tissue at the base of the

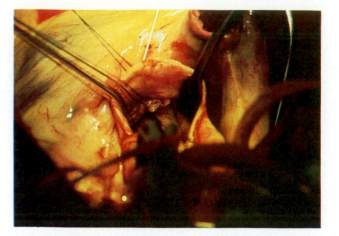

Fig. 14-16 The aortic root is exposed through a transverse aortotomy. (Courtesy Edward A. Lefrak, MD; Doug Yarnold, CRNA, photographer.)

cusp (Fig. 14-15, *C*). When calcification is present, rongeurs may be used to remove calcified particles. A small round cup with saline is placed in a location where the surgeon can rinse debris from the rongeur tips. The rongeur and other instrument tips are wiped with a moist sponge to remove remaining particles. Care is taken to remove all loose tissue and other debris. (Some surgeons place a small radiopaque sponge into the left ventricular cavity to catch loose material.) Irrigation followed by suction helps to remove debris as well.
3. The surgeon sizes the annulus with obturators specific to the prosthesis desired and requests the appropriate-size valve. Occasionally, anatomic conditions necessitate a different type of valve; because this is a possibility, there should be a table with basins for rinsing a bioprosthesis even if a mechanical valve was the original valve of choice.
4. The valve selected is delivered to the field after the type and size are verified by circulating and sterile nurses. Identification tags attached to the prostheses are cut with scissors, taking care not to injure the valve.
   a. **Mechanical valve:**
      (1) Starr-Edwards—the poppet is removed and placed in a dish with heparinized saline; the valve handle is attached by engaging the top of the cage, and the prosthesis is placed on the back table until needed.
      (2) Medtronic-Hall—the prosthesis and attached handle are taken from the package and placed on the back table until needed.
      (3) St. Jude Medical—the valve within its valve stand is removed from the container; the handle is screwed into the holder preattached to the prosthesis, and the prosthesis is removed from its valve stand. The prosthesis is placed on the back table until needed.

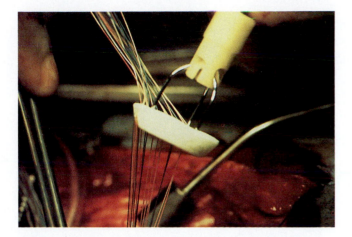

Fig. 14-17 Nonpledgeted interrupted sutures are passed through the sewing ring of a Starr-Edwards 1260 aortic valve. Note that the poppet has been removed to facilitate insertion of the sutures. (Courtesy Edward A. Lefrak, MD; Doug Yarnold, CRNA, photographer.)

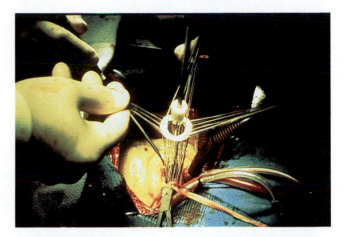

Fig. 14-18 All the stitches have been inserted into the native annulus and the sewing ring; they are grouped into three sets to correspond with the aortic commissures. (Courtesy Edward A. Lefrak, MD; Doug Yarnold, CRNA, photographer.)

b. **Biologic valve:**
  (1) Carpentier-Edwards porcine and pericardial aortic valve (Model 2700)—the valve is transferred with forceps from the container to the table prepared with basins of saline. The valve handle is screwed into the preattached valve holder. Any packing material is removed, and the bioprosthesis is placed in the first of three basins containing normal saline. The valve is gently agitated (holding the handle) for a minimum of 2 minutes. The valve is placed in the second basin for 2 minutes and in the third basin for 2 minutes. Cultures may be taken of the last bath solution (or all three basins) with a 10 ml syringe and sent to the laboratory. A separate syringe is used for drawing up a sample from each bath culture. After the valve has been adequately rinsed free of the glutaraldehyde storage solution, it is placed in a saline-moistened sponge and placed on the back table until needed. The prosthesis should not be allowed to dry.
  (2) Hancock porcine valve—the procedure is similar to that for the Carpentier-Edwards valve.
5. Pledgeted (or nonpledgeted) sutures are passed through the valve annulus and then into the prosthetic sewing ring (Figs. 14-15, *D*, and 14-17). Some surgeons prefer to place the annular stitches first, followed by insertion of the sewing ring sutures (Harlan, Starr, and Harwin, 1980). Felt-pledgeted sutures provide a good seal between the skirt of the prosthesis and the annulus, thereby helping to prevent the development of perivalvular leaks (Walhausen and Pierce, 1985).
6. The valve is threaded into the annulus, and the stitches are tied and cut (Figs. 14-15, *E*, 14-18, and 14-19).

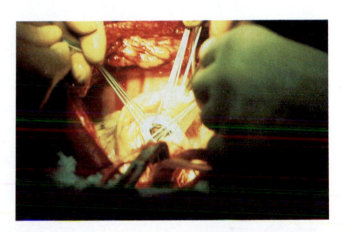

Fig. 14-19 The prosthesis is seated into the annulus. After the stitches are tied and cut, the poppet is replaced into the cage. (Courtesy Edward A. Lefrak, MD; Doug Yarnold, CRNA, photographer.)

7. The aortotomy is closed with a single or double running suture. To close a transverse aortic incision without tension, a folded towel may be placed under the handle of the cross-clamp to tilt it forward slightly, thereby bringing the edges of the aortotomy into closer approximation. If the aortic tissue is of poor quality, felt buttressing of the suture line may be performed (Waldhausen and Pierce, 1985).
8. The left ventricle is deaired, and the cross-clamp is removed.

Operative procedures: enlargement of the small aortic root

The following procedures are intended to enlarge the diameter of the annulus by 2 to 3 mm, allowing insertion of at least a 19 mm aortic valve prosthesis.

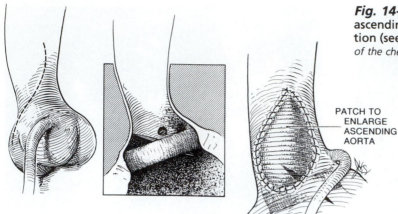

Fig. 14-20 Patch enlargement of a narrowed proximal ascending aorta producing supravalvular outflow obstruction (see text). (From Waldhausen JA, Pierce WS: *Johnson's surgery of the chest*, ed 5, St Louis, 1985, Mosby.)

Patch enlargement of the proximal ascending aorta (Fig. 14-20). When narrowing of the aorta is confined to the proximal ascending aorta, patch repair can be performed by making an oblique aortotomy and extending it into the noncoronary cusp. A diamond-shaped patch of preclotted woven Dacron or glutaraldehyde-preserved pericardium is sewn to the edges of the aortotomy. The size of the graft determines by how much the aorta is enlarged (Waldhausen and Pierce, 1985).

Nicks procedure (Fig. 14-21). An oblique incision is made in the aortic root. The valve leaflets are excised, and the annulus is measured. The incision is continued downward to the noncoronary sinus, dividing the aortic annulus, and extended only to the origin of the anterior mitral leaflet. A wedge-shaped Dacron patch is fashioned and sutured from the apex of the aortotomy to just beyond the annulus with 4-0 polypropylene. Felt pledgets may be needed (Waldhausen and Pierce, 1985).

Manouguian procedure (Fig. 14-22). The incision is more medial than that of the Nicks procedure. The

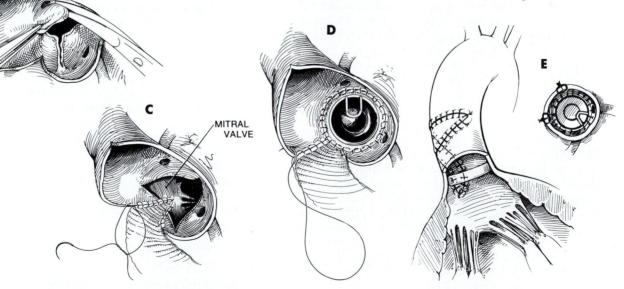

Fig. 14-21 Nicks procedure for aortic root enlargement (see text). Note the relationship between the aortic valve and the anterior leaflet of the mitral valve. (From Waldhausen JA, Pierce WS: *Johnson's surgery of the chest*, ed 5, St Louis, 1985, Mosby.)

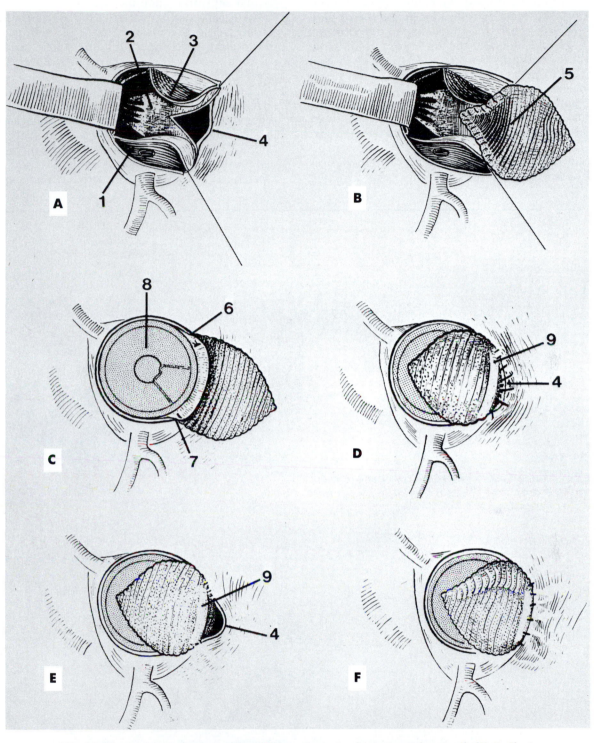

Fig. 14-22 Manouguian procedure for aortic root enlargement (see text). (Note that the prosthesis—the Bjork-Shiley—is no longer available in the United States). *1,* Left semilunar cusp; *2,* anterior mitral leaflet; *3,* noncoronary semilunar cusp; *4,* left atrial wall; *5,* patch; *6-7,* enlargement of the aortic valve ring; *8,* aortic valve prosthesis; *9,* sewing ring of the prosthesis. (From Manouguian A, Seybold-Epting W: Patch enlargement of the aortic valve ring, *J Thorac Cardiovasc Surg* 78[3]:402, 1979.)

transverse aortotomy is made into the commissure between the left coronary cusp and the noncoronary cusp and extended toward the center of the fibrous origin of the anterior mitral leaflet. A Dacron or pericardial patch is sutured to the V-shaped defect in the anterior mitral leaflet and the aortic root, thereby reestablishing continuity between the two (Manouguian and Seybold-Epting, 1979).

Konno-Rastan procedure (Fig. 14-23). The left ventricular outflow tract (LVOT) is enlarged by opening and enlarging the right ventricular outflow tract through the septum, creating a ventricular septal defect.

The aorta is incised vertically, and the incision is carried down into the right coronary cusp, avoiding the coronary orifice. The right ventricle is incised transversely below the pulmonary valve, and the ventricular septum is then incised.

A Dacron patch is cut to fit the area from the septotomy, across the annulus, to the ascending aorta. At the location of the annulus, the patch needs to be cut large enough to accept a sufficiently large prosthesis.

The patch is sutured to the septum and then to the edges of the annulus. A valve prosthesis is brought to the field and sutured to the native annulus and to the patch graft. Finally, the patch is sutured to the aortotomy. The ventriculotomy is closed with a pericardial patch or Dacron patch. Another method is to use a patch to close just the septal defect and then insert

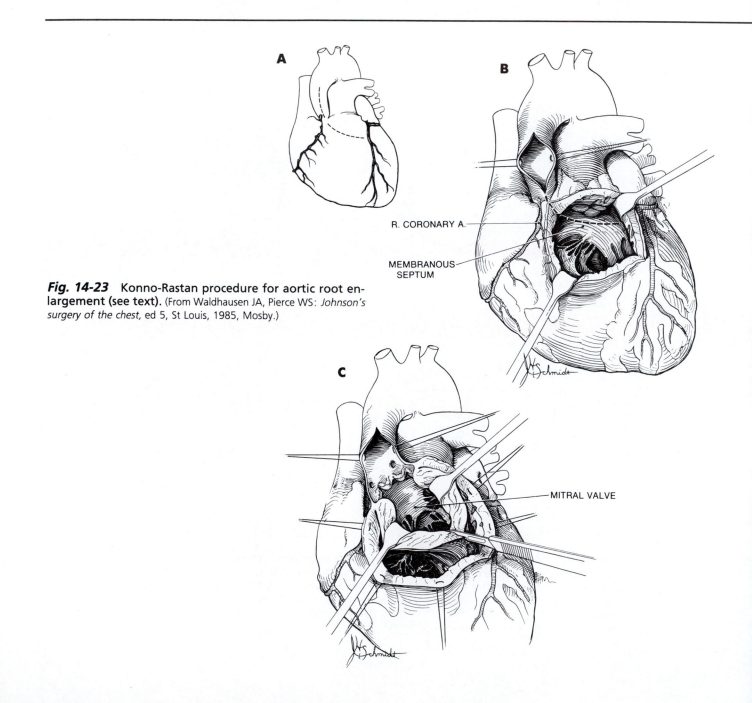

Fig. 14-23 Konno-Rastan procedure for aortic root enlargement (see text). (From Waldhausen JA, Pierce WS: *Johnson's surgery of the chest,* ed 5, St Louis, 1985, Mosby.)

the larger patch to close the aortotomy and ventriculotomy (Cooley, 1984).

This technique is particularly useful in children requiring an adult-size prosthesis. Complications include injury to the right coronary artery or the pulmonary valve, transection of a major left coronary artery septal perforator, complete heart block, and bleeding (Wisman and Waldhausen, 1991).

Left ventricular apicoabdominal aortic conduit (Fig. 14-24). Patients with a congenital, diffusely obstructed left ventricular outflow tract may benefit from this procedure (Cooley, 1984).

The left ventricular apex is exposed through a median sternotomy. The apex is stabbed well to the left of the anterior descending coronary artery with a

blade. A plug of myocardium is excised, and a specially made flanged cannula is inserted into the ventriculotomy. Interrupted pledgeted sutures are placed around the cannula to secure it to the myocardium. The cannula tip must penetrate the entire myocardial wall in order to avoid obstruction of the cannula tip.

The proximal end of a valved conduit is anastomosed end-to-end to the ventricular cannula; the distal end of the conduit is attached end-to-side to the descending thoracic or abdominal aorta. The advantage of sewing the conduit to the abdominal aorta is that if the valve within the conduit must be replaced, it is more easily accessible by laparotomy than by sternotomy (which would require dissection of sternal adhesions).

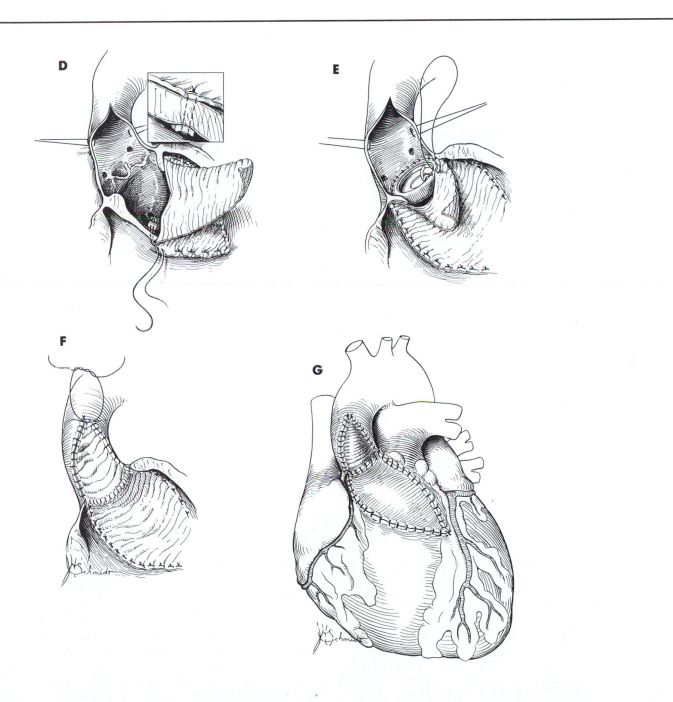

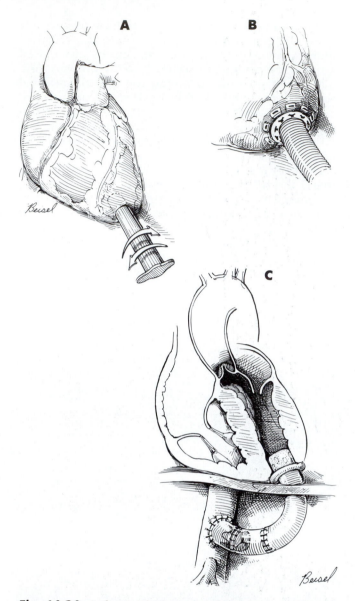

Fig. 14-24 Left ventricular apicoabdominal aortic conduit (see text). (From Waldhausen JA, Pierce WS: *Johnson's surgery of the chest*, ed 5, St Louis, 1985, Mosby.)

Operative procedure: allograft (homograft) replacement of the aortic valve, aortic root

Allografts are most commonly used in the aortic position. Because of the more complex structure of the mitral and tricuspid apparatus, allografts are infrequently used to replace these valves. Less commonly, the graft is mounted on a stent and used for tricuspid valve replacement (see Chapter 15).

Unmounted aortic allografts consisting of only the valve (or the valve and a portion of the attached aorta) are used to replace the excised native valve or, more commonly, the aortic root of the patient. Occasionally the graft is mounted onto a stent for aortic valve replacement, but this reduces the orifice area that is gained with the freehand insertion technique (Ross, 1987).

Supplies for allograft thawing include a sterile field prepared on a separate table, three 300 ml basins, a 50 ml syringe, two pairs of straight suture scissors, a Kelly clamp, vascular forceps, dissecting scissors (Metzenbaum or Cooley My scissors), and a specimen cup containing 10 ml of sterile saline (Graf and Gonzales-Lavin, 1988).

Procedure

1. A supply of cryopreserved grafts is transported to the operating room in a portable liquid nitrogen storage cylinder.

   In some institutions, fresh allografts are procured on the premises. They are measured, immersed in antibiotic solution and a preservative, and implanted. Cryopreservation is more common.

2. After the heart is arrested, a transverse, vertical, or semivertical incision is made in the aorta (O'Brien, McGriffin, and Stafford, 1989; Ross, 1991).

3. The recipient aortic root is sized with standard valve obturators or special cylindric sizers as described by Ross (1991). The appropriate-size allograft is selected, and if it is cryopreserved, it is taken from the portable freezer.

4. During thawing and reconstitution, concomitant procedures such as coronary artery bypass grafting may be performed.

5. Using insulated gloves, the circulating nurse (or a technician) removes the selected frozen valve from the container and places the bag holding the graft into a basin of warm (about 42° C [108° F]) water. Once the bag is pliable enough to open, it is dried, and the top of the bag is cut with sterile scissors, exposing the inner storage bag. The sterile nurse removes the inner bag with the sterile clamp and transfers it to a warm sterile water bath; the transferring forceps are removed from the field (Graf and Gonzales-Lavin, 1988).

   After a few minutes the inner bag is opened, and the contents are placed in the first of four basins filled with nutrient medium. The graft is rinsed in each basin for 2 minutes (total time: 8 minutes) and delivered to the field (O'Brien, McGriffin, and Stafford, 1989). This procedure will vary according to the allograft supplier's protocol.

6. The lower muscular margin is trimmed in preparation for implantation. A piece of excess tissue may be sent to the laboratory for aerobic, anaerobic, and fungal cultures.

7. The graft requires both proximal and distal suture lines.

   a. Proximal suture line (Fig. 14-25, *A*): Marking sutures help to align each allograft commissure and the corresponding point below the native valve annulus. The valve is inverted into the left ventricle, and each of these marking sutures is tied. The suture line is then performed with interrupted or continuous sutures (Fig. 14-25, *B*). Special caution is taken in the area of the membranous septum to avoid injury to bundle of His conduction tissue.

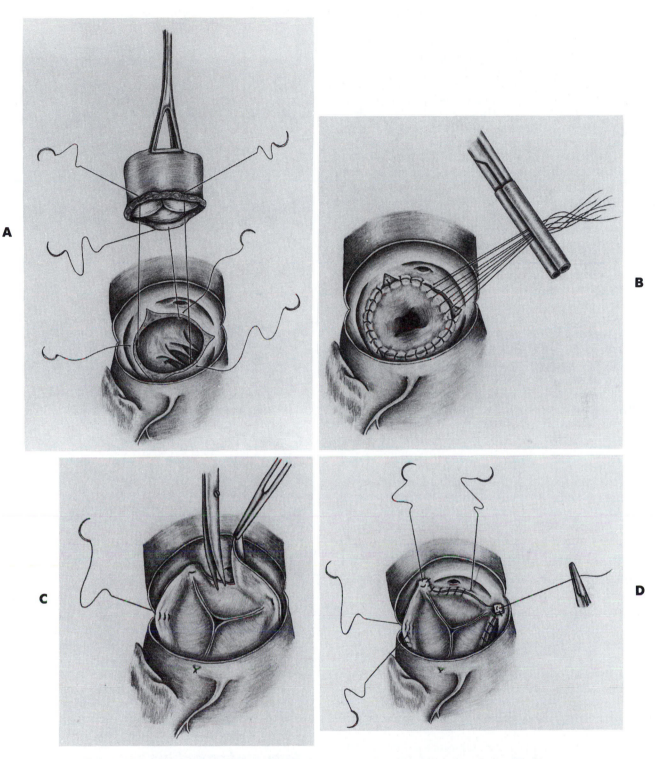

Fig. 14-25 Allograft (homograft) aortic valve replacement (see text). **A,** Marking sutures are placed from the base of the sinuses of both the aortic root and the allograft. The proximal suture line begins with sutures at the midpoint of each sinus of Valsalva. **B,** The allograft has been inverted and sewn below the native annulus with continuous or interrupted sutures. **C,** The valve is everted, and the commissures are anchored. The sinuses containing the right and left coronary ostia are scalloped to allow blood to enter the coronary circulation. **D,** The noncoronary sinus is left intact, and the distal suture line is a running suture below the coronary orifices. (From Randolph JD and others: Aortic valve and left ventricular outflow tract replacement using allograft and autograft valves, *Ann Thorac Surg* 48:345, 1989; drawing by M. LaWaun Hance, SA, PA-C.)

b. The graft is everted and brought back up into the aorta.

c. The allograft is then scalloped so that when it is in position it will expose the native coronary ostia (Fig. 14-25, *C*).

d. Distal suture line (Fig. 14-25, *D*): Three double-armed sutures are used for the distal suture line using the knots of the previous proximal sutures as a guide. Each suture is passed through the graft and the adjacent native sinus using a continuous over-and-over technique. The suture is run along the edge of the graft to the top of the pillar, passed through the pillar and the aortic wall, and then tied outside the aorta. The other two pillars are sutured in the same way (O'Brien, McGriffin, and Stafford, 1989; Randolph and others, 1989).

8. When the suture lines are completed, the surgeon tests the valve for competency. Saline is instilled into the left ventricle, and the valve leaflets are tested for competency (Graf and Gonzales-Lavin, 1988).

9. The aorta is closed.

Aortic valve replacement may be performed with the patient's pulmonary valve (autograft). The autograft is harvested from the right ventricular outflow tract and implanted into the native aortic root as described above. The right ventricular outflow tract is reconstructed with a pulmonary allograft (Randolph and others, 1989).

When the native annulus is 21 mm or less, patch enlargement may be performed first. The allograft proximal suture line is then performed without the inversion technique, because it takes up too much space in the annulus. The distal continuous suture line is performed in the same manner as described above (O'Brien, McGriffin, and Stafford, 1989).

Operative procedure: myomyectomy for hypertrophic subaortic stenosis (Morrow and others, 1975)

A bar or wedge of hypertrophic septal muscle is excised in order to relieve left ventricular outflow obstruction (Fig. 14-26).

Procedure

1. An incision is made in the ascending aorta and extended down into the noncoronary cusp sinus of Valsalva.

2. The (normal) aortic valve leaflets are retracted and protected from injury.

3. Bulging hypertrophic septal muscle beneath the right coronary leaflet is assessed. The anterior leaflet of the mitral valve may be thickened and opaque.

4. A flat narrow ribbon retractor is passed through the aortic valve annulus to displace and protect the anterior mitral leaflet.

5. A knife with a No. 10 or 12 hook blade is used to shave excess septal tissue. (An angled knife handle facilitates this maneuver). A second myotomy is made parallel to the first incision so that a generous

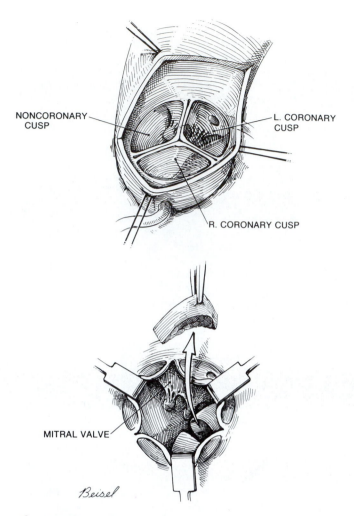

Fig. 14-26 Morrow procedure for resection of septal hypertrophy (see text). (From Waldhausen JA, Pierce WS: *Johnson's surgery of the chest*, ed 5, St Louis, 1985, Mosby.)

wedge can be excised. Cutting to a depth of more than 15 to 20 mm into the hypertrophied septum can cause a ventricular septal defect (Cooley, 1984).

6. Resection of the muscle bar may be completed with scissors, a rectangular knife, or, if necessary, an angled rongeur. Loose myocardial fragments are removed. Care is taken to avoid injury to conduction tissue under the right and noncoronary cusps.

7. The incision is closed. If a ventricular septal defect was created, it is closed and the repair is evaluated by transesophageal echocardiography (TEE).

Associated procedures

Aortic valve endocarditis. Surgery for aortic valve endocarditis is performed when there is evidence of recurrent septic emboli, the appearance of new or more serious dysrhythmias, resistance to antibiotic therapy, or profound hemodynamic deterioration. Valve replacement is performed in the usual manner unless there is extension of the infection onto the annular or subannular structures. An allograft may be considered.

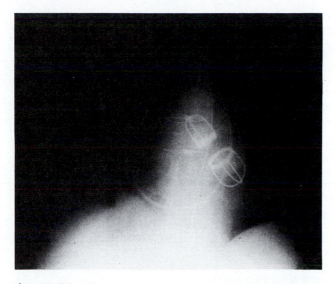

Fig. 14-27   Chest x-ray film of a patient after a double valve replacement with a Starr-Edwards 1260 aortic valve (smaller cage) and a 6120 mitral valve prosthesis. (Courtesy Edward A. Lefrak, MD.)

Abscess cavities must be obliterated, and if necessary, the prosthetic valve is translocated above the coronary ostia. In this case bypass grafts are performed to vascularize the heart. Allografts or composite valve grafts with coronary ostial reimplantation (see Chapter 16) are additional alternatives.

Aortic valve replacement with coronary artery bypass grafting. The procedure is similar to mitral valve replacement and coronary artery bypass grafting as described in Chapter 13. Distal anastomoses can be accomplished prior to valve replacement; the proximal grafts are usually attached after the aortotomy is closed and the patient is being rewarmed. The distal anastomoses are routinely done first so that elevation of the heart after valve insertion (with possible injury to the myocardium) can be avoided.

Double valve replacement. Double valve replacement of the aortic and mitral valves is described in Chapter 13. The relationship between the mitral and aortic valves and the relative differences in size can be seen radiologically in Fig. 14-27.

COMPLETION OF THE PROCEDURE

Once the valve is implanted, measures are taken to evacuate air from the left ventricle. During closure of the aortotomy, the left ventricle is allowed to fill with blood. This is done by clamping (or turning off) the left ventricular vent. Just before the aortotomy suture

is tied, the aorta is allowed to fill with blood. The patient is placed in the Trendelenburg position, and the ascending aortic needle vent (that was previously tested to be sure it was suctioning and not infusing) is placed in the ascending aorta and turned on to remove air within the left ventricle.

The cross-clamp is then removed, and the ventricular vent is turned on again. It is important that the ventricle not be allowed to eject blood (and possibly a bolus of air) before deairing is accomplished. An additional maneuver is hypodermic needle aspiration of the left ventricular apex (cautiously elevated by the surgeon to avoid endocardial puncture by the prosthesis). A long (spinal) needle may be used for transseptal evacuation of air from the left ventricle if the surgeon wants to avoid elevating the apex.

The pulmonary venous venting catheter is removed, and the entry site is closed with a figure-eight or a pursestring suture. The operating bed is returned to a level position. The ascending aortic vent is left in place until the surgeon is satisfied that deairing has been completed (Wisman and Waldhausen, 1991).

After the left ventricle has been deaired and hemostasis of the suture lines has been achieved, cardiopulmonary bypass is terminated and the chest is closed. Temporary atrial and ventricular pacing wires are attached, and drainage tubes are inserted. As in most cardiac procedures, preoperative ventricular function is the strongest predictor of operative risk.

POSTOPERATIVE COMPLICATIONS

Prosthesis-related complications of thromboembolism, anticoagulation-related hemorrhage, and infection pose a risk for patients with prosthetic valves. Aortic valve surgery is associated particularly with risks of stroke or other neurologic deficit (from particulate or air emboli), persistent bleeding (from coagulation disorders), and myocardial infarction (from coronary atheroembolism). Complete heart block is uncommon unless concomitant procedures involving the conduction pathways within the ventricular septum or the area below the right and noncoronary cusps have been performed.

In patients with aortic valve allografts, leaflet prolapse may result from misalignment of the graft and the native annulus. The surgeon assesses the repair for signs of aortic regurgitation by palpating the aorta for thrills (vibrations of blood hitting against the aortic wall) and leaflet closure. Intraoperative TEE will usually detect the problem early enough for technical repair (Graf and Gonzales-Lavin, 1988). Table 14-3 lists problems and complications related to the intraoperative and postoperative periods.

Table 14-3 ■ *Perioperative problems and complications of aortic valve surgery*

Complication/problem	Interventions
Intraoperative	
Aorta and aortotomy	
Calcification of ascending aorta	Cannulation of femoral artery for CPB may be required
	If cross-clamp cannot be safely applied, may need to use deep hypothermia and circulatory arrest (see Chapter 9)
	When closure of aortotomy is difficult, may need to perform endarterectomy and decalcification, and use felt-buttressed suture closure
Bleeding from aortic suture line	Close approximation of aortotomy edges may be facilitated by using marking stitches to align aortic edges; when there is a transverse aortotomy, a folded towel placed under handle of cross-clamp will tip upper aortotomy edge forward and closer to lower edge
	If retracting aorta, avoid pulling too hard so that incision line is not torn
	Surgeon may want to use felt buttressing to close a friable aorta or reinforce suture line with an aortic circumferential collar of Dacron (e.g., 8 mm tube graft) or PTFE
	Repairs are best performed when systemic blood pressure against aortic suture line is low; avoid hypertension
Aortic valve annulus	
Detachment of anterior mitral leaflet from annulus	Repair mitral leaflet and annulus with pledgeted sutures
Perforation of annulus	Avoid vigorous removal of calcium deposits; repair with pledgeted sutures
Suture interference with prosthetic function	When pledgeted sutures are used, their position may be subannular or supraannular depending on where they will be less likely to interfere with opening or closing mechanism of prosthesis
Coronary arteries and their origin	
Injury to coronary ostia	Use caution with direct ostial infusion
	Avoid injury due to instrument manipulation of ostial and periostial tissue
Embolization of surgical debris	Give meticulous attention to removal of calcium and tissue particles, suture fragments, and other debris
	Open-tip suction catheters, copious irrigation, and sponges placed to occlude coronary openings (and also LV cavity) help to avoid this complication
Ostial obstruction	Signs of ischemia may indicate prosthetic obstruction of ostia; may need to reposition valve
	Caged-ball valves should not be placed in small aortas because of potential obstruction
Misorientation of prosthetic valve	Major orifice of disk valve should be oriented so that it opens in such a way that it enhances left coronary artery perfusion in diastole
Conduction pathways: heart block	Injury to AV node or bundle of His near commissure of noncoronary or right cusps may cause heart block; this should be distinguished from the transient block that may occur from edema and mechanical trauma of surgery
	Temporary atrial and ventricular pacing wires are used to pace heart for a few days; if conduction remains blocked, permanent transvenous leads and a generator may be inserted
Postoperative	
Valvular deterioration (allograft or bioprosthesis)	Process is usually gradual, not catastrophic; if bioprosthesis is damaged, a new murmur will appear; replacement is indicated
Prosthetic failure; thrombosed occluder (disk or ball)	Cessation of valve noise alerts patient or clinician, sternotomy, assessment of valve, and replacement may be required; can be catastrophic (but less likely than with mitral valve prosthesis); when thrombus obstructs valve opening, debridement may first be attempted; thrombolytic therapy can be tried as well
Prosthetic dehiscence perivalvular leak	A new murmur with decreased hematocrit (from hemolysis) alerts clinician; surgical exploration may result in placement of additional stitches or in prosthetic replacement
Prosthetic valve endocarditis with or without root abscess	Elevated temperature and positive blood cultures alert clinician; surgical debridement and drainage, reconstruction or patch repair of any defects, and/or valve replacement may be required
	Relatively independent of prosthesis used; high-dose antibiotics instituted
Inefficient hemodynamic performance or prosthesis	Inadequate cardiac output may require reoperation to replace prosthesis or implant an allograft in an effort to improve transvalvular flow
	Patient activity may require modification
Anticoagulation-related hemorrhage	Readjust warfarin (Coumadin) dosage; recommend more frequent laboratory studies until prothrombin time is within acceptable range
	Refer for additional teaching and family support
	Assess dietary, medication, and life-style habits for risk
Thromboembolism, embolism related to surgical intervention	Adjust anticoagulation dosage to prolong prothrombin time; report neurologic deficits
	Give meticulous attention to removal of surgical debris and intraoperative cleaning of instruments

Modified from Wisman CB, Waldhausen JA: Aortic valve surgery. In Waldhausen JA, Orringer MB: *Complications in cardiothoracic surgery*, St Louis, 1991, Mosby. *AV*, Atrioventricular; *LV*, left ventricular; *PTFE*, polytetrafluoroethylene.

References

Abramczyk EL, Brown MM: Valvular heart disease. In Kinney MR and others: *Comprehensive cardiac care*, ed 7, St Louis, 1991, Mosby.

Arom KV and others: Ten years' experience with the St. Jude Medical valve prosthesis, *Ann Thorac Surg* 47:831, 1989.

Assey ME, Usher BW, Hendrix GH: Valvular heart disease: use of invasive and noninvasive techniques in clinical decision-making. I. Aortic valve disease, *Mod Concepts Cardiovasc Dis* 58(10):55, 1989.

Barratt-Boyes BG: Homograft aortic valve replacement in aortic incompetence and stenosis, *Thorax* 19:131, 1964.

Block PC, Palacios IF: Clinical and hemodynamic follow-up after percutaneous aortic valvuloplasty in the elderly, *Am J Cardiol* 62:760, 1988.

Braunwald E: Valvular heart disease. In Braunwald E: *Heart disease*, ed 4, Philadelphia, 1992, WB Saunders.

Byrd RC, Cheitlin MD: Endocarditis. In Greenber BH, Murphy E, editors: *Valvular heart disease*, Littleton, Mass, 1987, PSG Publishing.

Cooley DA: *Techniques in cardiac surgery*, ed 2, Philadelphia, 1984, WB Saunders.

Cosgrove DM and others: Valvuloplasty for aortic insufficiency, *J Thorac Cardiovasc Surg* 102(4):571, 1991.

Frater RW and others: The Carpentier-Edwards pericardial aortic valve: intermediate results, *Ann Thorac Surg* 53:764, 1992.

Gibbon JH: Application of a mechanical heart and lung apparatus to cardiac surgery, *Minn Med* 37:371, 1954.

Graf D, Gonzales-Lavin L: The homograft: a new dimension for cardiac valve replacement, *AORN J* 48(5):911, 1988.

Harken DE and others: Partial and complete prostheses in aortic insufficiency, *J Thorac Cardiovasc Surg* 40(6):744, 1960.

Harlan BJ, Starr A, Harwin FM: *Manual of cardiac surgery*, vol 1, New York, 1980, Springer-Verlag.

Hazinski MF: *Nursing care of the critically ill child*, ed 2, St Louis, 1992, Mosby.

Hufnagel CA, Harvey WP: The surgical correction of aortic insufficiency, *Bull Georgetown Univ Med Center* 6:60, 1953.

Hurst JW: *The heart*, ed 7, vols 1 and 2, New York, 1990, McGraw-Hill.

Jacobs ML, Austen G: Acquired aortic valve disease. In Sabiston DC, Spencer FC: *Surgery of the chest*, ed 5, vols 1 and 2, New York, 1990, WB Saunders.

Jorgensen CR: The pathophysiology of aortic stenosis. In Emery RW, Arom KV: *The aortic valve*, Philadelphia, 1991, Hanley & Belfus.

King RM and others: Ultrasonic aortic valvuloplasty. In Emery RW, Arom KV: *The aortic valve*, Philadelphia, 1991, Hanley & Belfus.

Kirklin JW, Barratt-Boyes BG: *Cardiac surgery*, ed 2, New York, 1993, Churchill Livingstone.

Lange PL, Hopkins RA: Allograft valve banking: techniques and technology. In Hopkins RA: *Cardiac reconstructions with allograft valves*, New York, 1989, Springer-Verlag.

Lombardy JT, Selzer A: Valvular aortic stenosis: a clinical and hemodynamic profile of patients, *Ann Intern Med* 106(2):292, 1987.

Manouguian A, Seybold-Epting W: Patch enlargement of the aortic valve ring by extending the aortic incision into the anterior mitral leaflet, *J Thorac Cardiovasc Surg* 78(3):402, 1979.

Marshall WG, Kouchoukos NT: Aortic valve replacement. In Grillo HC and others, editors: *Current therapy in cardiothoracic surgery*, Philadelphia, 1989, BC Decker.

Matsuki O and others: Long-term performance of 555 homografts in the aortic position, *Ann Thorac Surg* 46:187, 1988.

McBride LR and others: Aortic valve decalcification, *J Thorac Cardiovasc Surg* 100(1):36, 1990.

Miller DC, Shumway NE: "Fresh" aortic allografts: long-term results with free-hand aortic valve replacement, *J Cardiac Surg* 1(3, suppl):185, 1987.

Mindich BP, Guarino T, Goldman ME: Aortic valvuloplasty for acquired aortic stenosis, *Circulation* 74(suppl 1):1-130, 1986.

Morgan RJ, Davis JT, Fraker TD: Current status of valve prostheses, *Surg Clin North Am* 65(3):699, 1985.

Morrow AG and others: Operative treatment in hypertrophic subaortic stenosis: techniques, and the results of pre and postoperative assessments in 83 patients, *Circulation* 52:88, 1975.

Morton MJ: The heart in pressure overload. In Greenberg BH, Murphy E: *Valvular heart disease*, Littleton, Mass, 1987, PSG Publishing.

Nolan SP, Muller WH: Acquired disorders of the aortic valve. In Sabiston DC: *Textbook of surgery*, ed 13, Philadelphia, 1986, WB Saunders.

O'Brien MF, McGriffin DC, Stafford G: Allograft aortic valve implantation: techniques for all types of aortic valve and root pathology, *Ann Thorac Surg* 48:600, 1989.

Pedersen WR, Goldenberg IF: The pathophysiology of aortic insufficiency. In Emery RW, Arom KV: *The aortic valve*, Philadelphia, 1991, Hanley & Belfus.

Randolph JD and others: Aortic valve and left ventricular outflow tract replacement using allograft and autograft valves: a preliminary report, *Ann Thorac Surg* 48:345, 1989.

Roberts WC: Anatomically isolated aortic valvular disease: the case against its being of rheumatic etiology, *Am Med J* 49:151, 1970.

Ross D: Homograft replacement of the aortic valve, *Lancet* 2:487, 1962.

Ross D: Application of homografts in clinical surgery, *J Cardiac Surg* 1(3, suppl):175, 1987.

Ross D: Technique of aortic valve replacement with a homograft: orthotopic replacement, *Ann Thorac Surg* 52:154, 1991.

Safian RD and others: Balloon aortic valvuloplasty in 170 consecutive patients, *N Engl J Med* 319:125, 1988.

Seifert PC, Auer JE: Surgical repair of annular disruption following percutaneous balloon aortic valvuloplasty, *Ann Thorac Surg* 46:242, 1988.

Selzer P: Changing aspects of the natural history of valvular aortic stenosis, *N Engl J Med* 317(2):91, 1987.

Sethig K and others: Clinical hemodynamic and angiographic predictors of operative mortality in patients undergoing single valve replacement, *J Thorac Cardiovasc Surg* 93:884, 1987.

Spencer FC: Acquired heart disease. In Schwartz SI: *Principles of surgery*, ed 5, New York, 1989, McGraw-Hill.

Spotnitz HM, Antunes ML: Effect of aortic and mitral regurgitation on left ventricular structure and function, *Adv Cardiac Surg* 2:85, 1990.

Starr A, Edwards ML: Mitral replacement: clinical experience with a ball-valve prosthesis, *Ann Surg* 154:726, Oct 1961.

Stelzer P, Elkins RC: Homograft valves and conduits: applications in cardiac surgery. In Wells SA, editor: *Curr Probl Surg* 26(6):385, 1989.

Subramanian R, Olson LJ, Edwards WD: Surgical pathology of pure aortic stenosis: a study of 374 cases, *Mayo Clin Proc* 59:683, 1984.

Titus JL, Edwards JE: The aortic root and valve: development, anatomy, and congenital anomalies. In Emery RW, Arom KV: *The aortic valve*, Philadelphia, 1991, Hanley & Belfus.

Walhausen JA, Pierce WS: *Johnson's surgery of the chest*, ed 5, St Louis, 1985, Mosby.

Walker WE: Acquired cardiac disorders. In Miller TA, editor: *Physiologic basis of modern surgical care*, St Louis, 1988, Mosby.

Whitman GR, Guzzetta CE: Cardiac surgery. In Dossey BM, Guzzetta CE, Kenner CV: *Critical care nursing: body-mind-spirit*, Philadelphia, 1992, JB Lippincott.

Whitman GJ, Harken AH: Acquired disorders of the aortic valve. In Sabiston DC: *Textbook of surgery*, ed 14, New York, 1991, WB Saunders.

Wisman CB, Walhausen JA: Aortic valve surgery. In Waldhausen JA, Orringer MB: *Complications in cardiothoracic surgery*, St Louis, 1991, Mosby.

15

Tricuspid and Pulmonary Valve Procedures

The three goals of a valvuloplasty are: to give a predictable result, to preserve normal valve function, and to provide a definitive repair.

Alain Carpentier, MD, 1974 (p. 344)

Surgical treatment for tricuspid valve disease remains a challenge. Of the four cardiac valves, the tricuspid is most likely to undergo surgical repair rather than replacement in order to avoid the risk of valve-related complications such as thromboembolism, thrombosis, and anticoagulation-related problems (Kratz and others, 1985).

Surgery on the pulmonary valve is rarely performed in adults but on occasion may be necessary. It is discussed later in this chapter.

TRICUSPID VALVE PROCEDURES

TRICUSPID APPARATUS

The tricuspid valve is the largest of the four cardiac valves and is similar to the mitral valve in form and function (see Chapter 13). It is situated so that it lies in a plane caudad to the mitral valve (Karp, 1990). Like the mitral apparatus, the tricuspid apparatus consists of the leaflets, annular tissue, chordae tendineae, papillary muscles, and the ventricular wall.

In addition to the lower pressures within the right side of the heart, there are other differences. One of these is that, unlike the bicuspid mitral valve, the tricuspid valve has three leaflets: the anterior, posterior, and septal (Fig. 15-1). Of surgical significance is that the penetrating portion of the conduction system, the bundle of His, and the atrioventricular node can be found at the base of the septal leaflet.

Another notable difference is that there is no discrete tricuspid annulus; rather, there is a relatively undefined ring of tissue to which the bases of the three leaflets are attached to the heart at the atrioventricular junction. (For ease of discussion, the term "annulus" will be used throughout the chapter.) Surrounding this ring of tissue is the base of the aortic valve, the

membranous septum, the central fibrous body (also known as the right fibrous trigone), the right coronary artery, the coronary sinus, and the bundle of His (Fig. 15-2).

Two-dimensional echocardiographic studies have shown that both mitral and tricuspid annular tissue change dynamically during the cardiac cycle. The tricuspid annulus reaches its maximum size in late diastole and its minimum size in midsystole; the annular area can change in size by as much as 39%. That the tricuspid valve demonstrates a greater reduction in circumference than the mitral valve (up to 31% reduction) is thought to be due to the fact that tricuspid annular tissue is largely composed of myocardium and thus exhibits greater reduction during ventricular systole when the myocardium contracts (Tei and others, 1982). Evaluating annular size and function is helpful in planning the surgical procedure and provides additional clinical data for the surgeon performing digital palpation of the tricuspid valve prior to instituting cardiopulmonary bypass.

TRICUSPID VALVE DISEASE

Tricuspid valve disease requiring surgery is rarely an isolated lesion except when there is a congenital malformation (Cohen and others, 1987a). More often it is a functional disorder secondary to valve disease in the left side of the heart. In contrast, organic tricuspid valve disease affects the valve itself and produces stenosis and/or regurgitation. It is due most often to infective endocarditis, congenital heart disease, or rheumatic fever (Hauck and others, 1988). Other organic factors include diffuse connective tissue disorders, right atrial tumors, carcinoid syndrome (distortion of the valve by endocardial fibrosis created by a metastasizing gastrointestinal carcinoma), congenital

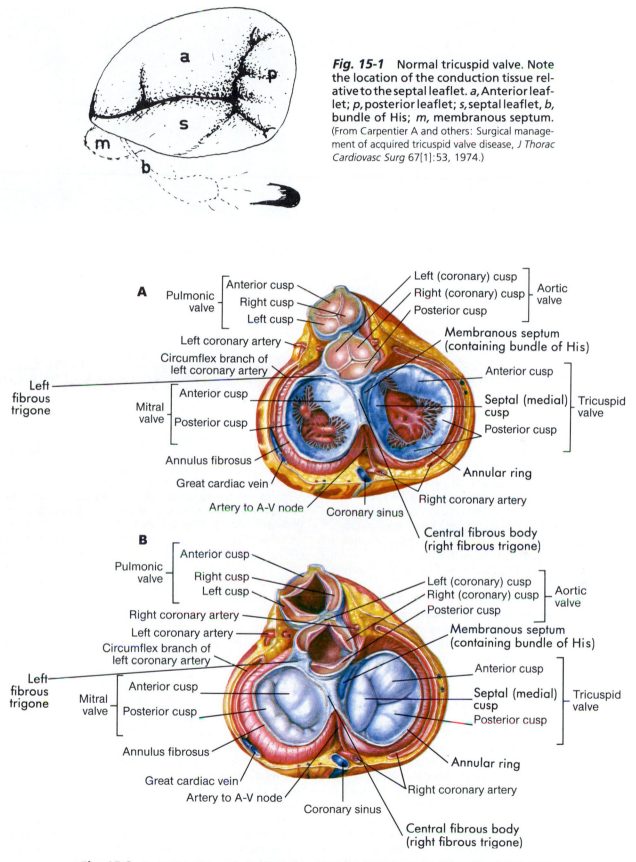

Fig. 15-1 Normal tricuspid valve. Note the location of the conduction tissue relative to the septal leaflet. *a,* Anterior leaflet; *p,* posterior leaflet; *s,* septal leaflet, *b,* bundle of His; *m,* membranous septum. (From Carpentier A and others: Surgical management of acquired tricuspid valve disease, *J Thorac Cardiovasc Surg* 67[1]:53, 1974.)

Fig. 15-2 Superior view of cardiac valves during diastole, **A,** and systole, **B.** Note the relationship of the tricuspid valve to the surrounding structures. (From Canobbio M: *Cardiovascular disorders,* St Louis, 1990, Mosby.)

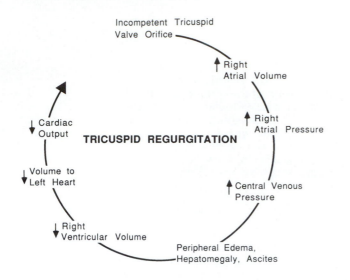

lesions such as Ebstein's anomaly (Alexander and O'Brien, 1991) or atrioventricular canal, and trauma (Braunwald, 1992; Brundage and others, 1987; Gayet and others, 1987; Kleikamp and others, 1992).

Tricuspid Regurgitation

Functional tricuspid regurgitation (insufficiency) is frequently caused by mitral or aortic valve disease producing left ventricular failure, which creates chronically elevated left atrial pressure. This leads to increased pulmonary vascular resistance, pulmonary hypertension, and, eventually, right ventricular failure, causing right ventricular dilatation, tricuspid annular dilatation, and subsequent valvular regurgitation (Spencer, 1989). In these cases the leaflets themselves may be relatively normal in appearance.

With the development of tricuspid insufficiency, increased right atrial volume raises right atrial pressure, which is reflected backward to the venous system. At the same time forward blood flow is reduced as a result of regurgitation of blood into the right atrium. Eventually, right-sided cardiac output is reduced (Fig. 15-3).

Rheumatic disease

Tricuspid rheumatic inflammatory changes are almost never seen in isolation; they commonly affect the mitral and/or the aortic valve as well. The process of fibrosis and contraction of the leaflets is similar to that affecting the mitral valve except that calcification is rarer on the tricuspid valve.

Marfan's syndrome

Patients with Marfan's syndrome may demonstrate annular dilatation unrelated to pulmonary hypertension (Braunwald, 1992). Marfan's syndrome and other connective tissue disorders (such as those associated

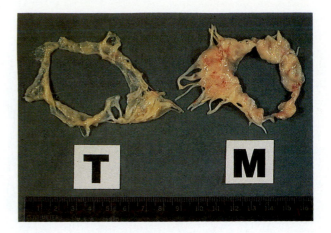

Fig. 15-4 Myxomatous proliferation of tricuspid *(left)* and mitral *(right)* valves producing valvular insufficiency. (Courtesy Edward A. Lefrak, MD.)

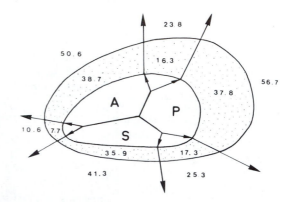

Fig. 15-5 Tricuspid insufficiency. Dilatation primarily affects the posterior *(P)* and anterior *(A)* leaflets. Numbers indicate the average lengths of the attachment of the leaflets in a normal *(central numbers)* and a dilated *(peripheral numbers)* orifice, S, Septal. (From Carpentier A and others: Surgical management of acquired tricuspid valve disease, *J Thorac Cardiovasc Surg* 67[1]:53, 1974.)

with mitral valve prolapse) may also affect the leaflets. The mucoid or myxomatous elements of the leaflets proliferate to a greater extent than the sturdier fibrosa element (Roberts, 1987). This produces excessive thinning and stretching of the leaflet tissue, thereby resulting in valvular regurgitation (Fig. 15-4).

Coronary artery disease

Acute thrombosis of the coronary arteries supplying the right ventricle and, in particular, the inferior wall are increasingly being recognized as an etiologic factor in the development of tricuspid insufficiency. Impaired contractility from right ventricular failure results in a reduction in the narrowing of the annulus during systole. Annular dilatation primarily affects the anterior and posterior leaflets; usually only a portion of the septal leaflet annulus becomes dilated (Fig. 15-5). Although pulmonary symptoms are common with

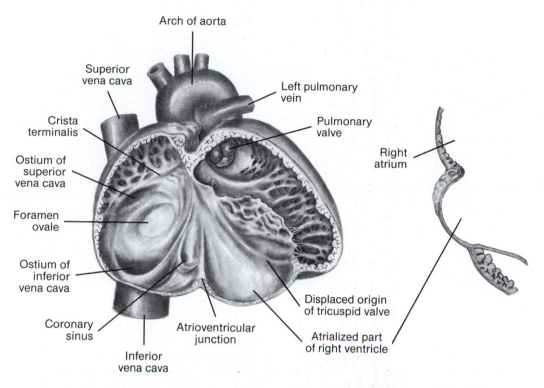

Fig. 15-6 Ebstein's anomaly. The "atrialized" portion of the right ventricle is shown on the right. (From Canobbio M: *Cardiovascular disorders*, St Louis, 1990, Mosby.)

left ventricular failure, they are often absent in primary right-sided heart failure, which causes congestion and distension of the venous system (Muirhead, 1989; Robison, 1987).

Endocarditis

Although the tricuspid valve is usually an uncommon source of infection, septic endocarditis is being seen with increasing frequency in patients who are intravenous drug users (Ginzton, Siegel, and Criley, 1982; Relf, 1993).

Ebstein's anomaly

Ebstein's anomaly (Fig. 15-6) is a congenital disorder that may not require surgical intervention until adulthood. The posterior, and often the septal, leaflets are adherent and tethered to the right ventricular wall. Although the anterior leaflet is normally attached to the annular ring, all three leaflets are usually malformed, being either enlarged or reduced in size, and thickened and distorted. The downward displacement of the posterior and septal leaflets in the right ventricle creates a division of the chamber into a proximal "atrialized" portion with a thin wall and pressures similar to those of the right atrium. The distal ventricular portion consists mainly of apical and infundibular portions of the ventricle. Tricuspid regurgitation is present and may be mild to severe, depending on the degree of leaflet displacement (Graham and Friesinger, 1987).

Although the anomaly manifests itself during in-

fancy, clinical symptoms may not appear until adolescence or adulthood. Cardiomegaly and hepatomegaly frequently accompany tricuspid regurgitation. Conduction delays, supraventricular tachycardia, and other rhythm disturbances are common and may pose an increased risk during cardiac catheterization. The type of surgery depends on the severity of the lesion and the presence of refractory congestive heart failure or conduction disorders. When feasible, valve repair is preferred (Carpentier and others, 1988), but replacement may be necessary if the valve is very deformed. Associated atrial septal defects are closed, and conduction disturbances are treated as necessary (Kirklin and Barratt-Boyes, 1993).

Tricuspid Stenosis

Pure tricuspid stenosis is unusual in the adult. When it occurs, it is usually due to rheumatic disease (which often produces a mixed stenotic and regurgitant lesion), mechanical obstruction by thrombus, bacterial vegetations, tumors (such as atrial myxomas), or metastatic carcinoid lesions (Braunwald, 1992; Rankin, 1991). Congenital absence of the tricuspid valve (tricuspid atresia) is uncommon, but there are reported cases of adults with this malformation (Jordan and Sanders, 1966). Survival depends on the presence of a shunt or a defect to provide an alternative route for blood flow (Perloff, 1987).

The pathologic changes in tricuspid stenosis are similar to those seen in mitral stenosis. The commis-

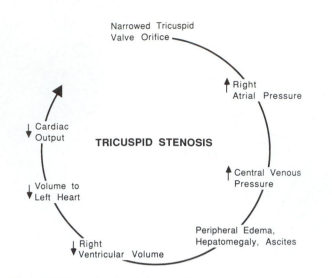

Fig. 15-7 Pathophysiology of tricuspid stenosis. (From Kinney MR and others: *Comprehensive cardiac care*, ed 7, St Louis, 1991, Mosby.)

sures fuse, thereby narrowing the central opening, and right atrial and central venous pressures become elevated (Fig. 15-7), producing symptoms of systemic venous congestion.

DIAGNOSTIC EVALUATION OF TRICUSPID VALVE DISEASE
Physical Examination

With both tricuspid valve regurgitation and stenosis, signs and symptoms of right-sided congestion appear (Fig. 15-8). These include hepatomegaly, ascites, right upper abdominal tenderness, increased abdominal girth, and anorexia from liver and intestinal engorgement. Jugular venous distension and edema result from elevated right atrial pressure, and fatigue occurs from low cardiac output (Cavallo, 1992). Hepatomegaly may be present; elevated bilirubin levels suggest hepatic congestion from severe right ventricular dysfunction or hepatic ischemia from a low output state (Baughman and others, 1984).

Tricuspid regurgitation is more common than stenosis and should be suspected in patients who continue to complain of symptoms despite optimal medical treatment with digitalis, sodium restriction, and diuretics (Cohen and others, 1987b). A moderate degree of tricuspid insufficiency can be tolerated quite easily for many years in some patients; this is in sharp contrast to the more adverse effects of mitral insufficiency.

In addition to the clinical features related to systemic venous congestion and reduced cardiac output, the physical examination generally reveals a systolic (regurgitant) or diastolic (stenotic) murmur along the left lower sternal margin and a prominent jugular venous pulse. The murmur is usually augmented during inspiration and reduced during expiration, particularly during the Valsalva maneuver, which may help to distinguish tricuspid murmurs from mitral murmurs. In patients with tricuspid regurgitation, there may be prominent right ventricular pulsations along the left parasternal region (Braunwald, 1991).

In patients with both stenotic and regurgitant valves, the electrocardiogram usually shows changes associated with enlargement of the right atrium, such as atrial fibrillation. If the right ventricle is enlarged, incomplete right bundle-branch block may also be evident. Chest roentgenograms commonly reveal an enlarged right atrium with tricuspid stenosis and/or re-

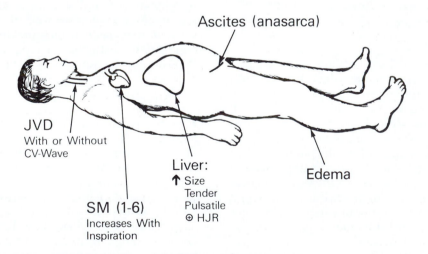

Fig. 15-8 Clinical signs of tricuspid insufficiency producing systemic venous congestion. *JVD,* Jugular venous distension; *SM,* systolic murmur; *HJR,* hepatojugular reflux. (From Cohen SR and others: Tricuspid regurgitation in patients with acquired, chronic, pure mitral regurgitation. I. Prevalence, diagnosis, and comparison of preoperative clinical and hemodynamic features in patients with and without tricuspid regurgitation, *J Thorac Cardiovasc Surg* 94[4]:481, 1987.)

gurgitation; the superior vena cava may be enlarged with tricuspid stenosis.

Clinical findings and hemodynamic data alone are often inadequate to make a diagnosis. The severity of the lesion often requires confirmation at surgery by noting the appearance of the right atrium, digitally palpating the valve before instituting cardiopulmonary bypass, and visually inspecting the valve structure and the size of the annulus (Cohen and others, 1987b).

Diagnostic Studies

Diagnosing tricuspid valve disease presents a number of challenges related to the techniques used, right-sided heart hemodynamics, and the left-sided lesions that are often present. Distinguishing tricuspid problems from aortic or mitral valve disease may be difficult, because many of the available diagnostic techniques are better at evaluating left-sided rather than right-sided problems.

Echocardiography

Color flow echocardiography is often used to make the diagnosis of tricuspid regurgitation; vegetations may be seen in patients with endocarditis. Doppler methods are used to estimate both the severity of the lesion and the pulmonary artery pressure. Doppler echocardiography has enhanced detection of even minor (and inaudible) amounts of tricuspid regurgitation in over half of patients with no symptoms or structural heart disease (Lee, Bhatia, and Sutton, 1989). However, no gold standard exists for measuring the severity of tricuspid regurgitation (Cohen and others, 1987a).

Doppler methods can also be used to compute the transvalvular pressure gradient with stenotic valves (normally there is no difference in pressure between the atrium and the ventricle during diastole). Usually a mean diastolic gradient exceeding 4 mm Hg will produce symptoms of systemic venous congestion (unless sodium intake has been limited and diuretics have been given). Because the pressures in the right side of the heart are already low, small variations between the right atrium and the ventricle become significant (Braunwald, 1991).

Cardiac catheterization

Invasive procedures such as cardiac catheterization may be unreliable, and false-positive results are not uncommon. One reason is that angiographic catheters are inserted into a systemic vein and threaded antegradely into the right atrium, across the tricuspid valve, and into the right ventricle, where dye is injected. Catheter-induced tricuspid regurgitation is easily produced when the catheter crosses the valve (Fig. 15-9). Even though such artifact may produce only a slight increase in the amount of regurgitation detected, in the low-pressure right side of the heart, even small increases may be suggestive of a more serious problem that actually exists.

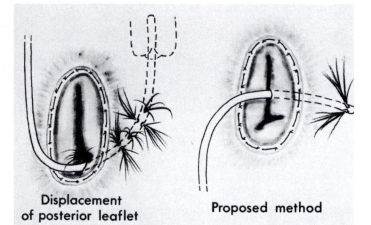

Displacement of posterior leaflet   **Proposed method**

Fig. 15-9 *Left:* Mechanism of catheter-induced regurgitation in a patient who has had a tricuspid annuloplasty. The same mechanism can cause artifacts during preoperative evaluation. *Right:* Alternative method for minimizing catheter-induced regurgitation. (From Grondin P and others: Carpentier's annulus and DeVega's annuloplasty, *J Thorac Cardiovasc Surg* 70[5]:852, 1975.)

In contrast, mitral valve studies are performed by passing the catheter retrogradely from the aorta into the left ventricle, where dye is injected to detect the presence of mitral valve regurgitation. The catheter does not need to cross the mitral valve, thereby minimizing the possibility of the catheter interfering with mitral leaflet function. In view of these difficulties, noninvasive techniques such as echocardiography are routine advocated for studying the tricuspid valve; cardiac catheterization is still used for evaluating other disorders such as coronary artery disease.

Another problem that may be encountered is catheter-induced premature ventricular contractions or catheter dislocation during the injection of contrast dye. Although these problems tend to increase the possibility of false-positive findings, right ventricular angiography probably remains the most objective standard for diagnosing tricuspid regurgitation (Curtius and others, 1985).

To improve the diagnostic accuracy of right-sided cardiac catheterization and angiography in grading tricuspid regurgitation, it has been suggested that small doses of contrast material be injected at low velocities (Cohen and others, 1987a).

Assessment of tricuspid stenosis is more accurate when right atrial and right ventricular pressures are measured simultaneously rather than sequentially with the pull-back technique (e.g., the catheter is advanced to the right ventricle and pressures are measured, after which the catheter is pulled back into the right atrium and pressures are measured). Left-sided cardiac catheterization is routinely performed to study associated lesions of the mitral and/or aortic valve, left ventricular function, and the severity and extent of existing obstructive coronary artery disease.

Table 15-1 ■ *Standards of nursing care for tricuspid valve surgery**

Nursing diagnosis	Patient outcome	Nursing actions
Anxiety related to disease, surgery, and perioperative events	Patient demonstrates acceptable levels of anxiety and is able to co-operate with therapeutic regimen	Elicit questions and concerns about tricuspid disease and treatment Identify learning needs; refer if necessary for later follow-up Institute measures to relieve systemic venous congestion: rest, cautious intravenous infusion, avoidance of pressure on abdomen; elevate head of stretcher
Knowledge deficit related to inadequate knowledge of planned surgery and perioperative events	Patient demonstrates knowledge of physiologic and psychologic responses to tricuspid valve surgery	Determine patient's understanding of tricuspid valve disease; possible surgical interventions (annuloplasty, replacement, excision, commissurotomy); types, benefits and risks of prostheses; and preferences if any Clarify patient's understanding of possible need for permanent pacemaker due to surgical proximity to conduction tissue If additional procedures are planned, refer to specific standards of care Assess mitral and/or aortic valve disease in addition to tricuspid valve disease; assess left ventricular and right ventricular function; note presence of pulmonary hypertension, liver dysfunction, other problems related to systemic venous congestion
High risk for injury related to use of valve retractor	Patient is free of injury from use of retraction devices	Use hand-held valve retractors with caution to avoid injury to conduction tissue, atrial septum, and surrounding tissue

Modified from Seifert PC: Cardiac surgery. In Rothrock JC: *Perioperative nursing care planning*, St Louis, 1990, Mosby.
*See also Chapter 13 on mitral valve surgery.

SURGERY FOR TRICUSPID VALVE DISEASE

Because operations for tricuspid valve disease are commonly related to left-sided valvular lesions, surgical outcome is affected by the perioperative status of the left side of the heart. In general, surgical outcome is more successful in patients without severe systemic venous hypertension or right ventricular dysfunction, fixed pulmonary hypertension, or incomplete repairs of left-sided problems (Duran and others, 1980; McGrath and others, 1990). In the presence of these derangements, tricuspid regurgitation may actually worsen after surgery.

Patient teaching considerations

Because tricuspid valve dysfunction is often related to left-sided valvular lesions, patient teaching considerations include learning needs associated with both the tricuspid valve disease and concomitant aortic or mitral valve disease (Table 15-1). The nurse can clarify how left-sided lesions affect the tricuspid valve and produce symptoms of systemic venous congestion. When pulmonary function has been affected by the valvular disorder, the patient can be informed about rehabilitative regimens that enhance both pulmonary and cardiac function.

Psychologic and social responses to the disease and the interventions can be investigated with the patient and family. When the etiology is related to intravenous drug use, referrals to addiction treatment programs should be considered. The risk of recurring endocarditis from continued drug use needs to be stressed.

Patients may undergo valve repair or replacement (or excision). As part of the consent process, the surgeon reviews the risks and benefits of the planned procedure, and the nurse can clarify this information and discuss the functional implications for postoperative activities of daily living.

When valve replacement is planned, patient teaching is directed toward the type of prosthesis (or allograft) to be used and its postoperative implications. Unlike bioprostheses and allografts, mechanical valves require chronic anticoagulation, and attendant risks and precautions should be part of the patient teaching (see Chapter 13 on mitral valve surgery).

Procedural considerations

Instrumentation and supplies (Box 15-1) are similar to those used for mitral valve surgery (see Chapter 13). If surgery on the mitral and/or aortic valve is planned, specialty items related to those procedures should be included.

Table 15-1 ■ *Standards of nursing care for tricuspid valve surgery—cont'd*

Nursing diagnosis	Patient outcome	Nursing actions
High risk for injury related to:	The patient is free of injury related to:	
Physical hazards	Physical hazards	Have available type and sizes of valvular prostheses desired by surgeon; store valves and annuloplasty rings in cool, dry location; have appropriate accessories to size and insert prostheses; have necessary suture available (pledgeted, nonpledgeted, multicolored); have tricuspid sizers for tricuspid rings; have appropriate bypass and cardioplegia cannulas/catheters Have double venous cannulas, right-angle cannulas (per surgeon's request); caval tourniquets or clamps Have left atrial line and suture for securing
Electrical hazards	Electrical hazards	Have temporary and permanent epicardial atrial and ventricular pacing leads; have temporary and permanent pacemaker generator per surgeon's request; check for kinks in leads Test pacer leads and generator to ensure they are working properly

High risk for self-care deficit related to inadequate knowledge of rehabilitation period	Patient demonstrates knowledge of rehabilitation period as it relates to self-care abilities	Assess patient's knowledge of signs/symptoms of tricuspid valve failure
		Assess patient's understanding of possible complications of surgery performed and knowledge of reportable signs and symptoms:
		  Heart block: slow pulse, fatigue, syncope
		  Regurgitation/stenosis: edema, jugular venous pulsation, abdominal discomfort, fatigue
		  Endocarditis: fever, anemia, murmur, chills, weight loss, microembolic petechiae
		Know complications of prosthetic valves (see Chapter 13 on mitral valve surgery and Chapter 14 on aortic valve surgery) and reportable signs and symptoms
		Refer for counseling if history of illicit drug use
		Refer for pulmonary and cardiac rehabilitation as needed

Intracardiac hemodynamic monitoring of the right side of the heart is performed with a central venous pressure line inserted prior to surgery. Because a pulmonary artery balloon catheter interferes with the surgical exposure, pressure monitoring of the left side of the heart may require insertion of a left atrial line after completion of the tricuspid repair.

Cardiopulmonary bypass for tricuspid valve surgery is achieved with separate venous cannulas inserted into the superior and inferior vena cavae (Box 15-1). A right-angle cannula in the superior vena cava provides an unobstructed operative site (Duran and others, 1980). Umbilical tapes (or caval clamps) are placed around the cavae and tightened with tourniquets. This forces all the systemic venous return to enter the openings in the distal ends of the cannulas

and prevents venous return from obscuring the right atrium and tricuspid valve. In the presence of longstanding tricuspid regurgitation and associated liver dysfunction, use of an inferior vena caval tourniquet may produce significant back pressure on the liver, leading to hepatocellular necrosis; some authors (Kay, 1992) suggest avoidance of caval snares. A cardiotomy suction is used to remove coronary sinus drainage.

Frequently the surgeon performs a digital examination of the tricuspid valve before inserting the superior vena caval cannula into the right atriotomy. The purpose of this is to detect the degree of tricuspid insufficiency. Because many factors contribute to the amount of insufficiency—blood volume, atrial fibrillation, pulmonary hypertension, cardiac insufficiency, and anesthesia—some authors have cautioned that overestimation or underestimation of the degree of insufficiency is possible (Carpentier, 1983). Studies have not demonstrated a statistical correlation between the degree of tricuspid regurgitation palpated at surgery and the severity of regurgitation by the patient history, physical examination, or preoperative hemodynamic data (although longer duration of preoperative symptoms of congestive heart failure does seem to correlate with more severe tricuspid regurgitation). More accurate assessments are likely to result when sodium restriction and diuresis have been instituted preoperatively (Cohen and others, 1987a).

Whether the tricuspid valve disease is isolated or occurs in combination with mitral or aortic valve disease, cold cardioplegic arrest is used to protect the entire heart. Retroplegia is valuable in these procedures for protecting the right side of the heart (especially in the presence of a right dominant coronary system) because there is often some degree of right ventricular dysfunction. With the right atrium opened, a retroplegia catheter can be inserted into the coronary sinus under direct vision. Surgeons may use a combined approach with both antegrade and retrograde protection of the right and left sides of the heart; when antegrade cardioplegia is given, coronary venous return exiting the coronary sinus will temporarily obscure the operative field.

One of the most serious complications associated with tricuspid valve procedures is the creation of heart block from injury to the atrioventricular node and the bundle of His located along the annular portion of the septal leaflet. Injury may be due also to edema from surgical manipulation or to a suture placed in the conduction pathway. Another potential danger is injury to the right coronary artery. Precautions include gentle handling of tissue, avoidance of unnecessary instrument manipulation of conduction tissue, and optimum exposure of the surgical site (Box 15-2).

Associated left-sided lesions are repaired first, followed by the tricuspid valve procedure (Mullany and others, 1987). With respect to myocardial revascularization procedures, if saphenous vein coronary bypass grafts are performed to the right coronary artery (or to the posterior descending branch of the right coronary artery), the proximal anastomosis to the aorta is done after the right atrium is closed.

Tricuspid Valve Repairs
Procedural considerations

A number of reparative procedures can be performed (Minale, Lambertz, and Messmer, 1987). The DeVega suture annuloplasty is a simple procedure that requires less operative time than other, more complex reparative techniques (Grondin and others, 1975; Rivera, Duran, and Ajuria, 1985). One of the complications of this technique is suture dehiscence (with resulting insufficiency).

Annuloplasty rings. Duran and Carpentier annuloplasty rings with specific sizers are available. Rings

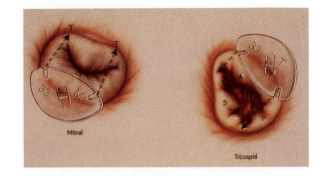

Fig. 15-10   One side of the Duran annuloplasty ring sizer is used for tricuspid valve repairs *(right)*, and the other side is used for mitral valve repairs *(left).* (Courtesy Medtronic, Inc., Minneapolis, Minn.)

and sizers should be differentiated from mitral valve devices, as well as from each other. Interrupted sutures are commonly used to insert annuloplasty rings, but a continuous suture technique can be used (Gay, 1990). In general, women require a smaller size than men.

Carpentier tricuspid rings are available in even-numbered sizes (e.g., 30, 32, 34, 36). The rings are similar to their mitral annuloplasty counterparts except that the tricuspid ring has a gap in that portion corresponding to the area adjacent to conduction tissue; the gap prevents the placement of sutures in this critical area. Obturators are made of nondisposable plastic and require sterilization prior to use; they are also different in shape from those for the mitral annuloplasty ring. The reusable metal obturator handle does fit both tricuspid and mitral rings (see Chapter 5). The ring itself is held by the assistant during implantation; no ring holder is available.

Duran annuloplasty rings with disposable sizers are available in odd-numbered sizes (e.g., 31, 33, 35) and can be used in either the tricuspid or mitral position. However, orientation of the ring and the sizers must be appropriate for the valve repaired (Fig. 15-10). When sizing the tricuspid valve, the obturator is held

with the side displaying the initial "T" for tricuspid (the reverse side, with the initial, "M" would be used to measure a mitral valve). A tonsil or Kelly hemostat is used to grasp the central bar of the obturator, and the sizer is lowered onto the valve. The notches are aligned with the commissures of the septal leaflet, and the anterior leaflet is extended to cover the surface of the selected obturator. The obturator with the surface area most nearly matching the anterior leaflet and commissural notch spacing corresponds to the size ring that should be used.

The Duran ring is supplied with an attached holder; a metal reusable handle is screwed into the plastic holder. The ring/holder assembly needs to be oriented so that the word "tricuspid" is at the upper side (the word "mitral" will appear upside down on the assembly). After the sutures have been placed and the prosthesis has been lowered into the annulus, the retaining sutures are cut to remove the holder.

Operative procedure: repair of the tricuspid valve

1. A median sternotomy is performed. Atrial pursestring sutures are placed in the appendage and the atrial wall for bypass cannulas. Before inserting the cannula into the appendage opening, the surgeon may place a finger through the atriotomy to palpate the tricuspid valve (Fig. 15-11) in order to determine the degree of valvular regurgitation.

2. Double venous cannulas are inserted so that they do cross one another in the right atrium. A right-angle cannula (Fig. 15-12) may be used in the superior vena cava. Occluding tapes or caval clamps (Fig. 15-13) are tightened around the cavae and cannulas to prevent venous return from obscuring the surgical site. Cardioplegia solution is infused antegradely through the aortic root.

3. The right atrium is opened longitudinally along the atrioventricular groove to expose the tricuspid valve, and retractors are inserted (see Chapter 13 on mitral valve surgery). Cardiotomy suctions are used to remove coronary sinus

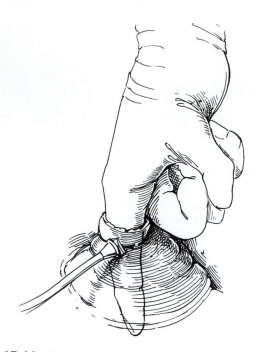

Fig. 15-11 Prior to insertion of the venous drainage cannula, the surgeon places a finger through the right atriotomy to palpate the tricuspid valve and to detect the degree of tricuspid regurgitation. (From Waldhausen JA, Pierce WS: *Johnson's surgery of the chest*, ed 5, St Louis, 1985, Mosby.)

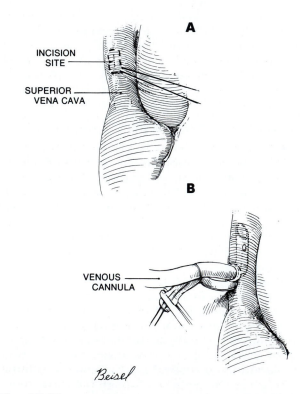

INCISION SITE

SUPERIOR VENA CAVA

VENOUS CANNULA

Beisel

Fig. 15-12 Insertion of a right-angle venous cannula. **A,** Pursestring suture in the superior vena cava. **B,** Right-angle venous cannula with a tourniquet. (From Waldhausen JA, Pierce WS: *Johnson's surgery of the chest*, ed 5, St Louis, 1985, Mosby.)

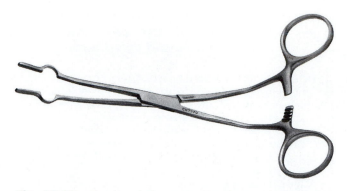

Fig. 15-13 The caval clamp is placed over the superior vena cava and venous cannula (see text). (Courtesy Baxter Healthcare Corp., V. Mueller Div., Chicago, Il.)

drainage. Retroplegia may be given under direct vision.

4A. **Kay bicuspidization technique** (Kay, 1992): This is one of the earliest reparative techniques developed for the tricuspid valve; it is now infrequently performed. The annulus of the posterior leaflet is plicated with sutures, producing a two-leaflet valve.

4B. **DeVega suture annuloplasty technique** (Rabago and others, 1980): A double-armed, felt-pledgeted suture is placed in or near the tricuspid valve ring, beginning at the anteroseptal commissure and continuing along the anterior and posterior leaflet annulus to the level of the coronary sinus in the area of the septal leaflet (Fig. 15-14, *A*). The suture is placed into a second pledget. The other arm of the suture is then similarly placed (in reverse), and the two ends of the suture are tied over the pledget at the anteroseptal commissure (Fig. 15-14, *B*). To achieve the correct size for the annulus, a valve obturator may be inserted into the annular opening; the suture is then pulled up against the sizer, and the stitch is tied.

This technique is used less frequently than the Carpentier and Duran annuloplasty repairs.

4C. **Carpentier annuloplasty ring technique** (Carpentier, 1983): Carpentier's (1974) goals of predictability, preservation of valve function, and definitive repair form the basis for the development of the ring annuloplasty technique that has become widely used to repair the tricuspid valve. (Lambertz and others, 1989). According to Carpentier (1975), predictability is achieved by precise measurement of the leaflets with sizing obturators, and valve function is preserved with restoration of a normal valve orifice using a preformed ring. If these goals are achieved, a definitive repair can be expected.

A prosthetic semirigid ring is inserted in a manner similar to that for a mitral valve ring annuloplasty. The annuloplasty ring itself dif-

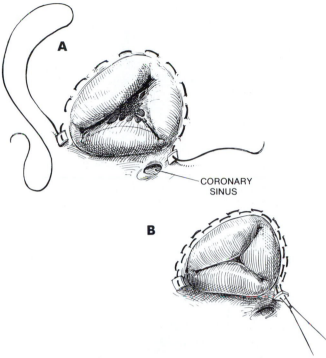

Fig. 15-14 DeVega annuloplasty. **A,** The pledgeted suture is started at the posteroseptal commissure and continued counterclockwise to the anteroseptal commissure, where another pledget is attached. **B,** The suture is brought back to the starting point, and the two ends are tied around an obturator to achieve the correct size. (From Waldhausen JA, Pierce WS: *Johnson's surgery of the chest,* ed 5, St Louis, 1985, Mosby.)

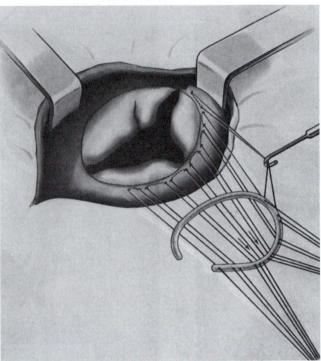

Fig. 15-16 Suturing of the prosthetic ring using mattress sutures. The interval between sutures is reduced at the commissures *(arrows).* (From Carpentier A: Cardiac valve surgery: "the French correction," *J Thorac Cardiovasc Surg* 86[3]:323, 1983.)

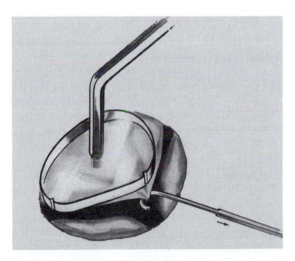

Fig. 15-15 Sizing is performed by measuring the anterior leaflet with obturators. The two notches in the edge of the obturator correspond with the commissures on either side of the septal leaflet. (From Carpentier A: Cardiac valve surgery: "the French correction," *J Thorac Cardiovasc Surg* 86[3]:323, 1983.)

fers, however, in that there is a gap in the ring corresponding to the annular area containing nodal and bundle conduction tissue. The size of the ring is determined with special tricuspid obturators (Fig. 15-15) that are used to measure the anterior leaflet. Another method is to select the obturator with notches corresponding to the commissures on either side of the septal leaflet (this technique is based on the finding that the septal leaflet is relatively unaffected by annular dilatation and tends to retain its normal size and shape).

Interrupted, alternately colored sutures are placed around the circumference of the annulus (except the conduction tissue portion of the septal leaflet) and then into the corresponding area on the prosthetic ring (Fig. 15-16). When the stitches are tied, the excess annular tissue is evenly drawn up against the prosthesis, thereby reducing the annular size and also remodeling the annulus (Fig. 15-17).

4D. **Duran annuloplasty ring technique** (Duran, 1989; Duran and others, 1980): A flexible circular ring (see Fig. 5-64) is used to reduce and selectively remodel the annulus (see Chapter 13 for illustration of the Duran ring in mitral repair). Obturators are used for sizing, and stitches are placed into the annulus in a manner similar

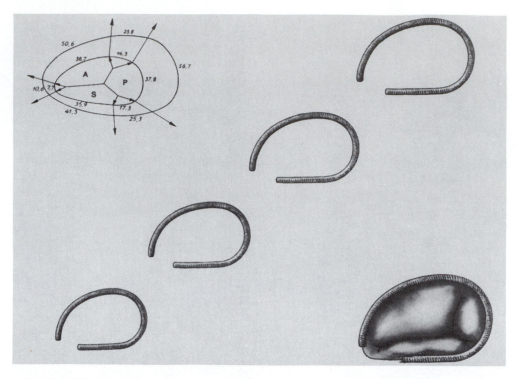

Fig. 15-17 Carpentier prosthetic tricuspid ring annuloplasty. Shown are dimensions (*left*), various sizes of rings (*middle*), and completed annuloplasty (*right*). (From Carpentier A: Cardiac valve surgery: "the French correction," *J Thorac Cardiovasc Surg* 86[3]:323, 1983.)

to that for the Carpentier technique. In the area of the septal leaflet, Duran recommends that sutures be placed superficially at the base of the septal leaflet rather than deep into the annulus in order to avoid creation of heart block.

5. The repairs are tested for residual insufficiency (a bulb syringe is often used), and the right atrium is closed.
6. A left atrial pressure monitoring line may be inserted and secured with a fine silk suture (Fig. 15-18).
7. Temporary atrial and ventricular pacing wires are attached, and the patient is weaned from cardiopulmonary bypass. Occasionally, permanent epicardial pacing leads are attached.
8. Hemostasis is achieved, chest tubes are inserted, and all incisions are closed.

Operative procedure: tricuspid valve commissurotomy for tricuspid stenosis

Open commissurotomy (Fig. 15-19) is performed for tricuspid valve stenosis. An annuloplasty ring is often inserted to remodel the annulus to create a more normal configuration and prevent residual insufficiency. When the posterior leaflet is retracted, it may be excluded on insertion of the annuloplasty ring, producing a bicuspid valve (Carpentier, 1983).

Procedure

1. All three commissures are sharply incised to mobilize the leaflets; some secondary chordae tendineae may require resection.

2. An annuloplasty ring is inserted. Occasionally bicuspidization is performed when the posterior leaflet is retracted (Fig. 15-19, *C*).

Tricuspid Valve Replacement

Even when replacement is performed for dysfunctional mitral or aortic valves, implantation of a tricuspid prosthesis is avoided when possible. The exception can occur in the presence of massive tricuspid regurgitation, destruction of the valvular apparatus, fixed pulmonary hypertension, and/or severe right ventricular dysfunction (Cohen and others, 1987b, Vlahakes and Austin, 1989). Valve replacement may also be necessary in patients with carcinoid disease of the heart producing either stenosis or regurgitation (Knott-Craig and others, 1992).

When valve replacement is indicated, the lower stresses found in the lower-pressure environment of the right ventricle (as compared with the left ventricle) favor the use of bioprosthetic valves (or aortic valve allografts mounted on a stent), whose leaflets do not seem to degenerate as quickly as they do under the higher pressures generated in the left side of the heart (Grattan, Miller, and Shumway, 1991).

Bioprostheses are also favored because they are less thrombogenic than mechanical valves, which have a significant incidence of thrombosis in the right side of the heart. The mechanism of thrombus formation is related to the presence of synthetic materials contacting blood (Edmunds, 1987); the process may be

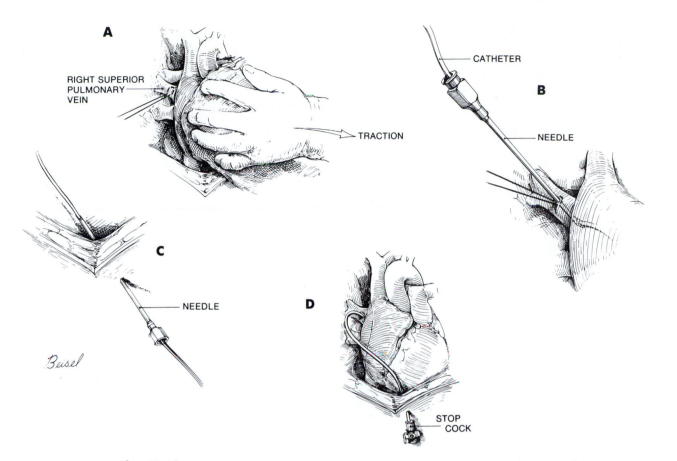

Fig. 15-18 Left atrial pressure monitoring line. **A,** The right atrium is retracted to expose the right pulmonary vein, and a pursestring suture is inserted. **B,** The monitoring catheter is inserted into the left atrium via a catheter introducer needle (some devices have a peel-away introducer). The introducer is removed, and the pursestring suture is tied. An additional suture may be used to attach the catheter to the pericardium. **C,** The catheter is threaded through a large-bore needle passed through skin and subcutaneous tissue into the pericardium. The catheter is brought out to the skin. **D,** A stopcock can be added, and the catheter is secured to the skin with a suture. Blood is aspirated to ensure proper placement of the catheter, which is then attached to pressure tubing connected to a transducer. (From Waldhausen JA, Pierce WS: *Johnson's surgery of the chest,* ed 5, St Louis, 1985, Mosby.)

accelerated in the right side of the heart because blood flow is slower and more apt to promote venous stasis (Thorburn, 1983). Optimum warfarin (Coumadin) anticoagulation is mandatory.

Another factor favoring bioprostheses is that the wedge-shaped right ventricular cavity conforms poorly to both disk and ball-and-cage valves. Residual tissue may interfere with disk movement, and the right ventricular endocardium may restrict ball movement (Harlan, Starr, and Harwin, 1981).

On occasion, a bioprosthesis may be considered unsuitable because of a high potential for late calcification, stenosis, or failure. If an allograft is unavailable, a mechanical valve must be used. Although the long-term results with most mechanical valves have been disappointing because of thrombosis, prosthetic endocarditis, and anticoagulation-related hemorrhage, the St. Jude Medical valve has shown good results. The advantages of this valve appear to be related to its central laminar flow pattern, rapid leaflet motion,

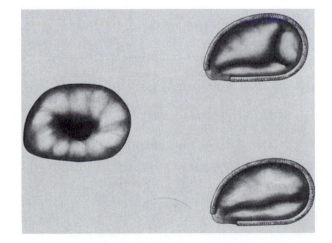

Fig. 15-19 Tricuspid valve commissurotomy and repair with an annuloplasty ring. (From Carpentier A: Cardiac valve surgery: "the French correction," *J Thorac Cardiovasc Surg* 86[3]323, 1983.)

and low residual gradient (Singh, Feng, and Sanofsky, 1992; Wellens and others, 1985).

Mechanical prostheses are also often used for patients with Ebstein's anomaly (see Fig. 15-6). Valve replacement can produce long-lasting clinical improvement (Abe and Komatsu, 1983), although reparative techniques (Carpentier and others, 1988) are available. Two technical problems are often encountered in these patients. One is the method of fixation of the prosthetic valve and the associated risk of heart block. Abe and Komatsu (1983) have experienced their best results when the prosthesis is placed in the anatomic annular ring (rather than above the coronary sinus).

The second technical difficulty involves the atrialized portion of the right ventricle. Some authors have suggested plicating the excess tissue to enhance right ventricular pumping postoperatively. Others have not favored plication of the atrialized wall, noting eventual reduction in the functional status of the right ventricular cavity, as well as less diminished paradoxical movement of the lateral atrialized wall (Abe and Komatsu, 1983; Bharati, Lev, and Kirklin, 1983).

Procedural considerations

Mitral valve prostheses are used for tricuspid valve replacement. During excision of the valve leaflets, a portion of the septal leaflet is retained. In this area, sutures are placed into the retained leaflet tissue rather than into the body of the annular ring. This aids in reducing the risk of injury to the conduction pathways.

Operative procedure: tricuspid valve replacement with a biologic or mechanical prosthesis

1. The tricuspid valve is exposed as described in step 3 of the procedure for repair of the tricuspid valve, and the leaflets are excised. A portion of the septal leaflet tissue where it joins the annulus is retained for placement of sutures in this section.
2. The valve ring is sized with obturators, and the appropriate (mitral) prosthesis is delivered to the field. If a bioprosthesis is used, it is rinsed with saline to remove the glutaraldehyde storage solution (see Chapter 13 on mitral valve surgery).
3. Individual, alternately colored sutures are placed in the valve annulus and the prosthetic sewing ring. The valve is seated, and the stitches are tied.
4. The atrium is closed, and the procedure is completed as described in step 8 of the procedure for repair of the tricuspid valve.

Operative procedure: allograft (homograft) replacement of the tricuspid valve

The advantages of central flow and freedom from anticoagulation, hemolysis, and prosthetic noise have made aortic (and pulmonary) allografts attractive for valvular lesions in the left side of the heart and for reconstruction of the right ventricular outflow tract (see Chapter 14 on aortic valve surgery). When tricuspid valve replacement is necessary, these advantages have been cited by those (Ross, 1987) who prefer the allograft to a prosthetic valve. Like tissue valves, allograft durability is enhanced by lower right-sided heart pressures (Kirklin and Barratt-Boyes, 1993; McKay, Sono, and Arnold, 1988; Ross, 1987).

Procedure

1. The aortic valve (or pulmonary valve) allograft is evaluated to confirm the absence of any structural abnormalities (Kirklin and Barratt-Boyes, 1993) and is prepared as described in Chapter 14.
2. The allograft is mounted onto a stent or frame (or attached to a segment of Dacron graft) and sewn to the tricuspid annular ring. If the graft is not used immediately, it can be stored in solution at 4° C (39.5° F), or it can be cryopreserved.

Tricuspid Valvulectomy

Special problems may be encountered in patients with intractable bacterial endocarditis (often caused by *Staphylococcus aureus* or *Pseudomonas aeruginosa*) that cannot be controlled with intensive antibiotic therapy (Relf, 1993). In these patients, who are often intravenous drug users, florid vegetations involving all three leaflets may make valve repair by debridement of the vegetations or valvuloplasty unfeasible. Replacement of the valve is associated with thrombotic complications and a significant incidence of reinfection leading to prosthetic valve endocarditis. In an effort to avoid continued sepsis and recurring infection (generally attributed to resumption of drug use), some researchers have performed initial valvulectomy, followed if necessary by a later second operation for tricuspid valve replacement (Arbulu and Asfaw, 1981; Barbour and Roberts, 1986; Karchmer, 1989). Others (Stern and others, 1986) have questioned the need for excision and prefer initial implantation of a bioprosthesis. Absence of the tricuspid (or pulmonary) valve can be hemodynamically tolerated by some patients, unlike aortic or mitral valve excision without replacement.

Indications for surgery generally include persistent sepsis, recurrent septic pulmonary emboli, and valvular insufficiency leading to acute right-sided heart failure (Stern and others, 1986).

Operative procedure

1. A median sternotomy and bicaval cannulation for cardiopulmonary bypass are performed. Cardioplegic arrest is used to protect the heart.
2. The right atrium is incised longitudinally.
3. The tricuspid valve is totally excised, with care taken to preserve the conduction tissue in the area of the septal leaflet. Portions of infected tissue may be cultured. (It may be advisable to confine and contain the instruments used to excise the infected valve.)
4. If the infectious process extends to the pulmonary valve, excision of that valve may be indicated. A supravalvular incision is made in the pulmonary artery, and the valve is excised.
5. The surgical field is irrigated, debris is removed, and all incisions are closed.

Table 15-2 ■ *Postoperative complications of tricuspid valve surgery*

Complication	Interventions
Rhythm Disturbances (Complete Heart Block)	
Early onset: may be due to edema; may be iatrogenically related to suture placement in conduction tissue; increased risk with combined tricuspid surgery and mitral valve replacement (compression of firm prosthetic sewing rings)	Permanent pacemaker may be inserted; usually epicardial lead is inserted via thoracotomy to avoid possible injury to valve prosthesis from transvenous insertion; occasionally epicardial leads are placed at time of surgery when heart block has been strongly suspected or confirmed.
Delayed onset: usually related to scar formation around prosthetic annulus; may be idiopathic degeneration of surrounding tissue	Same
Recurrent/Residual Tricuspid Regurgitation	
More likely in patients with irreversible pulmonary hypertension or continued mitral valve problems (prosthetic malfunction, endocarditis)	Repair left-sided lesion Replace mitral prosthesis Repair/replace tricuspid valve
Residual Tricuspid Diastolic Gradient	
May be related to tricuspid prosthetic (valve or ring) annulus being too small; residual stenosis	Replace with larger prosthesis
Persistent Right Ventricular Failure	
Related to dysfunctional right ventricle	Valve replacement may (or may not) improve condition Medical treatment includes diuretics, low-sodium diet, rest, and digitalis
Prosthesis-Related Complications	
Prosthetic valve endocarditis Anticoagulation-related hemorrhage Bioprosthetic degeneration: may occur later than with left-sided bioprosthesis because of lower stresses in right ventricle	See Chapter 13 on mitral valve surgery
Prosthetic dehiscence from torn suture or fractured ring	Repair annuloplasty
Prosthetic thrombosis: high risk in right side of heart; may occur early or late; is generally due to inadequate anticoagulation of mechanical valve	Intravenous thrombolysis can be useful when thrombosis first occurs; thrombectomy and valve replacement (with bioprosthesis)

Modified from Grattan MT, Miller DC, Shumway NE: Management of complications of tricuspid valve surgery. In Waldhausen JA, Orringer MB: *Complications in cardiothoracic surgery*, St Louis, 1991, Mosby.

Postoperatively valvulectomy patients require additional volume to maintain an adequate right atrial systolic pressure and right ventricular preload. Intravenous antibiotic therapy is continued for a number of weeks to eradicate the infection. With the valve excised, patients will display a pulsatile liver (from reflux), but in this case it does not necessarily indicate right-sided heart failure (Arbulu and Asfaw, 1981). A second operation may be undertaken for prosthetic valve replacement subsequent to a cure of the endocarditis or if medical treatment has failed to control hemodynamic derangements associated with right-sided or biventricular failure.

In patients habituated to the use of intravenous drugs, a more favorable outcome is likely if the addiction has been controlled. Counseling and rehabilitation should be available to the patient. Continued use of contaminated drug paraphernalia is likely to lead to recurrence of endocarditis.

POSTOPERATIVE CONSIDERATIONS

When tricuspid valve surgery is performed in conjunction with operations for aortic and mitral valve lesions, the results of surgery are dependent on the success of the operation for the left-sided lesions, the degree and reversibility of both left and right ventricular dysfunction, and the amount and reversibility of pulmonary hypertension (Duran, 1989). As with most cardiac operations, better results can be obtained if the operation is performed before the development of congestive heart failure (Karp, 1990). In addition to the benefits of cardiac rehabilitation, pulmonary rehabilitation may be helpful in these patients. If valve replacement with a mechanical prosthesis has been performed, warfarin anticoagulation is started approximately 48 to 72 hours after surgery (Kirklin and Barratt-Boyes, 1993).

Complications

The clinician is alert to the appearance of complete heart block throughout the postoperative hospital stay (Table 15-2), especially when valve replacement has been performed. Heart block may not become apparent until a few days after surgery, especially if temporary pacing has been used in the immediate postoperative period. ECG monitoring should be continued until a stable rhythm is established at an adequate rate (Kirklin and Barratt-Boyes, 1993). If permanent pacing is indicated, transvenous leads may be avoided because of the possibility of injuring the native valve or bioprosthesis, or of becoming entrapped in a mechanical prosthesis. When late heart block appears, it can be corrected with an epicardial lead placement through a thoracotomy approach (Grattan, Miller, and Shumway, 1991).

Complications related to annuloplasty techniques include residual regurgitation or stenosis. The former is commonly due to irreversible pulmonary hypertension, although suture dehiscence may be a cause. The latter may be the result of too small a prosthesis being inserted. Prosthetic valve replacement is associated with a number of complications described in Chapters 13 and 14 on aortic and mitral valve surgery.

PULMONARY VALVE PROCEDURES

PULMONARY VALVE DISEASE

The pulmonary valve, the smallest of the cardiac valves, has three leaflets and is similar to the aortic valve. It is situated between the distal right ventricular outflow tract and the entrance to the main pulmonary artery. When the pericardium is opened during median sternotomy, the bulging outline of the anterior sinuses surrounding the valve leaflets can be seen on the front of the heart at the entrance to the main pulmonary artery. They are even more apparent when the right ventricular outflow tract is distended.

Acquired lesions of the pulmonary valve are rare, and this is probably related to the conditions within the right side of the heart, such as lower pressures and less turbulent blood flow, which subject the valve to less stress as compared with the valves in the left side of the heart. Rheumatic fever and infective endocarditis are less likely to affect the pulmonary valve than they are the other valves of the heart (Braunwald, 1991). When pulmonary valve disorders do exist, they are usually associated with primary pulmonary hypertension, or they develop secondary to lesions in the left side of the heart (e.g., mitral or aortic valve disease) that produce pulmonary hypertension leading to pulmonary valvular regurgitation (Fig. 15-20). Correction of the left-sided lesion often reduces the degree of regurgitation.

Other causes of pulmonary insufficiency are dilatation of the pulmonary valve ring or the pulmonary artery secondary to pulmonary hypertension or connective tissue disorders such as Marfan's syndrome. Infective endocarditis, valvular damage due to the prolonged use of pulmonary artery monitoring catheters, carcinoid syndrome, direct trauma to the heart, and previous valvulotomy for pulmonary stenosis may also be etiologic factors (Ansari, 1991; Braunwald, 1992; Wynne and Braunwald, 1992).

Symptoms of pulmonary regurgitation include dyspnea and fatigue, but these are not usually apparent unless there is coexisting pulmonary hypertension (Abramczyk and Brown, 1991).

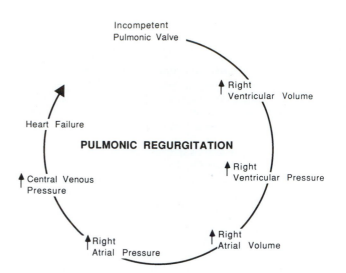

Fig. 15-20 Pathophysiology of pulmonary regurgitation. (From Kinney MR and others: *Comprehensive cardiac care*, ed 7, St Louis, 1991, Mosby.)

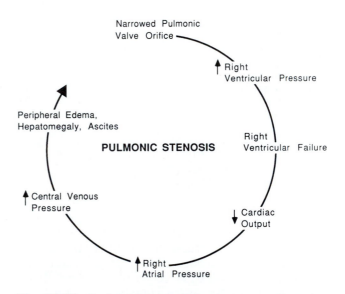

Fig. 15-21 Pathophysiology of pulmonary valve stenosis. (From Kinney MR and others: *Comprehensive cardiac care*, ed 7, St Louis, 1991, Mosby.)

Stenotic lesions causing obstruction to flow may result from infectious or inflammatory processes, tumors, carcinoid plaques or atheromas (Issenberg, 1987). Although acute rheumatic fever does involve the pulmonary valve, as well as the other valves of the heart, it rarely causes appreciable chronic fibrosis or dysfunction (Altrichter and others, 1989).

Typically, pulmonary valve stenosis is a congenital lesion. The valve may be bicuspid or tricuspid; it may be accompanied by infundibular muscular stenosis causing right ventricular outflow tract obstruction. Depending on its severity, pulmonary stenosis may not be recognized until childhood or adulthood (Fig. 15-21). Symptoms include dyspnea on exertion, fa-

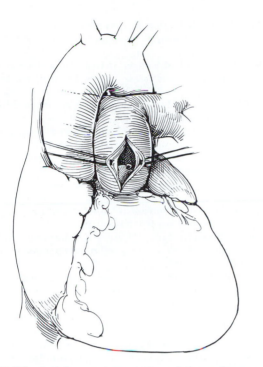

Fig. 15-22 Incision and retraction of the pulmonary artery for exposure of the pulmonary valve. (From Waldhausen JA, Pierce WS: *Johnson's surgery of the chest*, ed 5, St Louis, 1985, Mosby.)

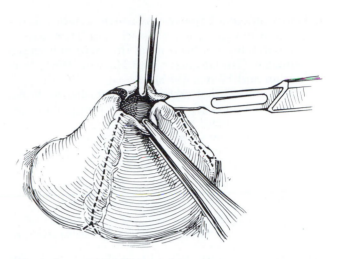

Fig. 15-23 Commissurotomy for pulmonary stenosis. Incisions are made along the dotted lines. (From Waldhausen JA, Pierce WS: *Johnson's surgery of the chest*, ed 5, St Louis, 1985, Mosby.)

tigue, and occasionally cyanosis (Harlan, Starr, and Harwin, 1981). These are manifestations of congestive failure due to chronic pressure overloading of the right ventricle, reduced cardiac output from obstruction to flow, and an inadequate supply of oxygenated blood to the systemic circulation.

DIAGNOSTIC EVALUATION OF PULMONARY VALVE DISEASE

In addition to a thorough medical history, diagnostic evaluation includes an electrocardiogram to identify the presence right ventricular hypertrophy, right atrial dilatation, and conduction disturbances; a chest x-ray film to detect right ventricular enlargement, pulmonary artery dilatation, and pulmonary vascular changes; and color flow Doppler echocardiography to visualize and quantify valvular hemodynamic changes. Cardiac catheterization is used for surgical candidates to assess pulmonary artery/right ventricular pressure gradients, the degree of regurgitation, left-to-right shunts, and other possible anomalies or lesions (Ansari, 1991).

SURGERY FOR PULMONARY VALVE DISEASE

Percutaneous balloon valvuloplasty is commonly performed for isolated pulmonary valve stenosis. The success of balloon dilatation procedures is due in part to the frequent absence of calcification on the pul-

monary valve, in contrast to that on valves in the left side of the heart (Altrichter and others, 1989).

When valves are dysplastic or hypoplastic, surgical treatment may be performed to repair or, rarely, to replace the valve. Surgery for acquired pulmonary regurgitation is uncommon. If pulmonary valve replacement is indicated, aortic valve prostheses are used. Increasingly, allografts are being used in preference to mechanical or bioprosthetic valves. They are widely used in children to replace the pulmonary valve or to reconstruct the right ventricular outflow tract (Ross, 1987).

Open commissurotomy remains the most commonly performed procedure for pulmonary stenosis; in the acyanotic patient, operative mortality is less than 1% (Harlan, Starr, and Harwin, 1981).

Operative procedure: open commissurotomy for pulmonary valve stenosis

1. A median sternotomy is performed, and cardiopulmonary bypass is established using double venous cannulation to keep venous return from obscuring the surgical site. The heart is arrested with cardioplegia solution or fibrillated with an alternating-current (AC) fibrillator so that air cannot be ejected into the left side of the heart.
2. The pulmonary artery is opened transversely or longitudinally (Fig. 15-22) to expose the pulmonary valve. Traction sutures may be used to facilitate exposure.
3. The valve is inspected, and the commissures are incised to the annulus with a knife (No. 11 blade) (Fig. 15-23). Hegar dilators may be used to calibrate the valve orifice and the infundibulum.
4. If annular enlargement is indicated, a patch (autologous pericardium or prosthetic patch material) is used to enlarge the annulus and at the same time close the incision).

5. If infundibular hypertrophy restricts right ventricular outflow, part of the muscle can be resected.
6. If a patch has not been used, the incision is closed primarily (Harlan, Starr, and Harwin, 1981; Walhausen and Pierce, 1985).
7. To resume cardiac action in the fibrillating heart, direct-current (DC) countershock is applied to defibrillate the heart.
8. Incision sites are inspected for hemostasis, cardiopulmonary bypass is terminated, chest tubes are inserted, and all incisions are closed.

REFERENCES

Abe T, Komatsu S: Valve replacement for Ebstein's anomaly of the tricuspid valve: early and long-term results of eight cases, *Chest* 84(4):414, 1983.

Abramczyk EL, Brown MM: Valvular heart disease. In Kinney MR and others, *Comprehensive cardiac care,* ed 7, St Louis, 1991, Mosby.

Alexander JA, O'Brien DJ: Ebstein's anomaly. In Sabiston DC, editor: *Textbook of surgery,* ed 14, Philadelphia, 1991, WB Saunders.

Altrichter PM and others: Surgical pathology of the pulmonary valve: a study of 116 cases spanning 15 years, *Mayo Clin Proc* 64:1352, 1989.

Ansari A: Isolated pulmonary valvular regurgitation: current perspectives, *Prog Cardiovasc Dis* 33(5):329, 1991.

Arbulu A, Asfaw I: Tricuspid valvulectomy without prosthetic replacement, *J Thorac Cardiovasc Surg* 82(5):684, 1981.

Barbour DJ, Roberts WC: Valve excision only versus excision plus replacement for active infective endocarditis involving the tricuspid valve, *Am J Cardiol* 57:475, 1986.

Baughman KL and others: Predictors of survival after tricuspid valve surgery, *Am J Cardiol* 54:137, 1984.

Bharati S, Lev M, Kirklin JW: *Cardiac surgery and the conduction system,* New York, 1983, John Wiley & Sons.

Braunwald E: Valvular heart disease. In Wilson JD and others: *Harrison's principles of internal medicine,* ed 12, New York, 1991, McGraw Hill.

Braunwald E: Valvular heart disease. In Braunwald E: *Heart disease,* ed 4, Philadelphia, 1992, WB Saunders.

Brundage BH and others: Acquired tricuspid valve disease. In Greenberg BH, Murphy E, editors: *Valvular heart disease,* St Louis, 1987, Mosby.

Carpentier A: Discussion of Boyd AD and others: Tricuspid annuloplasty: five and one-half years' experience with 78 patients, *J Thorac Cardiovasc Surg* 68(3):344, 1974.

Carpentier A: Discussion of Grondin P and others: Carpentier's annulus and DeVega's annuloplasty: The end of the tricuspid challenge, *J Thorac Cardiovasc Surg* 70(5):852, 1975.

Carpentier A: Cardiac valve surgery: "the French correction," *J Thorac Cardiovasc Surg* 86(3):323, 1983.

Carpentier A and others: A new reconstructive operation for Ebstein's anomaly of the tricuspid valve, *J Thorac Cardiovasc Surg* 96(1):92, 1988.

Cavallo GA: The person with valvular heart disease. In Guzzetta CE, Dossey BM: *Cardiovascular nursing practice,* St Louis, 1992, Mosby.

Cohen SR and others: Tricuspid regurgitation in patients with acquired, chronic, pure mitral regurgitation. I. Prevalence, diagnosis, and comparison of preoperative clinical and hemodynamic features in patients with and without tricuspid regurgitation, *J Thorac Cardiovasc Surg* 94(4):481, 1987a.

Cohen SR and others: Tricuspid regurgitation in patients with acquired, chronic, pure mitral regurgitation. II. Nonoperative management, tricuspid valve annuloplasty, and tricuspid valve replacement, *J Thorac Cardiovasc Surg* 94(4):488, 1987b.

Curtius JM and others: Doppler versus contrast echocardiography for diagnosis of tricuspid regurgitation, *Am J Cardiol* 56:333, 1985.

Duran CM: Tricuspid valve repair. In Grillo HC and others, editors: *Current therapy in cardiothoracic surgery,* Philadelphia, 1989, BC Decker.

Duran CM and others: Is tricuspid valve repair necessary? *J Thorac Cardiovasc Surg* 80(6):849, 1980.

Edmunds LH: Thromboembolic and bleeding complications of prosthetic heart valves. In Rabago G, Cooley DA, editors: *Heart valve replacement: current status and future trends,* Mt Kisco, NY, 1987, Futura Publishing.

Gay WA: *Atlas of adult cardiac surgery,* New York, 1990, Churchill Livingstone.

Gayet C and others: Traumatic tricuspid insufficiency: an underdiagnosed disease, *Chest* 92(3):429, 1987.

Ginzton LE, Siegel RJ, Criley JM: Natural history of tricuspid valve endocarditis: a two dimensional echocardiographic study, *Am J Cardiol* 49:1853, 1982.

Graham TP, Friesinger CG: Complex cyanotic congenital heart disease. In Roberts WC: *Adult congenital heart disease,* Philadelphia, 1987, FA Davis.

Grattan MT, Miller DC, Shumway NE: Management of complications of tricuspid valve surgery. In Walhausen JA, Orringer MB: *Complications in cardiothoracic surgery,* St Louis, 1991, Mosby.

Grondin P and others: Carpentier's annulus and DeVega's annuloplasty: the end of the tricuspid challenge, *J Thorac Cardiovasc Surg* 70(5):852, 1975.

Harlan BJ, Starr A, Harwin FM: *Manual of cardiac surgery,* vol 2, New York, 1981, Springer-Verlag.

Hauck AJ and others: Surgical pathology of the tricuspid valve: a study of 363 cases spanning 25 years, *Mayo Clin Proc* 63:851, 1988.

Issenberg HJ: Pulmonic valve disease. In Greenberg BH, Murphy E, editors: *Valvular heart disease,* St Louis, 1987, Mosby.

Jordan JC, Sanders CA: Tricuspid atresia with prolonged survival, *Am J Cardiol* 18:112, 1966.

Karchmer AW: Prosthetic and native valve endocarditis. In Grillo HC and others, editors: *Current therapy in cardiothoracic surgery,* Philadelphia, 1989, BC Decker.

Karp RB: Acquired disease of the tricuspid valve. In Sabiston DC, Spencer FC: *Surgery of the chest,* ed 5, vols 1 and 2, New York, 1990, WB Saunders.

Kay JH: Surgical treatment of tricuspid regurgitation, *Ann Thorac Surg* 53:1132, 1992.

Kirklin JW, Barratt-Boyes BG: *Cardiac surgery,* ed 2, New York, 1993, Churchill Livingstone.

Kleikamp G and others: Tricuspid valve regurgitation following blunt thoracic trauma, *Chest* 102(4):1294, 1992.

Knott-Craig CJ and others: Carcinoid disease of the heart: surgical management of ten patients, *J Thorac Cardiovasc Surg* 104(2):475, 1992.

Kratz JM and others: Trends and results in tricuspid valve surgery, *Chest* 86(6):837, 1985.

Lambertz H and others: Long-term follow-up after Carpentier tricuspid valvuloplasty, *Am Heart J* 117(3):615, 1989.

Lee RT, Bhatia SJ, Sutton MG: Assessment of valvular heart disease with Doppler echocardiography, *JAMA* 262(15):2131, 1989.

McGrath LB and others: Tricuspid valve operations in 530 patients: twenty-five-year assessment of early and late phase events, *J Thorac Cardiovasc Surg* 99(1):124, 1990.

McKay R, Sono J, Arnold RM: Tricuspid valve replacement using an unstented pulmonary homograft, *Ann Thorac Surg* 46:58, 1988.

Minale C, Lambertz H, Messmer BJ: New developments for reconstruction of the tricuspid valve, *J Thorac Cardiovasc Surg* 94(4):626, 1987.

Muirhead J: Right ventricular infarction. In Underhill SL and others: *Cardiac nursing*, ed 2, Philadelphia, 1989, JB Lippincott.

Mullany CJ and others: Repair of tricuspid valve insufficiency in patients undergoing double (aortic and mitral) valve replacement: perioperative mortality and long-term (1 to 20 years) follow-up in 109 patients, *J Thorac Cardiovasc Surg* 94(5):740, 1987.

Perloff JK: Potential longevity in unoperated adults. In Roberts WC: *Adult congenital heart disease*, Philadelphia, 1987, FA Davis.

Rabago G and others: The new DeVega technique in tricuspid annuloplasty: results in 150 patients, *J Cardiovasc Surg* 21:231, 1980.

Rankin JS: Mitral and tricuspid valve disease. In Sabiston DC, editor: *Textbook of surgery*, ed 14, Philadelphia, 1991, WB Saunders.

Relf MV: Surgical intervention for tricuspid valve endocarditis: vegetectomy, valve excision, or valve replacement? *J Cardiovasc Nurs* 7(2):71, 1993.

Rivera R, Duran E, Ajuria M: Carpentier's flexible ring versus DeVega's annuloplasty: a prospective randomized study, *J Thorac Cardiovasc Surg* 89(2):196, 1985.

Roberts WC: Congenital cardiovascular abnormalities usually silent until adulthood. In Roberts WC: *Adult congenital heart disease*, Philadelphia, 1987, FA Davis.

Robison JS: Acute right ventricular infarction: recognition, evaluation, and treatment, *Crit Care Nurse* 7(4):42, 1987.

Ross D: Application of homografts in clinical surgery, *J Cardiac Surg* 1(3, suppl):175, 1987.

Singh AK, Feng WC, Sanofsky SJ: Long-term results of St. Jude Medical valve in the tricuspid position, *Ann Thorac Surg* 54:538, 1992.

Spencer FC: Acquired heart disease. In Schwartz SI, editor: *Principles of surgery*, ed 5, New York, 1989, McGraw-Hill.

Stern HJ and others: Immediate tricuspid valve replacement for endocarditis, *J Thorac Cardiovasc Surg* 91(2):163, 1986.

Tei C and others: The tricuspid valve annulus: study of size and motion in normal subjects and in patients with tricuspid regurgitation, *Circulation* 66(3):665, 1982.

Thorburn CW and others: Long-term results of tricuspid valve replacement and the problem of prosthetic valve thrombosis, *Am J Cardiol* 51:1128, 1983.

Vlahakes GJ, Austen WG: Tricuspid valve replacement. In Grillo HC and others, editors: *Current therapy in cardiothoracic surgery*, Philadelphia, 1989, BC Decker.

Waldhausen JA, Pierce WS: *Johnson's surgery of the chest*, ed 5, St Louis, 1985, Mosby.

Wellens F and others: Tricuspid valve replacement: a comparative experience with different valve substitutes. In Matloff JM, editor: *Cardiac valve replacement: current status*, Boston, 1985, Martinus Nijhoff Publishing.

Wynne J, Braunwald E: The cardiomyopathies and myocarditides: toxic, chemical, and physical damage to the heart. In Braunwald E: *Heart disease*, ed 4, Philadelphia, 1992, WB Saunders.

16

Surgery on the Thoracic Aorta

The operation now proposed by the writer is applicable to . . . all fusiform and saccular aneurisms, whether traumatic or idiopathic, in which the conditions for securing provisional haemostasis can be obtained . . . These cases offer admirable opportunities for the conservative application of ateriorrhaphy, with the view of preserving the lumen of the injured vessel, and thus maintaining their functional value as blood carriers.

Rudolph Matas, MD, 1903

Matas' treatment of aneurysms was limited to the peripheral vascular system because in the early twentieth century there were no methods to provide circulatory support or prosthetic grafts to replace the diseased aorta. Most aneurysms of the thoracic aorta were inoperable. Occasionally, saccular aneurysms could be treated by clamping the neck of the lesion, excising the aneurysmal sac, and suturing the remaining edges of the aorta (Cooley, 1989). The contributions of Matas were significant nonetheless, because he was one of the first to suggest techniques that have become commonplace today: obtaining proximal and distal control of the artery, performing minimal dissection of adjacent structures, and restoring normal, unobstructed flow through the vessel (Cooley, 1984; Kirklin and Barratt-Boyes, 1993).

THE AORTA

The normal aorta is a remarkably strong conduit that can withstand the impact of 2.5 to 3 billion heartbeats in an average lifetime. The aorta is the primary blood conductor and, with its major branches, supplies blood to all the major organs of the body (see Fig. 4-19). When surgery requires temporary occlusion of a portion of the aorta, tissues receiving blood from that segment are deprived of oxygen, nutrients, and the other metabolic requirements. In procedures on the heart, measures are instituted to protect the myocardium and the brain from the effects of ischemia. In procedures on the thoracic aorta, one has to be especially concerned about the neurologic effects of ischemia not only on the brain, but also on the spinal cord. In treating lesions of the ascending aorta, and in particular of the aortic arch, which necessitates temporary interruption of cerebral blood flow, there is a risk for stroke. When disorders of the descending thoracic aorta or thoracoabdominal aneurysms are being treated, interruption of aortic blood flow between the eighth thoracic and fourth lumbar vertebrae can result in paraplegia, because the spinal cord receives its most important blood supply within this area. Prevention of these complications is a major consideration during surgery on the thoracic aorta (Box 16-1).

THE AORTIC WALL

Like all arteries, the aortic wall consists of three layers (Fig. 16-1). The **tunica intima** is the thin inner layer made up of endothelial cells; the thick middle layer, the **tunica media,** consists of relatively little smooth muscle (as compared with the peripheral arteries) but contains a large amount of laminated and intertwining sheets of elastic tissue arranged in spiral fashion; and the outermost layer, the **tunica adventitia,** contains mainly collagen but also the vasa vasorum and lymphatics, which nourish the aortic wall. The structure of the aortic wall facilitates both the forward propulsion of blood and its circulation throughout the body.

When blood is ejected by the left ventricle, the aorta distends and then recoils, propelling the blood distally into the arterial bed. As the patient ages, smooth muscle and elastic tissue in the aorta and its branches tend to stiffen, producing an increase in the systolic blood pressure and a reduction in the distensibility of the aortic wall. The development of arteriosclerosis and hypertension associated with aging, as well as the existence of inherited or acquired disorders such as infection, inflammation, atherosclerosis, or autoimmune diseases, can produce pathologic changes in the

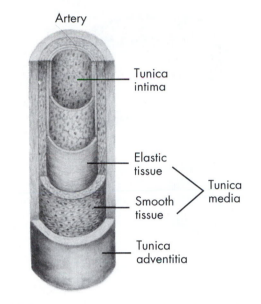

Fig. 16-1   The aortic wall consists of three layers: the inner tunica intima, the tunica media composed of elastic and muscular tissue, and the tunica adventitia. (From Canobbio MM: *Cardiovascular disorders,* St Louis, 1990, Mosby.)

aortic wall, leading to the formation of aortic aneurysms and other disorders of the thoracic aorta (Eagle and DeSanctis, 1992).

AORTIC ANEURYSMS AND AORTIC DISSECTIONS
Aneurysm

An aneurysm is a localized or diffuse dilatation of the arterial wall occurring with increasing frequency between the fifth and seventh decades of life (Webb and Kelly, 1986). Thoracic (and abdominal) aortic aneurysms are characterized by weakening and degeneration of the medial layer, which leads to progressive enlargement of all layers of the vessel. There is compression of the surrounding structures and, if untreated, eventual rupture with exsanguination. When thoracic aneurysms rupture into the pericardium, death is usually caused by cardiac tamponade. The standard treatment for aneurysms is the surgical restoration of vascular continuity by relining or replacing the diseased aorta with a prosthetic graft.

Aortic Dissection

Aortic dissection is a unique entity affecting the aortic media. It is the most common catastrophe involving the aorta and occurs two to three times more often than the acutely rupturing abdominal aortic aneurysm (Wheat, 1990). Repeated biomechanical stress, often in combination with hypertension and a congenital predisposition, produces an intimal tear (Fig. 16-2) through which blood enters and creates a dissecting hematoma of variable distance within the tunica media (Weiland and Walker, 1986). As blood continues to enter the false lumen, it enlarges and impinges on the true lumen. Eventually this causes compression of the arterial branches of the aorta. The torn intima may create a flap of tissue or progress to create a circumferential dissection with intussusception of the intima into the distal portion of the aorta (Reitknecht, Bhayana, and Lajos, 1988).

The intimal tear may originate in any portion of the aorta but is most often found in the ascending thoracic aorta just above the coronary ostia and in the descending thoracic aorta just distal to the subclavian artery. It can occur in the presence of an atherosclerotic aorta. Interestingly, progression of an ascending aortic dissection may be prevented or halted by severe atherosclerosis of the aortic arch, which causes atrophy and fibrosis of the underlying media (Roberts, 1986).

Although the term "dissecting aortic aneurysm" is often applied to all of these lesions, it is appropriate only for those dissections that are superimposed on preexisting fusiform aneurysms (Crawford and others, 1988). "Aortic dissection" is considered a more

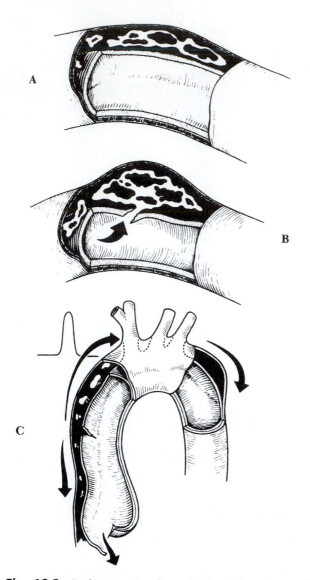

Fig. 16-2 Pathogenesis of aortic dissection. **A,** Medial and intimal degeneration in the aortic wall predispose the vessel to injury. **B,** Hemodynamic forces acting on the aortic wall produce an intimal tear, directing the bloodstream into diseased media. **C,** The resulting dissecting hematoma is propagated in both directions by a pulse wave produced by each myocardial contraction. (From Wheat MW: Acute dissecting aneurysms of the aorta. In Goldberger E: *Treatment of cardiac emergencies,* ed 5, St Louis, 1990, Mosby.)

accurate designation when the affected aorta was not previously aneurysmal. Dilatation of the vessel is due mainly to the dissecting hematoma rather than to a transmural dilatation of all layers of the aortic wall. The dissection may be classified as acute if it is less than 2 weeks in duration; chronic dissections are those present for more than 2 weeks (Bourland, 1992).

Surgery is recommended for all patients with dissections of the ascending aorta and the transverse aortic arch (Svensson and others, 1990). Dissections of the descending thoracic aorta are surgically treated when there is continuing enlargement of the vessel,

danger of imminent rupture, or other complications, usually related to interruption of blood flow through branching blood vessels. Uncomplicated descending thoracic aortic aneurysms are often treated medically with antihypertensive and beta-adrenergic–blocking medications, analgesics, sedatives, and rest.

CLASSIFICATION OF AORTIC ANEURYSMS AND AORTIC DISSECTIONS

Aneurysms and dissections of the thoracic aorta may be classified according to location, morphology, and etiology. Consideration of all three factors is critical to perioperative nurses and surgeons alike for preparing and executing the surgical plan. In particular, this knowledge provides the most meaningful information for determining the indications for operation, the surgical approach (including positioning and instrumentation), and the technique of circulatory support.

Location

For simplicity, aortic disease is typically described according to the principal structural region in which it occurs (i.e., ascending, transverse, or descending aorta) (Fig. 16-3), although the disease process or injury often crosses these anatomic boundaries. Descending aortic aneurysms may be confined to the thoracic section of the aorta (above the diaphragm), or they may occupy both thoracic and abdominal sections of the aorta (thoracoabdominal aneurysms).

Aortic dissection has prompted distinctive classification systems based on the portion of the aorta affected. It is especially important to ascertain whether the dissection involves the ascending aorta, because there is a high risk of rupture in this region. DeBakey and colleagues (1965) were the first to place dissections into three categories: types I, II, and III (Fig. 16-4). In type I dissections, the intimal tear originates in the ascending aorta and the dissecting hematoma extends to the descending thoracic aorta or beyond. Type II dissections involve the ascending aorta only. Type III dissections occur in the descending thoracic aorta. The other most commonly used classification system is the one devised at Stanford by Miller, Shumway, and their associates (Miller and others, 1971) (Fig. 16-4). It divides dissections into two types: type A, located in the ascending aorta, and type B, involving the descending aorta.

Morphology

Morphologically, aneurysms are commonly described as true or false (Fig. 16-5). **True aneurysms** involve all three layers of the arterial wall: intima, media, and adventitia; the full thickness is dilated beyond normal limits. Aneurysms can be further subdivided into saccular or fusiform aneurysms. The former is a localized outpouching from the vessel wall, frequently attached

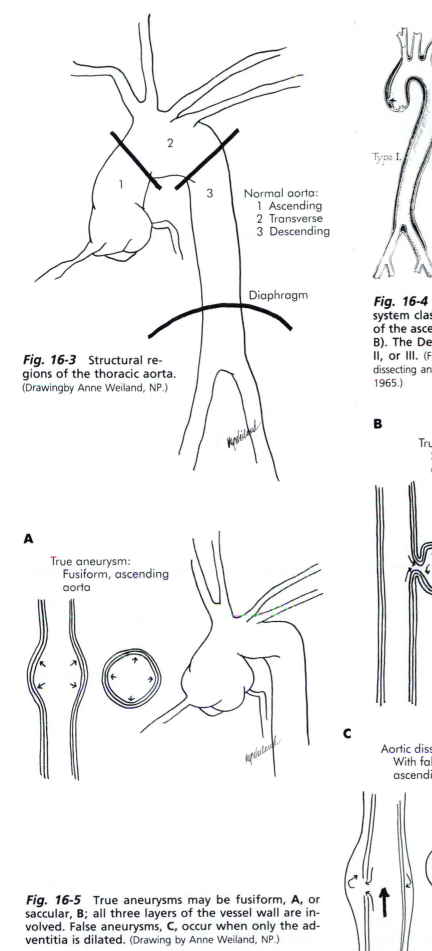

Fig. 16-3 Structural regions of the thoracic aorta. (Drawing by Anne Weiland, NP.)

Normal aorta:
1 Ascending
2 Transverse
3 Descending

Diaphragm

A

True aneurysm:
Fusiform, ascending aorta

Fig. 16-5 True aneurysms may be fusiform, A, or saccular, B; all three layers of the vessel wall are involved. False aneurysms, C, occur when only the adventitia is dilated. (Drawing by Anne Weiland, NP.)

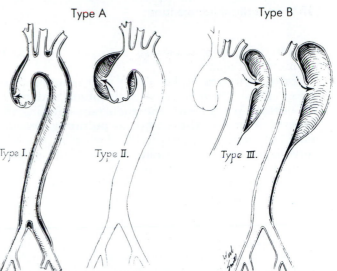

Type A

Type B

Type I.

Type II.

Type III.

Fig. 16-4 Location of aortic dissections. The Stanford system classifies aortic dissections based on involvement of the ascending aorta (type A) or noninvolvement (type B). The DeBakey system classifies dissections into type I, II, or III. (From DeBakey ME and others: Surgical management of dissecting aneurysms of the aorta, *J Thorac Cardiovasc Surg* 49:130, 1965.)

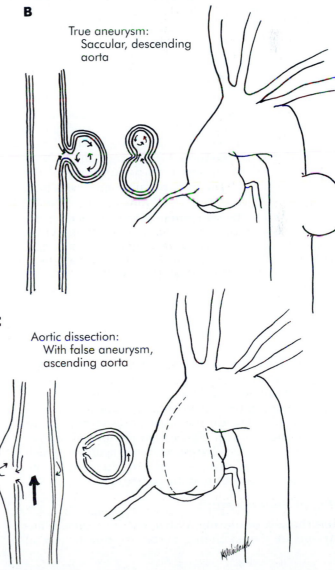

B

True aneurysm:
Saccular, descending aorta

C

Aortic dissection:
With false aneurysm, ascending aorta

by a neck of tissue. Fusiform aneurysms involve circumferential dilatation.

False aneurysm implies a separation of intima from outer layers. The innermost aortic intimal width may be normal in size, with the aneurysm affecting the outermost layers. Also known as **pulsating hematomas,** false aneurysms are produced when injury to the inner layers causes extravasation of blood through the intimal and medial layers, but the hematoma is contained by the adventitial layer (Sabiston, 1991). Aortic dissections are a form of false aneurysm.

Etiology

Lesions may be either congenital or acquired. Acquired diseases may be complicated by underlying inherited histologic disorders that compromise vascular integrity and accelerate the degenerative process.

Congenital aneurysms

Congenital forms are rare. When they do occur, they are often related to anatomic anomalies or inherited metabolic disorders. Coarctation of the aorta produces hypertension and increased pressure on the aortic wall proximal to the coarctation. A bicuspid aortic valve increases turbulent blood flow and reduces laminar flow, thereby placing greater lateral stress on the aorta and causing local injury (Bourland, 1992).

Abnormalities of the aortic root sinuses may first become apparent when they rupture. If they are detected earlier, it is often an incidental finding at cardiac catheterization for coronary artery disease. Although other sinuses can be involved, they commonly affect the right sinus of Valsalva, which usually ruptures into the right ventricle or the right atrium, creating a fistula that produces a left-to-right shunt. Noncoronary sinus aneurysms tend to rupture into the right atrium, and left coronary sinus aneurysms have been known to rupture into all four chambers of the heart, as well as the pulmonary artery. Treatment depends on the lesion and consists of closing small fistulas primarily and patching larger fistulas and, if present, septal defects of the ventricle. If aortic root dilatation has made the aortic valve incompetent, valve replacement may be necessary (Grover and Calhoun, 1991).

Acquired aneurysms/dissections

Acquired aneurysms and dissections of the thoracic aorta are associated with medial degeneration ("cystic medial necrosis"), arteriosclerosis, atherosclerosis, and trauma. Hypertension is a common finding in these patients and can further weaken an aortic wall already damaged by other causes. Aneurysms tend to occur in older patients with atherosclerotic disease, but patients with inherited connective tissue disorders, which can aggravate an existing problem, may acquire an aneurysm or dissection at an earlier age.

Medial degeneration

Most thoracic aortic aneurysms, and in particular aneurysms of the ascending aorta, are due to medial degeneration. "Cystic medial necrosis" is often used to describe this condition, but the term is a misnomer, because true cysts and necrosis of the smooth muscle cells are absent. Rather, there is degeneration and loss of smooth muscle cells and elastic tissue with scarring and fibrotic changes.

The causes of this degenerative process are unknown but are thought to be related to biochemical defects in the synthesis or degradation of collagen, elastin, or mucopolysaccharides within the medial layer of the wall. It is uncertain whether this is a primary medial defect producing dilatation (and occasionally dissection), or whether it is an ongoing process of repetitive aortic injury and repair (Schlatmann and Becker, 1977). There is often a history of hypertension, and this is significant because of the additional constant stress it places on the vessel wall. Over a period of time, the aortic wall weakens and dilates, and a vicious cycle of further weakening and dilatation eventually produces rupture or dissection.

Marfan's syndrome

Patients with Marfan's syndrome demonstrate similar degenerative changes in the elastic fibers of the aortic media and have a characteristic constellation of signs. These are musculoskeletal characteristics that are the result of skeletal overgrowth: excessive height, kyphoscoliosis, slender spiderlike fingers and toes, chest wall deformities such as pectus excavatum (funnel chest) or pectus carinatum (pigeon chest), weak joint capsules, and elongated facial features. Ocular manifestations include exophthalmos, dislocated lens, shallow anterior chamber, detached retina, cataracts, and myopia (Anderson, 1991).

It is thought that an additional inherited connective tissue disorder produces a deficiency of the microfibrillar fibers forming the scaffolding for elastin, which is one of the primary components of the tunica media. Abnormalities in the development of these fibers cause them to elongate progressively over time and fragment the elastic lamellae of the media, thereby affecting the aorta's ability to withstand the constant stress of pulsatile blood flow and other biomechanical forces (Hollister and others, 1990).

These changes accelerate the degenerative process, resulting in the appearance of cardiovascular lesions at an early age and often in an emergency setting. The most frequently encountered of these problems are dilatation of the aortic root (complicated by aortic dissection) and rupture, aortic valve regurgitation, and mitral valve prolapse. These cardiovascular problems form part of the triad of signs and symptoms that also include musculoskeletal deformities and ocular abnormalities (Pyeritz, 1990). Patients who do not display the external stigmata associated with Marfan's syndrome but who have a positive family history and display annuloaortic dilatation are said to have an incomplete form ("forme fruste") of the disorder.

Annuloaortic ectasia

Annuloaortic ectasia is a pathoanatomic description for a combination of aneurysm of the aortic root, dilatation of the aortic annulus, and subsequent aortic valve insufficiency. The lesion, named by Ellis, Cooley, and DeBakey in 1961, is associated with aortic medial degeneration (with or without Marfan's syndrome) that is idiopathic or attributable to the aging process. Aortic dissection and rupture may complicate annuloaortic ectasia.

Usually there is cephalad displacement of the coronary orifices with aneurysms that involve the sinuses of Valsalva. Composite replacement of the aortic valve and the aortic root (with coronary reimplantation) is often required, as it is for most lesions involving the aortic root and valve. Ironically, the upward displacement of the coronary ostia seen in ectatic lesions makes their reimplantation into the graft somewhat easier because there is more room for the surgeon to perform the ostial anastomoses. Normally placed coronary artery ostia are more difficult to implant directly into a combined valve-graft prosthesis (Cooley, 1991a, 1991b).

Atherosclerosis

Atherosclerotic lesions are more commonly found in the descending thoracic and abdominal aorta but may also affect the ascending aorta or aortic arch. They generally occur in older patients. The media undergoes atrophy and fibrous replacement with avascular connective tissue. Aortic dilatation compromises the ability of the vasa vasorum to nourish the vessel wall. As the wall is exposed to both greater tension and diminishing nutrition, the aneurysm enlarges, resulting in eventual rupture if untreated (Webb and Kelly, 1986).

Trauma

Blunt chest trauma such as that occurring from automobile and motorcycle accidents, can cause creation of false aneurysms in the younger age group (Wolfe, 1991). Mortality can be more than 90% (Kram and others, 1989). The most common mechanism of injury is related to the acceleration-deceleration of the body when it contacts an immovable object (e.g., dashboard or steering wheel) and the continued movement of internal organs, specifically the heart and great vessels. As these internal organs continue to move forward, the aorta tears at those points where it is attached within the chest. Most commonly this is the aortic **isthmus,** where the aorta is attached to the ligamentum arteriosum, and the left subclavian artery (see Chapter 21), where the ligamentum arteriosum (the remnant of the fetal ductus arteriosus) connects the aorta and the pulmonary artery. It can also occur before the takeoff of the innominate artery where the right side of the aortic arch is fixed.

Direct trauma, rather than acceleration-deceleration injury, is more likely to injure the ascending aorta and the aortic arch. When all layers of the aortic wall are transected, exsanguination is rapid, and survival rates are very low.

Survival of traumatic transection of the aorta initially depends on the formation of a false aneurysm whereby the adventitia remains intact and contains the hematoma with support from surrounding mediastinal structures. Without the creation of this false aneurysm, there would be rapid extravasation of the blood volume, allowing insufficient time for prevention or repair of the rupture.

A widened mediastinum or a suspicious shadow may be seen on the chest x-ray film. Early diagnosis and prompt surgical treatment may be delayed, however, because there may be little or no external evidence of chest trauma, or additional injuries may divert attention from the aortic tear. Also, patients may be unable to describe symptoms when head trauma affects their mental status (Kram and others, 1989).

Other causes

Now rare, but at one time the most common cause of thoracic aneurysms, **syphilis** produces inflammatory changes, with scarring and destruction of the aortic wall, leading to fusiform or saccular aneurysms. Also seen with less frequency are aneurysms caused by infection, commonly termed **mycotic aneurysms.** These tend to be saccular and are found mainly in intravenous drug abusers and patients who are immunosuppressed. Surgical excision is often necessary to prevent rupture and to remove the lesion, which tends to be highly resistant to antibiotic treatment.

Ehlers-Danlos syndrome is a connective tissue disorder affecting collagen formation. Aortic dissection is one of the internal complications of the syndrome. **Takayasu's disease** produces an arteritis that affects all layers of the arterial wall and is associated with the formation of fusiform or saccular aneurysms.

The hemodynamic stresses of pregnancy may contribute to acute dissection and rupture of the aorta, but usually there is some underlying predisposition for this to occur. Intraoperative aortic dissections or postoperative false aneurysms (pseudoaneurysms) may occur at aortic cannulation sites, in areas where arterial anastomoses are performed, and at the femoral (or brachial) artery entry site of cardiac angiographic catheters. Dissections of the aorta or the coronary arteries may occur during angiography or angioplasty.

DIAGNOSTIC EVALUATION OF THORACIC AORTIC DISEASE
Signs and Symptoms

Improved survival and reduced morbidity in patients with thoracic aortic lesions is dependent on early diagnosis. The presence of a thoracic aneurysm or dissection is often first suggested by symptoms related to compression or obstruction of surrounding mediastinal structures, dissection, or rupture (Table 16-1).

The pain of dissection is the classic symptom. It is often described as "ripping," "tearing," or "splitting" (Crawford, 1990). It is frequently intense from onset. When the pain persists despite large doses of analgesics, it is thought to indicate progression of the dissection. Abrupt cessation of pain, followed by recurrence, may signal impending rupture. In patients with proximal aortic dissections, the pain may be located

Table 16-1 ■ *Signs, symptoms, and findings of thoracic aortic disease*

Ascending aorta	Aortic arch	Descending aorta
Signs and Symptoms		
Acute aortic valve insufficiency: new murmurs, pulmonary edema, congestive heart failure	Hoarseness from pressure on recurrent laryngeal nerve	
Angina	Cough, dyspnea, bloody sputum	
Severe, unremitting chest or back pain with dissection	Same	Same
Pain related to pressure on adjacent structures	Same	Same
Unequal peripheral pulses with dissection	Same	Same
Marfan's syndrome stigmata: excessive height, slender spiderlike fingers and toes	Same	Same
Brachiocephalic venous distension from compression of superior vena cava	Dysphagia from esophageal compromise	Nausea and vomiting from duodenal pressure
Changes in mentation	Same	
Reduction in urinary output	Same	
Chest X-Ray Film		
Dilated ascending aorta	Dilated aortic arch	Dilated descending aorta
Possible hemopericardium	Same	Same
Possible hemothorax	Same	Same
Pulmonary edema	Same	
Widened mediastinum	Same	
	Deviated trachea or esophagus	Same
Electrocardiogram		
Dysrhythmias		
Ischemic changes from impaired coronary perfusion		
Usually not diagnostic	Same	Same
Echocardiography		
Visualizes aneurysm	Same	Same
Aortography		
Identifies location of aortic tear in dissection; extent of dissection; true and false lumen	Same	Same
Notes blood flow to branches of aorta; compression of major branches	Same	Same
Detects aortic valve insufficiency		
Computed Tomographic Scanning		
Notes location, size, and extent of aneurysm/dissection	Same	Same
Cardiac Catheterization		
Detects coronary artery disease, cardiac or pulmonary shunts, aortic insufficiency		

Modified from Miller DC: Surgical management of acute aortic dissection: new data, *Semin Thorac Cardiovasc Surg* 3(3):225, 1991; and Weiland AP, Walker WE: Thoracic aneurysms, *Crit Care Q* 9(3):20, 1986.

in the anterior part of the chest; descending aortic dissections may produce pain in the posterior part of the thorax, although such specificity is not always present.

Compression of adjacent nerves can produce voice changes; obstruction of the tracheobronchial tree can cause dyspnea or cough. Bloody sputum may be a sign of rupture. If dilatation of the aortic root is present, the valve leaflets are unable to coapt, and acute insufficiency with congestive heart failure ensues (Webb and Kelly, 1986).

Patients with aortic dissections may present emergently, and signs and symptoms are assessed. Difficulty breathing or swallowing is suggestive, especially when associated with complaints of excruciating pain. If the false lumen of the dissection obstructs vital branches as a result of the false lumen's compressing the true lumen, symptoms may be apparent. These include mental status changes from cerebral ischemia, reduced urinary output from renal artery compression, and abdominal pain from mesenteric obstruction. Other symptoms include pulse deficits producing

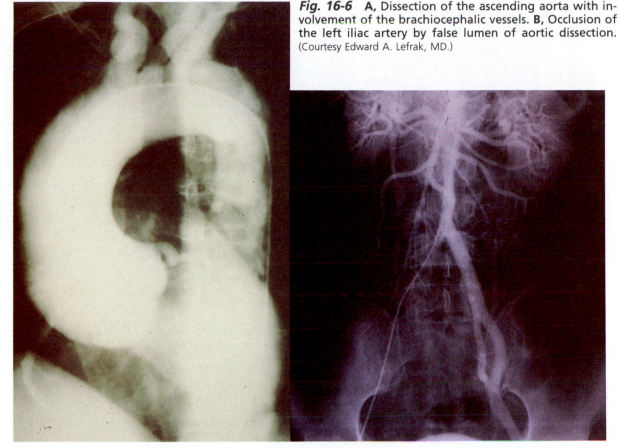

Fig. 16-6 **A,** Dissection of the ascending aorta with involvement of the brachiocephalic vessels. **B,** Occlusion of the left iliac artery by false lumen of aortic dissection. (Courtesy Edward A. Lefrak, MD.)

unequal bilateral radial, brachial, carotid, and/or femoral pulses if the artery on one side has been obstructed by the hematoma (Fig. 16-6).

Not infrequently, signs and symptoms may alert the clinician to consider a diagnosis of acute myocardial infarction. Differentiating between dissection and infarction usually focuses on the quality, location, and duration of the pain, and on the presence (infarction) or absence (dissection) of electrocardiographic or enzymatic evidence of infarction. Myocardial pain usually builds up more gradually, has a squeezing quality to it, and is located in the anterior part of the chest with or without radiation to the jaw and arms. In the age of thrombolytic therapy for acute myocardial infarction, administration of such agents can have disastrous consequences for patients with aortic dissection (Cigarroa and others, 1993).

Diagnostic Tests

Routine laboratory tests may provide little useful information unless massive hemorrhage has reduced the level of hemoglobin. When there is ischemia to major branches of the aorta due to a dissection, the clinician may see abnormal liver, kidney, or gastrointestinal function studies.

The electrocardiogram may show hypertrophy of the left ventricle in patients with chronic hypertension and may be used to rule out myocardial infarction. It may also be helpful in the presence of a dissection that extends retrogradely and occludes the entrance to the coronary artery (producing ischemia or infarction) or affects the interatrial septum (producing heart block). A chest roentgenogram usually shows a mediastinal mass associated with the aortic shadow. A widened mediastinum and pleural fluid may be evident.

Transesophageal echocardiography (TEE) using Doppler color flow mapping has significantly improved prompt diagnosis by displaying the entire aorta and the presence of pericardial fluid and by demonstrating specific lesions such as aortic valve insufficiency and an aortic flap if dissection is present (Simon and others, 1992). The test is noninvasive, widely available, and easily and quickly performed. It may be contraindicated in patients with esophageal disease, but important side effects are rare (Cigarroa and others, 1993).

Aortography (see Fig. 16-6) confirms the diagnosis and best defines the location and condition of the aortic arch branch vessels and the function of the aortic valve (Crawford, 1990). It is particularly useful for detecting involvement, such as occlusion, of one or more major branches of the aorta and remains one of the definitive methods of diagnosing dissections of the thoracic aorta (Cigarroa and others, 1993).

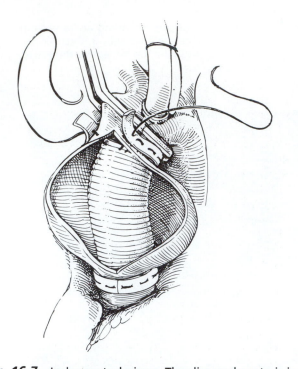

Fig. 16-7 Inclusion technique. The diseased aorta is incised, a graft is placed within the wall, and vascular continuity is restored with anastomoses to the proximal and distal portions of the aorta. The remnant wall may be wrapped around the graft. (From Waldhausen JA, Pierce WS: *Johnson's surgery of the chest,* ed 5, St Louis, 1985, Mosby.)

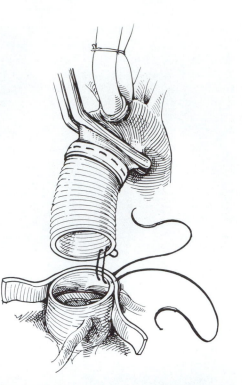

Fig. 16-8 Excision technique. The diseased aorta is resected and replaced with a graft. (From Waldhausen JA, Pierce WS: *Johnson's surgery of the chest,* ed 5, St Louis, 1985, Mosby.)

Cardiac catheterization with aortography and left ventriculography may be performed to determine aortic valve function and to identify shunts when there is a sinus of Valsalva rupture into a cardiac chamber, but cardiac catheterization may be unnecessary (or unsafe) for diagnosis. In patients with involvement of the ascending aorta, the possibility of catheter-induced injury to the vessel wall may preclude selective coronary angiography or other procedures that pose a risk to the patient.

Computed tomographic (CT) scanning with or without contrast enhancement has been very useful for diagnosing aortic dissection and for determining the size of aneurysmal dilatation. It is noninvasive (although contrast material must be injected) and is usually available in many hospitals. Disadvantages include its inability to detect the involvement of branch vessels or delineate the coronary arteries. Magnetic resonance imaging (MRI) provides extraordinary accuracy, but there are important disadvantages, including the amount of time required to obtain and compute the images (Bourland, 1992) and the relative inaccessibility of patients (who are often hemodynamically unstable) when they are inside the MRI tube. In addition, there is the danger of the effect of the strong magnetic field on metallic implants such as pacemakers, aneurysm clips, and possibly certain metallic prosthetic heart valves (Cigarroa and others, 1993).

When aortic dissection is diagnosed, the point of origin must be determined. Dissections originating in the ascending aorta are true surgical emergencies because of the danger of rupture with intrapericardial hemorrhage and death from cardiac tamponade (Cooley, 1991a).

SURGERY ON THE THORACIC AORTA

In general, saccular aneurysms with a narrow neck may be tangentially excised using a partial-occlusion clamp. Where there is greater involvement of the vessel, total-occlusion clamps may be required to control the aorta proximally and distally. Occasionally, direct closure of the aorta may be performed when the defect is not too large (and the tissue is relatively sturdy), but patch repair is usually necessary to avoid tension on the suture line, especially with fragile tissue.

Fusiform aneurysms require circumferential replacement to restore vascular continuity. Two techniques can be used. The inclusion technique is one wherein the aorta is incised longitudinally and a prosthetic graft is inserted within the lumen of the vessel and anastomosed proximally and distally to healthy aorta; the remnant aortic wall may then be closed around the graft for hemostasis (Fig. 16-7). The other technique is to excise the diseased portion of the aorta entirely, interpose the synthetic graft, and perform proximal and distal end-to-end anastomoses (Fig. 16-8). Other technical considerations depend on the location and cause of the lesion (Crawford and Crawford, 1984).

Initial Therapy

Whether medical or surgical therapy is planned, initial treatment for dilatation of the thoracic aorta, and in particular aortic dissections, consists of lowering intravascular pressures in order to forestall rupture and retard progression of the dissecting hematoma. This includes treating not only the absolute blood pressure in the aorta, but also the force with which the aortic pressure rises with left ventricular ejection (dP/dt). This is reflected by the steepness of the pulse wave that is generated by each contraction, and it is this that is especially damaging to the dissecting aorta. Treatment is aimed at modifying the strength of the contractions, decreasing the cardiac impulse, and lowering systemic blood pressure.

Because the increased shearing force can extend the dissection, pharmacologic therapy is instituted promptly. Medications to reduce contractility of the left ventricle and lower blood pressure include beta-adrenergic blockers (such as propranolol, a negative inotrope), vasodilators (such as sodium nitroprusside), and antihypertensive agents (such as trimethaphan camsylate, which decreases left ventricular work and stroke volume).

Patient Teaching Considerations

The gradual or sudden onset of symptoms related to thoracic aneurysm, as well as the excruciating pain associated with aortic dissection, makes these lesions particularly stressful to patients both physically and emotionally. Because of the frequent emergent need for surgery, extensive preoperative teaching is usually not possible. The preoperative interview may be limited to a quick assessment of the patient's status, and significant information about the location and type of disorder is communicated to perioperative nurses preparing for surgery (Table 16-2).

If the patient is conscious and is attended by family or friends, the perioperative nurse may provide a brief overview of the planned procedure, the expected length of surgery (this can be highly variable), and information about how (and when) progress reports will be communicated during surgery. Under the circumstances, reassuring the patient and family with a gentle handgrip and calm efficiency may be more beneficial than detailed explanations. The family should be directed to a waiting area where they can be contacted during surgery. More extensive teaching may need to be deferred to the postoperative period.

Table 16-2 ■ *Standards of nursing care for surgery on the thoracic aorta*

Nursing diagnosis	Patient outcome	Nursing actions
Anxiety/fear related to lack of understanding of pathologic lesion and surgery	Patient demonstrates reduced anxiety and fear as a result of sufficient understanding of lesion and surgical treatment	Assess patient's/family's understanding of lesion and proposed surgery Describe events that are taking place in understandable terms Clarify misconceptions, provide reassurance, offer comfort measures Briefly describe proposed surgery and anticipated length of time in OR (may vary widely) Determine where family will be waiting and where they can receive patient progress reports
Knowledge deficit related to inadequate knowledge of planned surgery and perioperative events	Patient demonstrates knowledge of physiologic and psychologic responses to surgery on thoracic aorta	Determine patient's understanding of aortic lesion, possible surgical interventions (replacement of aortic segment, with or without aortic valve replacement, coronary artery bypass grafts); see standards for aortic valve surgery (Chapter 14) and coronary artery bypass (Chapter 12) Determine patient's understanding of surgery for ascending, arch, descending, or thoracoabdominal aortic lesion; describe immediate preoperative events (while patient is awake); reinforce or clarify what patient (and family) has been told by surgeon; elicit expected outcome of surgery
High risk for infection related to surgery	Patient is free of infection related to aseptic technique	Prepare leg at least to knees to expose leg vein Refer to aortic valve (Chapter 12) and coronary artery bypass (Chapter 12) for procedural considerations Keep instruments free of debris Document lot and serial numbers of grafts, valves, Teflon felt strips and pledgets, and other implants; maintain sterility of graft during preclotting procedures

Modified from Seifert PC: Cardiac surgery. In Rothrock JC: *Perioperative nursing care planning*, St Louis, 1990, Mosby.   *Continued.*

Table 16-2 ■ *Standards of nursing care for surgery on the thoracic aorta—cont'd*

Nursing diagnosis	Patient outcome	Nursing actions
High risk for altered skin integrity	Patient's skin integrity is maintained	Prepare chest cautiously to avoid traumatizing enlarged aorta Protect lower extremities with anesthesia screen over feet If deep hypothermia is to be used, pad face to prevent frostbite; pad extremities
High risk for injury from positioning	Patient is free of injury from positioning	When using lateral position, avoid nerve/pressure injury by padding extremities, using axillary roll, placing pillows between legs, and supporting head, feet, hands, and arms; stabilize patient anteriorly and posteriorly (tape, vacuum positioning devices) For semilateral position, have rolled towel (or similar device) to elevate left side of chest Follow standard for supine position (see Chapter 8)
High risk for injury related to: Retained foreign objects	Patient is free of injury related to: Retained foreign objects	Account for all prosthetic material Keep instruments free of tissue and suture debris
Chemical hazards	Chemical hazards	Label syringes and basins containing antibiotic solutions, fibrin glue, blood components, and other solutions/fluids Follow standard for aortic valve surgery (see Chapter 14) if valve replacement is to be performed
High risk for self-care deficit related to inadequate knowledge of rehabilitation period	Patient demonstrates knowledge of rehabilitation period as it relates to self-care abilities	Assess patient's knowledge of signs/symptoms of recurring aneurysm or dissection If patient has Marfan's syndrome, refer for education and follow-up, including counseling Refer for counseling and education if patient has history of hypertension Provide name of person if there are questions or concerns If aortic valve has been replaced, refer to standards for aortic valve surgery (Chapter 14); if coronary bypass has been performed for coronary artery disease, refer to standards for coronary artery bypass (Chapter 12)

Surgery on the Ascending Thoracic Aorta

Procedural considerations

Knowledge about the type of lesion and its treatment will assist the perioperative nurse in planning care. Of critical importance is an awareness of the aortic region involved (Seifert, 1986a). Because of the emergency nature of many of these cases (often at night or on weekends), the period of time between diagnosis and surgery may be very short. All too often the operating room (OR) team is told that the patient has a "thoracic aneurysm" without being told the location of the aneurysm. Valuable time can be wasted if preparations have been made on the assumption that a patient has an aneurysm in the descending aorta when the aneurysm is in fact in the ascending aorta. Prompt communication to the OR team about the status of

the patient and the location of the aneurysm is invaluable when one is trying to prepare for surgery as quickly as possible (Box 16-2).

Aneurysms or dissections of the ascending aorta are best approached with the patient in a supine position; sternotomy instruments and supplies will be required (Table 16-3). Graft prostheses and sizers should be available so that the correct-size graft can be readily opened when requested. Because the patient is systemically heparinized, low-porosity woven grafts are used; they demonstrate the least amount of bleeding through the interstices of the fabric, as compared with standard woven or knitted grafts (see Chapter 5). Preclotting the graft further reduces bleeding (Table 16-4). If the protocol for preclotting the graft requires the use of blood bank products (e.g., albumin or plasma), these should be ordered early enough to ensure that they will be in the operating room and on

Box 16-2 *Comments on nursing considerations related to dissections of the thoracic aorta*

Bridgit Schall, RN
Washington Hospital Center
Washington, D.C.

There is a saying that thoracic aortic dissections always come in threes and that they always occur in the middle of the night. I have found this to be usually true.

Thoracic aortic dissections present their own special problems for the cardiac team. A good time to sort through potential problems, organize priorities, and plan your course of action is during the ride into the hospital after you have been called in.

The first thing you should consider is the approach. A type I or II ascending aortic dissection requires a mediastinal approach, the use of the heart-lung machine, and different instrumentation than the type III descending thoracic aortic dissection.

Type III dissections require a thoracotomy and different instrumentation, and they may not need a heart-lung machine.

When you arrive in the OR and discover that it is a type I or II dissection, it would also be helpful to know whether or not there is aortic valve involvement. Arterial cannulation will be femoral. Repair material may include the use of felt, low-porosity woven patch material, and/or aortic graft valve conduits (either mechanical, porcine, or cryopreserved homografts). A quick but thorough check on sizes available is a must.

The procedure may be lengthy. The patient may require deep hypothermia, use of multiple blood products, and a long time to rewarm. It is essential to stay organized, set priorities, anticipate the needs of the team, and give a comprehensive report to the ICU.

Table 16-3 ■ *Surgery on the thoracic aorta: special considerations*

Ascending aorta	Aortic arch	Descending aorta
Instrumentation		
Sternotomy setup	Sternotomy setup	Thoracotomy setup
Vascular clamps	Vascular clamps	Vascular clamps
Femoral bypass instruments	Femoral bypass instruments	For femoral bypass with thoracoabdominal procedure: abdominal instruments and retractors
Aortic valve instruments		
Coronary bypass instruments		
Prostheses and Accessories		
Woven tube grafts and sizers	Same	Same
Aortic graft-valve prostheses, sizers, and holders		Intraluminal devices
Heart valves (See procedural considerations for aortic valve surgery, Chapter 14)		
Aortic allografts		
Supplies		
Anastomotic suture, long (36 inches) for continuous technique or multipack for interrupted stitches; polypropylene or polyester	Same	Same
Valve suture, single and multipack (multicolored), pledgeted and nonpledgeted		Suture to ligate/anastomose intercostal branches
Suture organizer (if used)		
Free pledgets, precut or cut to size	Same	Same
Felt strips (cut from patch)	Same	Same
Knitted grafts for collars (6, 8, or 10 mm)	Same	Same
Basins for preclotting grafts and needles, syringes	Same	Same
Supplies for coronary artery bypass (see Chapter 12) and aortic valve replacement (see Chapter 14)		
Eye cautery to cut opening into graft for anastomosis of bypass grafts, arterial branches, etc.	Same	Same

* LA, left atrium; LV, left ventricle.

Continued.

Table 16-3 ■ *Surgery on the thoracic aorta: special considerations—cont'd*

Ascending aorta	Aortic arch	Descending aorta
Circulatory Support		
Single or double venous cannulas for atrial cannulation	Same	Variable; may use left-sided heart bypass (LA or LV* to aorta), Gott shunt, or femoral vein–femoral artery bypass (with oxygenator)
Femoral bypass supplies, extra tubing and connectors to attach atrial cannula to femoral venous line	Same	
Antegrade cardioplegia supplies (hand-held coronary ostial perfusers)	Same	Very rarely used
Retrograde cardioplegia supplies	Same	Very rarely used
Supplies for deep hypothermia (topical ice bags for head, padding to protect facial prominences and extremities)	Same	Very rarely used
Venting needles, suction catheters for removing air from heart or aorta	Same	Same as for venting aorta
Positioning		
Supine	Proximal arch	Lateral: may use positioning device (beanbag)
Groin exposed	Supine	Groin exposed
	Distal arch	Thoracoabdominal aneurysm: semilateral
	Semilateral	
	Groin exposed	
Skin Preparation		
Midline of chest, inner aspect of both legs shaved	Same	Same, except chest shave not necessary unless hair interferes with incision
Legs washed at least to knees		
Draping		
Anterior chest exposed	Same	Left lateral area of chest and groin exposed
Legs exposed from groin to knees (can be covered with a towel if access is not required)	Same	
Anesthesia screen placed over lower legs to keep drapes off feet	Same	Same
Special Infection Control Measures		
Maintain sterility of graft with preclotting methods that use flash sterilization (see Table 16-4)	Same	Same
Keep instruments free of debris	Same	Same
Document lot and serial numbers of all impants	Same	Same
(See procedural consideration for aortic valve surgery, Chapter 14; coronary artery bypass, Chapter 12)		
Special Safety Measures		
Keep blood bank informed of need for blood/blood products	Same	Same
Have autotransfusion system ready for use	Same	Same
Label syringes and containers of solutions, medications: antibiotic solution, glutaraldehyde, etc.	Same	Same
Account for all sizers, handles, holders used for prostheses; pledget material, suture, needles	Same	Same
Documentation/Report to Cardiac Surgical Intensive Care Unit*		
Preoperative diagnosis	Same	Same
Procedure, location, and type of repair	Same	Same
Renal function, urinary output, neurologic status	Same	Same

*In addition to standard documentation/postoperative report; see Chapter 9.

Table 16-4 ■ *Preclotting techniques for vascular grafts*

Technique	Indication	Considerations
Unheparinized venous blood	Patient partially heparinized (abdominal aortic aneurysm, peripheral vascular surgery)	Syringe and needle to draw 10 ml of venous blood from large vein before patient is heparinized; place blood into clean, dry basin and massage into graft
Autoclaved plasma-moistened graft (Cooley and others, 1981) (Albumin, or a combination of cryoprecipitate and topical thrombin also has been used)	Patient totally heparinized (cardiopulmonary bypass, surgery on thoracic aorta)	Autologous or blood bank plasma placed in basin and massaged into graft, which is placed in sterile autoclave pan and flash sterilized for 3 minutes (in sterilizer that has just completed a 3-minute cycle); graft returned to field in sterile manner and implanted (Seifert, 1986b)

the sterile field when they are needed. Collagen-impregnated grafts are now available that do not require preclotting before use in systemically heparinized patients.

When there is evidence of significant aortic valve insufficiency, valve instruments and supplies (including prostheses) should be immediately accessible. If the patient has concomitant coronary artery disease, or if the aortic root containing the coronary ostia must be excised, then coronary bypass instruments should also be available. Aortic valve replacement with graft replacement of the aortic root and reimplantation of the coronary ostia (The Bentall-Bono procedure, described below) requires a special conduit that is composed of a low-porosity woven graft with an aortic valve prosthesis attached to the proximal end.

The operative procedure may be staged when there is diffuse disease of the aorta involving both proximal and distal segments. The most symptomatic and life-threatening segment is replaced first, and the other is removed 6 weeks to 3 months later. If both segments require simultaneous surgery, two incisions may be used to provide access to the lesions (Crawford and others, 1988).

Perfusion of the heart and other vital organs

Cannulation for cardiopulmonary bypass is usually performed via the right atrium and the femoral artery, because the aorta may be too fragile to cannulate. If the aorta is greatly dilated, posing a high risk of rupture, the femoral artery may be cannulated before the sternum is opened.

On rare occasions the femoral vein may be cannulated for venous return of the lower extremities. Long venous drainage cannulas are available that can be inserted into the femoral vein and advanced to the right atrium, but venous return may be inadequate (with disastrous consequences) if it drains by gravity alone (passive drainage). The cannulas work best when venous return is actively drained with a centrifugal pump. Because femoral venous drainage is incomplete, the right atrium is cannulated to receive blood returning from the superior vena cava after the chest is opened. After the aorta is controlled, a cannula

is inserted into the right atrium or superior vena cava and connected to tubing that is "Y'd" into the femoral venous line. Complete venous drainage can then be achieved.

In aortic dissections, one of the potential dangers of femoral artery (retrograde) cannulation and perfusion of the aortic branches is cannulation of the false lumen rather than the true lumen of a dissected aorta, with a resulting malperfusion. Griepp (1991) has suggested first partially or totally occluding the venous line while gradually initiating femoral arterial inflow. This is done so that there is not a rapid change from the antegrade flow, produced by the contracting ventricle through the aortic valve, to the retrograde flow, produced by the bypass pump via the cannula in the femoral artery. Venous return is then allowed to drain freely. (If retrograde flow was initiated suddenly, the force of the blood could propel an existing intimal flap up against a major aortic branch or extend the dissection.) Transesophageal or epicardial color flow echocardiography can also be used to ensure that the correct lumen has been entered, that perfusion of the vital organs is occurring, and that the dissection is not being extended (Kouchoukos and Wareing, 1991; Simon and others, 1992).

The perfusionist initiates arterial pump flow slowly, comparing the arterial line pressure with the patient's (radial) arterial blood pressure (Borst, Laas, and Heinemann, 1991). If there is too large a discrepancy between the two, malperfusion is suspected. Renal and cardiac function are also monitored for signs of diminished perfusion. Another method, suggested by Eleftteriades and colleagues (1992), to ensure perfusion of the true lumen is to perform a fenestration procedure in the abdominal aorta or iliac artery. An opening is created in a nondissected portion of the vessel. This allows blood in the false lumen to exit antegradely into the true lumen, thereby decompressing the false lumen. (This method may be more applicable in dissections of the descending aorta.)

Sternotomy

The period during which the chest is opened and the aorta is clamped can be characterized as one of controlled tension and anticipation in the OR. Often there is only a thin layer of adventitia confining an aortic dissection, and blood can be seen swirling beneath tissue. Extreme caution must be taken to avoid any injury that could produce a ruptured aorta (Box 16-3).

The quality of the tissue has other implications for surgical repair. In aortic dissections, for example, chronic lesions have tissue that is often sturdier and can be repaired more easily than that in aortas that have dissected acutely. In the latter case the tissue tends to be fragile, delicate, and prone to tearing (Cooley, 1991b). This has prompted some researchers to treat aortic tissue with biologic glue (composed of gelatin, resorcin, and formaldehyde) to strengthen the tissue (Carpentier, 1991; Weinschelbaum and others, 1992). When tissue is weak, it is more difficult to achieve adequate hemostasis, and the perioperative nurse can anticipate the use of buttressing felt strips, reinforcing wraps, and other methods to secure the suture line in these situations.

Operative procedure: repair of an ascending aortic aneurysm

Consideration is given to the extent of the lesion proximally and distally, and to involvement of the aortic valve. The following procedure is performed when the aneurysm is limited to a segment of the ascending aorta and there is minimal or no aortic valve insufficiency. Significant aortic valve incompetence and aortic root enlargement are usually indications for replacement of these structures with a composite graft (see following discussion of Bentall-Bono procedure).

Procedure

1. The patient is placed in the supine position, and a median sternotomy is performed.
2. Cardiopulmonary bypass is instituted.
   a. If the distal portion of the ascending aorta is normal, it may be cannulated for arterial inflow; the proximal transverse aortic arch may also be used. The right atrium is cannulated with single or double cannulas for venous drainage.
   b. If there is no suitable place to cannulate the ascending aorta for arterial inflow or the right atrium for venous return, or if there is a high risk of injury to the aorta during sternal opening, femoral vein–femoral artery cannulation may be performed prior to opening the chest. Following systemic heparinization the cannulas are inserted into the exposed vein and artery. Bypass is initiated after the chest is opened to perfuse the body and achieve systemic hypothermia.

   When feasible, a cannula is inserted into the superior vena cava and connected by tubing to the femoral venous line after the sternum is opened.
3. After the aorta is clamped (across healthy tissue,) the aneurysm is incised longitudinally to a point above the entrance to the coronary ostia, and the aortic wall is preserved for later wrapping or is excised. Minimal dissection of surrounding tissue is performed.
4. Retrograde cardioplegia is infused. The left ventricular venting catheter is inserted into the right superior pulmonary vein and threaded through the mitral valve into the left ventricle (see Chapter 14).
5. The aneurysmal aortic wall and the aortic valve are inspected.
   a. If there is minimal aortic valve incompetence and the valve is morphologically normal (and there is no underlying connective tissue disorder), it may be resuspended (Fig. 16-9) with pledgeted mattress sutures placed at the level of the commissures and passed through the layers of the aortic wall. Aortic root reconstruction with felt reinforcement is another, less common, technique to salvage the native valve (Miller, 1991).
   b. If the valve requires replacement, this is done in the standard fashion (see Chapter 14). A collar of aorta is retained for anastomosis of the graft.
6. The aorta is sized, and the appropriate low-porosity woven graft is delivered to the field, where it is preclotted per protocol (if necessary).
7. The proximal and distal anastomoses are made to healthy aorta with a running 2-0 or 3-0 polypropylene or polyester suture. The suture line may be reinforced with a strip of felt or a small knitted

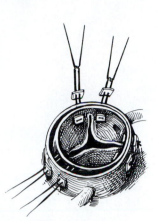

Fig. 16-9 Resuspension of the aortic valve commissures with pledgeted sutures to restore aortic valve competence. (From Waldhausen JA, Pierce WS: *Johnson's surgery of the chest,* ed 5, St Louis, 1985, Mosby.)

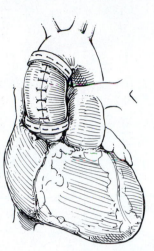

Fig. 16-11 The remnant aorta is wrapped around the graft and closed. Additional reinforcing strips of felt or knitted grafts may be attached. (From Waldhausen JA, Pierce WS: *Johnson's surgery of the chest,* ed 5, 1985, Mosby.)

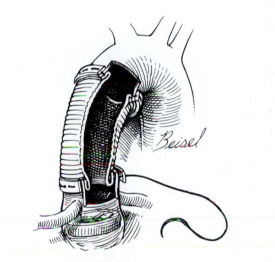

Fig. 16-10 Cut-away showing completed aortic valve replacement and prosthetic repair of the ascending aorta. (From Waldhausen JA, Pierce WS: *Johnson's surgery of the chest,* ed 5, St Louis, 1985, Mosby.)

tube graft (8 or 10 mm); a long, angled clamp is used to bring the reinforcing material around the aorta. A Kelly clamp can be used to hold the felt or graft collar around the anastomosis while the surgeon sews it together. Excess material is trimmed (Fig. 16-10).

8. The remaining aorta (if not excised) is trimmed and wrapped around the completed repair, and the edges are oversewn with a continuous suture (Fig. 16-11). The remnant aorta may be wrapped loosely, or if the objective is hemostasis, it is tightly wrapped. Some authors suggest an additional strip of felt around the aorta at the location of the proximal and distal anastomoses (Waldhausen and Pierce, 1985).

9. Air is removed from the left side of the heart through the right superior pulmonary venous venting catheter, needle aspiration of the left ventricular apex, and/or needle venting of the ascending aorta with the patient in the deep Trendelenburg position. The cross-clamp is removed, the patient is rewarmed, and cardiopulmonary bypass is discontinued.

Bentall-Bono procedure

Annuloaortic ectasia or aortic dissection involving the aortic root and aortic valve generally require their replacement, especially in patients with Marfan's syndrome or other degenerative disorders.

The procedure described by Bentall and deBono (1968) involves the use of a valved conduit to replace the aortic valve and ascending aorta (see Chapter 5). The coronary ostia are reimplanted into openings made in the graft, and the remnant aortic wall is then wrapped around the graft.

A number of modifications have been made to the operation to reflect technical improvements, such as methods to preclot grafts and to rectify problems seen with the original procedure. Some of these problems include hemorrhage from anastomotic suture lines, disruption of the coronary ostia, pseudoaneurysm formation at the coronary ostial or aortic suture lines, and injury from clamping the fragile aortic wall (Kouchoukos, 1991; Kouchoukos, Marshall, and Wedige-Stecher, 1986; Kouchoukos and Wareing, 1991; Lewis and others, 1992).

Conduit size. An important consideration in these procedures is proper sizing of both the proximal end of the conduit (containing the prosthetic valve) and the distal graft portion of the conduit. The distal end can be sized with graft sizers; the graft may be beveled to better fit the aorta.

In sizing the proximal end, the surgeon considers

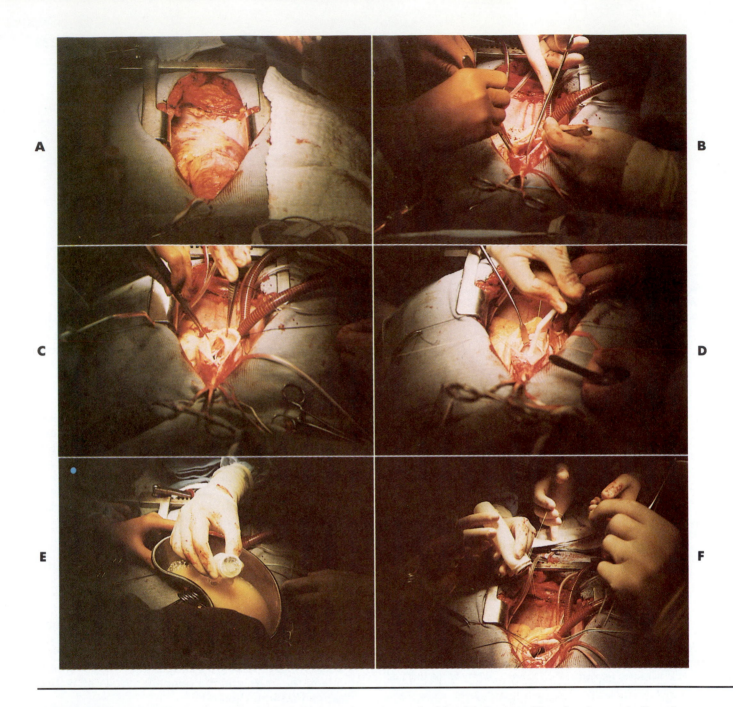

the graft and the valve contained within it. In commercially manufactured conduits the process of sewing the graft to the valve adds 2 mm to the diameter of the valve contained within the conduit. Thus when the surgeon sizes the annulus, the size obturator that fits best (rather than the size of the valve within the conduit) determines the size of the conduit. A 23 mm annulus will have a 23 mm conduit (containing a 21 mm valve prosthesis) implanted. If the surgeon determines that a 25 mm obturator fits best into the annulus, the surgeon should be given a 25 mm conduit, which contains a 23 mm valve. The obturators should correspond to the type of conduit used (e.g., St. Jude Medical obturators to determine the appropriate St. Jude Medical conduit).

Another consideration related to conduits is that a low-profile valve is commonly used because it is technically easier to reimplant the coronary ostia, as compared with a higher-profile valve (e.g., a ball-and-cage valve). Also, mechanical valves tend to be favored because of their greater durability as compared with bioprostheses, which could require difficult reoperation. Aortic allografts and pulmonic autografts (with pulmonary allografts to replace the pulmonic valve and pulmonary artery) may become suitable alternatives to the composite graft (Kouchoukos, 1991).

Cannulation and sternotomy are similar to the procedure just described for an ascending aortic aneurysm.

Operative procedure: annuloaortic ectasia or aortic dissection—modified Bentall-Bono technique *(Fig. 16-12)*

1. The sternum is divided, and the pericardium is opened. The aneurysm is inspected. The femoral

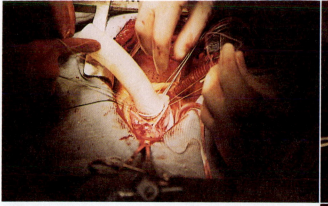 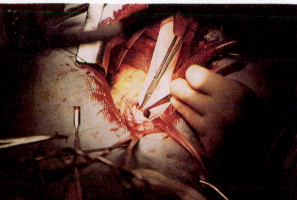

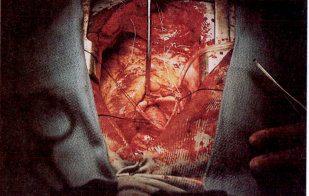

Fig. 16-12 Modified Bentall-Bono procedure. **A,** The aneurysm is exposed through a median sternotomy (head is at bottom of picture). **B,** The aneurysm is incised. **C,** The aortic valve is inspected. **D,** The aortic annulus is sized with an obturator. Note the aortic leaflet retractor. **E,** The graft is immersed in clotting medium, and the medium is massaged into the material. **F,** After stitches have been inserted into the aortic annulus, stitches are placed in the sewing ring of the valve end of the conduit. Another technique is to place stitches into the annulus and prosthesis sewing ring at the same time. **G,** After all the stitches have been inserted, the prosthesis is seated and the stitches are tied. **H,** The left coronary ostium is reimplanted into the graft. **I,** The completed repair. The aortic wall will be closed around the graft after protamine has been infused to reverse the heparin and hemostasis has been achieved. Note that the patient is off bypass and that the venous cannulas have been removed. (Courtesy Edward A. Lefrak, MD; Doug Yarnold, CRNA, photographer.)

artery is cannulated for arterial inflow; a two-stage venous cannula is inserted for venous drainage.

2. The distal ascending aorta is clamped (Fig. 16-13). If there is a dissection involving the proximal aortic arch, hypothermic circulatory arrest may be used (see later section) in order to avoid clamping (and possibly further injuring) the dissected aorta (Cooley, 1991a).

3. The aorta is incised transversely or longitudinally. If dissection is present, the location of the intimal tear is noted. Cardioplegia solution is infused retrogradely. Rarely, the coronary ostia are infused with cardioplegia solution. Stitches may be placed into each side of the aneurysmal aortic wall for retraction.

4. The aortic valve and the sinuses of Valsalva are inspected. The openings to the coronary arteries are identified, and their position relative to the annulus is noted (elevated or in the normal position).

5. The aortic valve leaflets are excised, and the annulus is measured with obturators of the type of prosthetic valve contained in the valved conduit.
   a. Conduit: The appropriate-size conduit is delivered to the field and preclotted. When the conduit is being preclotted, the valve portion should not be immersed in the preclotting medium; the valve occluder mechanism should be checked to ensure that it is moving freely. If a prosthesis handle is available and the surgeon elects to use it, it should be attached to the conduit (Fig. 16-14).
   b. Allograft: An aortic allograft (e.g., homograft) may be inserted as described in Chapter 14 on aortic valve surgery.

6. The proximal (valve) end of the conduit is inserted into the annulus (Fig. 16-15). The interrupted or continuous suture technique is used (see Chapter 14). Pledgets may be used to buttress the annulus. Cardioplegia solution is infused before entry to the coronary arteries is reestablished.

7. Coronary circulation is restored. No matter which of the following techniques is used for a synthetic graft, an opening must be made into the graft for the anastomosis. A battery-powered, hand-held (eye) cautery is helpful for making the opening and simultaneously heat-sealing the graft edges to prevent fraying.
   a. A button of aorta surrounding both the left and the right coronary ostia is retained and

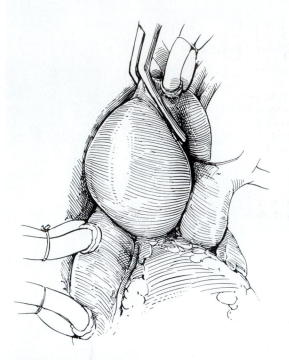

Fig. 16-13 The distal aorta is clamped. (From Waldhausen JA, Pierce WS: *Johnson's surgery of the chest*, ed 5, St Louis, 1985, Mosby.)

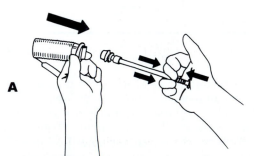

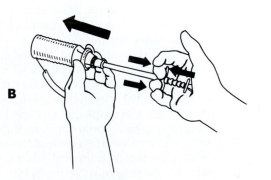

Fig. 16-14 **A,** The conduit handle (specific to the prosthesis) is inserted. The handle jaws are aligned with the lateral openings in the St. Jude Medical valve; the end of the handle is depressed, and the jaws are inserted into the prosthesis. **B,** Removal of the handle from the prosthesis. (Courtesy St. Jude Medical Center, Inc., Minneapolis, Minn.)

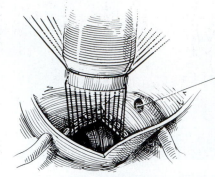

LEFT CORONARY OSTIUM

Beisel

Fig. 16-15 The valve end of the graft-valve conduit is sewn into the aortic annulus. (From Waldhausen JA, Pierce WS: *Johnson's surgery of the chest*, ed 5, St Louis, 1985, Mosby.)

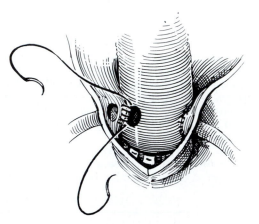

Fig. 16-16 Anastomosis of the right coronary ostium to the prosthetic graft. The left coronary ostial reimplantation has been completed. (From Waldhausen JA, Pierce WS: *Johnson's surgery of the chest*, ed 5, St Louis, 1985, Mosby.)

anastomosed to the respective openings made in the graft using a continuous 4-0 polypropylene suture (Lewis and others, 1992). Cephalad displacement of the coronary ostia, commonly found in annuloaortic ectasia, facilitates this method of reimplanting the coronary ostia (Cooley, 1991a, 1991b). The anastomosis can incorporate the remnant aortic wall as well (Fig. 16-16). Some authors (Crawford and Coselli, 1988; Miyamoto, 1992) use a "washer" of Teflon felt around each ostial anastomosis to buttress the tissue.

b. Cabrol, Pavie, and Mesnildrey (1986) devised a reimplantation technique (Fig. 16-17) aimed at reducing tension on the coronary ostial suture line. One end of a preclotted 8 or 10 mm woven tube graft is anastomosed end-to-end to the origin of the left coronary artery. The graft is brought across the anterior aspect of (or behind) the aortic graft to the right coro-

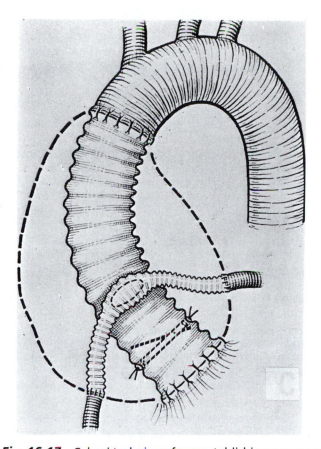

Fig. 16-17 Cabrol technique for reestablishing coronary circulation. The ends of the graft are anastomosed to each coronary ostium, and a side-to-side anastomosis of the transverse graft is made to the graft-valve conduit. (From Cabrol C and others: Long-term results with total replacement of the ascending aorta and reimplantation of the coronary arteries, *J Thorac Cardiovasc Surg* 91:17, 1986.)

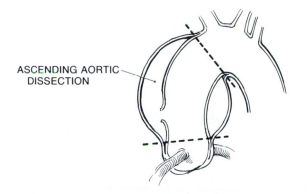

Fig. 16-18 The dissected portion of the aorta must be identified and excluded during the repair to avoid redissection. (From Waldhausen JA, Pierce WS: *Johnson's surgery of the chest,* ed 5, St Louis, 1985, Mosby.)

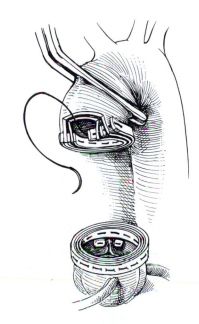

Fig. 16-19 Sandwiching the layers of the dissected aorta with felt to obliterate the false lumen. (From Waldhausen JA, Pierce WS: *Johnson's surgery of the chest,* ed 5, St Louis, 1985, Mosby.)

nary ostium, where it is cut and anastomosed end-to-end to the right ostium. An opening is cut into the coronary graft and into the aortic graft at a level above the prosthetic valve, and a side-to-side anastomosis is performed. Arterial blood flows into the aortic graft opening and then into both coronary ostia.

   c. Saphenous vein or a 6 to 8 mm prosthetic (Dacron or PTFE) graft is interposed between the coronary ostia and the aortic graft (Kouchoukos, 1991).

   d. In patients with obstructive coronary artery disease, saphenous vein bypass grafts are anastomosed distally to the heart and proximally to the aortic graft.

8. After coronary continuity is reestablished, cardioplegia solution may be infused through the graft and into the coronary openings (this may be technically difficult) or given retrogradely.

   The graft is brought up to the location of the distal anastomosis, and excess graft is cut. If the aorta is dissected, the location of the intimal tear must be excluded from the remaining aorta, or redissection will occur (Fig. 16-18). In addition, circumferential strips of Teflon felt may be used to sandwich the distal edges of the transected aorta to obliterate the false lumen. (When available, biologic glue may be used to seal the edges together prior to suturing the aorta.

9. The distal anastomosis is performed with a running 2-0 or 3-0 polypropylene or polyester suture incorporating all layers of the felt (Fig. 16-19).

10. The patient is placed in the Trendelenburg position, and a venting needle is placed in the most anterior portion of the aorta (Waldhausen and Pierce, 1985). Air is removed from the left ventricle with a needle or with a venting catheter in the right superior pulmonary vein.

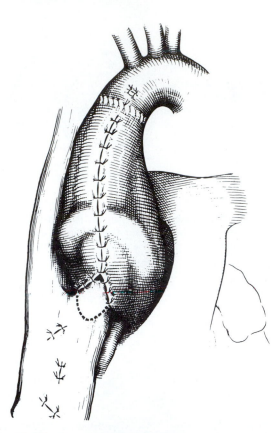

Fig. 16-20 Cabrol technique to close the aneurysmal wall over the prosthesis. A fistula is created between the periprosthetic space and the right atrial appendage. (From Cabrol C and others: Long-term results with total replacement of the ascending aorta and reimplantation of the coronary arteries, *J Thorac Cardiovasc Surg* 91:17, 1986.)

11. The cross-clamp is removed, and the anastomoses and graft are inspected for bleeding. Pledgeted or nonpledgeted sutures are used to reinforce suture lines as necessary.

12. If oozing from the graft or suture lines persists, some authors favor the "inclusion wrap technique": tightly wrapping the graft with the remaining aortic wall and oversewing the approximated aortic edges. Additional felt strips or graft wraps may be used.

    a. Some authors prefer to leave the repair unwrapped or loosely wrapped (Kouchoukos, 1991), because tight wrapping may place stress on the suture lines. This preference stems from an attempt to avoid disruption of the ostial graft anastomoses and formation of a pseudoaneurysm at the coronary ostial anastomoses when there is tension on the suture line from accumulated blood between the aortic wrap and the graft (Kouchoukos, Marshall, and Wedige-Stecher, 1986).

    b. Another technique developed by Cabrol, Pavie, and Mesnildrey (1986) is used to decompress the perigraft space when the inclusion-wrap technique is being used. A fistula is cre-ated between the aortic wrap and the right atrium (Fig. 16-20). This allows collected blood to drain into the right side of the heart. If the fistula does not close spontaneously and bleeding persists, reoperation may be necessary.

13. After removal of air from the left side of the heart and the aorta, the OR bed is brought to a level position. While rewarming is completed, temporary pacing wires and chest tubes are inserted.

14. Cardiopulmonary bypass is discontinued, and the chest is closed.

Surgery on the Aortic Arch
Procedural considerations

In aneurysms involving the ascending aorta, adequate circulatory support of the brain is achieved by cross-clamping the aorta proximal to the origin of the branches of the aortic arch and allowing femoral artery retrograde perfusion of the head and upper body. In aneurysms involving the transverse aortic arch, unless each branch vessel is selectively cannulated (as was performed in the past with generally unsatisfactory results), cerebral perfusion must be temporarily interrupted while the arch is repaired.

Blood flow can be interrupted by placing an occluding clamp on the aorta distal to the arch or by stopping the blood flow altogether. In either technique, irreversible brain injury can occur if protective measures are not taken.

Another consideration is the risk of injury to the phrenic nerve and the recurrent laryngeal branch of the vagus nerve, which cross the aortic arch. Injury to the former can affect diaphragmatic movement, and injury to the latter can produce vocal cord paralysis on the side of the affected nerve.

Hypothermic circulatory arrest

Protection of the brain remains the most serious concern. Although a number of methods to protect the brain (cerebroplegia) have been under investigation (Bachet and others, 1991; Swain and others, 1991), bringing the patient to lower levels of hypothermia (20° to 24° C (68° to 75.2° F), or down to 12° to 18° C (53.6° to 64.4° F) in some instances) with circulatory arrest remains the most widely used method of protecting cerebral tissue since the introduction of the technique by Griepp and colleagues in 1975 (see Chapter 11).

It is essential that all team members be familiar with the procedure and have all necessary equipment and supplies readily available to avoid prolonging the period of circulatory arrest unnecessarily. The procedure should be performed as rapidly as possible because of the danger of cerebral injury.

The patient is cooled internally with cardiopulmonary bypass. External cooling is performed with a cooling blanket and with ice packs to the head and, on occasion, to the entire body surface (Griepp and others, 1991). Because of the increased risk of lethal dysrhythmias with hypothermia from body surface

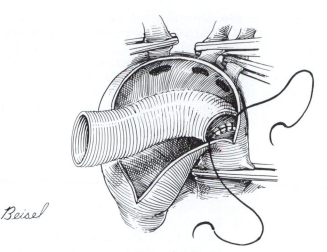

Fig. 16-21 Distal anastomosis for an aortic arch aneurysm. (From Waldhausen JA, Pierce WS: *Johnson's surgery of the chest*, ed 5, St Louis, 1985, Mosby.)

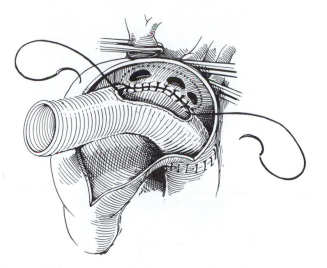

Fig. 16-22 The brachiocephalic arteries are anastomosed as an island to the prosthetic graft. (From Waldhausen JA, Pierce WS: *Johnson's surgery of the chest*, ed 5, St Louis, 1985, Mosby.)

cooling, all members of the cardiac team should observe the electrocardiogram for signs of ventricular irritability and/or fibrillation and be ready to institute appropriate measures if this occurs.

Another concern of team members should be avoidance of inadvertent rewarming of the patient. Internal cooling is achieved by the circulation of blood cooled with the heat exchanger within the bypass circuit. When the patient is under circulatory arrest and the bypass pump is turned off, internal cooling cannot be maintained with perfusion of cold blood, because circulation has been arrested. Cooling must be maintained by other methods. The room temperature setting should remain low (13° to 15° C [55° to 60° F]), and the cooling blanket should be set appropriately. If bags of ice are applied around the patient's head, these should be checked by the circulating nurse and replenished with additional ice as necessary.

Additional measures that have been used to protect the brain include avoidance of hyperglycemia (which can generate increased amounts of lactate and lower intracellular pH), the use of pharmacologic agents such as corticosteroids and barbiturates, and hemodilution (to reduce blood viscosity). (A common rule of thumb is that the hematocrit should equal the centigrade temperature.) The electroencephalogram (EEG) can be used to monitor brain activity, which is considered to be minimal with adequate hypothermia (Crawford and Coselli, 1988; Svensson and Crawford, 1992).

Once the desired temperature is reached (by monitoring, for example, esophageal, nasopharyngeal, rectal, and jugular venous temperatures), the bypass pump is turned off and the distal and arch anastomoses are performed. At 20° C (68° F), the metabolic rate is approximately 18% of normal (Cooley, 1991a), thus providing a relatively safe period of time to perform the distal repairs. Determination of a safe interval is difficult to judge, but arrest periods of 59 min-

utes (Griepp and others, 1975) and 104 minutes (Coselli and others, 1988) without neurologic injury have been reported.

After these anastomoses are completed, the graft is clamped proximal to the arch branches, air is removed, and cardiopulmonary bypass is reestablished. The proximal anastomosis is then performed while the patient is rewarmed. Rewarming is performed slowly at a rate of 1° C every 2 to 3 minutes; differences between the temperature of the circulating blood and the core body temperature (as measured by the esophageal temperature) should not be greater than approximately 8° C (46.4° F). A larger temperature gradient could injure blood cells and tissue.

Operative procedure: repair of a transverse aortic arch

1. The patient is placed in the supine position, and median sternotomy is performed. External and internal cooling to the desired temperature is achieved with topical cold applications and femoral vein–femoral artery cardiopulmonary bypass, respectively. A retroplegia catheter is inserted.

2. Once the patient is cooled, the aorta may be clamped or the pump turned off to create circulatory arrest (and a bloodless field). The aneurysm is incised, and a low-porosity woven tube graft is selected and preclotted per protocol. Atherosclerotic material, formed thrombus, and other debris is removed from the aorta and arch vessels.

3. The distal anastomosis (Fig. 16-21) to the descending thoracic aorta is performed with a continuous 2-0 or 3-0 polypropylene or polyester suture.

4. Implantation of the brachiocephalic arteries (Fig. 16-22) is done by making an oval opening (with an eye cautery) in the convex portion of the graft (Cooley, 1986). The graft is anastomosed to the

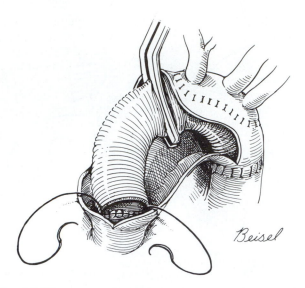

Fig. 16-23 The graft is clamped, cardiopulmonary bypass is resumed, and the proximal anastomosis is performed. (From Waldhausen JA, Pierce WS: *Johnson's surgery of the chest*, ed 5, St Louis, 1985, Mosby.)

common origin of the arch branch vessels (rather than to each individual artery).

5. After the distal anastomoses are completed, an occlusion clamp is placed on the graft proximal to the arch vessels (Fig. 16-23). With the patient in the deep Trendelenburg position, air is evacuated from the arch and its branches, and blood is allowed to fill the aortic arch and branch vessels. Cardiopulmonary bypass is slowly resumed, the perfusion flow rate is gradually increased, and rewarming is initiated (Cooley, 1986).

6. The proximal anastomosis is performed with a continuous 2-0 or 3-0 polypropylene or polyester suture. Retroplegia is infused as necessary.

7. The suture lines are inspected for hemostasis, and air is removed from the left side of the heart and aorta. Rewarming is completed, and bypass is terminated. Temporary pacing wires and chest tubes are inserted, and all incisions are closed.

Extension into the descending aorta

When the arch lesion extends into the descending thoracic aorta, the procedure may have to be modified. The patient can be placed in a semilateral position, and a transverse bilateral thoracotomy incision is made. The femoral artery is cannulated for arterial infusion; venous drainage may be obtained from the right atrium or right ventricle. The surgeon first stands to the left of the patient for the distal anastomosis and then moves to the right side to perform the arch and proximal anastomoses (Cooley, 1986).

The "elephant trunk" technique devised by Borst, Frank, and Schaps (1988) can be used to repair extensive aortic aneurysms and dissections, especially those requiring staged operations. The aortic arch is replaced, but instead of a conventional anastomosis

being done between the distal end of the arch graft and the origin of the descending aorta, an appropriate length of the terminal graft is first invaginated. The circular reflection fold thus created is then sutured end-to-end to the descending aorta. Before the anastomotic suture is tied, the invaginated portion of the graft is advanced into the downstream portion of the aorta (where it is suspended freely like an elephant trunk). Air is removed from the aorta and the space between the graft and the aneurysm by retrograde perfusion. If another operation is needed to repair the aorta downstream from the first repair, the distal end of the "elephant trunk" can be exposed through a left thoracotomy and anastomosed to another graft to replace the descending thoracic aorta. This technique allows graft-to-graft anastomoses for subsequent repairs on the descending (and abdominal) aorta and obviates the need for proximal graft-to-aorta anastomoses (thus avoiding having to sew on aneurysmal aortic tissue, which may not hold sutures securely).

Sacciform aneurysms

Sacciform aneurysms of the aortic arch may be excised at their neck and patch repaired during moderate hypothermia and a brief period of circulatory arrest (Cooley, 1986).

Surgery on the Descending Thoracic Aorta

Although surgery is the standard treatment for dissections and aneurysms of the ascending aorta and the transverse aortic arch, there is no single standard treatment for lesions of the descending thoracic aorta. In particular, surgery for dissections of the descending aorta may not always be indicated.

Reports (Daily and others, 1970; Wheat and others, 1969) of improved survival with medical versus surgical therapy in uncomplicated descending thoracic aortic dissections prompted clinicians to reserve surgery for patients whose aorta had ruptured or who demonstrated expansion of the dissection, continuing pain, and ischemia of visceral organs. These findings have been reconfirmed more recently by Glower and colleagues (1990) and by Elefteriades and associates (1992). As with other dissections, initial therapy is directed toward lowering blood pressure and myocardial contractility to retard progression of the intimal tear.

Procedural considerations

When surgery is being planned, the need for circulatory support must be considered. The heart is not arrested; it continues beating to perfuse the upper body. Thus myocardial protection techniques, such as systemic hypothermia and cardioplegia, are not used. Surgery is performed under normothermic conditions. Circulatory support may be used, however, to perfuse the kidneys, spinal cord, and lower extremities while the descending thoracic aorta is occluded.

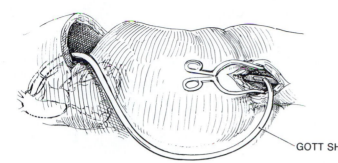

Fig. 16-24 Gott shunt. The proximal end is in the descending aorta just beyond the take-off of the subclavian artery. The distal end is in the left common femoral artery. (From Waldhausen JA, Pierce WS: *Johnson's surgery of the chest*, ed 5, St Louis, 1985, Mosby.)

Spinal cord injury. Of major concern during the period of aortic clamping is ischemic injury to the spinal cord, resulting in paresis or paraplegia. The most important blood supply to the spinal cord arises between the eighth thoracic and the fourth lumbar vertebrae. It has been suggested that intercostal arteries not involved in the aneurysmal or dissected aorta be preserved, with reimplantation of large intercostals into the prosthetic graft (especially in acute situations where collateral circulation has not had time to form). Other considerations include minimal excision of the aorta (consistent with adequate removal of diseased tissue), avoiding hypotension, and minimizing aortic occlusion time (Webb and Kelly, 1986). Because no one method of circulatory support has been shown to prevent postoperative spinal cord damage, many surgeons use the "clamp and go" technique without additional supportive procedures. There may be some benefit, however, in protecting the kidneys, especially when there is preexisting renal dysfunction. There may also be advantages for patients with impaired left ventricular function, because the increased afterload seen when the aorta is clamped can be modified (Cartier and others, 1990). Debate continues as to whether to shunt or bypass, or use the "clamp and go" technique; some authors (Svensson and others, 1990) have seen no conclusive evidence that distal perfusion reduces the incidence of paraplegia or paresis.

Circulatory support. When methods of support are instituted, the most commonly used are the Gott shunt, left atrial-distal aorta bypass, and femoral vein–femoral artery bypass.

The **Gott shunt** (Fig. 16-24) is a heparin-coated catheter, one end of which is inserted into the proximal portion of the descending thoracic aorta (or the left ventricular apex) and the other end into the common femoral artery (or the distal aorta). Pursestring sutures and tourniquets are used to secure the shunt proximally and distally. The heparin coating eliminates the need for systemic heparinization. Blood flow through the shunt is passive and dependent on cardiac output.

Left atrial–distal aorta bypass is achieved with a cannula in the left atrium receiving oxygenated blood, which travels through tubing to a cannula in the distal aorta. A blood pump is interposed in the tubing to actively propel the blood into the distal vascular bed. This is considered a form of left heart bypass and does not require an oxygenator in the circuit, because blood from the left atrium is freshly oxygenated. Systemic heparinization is not always required with this method of support.

Femoral vein–femoral artery bypass also can be instituted. An oxygenator is necessary to oxygenate femoral venous return before returning it to the femoral artery. A roller pump or centrifugal pump can be used to propel the blood. Systemic heparinization is required.

Nursing considerations

The lesion is approached via a left posterolateral thoracotomy through the fouth or fifth intercostal space; if the lesion is extensive, a proximal incision and a distal incision may be required. Equipment and supplies for placing the patient in a lateral position need to be available, as well as thoracotomy instruments and vascular clamps. Instruments and supplies for insertion of shunts or institution of bypass are readied, depending on the surgeon's preference.

Operative procedure: repair of a descending thoracic aortic aneurysm/dissection

1. The patient is positioned for lateral thoracotomy, and the skin is prepared from the shoulder to the knees. Access to the groin must be maintained for possible cannulation.
2. An incision is made in the left fourth intercostal space, and a rib retractor is inserted. (If necessary for exposure, a second incision can be made.)
3. If indicated, circulatory support is instituted.
   a. Gott shunt: double pursestring sutures (3-0 polyester) with tourniquets are placed in the proximal portion of the descending aorta and the distal aorta or common femoral artery. The proximal and distal ends of the shunt (7 or 9 mm) are inserted through stab wounds into the aorta and/or femoral artery.
   b. Left atrial–distal aorta bypass: a pursestring suture with a tourniquet is placed in the left atrium, and a cannula is inserted through a stab wound. The cannula is connected to tubing attached to a centrifugal pump or threaded through a roller pump. The distal end of the tubing is connected to a cannula that has been inserted through a pursestring into the femoral artery.
   c. Femoral vein–femoral artery bypass: institution of bypass is performed as described in Chapter 9.
4. The aneurysm/dissection is assessed and isolated between vascular clamps. A low-porosity woven tube graft is selected, delivered to the field, and preclotted.

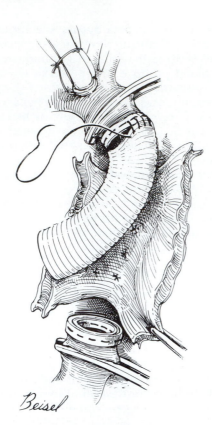

Beisel

Fig. 16-25 Proximal anastomosis for repair of the descending thoracic aorta. (From Waldhausen JA, Pierce WS: *Johnson's surgery of the chest,* ed 5, St Louis, 1985, Mosby.)

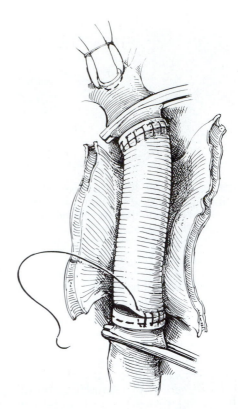

Fig. 16-26 Distal anastomosis for repair of the descending thoracic aorta. (From Waldhausen JA, Pierce WS: *Johnson's surgery of the chest,* ed 5, St Louis, 1985, Mosby.)

5. The aneurysm is opened longitudinally. Intercostal artery orifices are closed with suture ligatures for hemostasis; larger intercostals may be anastomosed end-to-side to the graft for spinal cord protection (Fig. 16-25).

6. The graft is anastomosed end-to-end to the aorta proximally with a 3-0 polypropylene double-armed suture and distally with a 3-0 or 4-0 suture. If the suture is 36 inches or more, the need for additional stitches to complete the anastomosis may be avoided. If the aorta is dissected, felt strips may be used to obliterate the false lumen (Fig. 16-26).

7. After the anastomoses are completed and the graft is deaired, the distal clamp is removed. The proximal clamp is then slowly removed (to avoid sudden hypotension), and the graft is inspected for hemostasis. The remnant aortic wall may be wrapped around the completed repair.

8. Shunts or cannulas are removed, and insertion sites are repaired.

Use of intraluminal prostheses

The construction of conventional suture anastomoses may be problematic when there is acute dissection of the aorta and the tissue is friable and easily torn. Preexisting multisystem organ impairment may be aggravated by prolonged cross-clamp times and metabolic derangements related to ischemia (Berger and others, 1992). Because of these problems, Dureau and

colleagues (1978) and Ablaza, Ghosh, and Grana (1978) introduced the use of a sutureless graft prosthesis that can be quickly inserted with tape ligatures (Fig. 16-27).

The prosthesis consists of a standard low-porosity woven Dacron tube graft with rigid velour-covered rings at each end. An array of diameter widths and lengths is available (see Chapter 5). There are tapered versions for use in locations where there is a great disparity between the proximal and distal vessel lumen. There is also a variable-length prosthesis that uses a movable fixation ring. Occasionally a conventional anastomosis is preferred, and this can be accomplished by removing the ring from one end of the prosthesis.

The initial enthusiasm for this technique has been dampened by reports describing poor results (Cooley, 1991b; Crawford, 1990). Present use of these devices is commonly restricted to the descending thoracic aorta; conventional suture techniques are preferred in the ascending aorta and transverse aorta.

Operative procedure: insertion of an intraluminal sutureless prosthesis

1. After the aorta is occluded and the wall is opened, the surgeon determines the appropriate prosthesis by measuring the diameter and length required. The prosthesis is delivered to the field.

2. The graft is placed into the true lumen proximally

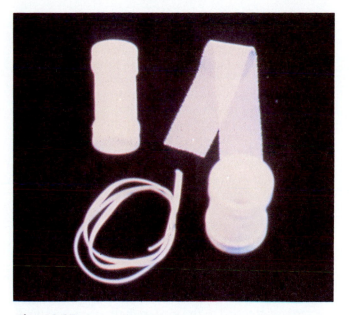

Fig. 16-27 Intraluminal graft with tapes (and mesh for reinforcement). (Courtesy Bard Vascular Systems Div., Billerica, Mass.)

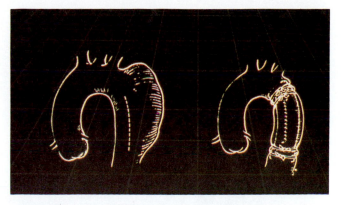

Fig. 16-28 Intraluminal prosthesis positioned in the descending thoracic aorta. (Courtesy Bard Vascular Systems Div., Billerica, Mass.)

and distally. The aortic wall is wrapped around the prosthesis, and Dacron tapes are placed around the aorta and the proximal and distal rings of the prosthesis. The tapes are tied, securing the prosthesis (Fig. 16-28). Stay sutures may be inserted for additional fixation.

3. If the ring is removed from one end, standard suture techniques are used for the anastomosis.
4. The repair is inspected for hemostasis, and all incisions are closed.

Surgery for Thoracoabdominal Aneurysms

Lesions involving the thoracic and abdominal aorta pose a significantly increased risk of morbidity and mortality. They usually occur in older patients with atherosclerotic disease and may attain considerable size before they are discovered. If the aneurysm is detected, operative treatment is considered when the diameter is twice that of the uninvolved proximal aortic segment (Crawford and others, 1986). Of major importance during surgery is revascularization of the major visceral organs supplied by the celiac artery and the superior and inferior mesenteric arteries, restoration of renal blood flow, and preservation of the spinal cord. Spinal cord and renal injury are the most frequent complications of surgery. Circulatory support such as that described for repairs of descending thoracic lesions may be used. Generally, cardiopulmonary bypass is not used, but some authors have suggested that the use of hypothermic circulatory arrest may be beneficial in preserving spinal cord function (Kouchoukos and others, 1990).

Diagnosis is confirmed with aortography. The use of aortography is essential for determining the pa-

tency of the major visceral arteries and planning the operation. Vessels occluded by the aneurysmal process (often the inferior mesenteric artery) may not benefit from reimplantation (Cooley, 1986).

Procedural considerations

To provide access to both the descending thoracic and abdominal aortic segments, the patient is placed in the supine position with a roll or pillow under the left side of the chest to achieve a 45-degree modified lateral position. Both thoracotomy and laparotomy instrumentation is added to the vascular clamps and other instruments required for the repair.

Operative procedure: repair of a thoracoabdominal aortic aneurysm

1. The patient is positioned, and the initial thoracic incision is made through the intercostal space, allowing the best access to the proximal portion of the thoracic aortic lesion. (This may be between the sixth or seventh intercostal space or lower [Fig. 16-29].) The incision is continued to the midline of the abdomen and down the linea alba to a point below the umbilicus.
2. If circulatory support is being used, it is instituted (as described previously).
3. A thoracotomy retractor is inserted into the thoracic incision; rib cutters may be needed.
4. The diaphragm is opened a few centimeters to expose the proximal abdominal aorta. Care is taken to avoid injury to the phrenic nerve, the lung, the liver, and other organs. An abdominal retractor is inserted.
5. The aneurysm is inspected, and the extent of the lesion proximally and distally is determined. If separate proximal and distal lesions are present, the operation can be performed in two stages (Crawford and others, 1986) (Fig. 16-30).
6. For aneurysms involving one segment the thoracoabdominal aorta only, repair is done in one operation. The abdominal viscera are mobilized and retracted to the right. The distal aorta or

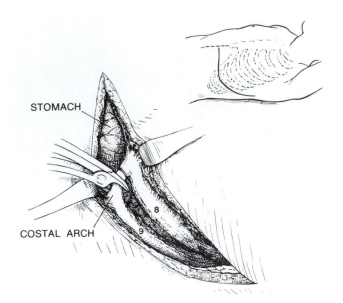

STOMACH

COSTAL ARCH

8

9

Fig. 16-29 Incision line for a thoracoabdominal aneurysm. The thoracotomy incision is carried to the midline and extended to beyond the umbilicus. Not shown is the roll or pillow placed under the left side to elevate the chest for exposure of the descending thoracic aorta. (From Waldhausen JA, Pierce WS: *Johnson's surgery of the chest,* ed 5, St Louis, 1985, Mosby.)

iliac arteries are dissected; if the spleen is injured, it should be removed (Cooley, 1986).

7. Prior to cross-clamping the aorta, heparin may be given (1 mg/kg of body weight [1000 units]) to prevent thrombosis or microemboli (Cooley, 1986). Some authors (Crawford and others, 1986) do not always use heparin.

Pharmacologic agents are used to control blood pressure and maintain hemodynamic stability. The aorta is cross-clamped proximally. The distal aorta or iliac arteries may be occluded or may be allowed to back bleed (Crawford and others, 1986). Occasionally, balloon occlusion catheters, gauze packing, or clamps are used to control profuse back bleeding.

8. The aorta is incised longitudinally, the lumen is measured, and the desired graft is delivered to the field and preclotted. The proximal anastomosis is performed with a continuous 3-0 or 4-0 suture. Large intercostal and lumbar arteries are reattached to the graft to help preserve spinal cord integrity (Fig. 16-30, *B*).

9A. When the visceral vessels and renal arteries are involved, the celiac and superior mesenteric arteries are anastomosed to openings made in the graft with a battery-powered hand-held cautery. If possible, they are reimplanted as a unit along

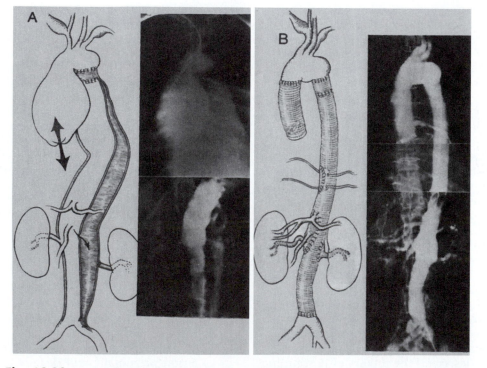

Fig. 16-30 **A,** Fusiform aneurysm of the ascending aorta and separate chronic dissecting aneurysm involving the entire descending thoracic and abdominal aorta (the patient had already undergone a graft replacement for a descending thoracic aneurysm). **B,** Drawing of staged operations showing graft replacement of the ascending aorta. Note reimplantation of intercostal arteries, visceral vessels, and both renal arteries. (From Crawford ES and others: Thoracoabdominal aortic aneurysms: preoperative and intraoperative factors determining immediate and long-term results of operations in 605 patients, *J Vasc Surg* 3:389, 1986.)

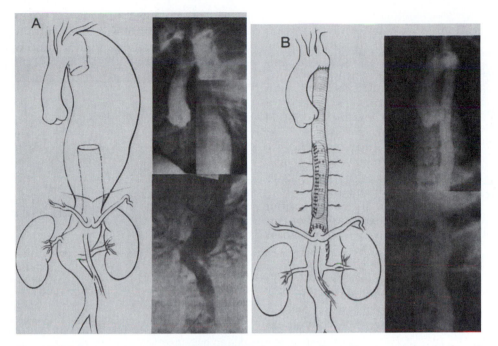

Fig. 16-31 **A,** Aneurysm of the descending thoracic aorta and upper abdominal aorta. **B,** Intercostal arteries are reimplanted into the graft. The visceral vessels and renal arteries are excluded from the repair. (From Crawford ES and others: Thoracoabdominal aortic aneurysms: preoperative and intraoperative factors determining immediate and long-term results of operations in 605 patients, *J Vasc Surg* 3:389, 1986.)

with the right renal artery (Crawford and others, 1986).

If the inferior mesenteric artery is patent, it is anastomosed to the graft. The left renal artery is reattached directly or with a short segment of 6 or 8 mm Dacron graft (or splenic artery if the spleen has been removed) (Fig. 16-30, *B*).

9B. If the visceral vessels and renal arteries are not involved, they can be excluded from the repair. The graft is beveled to repair the posterior portion of the abdominal aorta (Crawford and others, 1986) (Fig. 16-31).

10. The distal anastomosis is made to the distal abdominal aorta. If the aneurysm extends to the iliac arteries, a bifurcated graft is used (a bifurcated segment of graft may need to be anastomosed end-to-end to the distal portion of the tube graft.)

11. Air is evacuated, and each anastomosis is tested for hemostasis after completion. The aneurysmal sac is closed around the graft, and the viscera are replaced in the peritoneum. If circulatory support has been used, it is discontinued and incision sites are repaired.

12. A chest tube is inserted into the thorax, and an abdominal drain is inserted if excessive bleeding is anticipated (Cooley, 1986).

13. Thoracic and abdominal incisions are closed.

COMPLETION OF THE PROCEDURE

Following completion of the surgery, patients are transported to the surgical intensive care unit. In procedures involving extensive dissection (e.g., thoracoabdominal aneurysms), bleeding may be greater than that anticipated with other types of surgery. In addition to monitoring cardiac performance, attention is also focused on renal and neurologic function, especially when blood flow to the brain and the spinal cord has been interrupted.

POSTOPERATIVE COMPLICATIONS

Complications associated with repairing the thoracic aorta are listed in Table 16-5. Complications and patient teaching considerations for aortic valve prostheses are discussed in Chapter 14.

Table 16-5 ■ *Perioperative problems and complications of surgery on the thoracic aorta*

Complication/problem	Interventions
Hemorrhage	

Excessive bleeding may be caused by technical problems, excessive blood transfusions, prolonged cardiopulmonary bypass runs, excessive hemodilution, and coagulation defects related to hypothermia or intrinsic bleeding disorders	Intervention depends on cause of bleeding
	  Hemorrhage at suture lines:
	    Use felt strips to bolster suture line
	    Use fibrin glue and other topical hemostatic agents
	    Use preclotted grafts (or those manufactured to minimize interstitial bleeding)
	    Wrap suture line with Dacron graft (8 or 10 mm)
	  Excessive blood transfusions:
	    Avoid unnecessary connections or kinks in bypass circuit (damages blood cells)
	    Use cardiotomy suction gently, in pooled blood
	    Use fresh bank blood
	    Use autotransfusion system
	  Prolonged bypass runs/excessive hemodilution:
	    Avoid unnecessary delays during procedure
	    May require clotting factors
	    Membrane oxygenators and centrifugal pumps have been shown to preserve cell integrity
	    Administer desmopressin (DDAVP) to enhance activation of clotting factors
	  Coagulation defects due to hypothermia; when rewarming:
	    Do not allow OR to become too cold
	    Restart warming mattress
	    Use warm irrigation
	    Cover exposed skin when access not required
	  Coagulation defects due to intrinsic bleeding disorder:
	    Provide appropriate replacement therapy
	    Platelets may be required if there is history of aspirin

Central Nervous System Injury	

Embolization of particulate matter or air can cause neurologic injury; spinal cord paralysis is a complication of operations on descending thoracic and thoracoabdominal aorta; phrenic and vagus nerve injury can cause, respectively, paralysis of left diaphragm and left vocal cord; perfusion of false lumen in dissections can cause brain damage	Intervention depends on the type of injury
	  Embolization:
	    Remove all atheromatous and other debris from instruments and surgical site
	    Evacuate air completely from heart, aorta, and arch vessels
	    Gently manipulate vessels and perform careful debridement
	    Place in deep Trendelenburg position before reestablishing arterial flow
	    Use hypothermic circulatory arrest; occasionally, selective perfusion of arch vessels may be used in repair of aortic arch
	    Monitor electroencephalogram (EEG) and temperature
	  Spinal cord paralysis:
	    Minimize ischemic time; avoid delay
	    Maintain adequate distal flow and perfusion pressure with shunt or bypass; avoid hypotension
	    Monitor spinal cord function with evoked potentials
	    Reimplant major intercostal and lumbar (in thoracoabdominal aneurysms) arteries
	    Limit amount of aorta resected
	  Phrenic and vagus nerve injury:
	    Avoid stretching or severing nerves during surgery or aortic arch or proximal descending aorta
	    Note location of retractors
	  Brain injury from perfusion of false lumen (as well as injury to viscera):
	    May need to use circulatory arrest and open technique
	    May need to cannulate graft for antegrade flow after completion of first anastomosis
	    Monitor EEG
	    Simultaneously monitor femoral and both radial pulses
	(See text for additional details)

Modified from Kouchoukos NT, Wareing TH: Management of complications of aortic surgery. In Waldhausen JA, Orringer MB: *Complications in cardiothoracic surgery,* St Louis, 1991, Mosby.

Table 16-5 ■ *Perioperative problems and complications of surgery on the thoracic aorta—cont'd*

Complication/problem	Prevention/interventions
Infection of Prosthetic Grafts	
1% to 2% of all patients develop infection of prosthetic graft; mortality can be 25% to 75%; most infections are result of intraoperative contamination; risk is increased when operative time is prolonged, reoperation is performed, or there is excessive infusion of blood products	Prompt reoperation may be needed with replacement of infected prosthesis; a pedicle flap of omentum may be placed over graft Use strict operative sterile technique Provide antibiotic treatment (may require lifetime maintenance) Perform preoperative antibiotic prophylaxis Chlorhexidine gluconate may be preferred to povidone-iodine as operative cleansing agent
Pulmonary Complications	
Diffuse interstitial edema with reduced pulmonary compliance and acute respiratory failure may occur postoperatively; possible causes include anaphylatoxins generated during cardiopulmonary bypass, injury to lungs during retraction, or infusion of drugs or blood products	Provide mechanical ventilation at low inspiratory pressures in combination with positive end-expiratory pressure (PEEP); maintain 90% or greater arterial oxygen saturation Use caution during surgery to avoid injury to lungs from retraction and manipulation Use ultrafiltration to avoid excessive hemodilution during bypass; use membrane oxygenation Provide judicious infusion of blood products during surgery; antihistamines
Formation of Pseudoaneurysm at Anastomosis, Recurrent Dissection	
Associated with composite graft replacement of ascending aorta and aortic valve, or supracoronary graft replacement of ascending aorta for aortic dissection; may be greater risk in patients with connective tissue disorders (e.g., Marfan's syndrome); attributed to tension on suture line, persistent bleeding at anastomoses or between graft and aortic remnant closed over graft, and pathologic condition of aorta; may be caused by infection	Avoid tension on suture lines (e.g., use interposition of vein or synthetic graft between aortic graft and coronary ostia; use Cabrol technique (see text) Use measures to reduce bleeding Use measures to prevent or treat infection (see above) May need to avoid inclusion technique of wrapping remnant aneurysmal sac around graft In patients with dissections and Marfan's syndrome, composite graft replacement may be preferable to supracoronary graft replacement (so that weakened tissue is excluded from repair) Reoperation to repair or replace graft and pseudoaneurysm should be done before it becomes too enlarged

REFERENCES

Ablaza SG, Ghosh SC, Grana VP: Use of a ringed intraluminal graft in the surgical treatment of dissecting aneurysms of the thoracic aorta, *J Thorac Cardiovasc Surg* 76:390, 1978.

Anderson JK: Marfan's syndrome, *Crit Care Nurse* 11(4):69, 1991.

Bachet J and others: Cold cereplegia: a new technique of cerebral protection during operations on the transverse aortic arch, *J Thorac Cardiovasc Surg* 102(1):85, 1991.

Bentall H, deBono A: A technique for complete replacement of the ascending aorta, *Thorax* 23:338, 1968.

Berger RL and others: Replacement of the thoracic aorta with intraluminal sutureless prosthesis, *Ann Thorac Surg* 53:920, 1992.

Borst HG, Frank G, Schaps D: Treatment of extensive aortic aneurysms by a new multiple-stage approach, *J Thorac Cardiovasc Surg* 95:11, 1988.

Borst HG, Laas J, Heinemann M: Type A aortic dissection: diagnosis and management of malperfusion phenomena, *Semin Thorac Cardiovasc Surg* 3(3):238, 1991.

Bourland MD: Aortic dissection. In Rosen P, editor: *Emergency medicine: concepts and clinical practice*, ed 3, St Louis, 1992, Mosby.

Bradley JC, Craden MR: Infrarenal abdominal aortic aneurysm. In Association of Operating Room Nurses: *Core curriculum for the RN first assistant*, Denver, 1990, AORN.

Cabrol C, Pavie A, Mesnildrey P: Long-term results with total replacement of the ascending aorta and reimplantation of the coronary arteries, *J Thorac Cardiovasc Surg* 91:17, 1986.

Carpentier A: "Glue aortoplasty" as an alternative to resection and grafting for the treatment of aortic dissection, *Semin Thorac Cardiovasc Surg* 3(3):213, 1991.

Cartier R and others: Circulatory support during cross-clamping of the descending thoracic aorta: evidence of improved organ perfusion, *J Thorac Cardiovasc Surg* 99(6):1038, 1990.

Cigarroa JE and others: Diagnostic imaging in the evaluation of suspected aortic dissection, *N Engl J Med* 328(1):35, 1993.

Cooley DA: *Techniques in cardiac surgery*, ed 2, Philadelphia, 1984, WB Saunders.

Cooley DA: *Surgical treatment of aortic aneurysms*, Philadelphia, 1986, WB Saunders.

Cooley DA: Evolution of surgical treatment of thoracic aortic aneurysms, *Ann Thorac Surg* 48:137, 1989.

Cooley DA: Experience with hypothermic circulatory arrest and the treatment of aneurysms of the ascending aorta, *Semin Thorac Cardiovasc Surg* 3(3):166, 1991a.

Cooley DA: Panel discussion: ascending aorta, *Semin Thorac Cardiovasc Surg* 3(3):184, 1991b.

Cooley DA and others: A method for preparing woven Dacron grafts to prevent interstitial hemorrhage, *Cardiovasc Dis Bull Tex Heart Inst* 8(1):48, 1981.

Coselli JS and others: Determination of brain temperatures for safe circulatory arrest during cardiovascular operation, *Ann Thorac Surg* 45:638, 1988.

Crawford ES: The diagnosis and management of aortic dissection, *JAMA* 264(19):2537, 1990.

Crawford ES, Coselli JS: Marfan's syndrome: combined composite valve graft replacement of the aortic root and transaortic mitral valve replacement, *Ann Thorac Surg* 45:296, 1988.

Crawford ES, Crawford JL: *Diseases of the aorta*, Baltimore, 1984, Williams & Wilkins.

Crawford ES and others: Thoraco-abdominal aneurysms: preoperative and intraoperative factors determining immediate and long-term results of operation in 605 patients, *J Vasc Surg* 3:389, 1986.

Crawford ES and others: Aortic dissection and dissecting aortic aneurysms, *Ann Surg* 208(3):254, 1988.

Daily PO and others: Management of acute aortic dissections, *Ann Thorac Surg* 10:237, 1970.

DeBakey ME and others: Surgical management of dissecting aneurysms of the aorta, *J Thorac Cardiovasc Surg* 49:130, 1965.

Dureau G and others: New surgical technique for the operative management of acute dissections of the ascending aorta: report of two cases, *J Thorac Cardiovasc Surg* 76:385, 1978.

Eagle KA, DeSanctis RW: Diseases of the aorta. In Braunwald E: *Heart disease*, ed 4, Philadelphia, 1992, WB Saunders.

Elefteriades JA and others: Long-term experience with descending aortic dissection: the complication-specific approach, *Ann Thorac Surg* 53:11, 1992.

Ellis PR, Cooley DA, DeBakey ME: Clinical considerations and surgical treatment of annuloaortic ectasia, *J Thorac Cardiovasc Surg* 42:363, 1961.

Glower DD and others: Comparison of medical and surgical therapy for uncomplicated descending aortic dissection, *Circulation* 82(suppl IV):IV-39, 1990.

Griepp RB: Discussion: aortic dissection, *Semin Thorac Cardiovasc Surg* 3(3):251, 1991.

Griepp RB and others: Prosthetic replacement of the aortic arch, *J Thorac Cardiovasc Surg* 70:1051, 1975.

Griepp RB and others: The physiology of hypothermic circulatory arrest, *Semin Thorac Cardiovasc Surg* 3(3):188, 1991.

Grover FL, Calhoun JH: Aneurysms of the sinus of Valsalva. In Sabiston DC, editor: *Textbook of surgery*, ed 14, Philadelphia, 1991, WB Saunders.

Hollister DW and others: Immunohistologic abnormalities of the microfibrillar-fibrin system in the Marfan syndrome, *N Engl J Med* 323(3):152, 1990.

Kirklin JW, Barratt-Boyes: *Cardiac surgery*, ed 2, New York, 1993, Churchill Livingstone.

Kouchoukos NT: Composite graft replacement of the ascending aorta and aortic valve with the inclusion-wrap and open techniques, *Semin Thorac Cardiovasc Surg* 3(3):171, 1991.

Kouchoukos NT, Marshall WG, Wedige-Stecher TA: Eleven-year experience with composite graft replacement of the ascending aorta and aortic valve, *J Thorac Cardiovasc Surg* 92(4):691, 1986.

Kouchoukos NT, Wareing TH: Management of complications of aortic surgery. In Walhausen JA, Orringer MB: *Complications in cardiothoracic surgery*, St Louis, 1991, Mosby.

Kouchoukos NT and others: Elective hypothermic cardiopulmonary bypass and circulatory arrest for spinal cord protection during operations on the thoracoabdominal aorta, *J Thorac Cardiovasc Surg* 99(4):659, 1990.

Kram HB and others: Diagnosis of traumatic thoracic aortic rupture: a 10 year retrospective analysis, *Ann Thorac Surg* 47:282, 1989.

Lewis CTP and others: Surgical repair of aortic root aneurysms in 280 patients, *Ann Thorac Surg* 53:38, 1992.

Matas R: An operation for the radical cure of aneurism based on arteriorrhaphy, *Ann Surg* 37:161, 1903.

Miller DC: Surgical management of acute aortic dissection: new data, *Semin Thorac Cardiovasc Surg* 3(3):225, 1991.

Miller DC and others: Operative treatment of aortic dissections: experience with 125 patients over a sixteen-year period, *J Thorac Cardiovasc Surg* 78:365, 1979.

Miyamoto AT: Technique for replacing the ascending aorta and aortic valve with a modified Bentall's operation, *Ann Thorac Surg* 53:1125, 1992.

Pyeritz RE: Marfan syndrome, *N Engl J Med* 323(14):987, 1990.

Reitknecht FL, Bhayana JN, Lajos TZ: Circumferential intimal tear causing obstruction of the aortic arch: an unusual complication of aortic dissection, *Ann Thorac Surg* 46:100, 1988.

Roberts WC: Cardiac rupture, abdominal aneurysmal rupture and dissecting aortic rupture: a preventive trio, *Am J Cardiol* 57:892, 1986 (editorial).

Sabiston DC: Aneurysms. In Sabiston DC, editor: *Textbook of surgery*, ed 14, Philadelphia, 1991, WB Saunders.

Schlatmann TJ, Becker AE: Pathogenesis of dissecting aneurysm of aorta, *Am J Cardiol* 39:21, 1977.

Seifert PC: Dissecting aortic aneurysms: a problem in Marfan's syndrome, *AORN J* 43(2):443, 1986a.

Seifert PC: Preclotting of grafts, *AORN J* 43(5):972, 1986b (response: letter to editor).

Simon P and others: Transesophageal echocardiography in the emergency surgical management of patients with aortic dissection, *J Thorac Cardiovasc Surg* 103(6):1113, 1992.

Svensson LG, Crawford ES: Aortic dissection and aortic aneurysm surgery: clinical observations, experimental investigations, and statistical analyses, part 1, *Curr Probl Surg* 29(11):818, 1992.

Svensson LG and others: Dissection of the aorta and dissecting aortic aneurysms, *Circulation* 82(suppl IV):IV-24, 1990.

Swain JA and others: Low-flow hypothermic cardiopulmonary bypass protects the brain, *J Thorac Cardiovasc Surg* 102(1):76, 1991.

Waldhausen JA, Pierce WS: *Johnson's surgery of the chest*, ed 5, St Louis, 1985, Mosby.

Webb WR, Kelly JP: Aneurysms of the thoracic aorta. In Sabiston DC, editor: *Textbook of surgery*, ed 13, Philadelphia, 1986, WB Saunders.

Weiland AP, Walker WE: Thoracic aneurysms, *Crit Care Q* 9(3):20, 1986.

Weinschelbaum EE and others: Surgical treatment of acute Type A dissecting aneurysm, with preservation of the native aortic valve and use of biologic glue, *J Thorac Cardiovasc Surg* 103(2):369, 1992.

Wheat MW: Acute dissecting aneurysms of the aorta. In Goldberger E: *Treatment of cardiac emergencies*, St Louis, 1990, Mosby.

Wheat MW and others: Acute dissecting aneurysms of the aorta: treatment of results in 64 patients, *J Thorac Cardiovasc Surg* 58:344, 1969.

Wolfe WG: Aneurysms of the thoracic aorta. In Sabiston DC, editor: *Textbook of surgery*, ed 14, Philadelphia, 1991, WB Saunders.

17

Ventricular and Other Circulatory Assist Devices

Inside the body, the pump faces a very hostile environment. It's a hot saltwater solution with enzymes whose job it is to dissolve matter . . . Then you have the problem of size constraints. There are no voids in the body, so there's a big challenge when you try to insert anything. And finally, you have to interface with blood, whose reaction to a foreign object is to encapsulate it and try to exteriorize it . . . That's why it has taken us so long. We've had to develop new materials, figure out how to deal with blood, and design systems that are compatible with the anatomy.

Victor Poirier, 1992

Mechanical and muscle-powered ventricular assist devices (VADs) have become an increasingly important addition to the cardiac surgical armamentarium for treating heart failure and cardiogenic shock. The feasibility of temporary circulatory support was shown with Gibbon's (1954) introduction of the heart-lung machine. Within a few years, use of cardiopulmonary bypass (CPB) technology was expanded to clinical situations associated with severe cardiac decompensation. These experiences generated interest in the development of cardiac support devices of varying duration, design, and complexity, culminating with the insertion of a temporary total artificial heart (TAH) by Cooley and associates in 1969 and implementation of a permanent TAH in 1982 by De Vries (1988) (Fig. 17-1).

The primary purpose of these devices is to maintain the circulation when the heart is incapable of performing this function because of reversible or irreversible injury. In patients with reversible myocardial insults, these devices can temporarily assume the cardiac workload, partially or totally, while the heart rests and recuperates. When irreversible injury is present, support systems can maintain organ perfusion until a donor heart can be transplanted.

However, the use of these support systems is associated with a number of problems. For example, although CPB is satisfactory as a short-term method to support the circulation, long-term management is unsuitable because of excessive blood trauma, the need for systemic heparinization (causing bleeding), a high risk of infection, and the cumbersomeness of the technique. More sophisticated VADs, including

the TAH, have been subject to similar complications, as well as to a significant incidence of stroke from thromboembolism.

These factors, along with the increasing incidence of heart failure and the introduction of cardiac transplantation, have prompted researchers to continue their investigations of alternative long-term methods of ventricular support. Among the advances spurring greater use of mechanical devices, three are especially noteworthy. One is the introduction of the immunosuppressive drug cyclosporine which, by improving

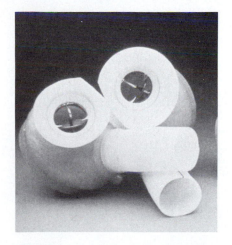

Fig. 17-1 Symbion Jarvik-7 total artificial heart. (From Quaal SJ, editor: *Cardiac mechanical assistance beyond balloon pumping,* St Louis, 1993, Mosby.)

349

survival after heart transplantation, has generated a growing demand for the use of these devices as a bridge to transplantation (Kolff, 1993). The second is the development of blood-contacting surfaces within the mechanical pumps, resulting in a significantly re-duced incidence of thrombus formation and emboli-zation, previously major limitations of VADs. Third, although the demand for heart transplantation has increased, the supply of donor hearts has leveled off during the past few years (Evans and others, 1986).

Box 17-1   Selected causes of heart failure

Mechanical Abnormalities

Increased Afterload
Aortic stenosis
Systemic arterial hypertension
Coarctation of aorta

Increased Preload
Valvular regurgitation
Shunts
Increased venous return

Altered Contractility
Myocardial infarction
Ventricular aneurysm

Obstruction or Impairment to Cardiac Chamber Filling
Mitral stenosis
Tricuspid stenosis
Pericardial constriction
Cardiac tamponade
Massive pulmonary embolus
Intracardiac tumor

Traumatic Injury
Myocardial contusion
Penetrating cardiac injury

Myocardial Abnormalities

Idiopathic Cardiomyopathies
Dilated
Hypertrophic
Restrictive

Neurovascular Cardiomyopathy
Duchenne's muscular dystrophy

Myocarditis
Bacterial
Viral
Mycotic
Protozoal

Metabolic Deficiencies
Diabetes mellitus
Beriberi
Acid-base imbalance
Electrolyte imbalance
Malnutrition

Cardiotoxic/Cardiodepressant Effect
Alcohol
Cocaine
Radiation exposure

Electrical shock
Tricyclic antidepressants
Chemotherapeutic agents
  Adriamycin
  Vincristine
Theophylline
Poison
  Plant
  Animal, insect
  Environmental
Effects of aging
Ischemia
  Acute
  Chronic
Infarction
Metabolic Disorders
  Acromegaly
  Hypoparathyroidism
  Pheochromocytoma
  Hyperthyroidism
  Cardiac glycogenesis
Other disease
  Amyloidosis
  Carcinoid heart disease
  Sarcoidosis
  Endocarditis
  Acute cardiac allograft rejection
  Crohn's disease
  Chronic obstructive pulmonary disease
  Connective tissue disorders
  AIDS-related cardiomyopathy
  Cocaine-induced heart disease
  Anaphylactic shock
  Septic shock

Conduction System Abnormalities

Bradydysrhythmias
Extreme sinus bradycardia
Junctional rhythm

Tachydysrhythmias
Prolonged supraventricular tachycardia
Ventricular tachycardia

Conduction Disturbance
High-grade heart block
Atrioventricular dissociation
Complete heart block

Fibrillation
Atrial
Ventricular

Modified from Rutan PM, Galvin EA: Adult and pediatric ventricular heart failure. In Quaal SJ, editor: *Cardiac mechanical assistance beyond balloon pumping,* St Louis, 1993, Mosby.

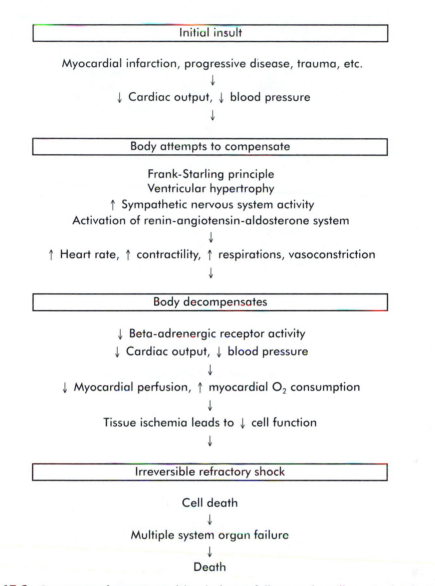

Initial insult

Myocardial infarction, progressive disease, trauma, etc.
↓
↓ Cardiac output, ↓ blood pressure
↓

Body attempts to compensate

Frank-Starling principle
Ventricular hypertrophy
↑ Sympathetic nervous system activity
Activation of renin-angiotensin-aldosterone system
↓
↑ Heart rate, ↑ contractility, ↑ respirations, vasoconstriction
↓

Body decompensates

↓ Beta-adrenergic receptor activity
↓ Cardiac output, ↓ blood pressure
↓
↓ Myocardial perfusion, ↑ myocardial O_2 consumption
↓
Tissue ischemia leads to ↓ cell function
↓

Irreversible refractory shock

Cell death
↓
Multiple system organ failure
↓
Death

Fig. 17-2 Sequence of events resulting in heart failure and cardiogenic shock. (From Quaal SJ, editor: *Cardiac mechanical assistance beyond balloon pumping,* St Louis, 1993, Mosby.)

CONGESTIVE HEART FAILURE

Although most cardiovascular disorders have decreased over the past decade, the incidence of congestive heart failure (CHF) has increased dramatically and now represents the most common medical discharge diagnostic category for patients over 65 years of age (Packer, 1987; Quaal, 1992). CHF may be caused by intrinsic heart disease or precipitating factors and in general can be categorized as a mechanical problem, myocardial abnormality, and/or conduction system problem (Schlant and Sonnenblick, 1990) (Box 17-1). It is frequently related to sequelae of ischemic heart disease. The resulting derangements produce systolic dysfunction leading to reduced stroke volume, diastolic impairment leading to elevated ventricular filling pressures and pulmonary congestion, or a combination of both (Rutan and Galvin, 1993). As heart failure worsens, systemic acidosis, hypoxia, vasoconstriction, hypotension, and decreased peripheral perfusion can lead to major organ dysfunction. If adequate coronary and systemic blood flow are not restored, multisystem organ failure and death occur (Fig. 17-2).

Myocardial "stunning," as described by Braunwald and Kloner (1982), is a myocardial abnormality related to ischemic heart disease that interferes with biochemical functions and the myocardial ultrastructure. Stunned myocardium is not infarcted, but it is severely ischemic and can produce prolonged ventricular dysfunction. It can occur adjacent to necrotic tissue after prolonged coronary occlusion and is also seen in patients with severely depressed hearts who have undergone ischemic cardiac arrest during CPB (Braunwald, 1990). These patients may demonstrate poorly

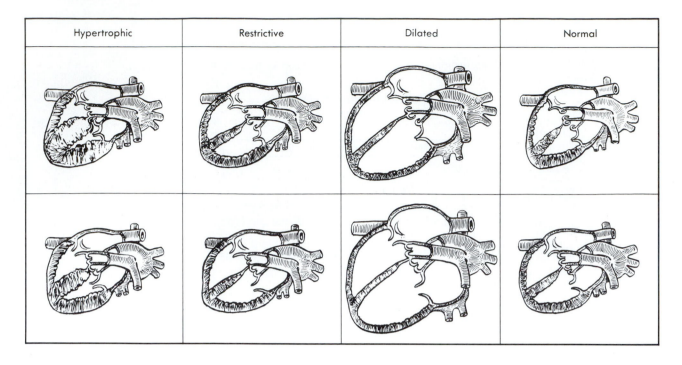

Hypertrophic	Restrictive	Dilated	Normal

Fig. 17-3   Types of cardiomyopathies compared with a normal heart. (From Thelan LA, Davie JK, Urden LD: *Textbook of critical care nursing: diagnosis and management,* St Louis, 1990, Mosby.)

contractile hearts requiring maximum inotropic support and intraaortic balloon pulsation (IABP) in order to wean the patient from CPB. More advanced forms of circulatory support may be required for prolonged postcardiotomy low-output syndrome.

The severity and duration of stunning are dependent on the length and intensity of the ischemia and the condition of the heart at the beginning of the ischemic episode. Myocardial reperfusion (thrombolysis, percutaneous transluminal coronary angioplasty, coronary bypass surgery) is necessary to reverse the injury, but the effects may not be evident for days or weeks after the intervention; during this period mechanical assistance may be necessary to allow the heart to recuperate. Repeated stunning can produce chronic left ventricular dysfunction, myocardial scarring, and ischemic cardiomyopathy (Braunwald and Sobel, 1992).

Acute Versus Chronic Failure

Reversal of myocardial and other major organ dysfunction is partially determined by whether failure is acute or chronic. The most frequent cause of acute CHF is myocardial infarction (MI), which leads to cellular death, producing intracellular acidosis and an accumulation of metabolic waste products. Other causes include sudden valvular regurgitation and pulmonary embolus. Reversal of acute failure can often correct systemic organ derangements before there is irreversible injury.

Chronic CHF may require several weeks of normal perfusion to improve organ function. It is frequently attributable to ischemic heart disease, longstanding valvular disease, chronic obstructive pulmonary disease, myocardial fibrosis, and changes in ventricular geometry that are known to produce heart failure (Quaal, 1992).

Cardiomyopathy (Fig. 17-3) is another major cause of chronic failure and may be due to neuromuscular or connective tissue disorders, alcohol abuse, viral infection, cardiotoxic substances, and a variety of other disorders (see Box 17-1). In the majority of cases the cause is unknown (idiopathic).

The most common form is **dilated cardiomyopathy,** in which the heart is enlarged and poorly contractile. Decreased ventricular contractility and increased end-diastolic pressure and volume lead to impaired ejection (systolic dysfunction). **Hypertrophic cardiomyopathy** is less common; increased wall thickness reduces ventricular compliance, producing elevated ventricular end-diastolic pressure. Diastolic filling (preload) is impaired, leading to systolic and diastolic dysfunction. Least common among the types of cardiomyopathy is that characterized as **restrictive.** End-diastolic volume and ventricular stretch are affected, leading to systolic and diastolic impairment. The cause may be unknown or related to disease processes that result in endomyocardial fibrosis (Rutan and Galvin, 1993).

Compensatory Mechanisms

When the heart is injured and is unable to eject a sufficient cardiac output, a variety of compensatory mechanisms are activated by the body in an attempt to enhance perfusion. These mechanisms can enhance cardiac output and major organ perfusion, but

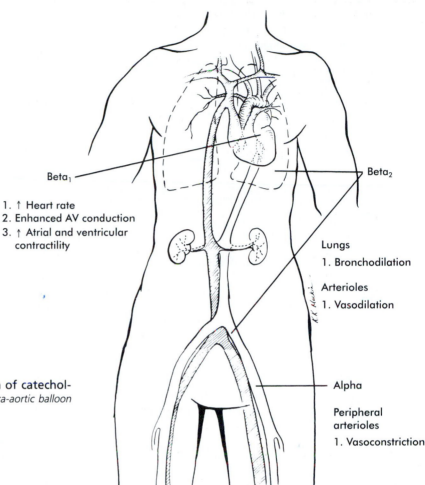

Beta₁

1. ↑ Heart rate
2. Enhanced AV conduction
3. ↑ Atrial and ventricular
   contractility

Beta₂

Lungs
1. Bronchodilation

Arterioles
1. Vasodilation

Alpha

Peripheral
arterioles
1. Vasoconstriction

Fig. 17-4 **Alpha- and beta-receptor action of catechol-amines.** (From Quaal SJ, editor: *Comprehensive intra-aortic balloon pumping*, St Louis, 1984, Mosby.)

only at the expense of other parts of the body (such as the peripheral organs) and only for a finite period of time (Braunwald, 1992). Eventually these mechanisms will also fail (Quaal, 1992; Rutan and Galvin, 1993).

Frank-Starling mechanism

One of the first mechanisms to be activated is the Frank-Starling mechanism whereby increasing diastolic filling pressures (preload) stretch the myocardial muscle fibers, which allows the ventricle to eject more forcefully and thereby produce a correspondingly larger stroke volume (Quaal, 1993). In the presence of progressive heart failure, however, the effectiveness of this mechanism is limited because the elevated preload increases ventricular wall tension, which increases myocardial oxygen consumption. Another limitation is that increasing ventricular diastolic pressure is transmitted to the pulmonary vascular system, producing congestion (Quaal, 1992).

Sympathetic nervous stimulation

Sympathetic nervous system (SNS) stimulation results in increased production of catecholamines by the car-diac adrenergic nerve endings and adrenal glands. Contractility and heart rate are increased, as is systemic vascular resistance. This allows perfusion of the heart and brain to be maintained, but only at the expense of other organs that receive insufficient blood flow.

Beta-adrenergic receptors

Beta-adrenergic receptors are found in the myocardium (beta-1) and in smooth muscle (beta-2). Beta-1 receptors increase heart rate, contractility, and conductivity of cardiac impulses (Fig. 17-4). Beta-2 receptors are primarily vasodilators. In heart failure, beta-1 receptors are "down regulated"; that is, they are reduced in density within the ventricle and become less active, with the result that myocardial contractility is inhibited. Presumably, this effect is due to high levels of circulating norepinephrine activated by the failing heart (Braunwald, 1992).

Renin-angiotensin activation

Hypoperfusion of the kidneys initiates another series of responses. Renin is released, stimulating the production of angiotensin-II, which produces vasocon-

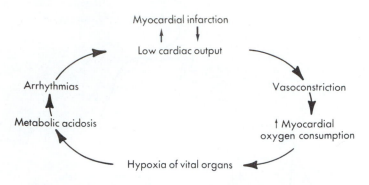

Fig. 17-5 Self-perpetuating cycle of cardiogenic shock. (From Quaal SJ, editor: *Comprehensive intra-aortic balloon pumping,* St Louis, 1984, Mosby.)

striction. Angiotensin-II stimulates aldosterone production, resulting in decreased sodium and chloride secretion and increased potassium excretion. Angiotensin-II also stimulates arginine vasopressin, another vasoconstrictor. The resulting increase in intravascular volume, preload, and afterload further stresses the heart.

Baroreceptors

When cerebral perfusion is decreased, carotid baroreceptors are activated. This causes an increase in sympathetic tone and stimulates the pituitary gland to release vasopressin.

Cardiac atrial baroreceptors respond to increased preload by releasing atrial natriuretic peptide (ANP), which produces arterial dilatation and venous dilatation, inhibits renin and aldosterone production, enhances sodium excretion, and reduces sympathetic vasoconstriction. Although ANP has the effect of regulating circulatory blood volume and lowering arterial blood pressure, other compensatory forces may override this mechanism (Rutan and Galvin, 1993).

Ventricular hypertrophy

Ventricular hypertrophy is stimulated by increased pressure and volume loading. Initially the increased muscle mass is capable of generating higher ejection pressures to maintain cardiac output, but worsening cardiac failure and increased myocardial oxygen consumption eventually result in refractory failure. The development of ventricular hypertrophy occurs with chronic overloading; when CHF occurs acutely, there is insufficient time for hypertrophy to develop.

Cardiogenic Shock

The most severe form of heart failure is cardiogenic shock, a state of progressive and severe circulatory deterioration that can lead to a self-perpetuating cycle of ischemic damage that results in irreversible myocardial dysfunction (Quaal, 1992). It can occur as a complication of acute myocardial infarction (Fig. 17-5) and may be apparent intraoperatively on termination of CPB. The high mortality associated with this condition is chiefly related to the inability of compensatory mechanisms to counteract the downward trend.

Clinical manifestations depend on the individual response to reduced blood flow and SNS stimulation. Heart rate is increased to perfuse vital organs. The skin is pale, cool, and clammy as a result of peripheral vasoconstriction; urinary output suffers from renal ischemia; and altered mentation occurs as a result of sympathetic stimulation, cerebral hypoxia, and respiratory alkalosis secondary to hyperventilation. When vasoconstriction is severe and prolonged, the resulting metabolic acidosis can produce cellular and systemic destruction (Quaal, 1992).

Intraoperatively, low cardiac output leading to CHF and shock becomes apparent when the surgical repair has been completed and weaning from CPB is attempted. The venous line is gradually occluded, forcing returning blood to enter the heart rather than being diverted to the bypass pump. This creates a volume and pressure load that the ventricles must overcome in order to eject blood. If a perioperative MI has occurred or the myocardium is stunned, for example, ventricular dysfunction prevents resumption of adequate stroke work, and evidence of failure is seen. Peripheral vascular resistance may be elevated, thereby increasing ventricular afterload. Impedance to ejection may also result from increased vascular volume, blood viscosity, and heart rate; these factors may be manipulated pharmacologically. Vascular stiffness may also contribute to increased afterload.

It is important to inspect the heart. One or both ventricles often appear distended, pale, and poorly contractile; manual palpation of the ascending aorta suggests hypotension. Hemodynamic measurements reflect systemic hypotension, the cardiac index is decreased, and pulmonary (filling) pressures are elevated.

Before diagnosis and treatment for low cardiac output syndrome is initiated, the surgeon must assess the overall adequacy and quality of the operation (e.g., valve repair or replacement, coronary artery bypass grafting) and correct any deficiencies. A bolus of air may have entered the coronary circulation, necessitating manual cardiac massage, inotropes, and high-pressure perfusion (e.g., partially occluding the aorta with a cross-clamp to increase coronary flow, which forces air downstream and out of the coronary bed). Retrograde coronary perfusion via the coronary sinus may also be used for this purpose (Wechsler, 1991).

The accuracy of hemodynamic readings must be confirmed. If there is a question about systemic blood pressure readings from a peripheral (e.g., radial) arterial pressure line, a central arterial monitoring line may be inserted via a femoral artery. Core blood pressure may also be determined with a small hypodermic needle placed in the ascending aorta; the needle is attached to pressure tubing, which is connected to a transducer. (When this method of pressure monitoring is no longer needed, the needle is removed and the entry site is closed with a fine suture.) In addition, all pressure line transducers should be recalibrated, and the tubing should be checked to confirm that there is no kinking or air in the line.

Initial Medical Management

Box 17-2 outlines the major principles of medical management in patients with low cardiac output syndrome. Initial treatment consists of expanding the circulatory blood volume with intravenous (IV) fluids. Pharmacologic reduction of peripheral vascular resistance with vasodilators and augmentation of myocardial contractility with inotropic agents is instituted to enhance blood flow to vital organs and increase cardiac output. Vasodilators reduce left ventricular afterload to further improve tissue perfusion.

Bradydysrhythmias causing hypotension are commonly treated with temporary epicardial pacemaker wires and external generators. Tachydysrhythmias resulting from hypovolemia, hypoxia, acidosis, and electrolyte disturbances may lead to lethal dysrhythmias. Antidysrhythmic drugs are generally ineffective unless the underlying volume deficit is replaced and arterial blood gas and electrolyte derangements are corrected with sodium bicarbonate and appropriate electrolyte replacement.

Often IABP counterpulsation is also instituted to augment systemic and coronary blood flow and to reduce the cardiac workload. If these interventions are insufficient, CPB is usually reinstituted while additional treatment options, such as the appropriateness of circulatory assist devices, are considered.

CIRCULATORY ASSIST DEVICES

Mechanical devices to support the heart and the circulation are used to reduce cardiac work, enhance myocardial oxygenation, and increase organ perfusion. Depending on the degree of cardiac dysfunction, devices are available that can partially or totally support ventricular stroke volume.

Table 17-1 ■ *Classifications of circulatory support devices*

Class	Selected examples
Availability	
FDA approval required	Novacor, Thoratec TCI HeartMate
FDA approval not required/commercially available	Centrifugal pump, Abiomed
Position of Pump	
External:	
Extracorporeal	Abiomed
Paracorporeal	Thoratec
Internal:	
Heterotopic	Novacor
Orthotopic	Utah 100 TAH
Intended Use	
Resuscitation	Hemopump
Short-term support	Centrifugal
Intermediate-term support	Abiomed
Long-term support (greater than 30 days)	TCI HeartMate
Source of Energy	
Pneumatic	Thoratec
Electrical	Novacor, TCI HeartMate
Flow Pattern	
Pulsatile	Abiomed, Nocacor, Thoratec, TCI HeartMate, TAH
Nonpulsatile	Centrifugal
Ventricle Supported	
Right	Abiomed, Thoratec
Left	Abiomed, Thoratec, Novacor, TCI HeartMate
Both	Abiomed, Thoratec
Reliance on Ventricular Stroke Volume	
Series: Functions in conjunction with native heart; augments existing CO; requires working heart	IABP, Hemopump
Parallel: Can provide stroke volume independent of cardiac function	Abiomed, Novacor, Thoratec, TCI HeartMate

Modified from Shiono M and others: Overview of ventricular assist devices. In Quaal SJ, editor: *Cardiac mechanical assistance beyond balloon pumping*, St Louis, 1993, Mosby.
CO, Cardiac output; *FDA*, Food and Drug Administration; *IABP*, intraaortic balloon pump; *TAH*, total artificial heart.

Multiple classification systems have been devised for assist devices in relation to their availability, position, intended use, source of energy, flow pattern, and reliance on native cardiac function (Table 17-1). The following sections discuss mechanical circulatory support devices according to categories suggested by Pennington and Swartz (1992) (Table 17-2).

Table 17-2 ■ *Mechanical circulatory support devices*

Category/name	Investigational*	Position	Support	Preferred application	Anticoagulation required	Duration
Resuscitative Devices						
IABP	No	Internal	Rt, L, Bi	P, R	Moderate	Short term
CPS System (Bard)	No	Extracorporeal	Bi	R	Full	Short term
ECMO	No	Extracorporeal	Bi	R	Full	Short term
Hemopump (Johnson & Johnson)	Yes	Internal	L	P, R	Moderate	Short, intermediate term
External Centrifugal and Roller Pump						
Centrifugal (Biomedicus, Sarns, St Jude Medical)	No	Extracorporeal	Rt, L, Bi	P, TX	Moderate	Short, intermediate term
Roller pump	No	Extracorporeal	Rt, L, Bi	P, R	Full	Short term
External Pulsatile VADs (Right, Left, Biventricular)						
Thoratec (Pierce-Donachy)	Yes	Paracorporeal	Rt, L, Bi	P, TX	Low	Intermediate, long term
Abiomed	No	Extracorporeal	Rt, L, Bi	P, TX	Moderate	Short, intermediate term
Implantable LVADs						
Novacor (Baxter)	Yes	Internal	L	TX	Low	Intermediate, long term
HeartMate (Thermocardiosystems)	Yes	Internal	L	TX	Low	Intermediate, long term
Total Artificial Heart						
Utah 100	Yes	Orthotopic	Bi	TX	Moderate	Intermediate, long term

Modified from Pennington DG, Swartz MT: Assisted circulation and mechanical hearts. In Braunwald E: *Heart disease,* ed 4, Philadelphia, 1991, WB Saunders.
*Investigational device exemption required from Food and Drug Administration (FDA).
Bi, Biventricular; *CPS,* proprietary name (Bard) for percutaneous cardiopulmonary bypass system; *ECMO,* extracorporeal membrane oxygenation; *L,* left; *LVAD,* left ventricular assist device; *P,* postcardiotomy; *R,* resuscitative; *RT,* right; *TX,* bridge to transplantation.

RESUSCITATIVE DEVICES

Resuscitative devices include the IABP and the Hemopump. Extracorporeal membrane oxygenation (ECMO) and percutaneous CPB (Bard CPS System) are also included in this category; they are described in Chapter 11.

Intraaortic Balloon Pump

One of the most widely used circulatory assist devices is the IABP. It has been used in patients with cardiogenic shock following MI, in patients with unstable hemodynamic status undergoing cardiac catheterization and angioplasty, and in patients with left and/or right ventricular heart failure following surgery (Maccioli, Lucas, and Norfleet, 1988).

Developed by Moulopoulos and colleagues in 1962 and first applied clinically by Kantrowitz and his associates in 1968 (Kantrowitz, 1990; Kantrowitz and others, 1968), the IABP provides short-term, temporary support to the failing heart. The balloon is commonly inserted percutaneously via the femoral artery, threaded retrogradely up the aorta, and positioned in the descending thoracic aorta distal to the left subclavian artery and proximal to the renal arteries (Fig. 17-6).

The device works on the principle of internal counterpulsation (Fig. 17-7). Balloon inflation (with helium or carbon dioxide gas) during diastole propels blood both antegradely to perfuse the distal organs and retrogradely to perfuse the brain and coronary arteries (Fig. 17-7, *A* and *B*). By propelling aortic blood flow both antegradely and retrogradely during diastole, coronary and systemic organ perfusion is enhanced and cardiac output is augmented; by deflating just before the following systole, the device also reduces the work of the heart and the myocardial oxygen demand by lowering the resistance to ejection (afterload) during systole (Fig. 17-7, *C;* Box 17-3).

Synchronization of balloon inflation and deflation is based on the arterial waveform and is dependent on a reliable ECG signal (Quaal, 1993). Both ECG electrodes and a pressure monitoring line are connected to the pump. Electrocautery can interfere with the ECG, as can dysrhythmias, artifact, and pacemaker spikes. When cautery is in use, pressure monitoring is used to time balloon inflation/deflation.

The major contraindication for IABP is aortic in-

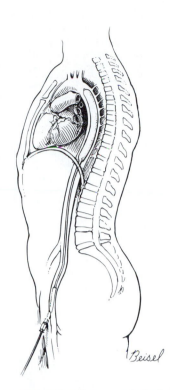

Fig. 17-6 Placement of an intraaortic balloon in the descending thoracic aorta. (From Waldhausen JA, Pierce WS: *Johnson's surgery of the chest*, ed 5, St Louis, 1985, Mosby.)

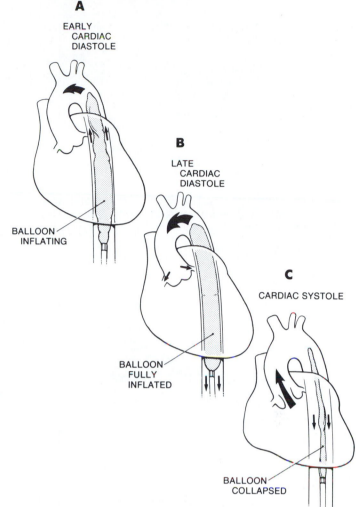

Fig. 17-7 **A,** Balloon inflating during early diastole. **B,** Balloon fully inflated during late diastole. **C,** Balloon collapsed during systole (see text). (From Waldhausen JA, Pierce WS: *Johnson's surgery of the chest*, ed 5, St Louis, 1985, Mosby.)

sufficiency, which would allow blood to preferentially enter the left ventricle rather than the coronary arteries, resulting in decreased coronary perfusion and increased ventricular distension. Aortic dissection or aneurysm is another contraindication because of the risk of aortic rupture.

Operative procedures: insertion of an intraaortic balloon pump
Femoral artery insertion *(Walhausen and Pierce, 1985)*

If pre- or post-CPB use of an IABP is anticipated for support of the left ventricle, the surgeon may insert a catheter (Fig. 17-8) into the femoral artery before the start of surgery for blood pressure monitoring and/or as an access route for the IABP. This is most easily performed before the start of the procedure and institution of CPB, because the patient will have a palpable pulse; after initiation of CPB (nonpulsatile flow), the femoral artery may be more difficult to locate by palpation, and a femoral artery cutdown may be necessary.

Box 17-3 *Desired effects of balloon inflation and deflation*

Balloon Inflation
Coronary blood flow is potentially increased.
Perfusion is augmented to aortic arch and distal systemic circulation.
Coronary collateral circulation is potentially increased.

Balloon Deflation
Reduction of aortic and end-diastolic pressure reduces afterload.
Myocardial oxygen consumption is decreased.
Cardiac output is increased.
Reduction in peak systolic pressure reduces left-to-right shunting in ventricular septal defects and regurgitant blood flow in mitral insufficiency.

Modified from Quaal SJ: *Comprehensive intra-aortic balloon pumping*, St Louis, ed 2, 1993, Mosby.

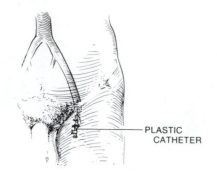

Fig. 17-8 Catheter inserted in the left femoral artery for later insertion of an intraaortic balloon. (From Waldhausen JA, Pierce WS: *Johnson's surgery of the chest,* ed 5, St Louis, 1985, Mosby.)

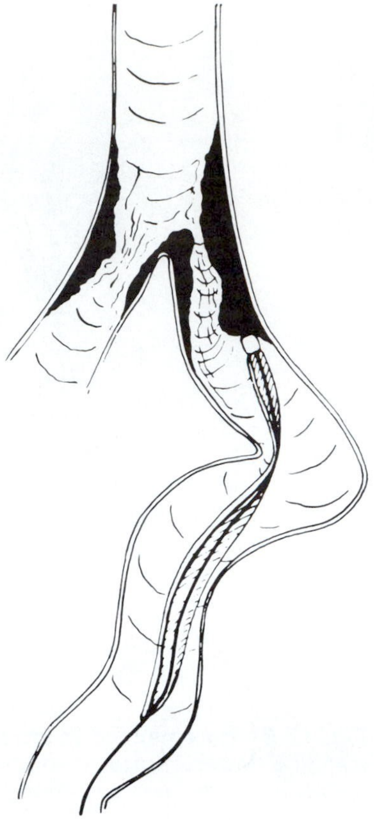

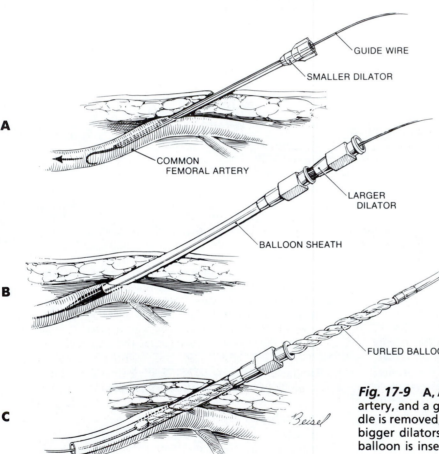

Fig. 17-10 Tortuous atherosclerotic artery impedes advancement of the balloon catheter. Use of a guidewire may help to direct the balloon past the obstruction. (From Quaal SJ: *Comprehensive intra-aortic balloon pumping,* St Louis, 1984, Mosby.)

Fig. 17-9 **A,** A Seldinger needle is inserted into the femoral artery, and a guidewire is threaded into the aorta. The needle is removed, and a small dilator is inserted. **B,** Increasingly bigger dilators are used to enlarge the tissue track. **C,** The balloon is inserted into the femoral artery. (From Waldhausen JA, Pierce WS: *Johnson's surgery of the chest,* ed 5, St Louis, 1985, Mosby.)

Procedure

1. An 18-gauge angiographic (Seldinger) needle is inserted percutaneously into the femoral artery; the obturator is removed, and a guidewire is threaded into the artery (Fig. 17-9, *A*). If there is extensive atherosclerotic disease of the aortoiliac junction or if the arteries are tortuous, passage of the guidewire (or the balloon) may be difficult (Fig. 17-10). Different guidewire shapes (straight or J shape) or Teflon-coated wires may ease insertion; entry via the opposite femoral artery may be necessary. Direct antegrade insertion (see following procedure) may be used on rare occasions.

2. The guidewire is advanced into the aorta. The needle is then removed, leaving the wire in place.

3. A series of dilators in increasingly larger sizes are used to enlarge the arteriotomy and surrounding tissue. Each dilator is threaded over the guidewire and then removed and replaced with the next larger size (Fig. 17-9, *B*).

4. The balloon is taken out of its package, and residual air within the balloon is removed with a syringe.

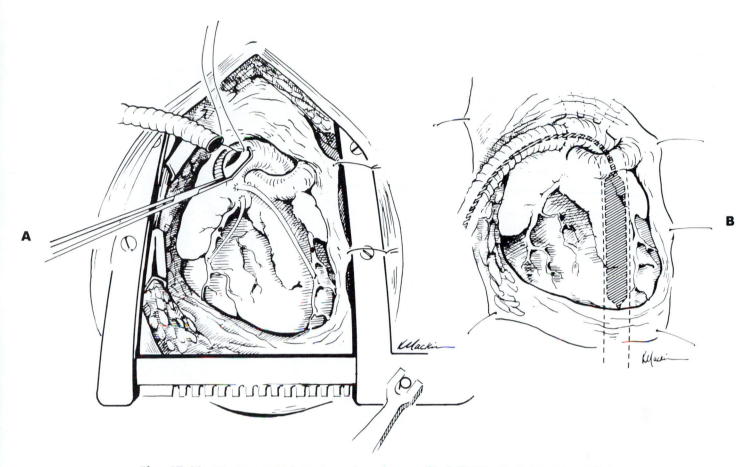

Fig. 17-11 Direct aortic insertion of an intraaortic balloon. **A,** A woven graft is anastomosed end-to-side to the ascending aorta. **B,** The balloon is inserted antegradely and positioned in the descending thoracic aorta. Heavy sutures are tied around the graft to close it around the balloon catheter for hemostasis. (From Quaal SJ: *Comprehensive intra-aortic balloon pumping,* St Louis, 1984, Mosby.)

The surgeon may place the balloon over the patient's chest to measure the distance from the left subclavian artery to the femoral artery entry site; a heavy silk tie may be used to mark the proximal end of the balloon where it would exit the femoral artery.

5. After the artery has been dilated, the balloon is inserted over the guidewire (Fig. 17-9, *C*) and advanced gradually until the guidewire is seen protruding from the proximal end of the balloon. (If excessive resistance is met, the balloon may have to be withdrawn.) The guidewire is removed, and the balloon is connected to the balloon pump. The pressure line coming off the balloon is connected to a transducer for blood pressure monitoring.

In the past, an introducer was usually inserted after dilatation, but the introducer may be omitted, with the balloon inserted directly over the guidewire in order to reduce the likelihood of compromising blood flow to the leg.

Complications. Complications of femoral insertion of IABP relate primarily to lower limb ischemia and thromboembolism, but sepsis and hemorrhage also pose risks. Aortic dissection and aortoiliac laceration or perforation have also been noted. To reduce the risk of complications, the balloon should be removed as quickly as possible to relieve leg ischemia. Thrombectomy and repair of the femoral artery may be required; in more severe cases of limb ischemia, fasciotomy or even amputation may be necessary (Frazier and Colon, 1988; Richenbacher and Pierce, 1991a). In patients with small femoral arteries, the end of an 8 mm Dacron graft can be anastomosed to the side of the femoral artery, with the balloon inserted through the graft into the artery. Heavy ties placed around the graft and balloon provide hemostasis. When the balloon is removed, the graft is trimmed and oversewn, and the incision is closed.

Direct ascending aorta insertion

When bilateral aortoiliac atherosclerotic disease prevents retrograde IABP insertion via the femoral artery, direct ascending aorta (or transverse arch) insertion may be considered (Fig. 17-11). The procedure requires application of a partial-occlusion clamp to the aorta and excision of a small portion of the aortic wall. A Dacron graft is anastomosed to the aortotomy, and the balloon is inserted antegradely through the graft into the artery. Because the prosthetic graft must first be anastomosed to the aorta, there is a time delay that may be poorly tolerated in a deteriorating patient. Moreover, placement of the graft may be difficult if the aorta is crowded with bypass grafts and the arterial infusion cannula. When the IABP is no longer needed, it is removed through the graft, which is then trimmed and oversewn (Bonchek and Olinger, 1981; Quaal, 1993).

Procedure

1. A partial-occlusion clamp is applied to the ascending aorta, and a segment of aorta is removed (Fig. 17-11, *A*).
2. An 8 or 10 mm Dacron graft is anastomosed end-to-side to the aortotomy.
3. As the partial-occlusion clamp is opened, the balloon is inserted into the aorta and threaded to the desired position in the descending thoracic aorta (Fig. 17-11, *B*).
4. Umbilical tapes are tied around the graft and the balloon.
5. The chest may be left partially open, with the incision covered with a sterile drape or dressing.
6. Removal of the IABP requires a return to the operating room, where the graft is trimmed and oversewn and the chest is closed in the routine manner (see Chapter 11).

Right ventricular intraaortic balloon pump

Direct insertion into the pulmonary artery for right ventricular support has also been used to promote pulmonary blood flow and decrease the right ventricular workload. Right ventricular failure may be due to perioperative MI, right coronary artery air embolism, right-sided volume overloading, and uneven myocardial protection producing ischemic injury. Biventricular failure may also be present (Holzum, 1990).

The procedure is similar to that for direct aortic insertion: a graft is anastomosed to the pulmonary artery, and the balloon is threaded through the graft and the artery (Fig. 17-12). Removal is similar to that for antegrade aortic IABP. Complications of direct aorta or PA insertion include vascular injury, air or thromboembolism, hemorrhage, and infection. It may not be possible to close the sternum without creating a mechanical tamponade (Richenbacher and Pierce, 1991a).

Hemopump Axial Flow Device

The Hemopump is another assist device that permits rapid placement and does not require an invasive, open chest surgical procedure for implantation (Fig. 17-13). Like other short-term cardiac support systems, its purpose is to rest the ventricle and allow it to recover by reducing preload, afterload, and ventricular wall stress, thereby decreasing myocardial oxygen con-

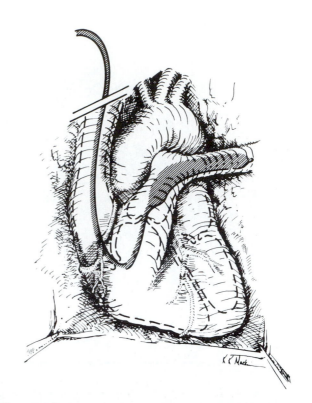

Fig. 17-12 Transvenous insertion of a pulmonary artery balloon. The balloon may also be inserted directly into the pulmonary artery via a graft anastomosed to the artery. (From Quaal SJ: *Comprehensive intra-aortic balloon pumping,* St Louis, 1984, Mosby.)

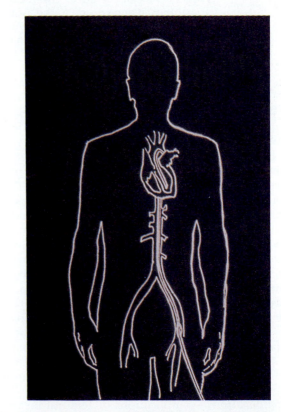

Fig. 17-13 Position of the Hemopump in the chest. (Courtesy Johnson & Johnson Interventional Systems Co., Warren, N.J.)

The cannula/pump assembly is inserted via the femoral artery and threaded retrogradely up the aorta, through the aortic valve, and into the apex of the left ventricle (Fig. 17-14). The device uses a rotating pump based on axial flow technology. The rotating portion of the pump turns at a high speed of up to 25,000 revolutions per minute (rpm) inside a tightly fitting metal container. Blood is drawn from the left ventricle through the distal silicone cannula to the pump, where it is propelled into the systemic circulation. The nonrotating part of the pump helps decrease the rotating of blood (reducing hemolysis) as it exits the device and maintains unidirectional blood flow (Fig. 17-15). The pump is connected to the sheath/drive cable, which is inserted into a motor magnet powered by the console. When the console is activated, it creates an alternating magnetic field within the motor, which turns the magnet and causes the pump blades to rotate. A pressure-controlled purge fluid system provides lubrication to the moving parts within the pump. Continuous, nonpulsatile blood flows of 0.5 to 3.0 L/min can be achieved (Rountree and others, 1993).

Severe aortic, iliac, or femoral vascular disease may prohibit insertion of the device and is the most common reason for failed insertion. Intraoperatively, alternate insertion routes, such as the ascending aorta, can be used.

Operative procedure: insertion of the Hemopump

1. The right or left femoral artery is exposed, and the patient is anticoagulated with heparin.
2. A 12 mm woven Dacron graft is anastomosed end-to-side to the artery.
3. The Hemopump is inserted through the graft into the artery.
4. The pump is advanced retrogradely up the aorta, across the aortic valve, and into the left ventricle. The distal tip of the cannula is positioned near the left ventricular apex, and the pump housing is sit-

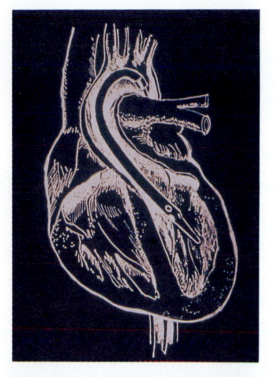

Fig. 17-14 Position of the Hemopump in the left ventricle. Blood is drawn from the ventricle and pumped into the aorta. (Courtesy Johnson & Johnson Interventional Systems Co., Warren, N.J.)

sumption. The device is indicated mainly in patients who cannot be weaned from CPB or who have sustained an MI. It is not indicated as a bridge to transplantation in the United States. Exclusion criteria are related to the transvalvular placement of the device within the left ventricle. These include the presence of a prosthetic aortic valve and severe aortic valve disease; other contraindications are aortic wall disease and thoracic or abdominal aortic aneurysm or dissection (Rountree and others, 1993).

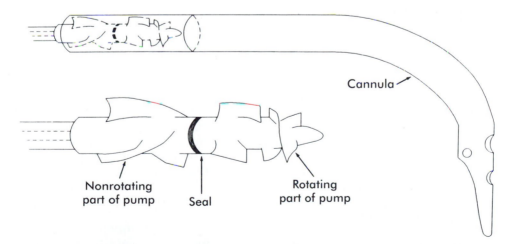

Nonrotating part of pump   Seal   Rotating part of pump   Cannula

Fig. 17-15 Hemopump cannula/pump assembly. The pump is contained within the cannula. (From Quaal SJ: *Cardiac mechanical assistance beyond balloon pumping,* St Louis, 1993, Mosby.)

uated in the descending thoracic aorta. Often this is done under fluoroscopy, but if this is unfeasible (and the chest is open), placement can be verified by palpation.

5. Hemostasis is achieved with the use of silicone plugs placed around the drive shaft and secured inside the graft. The pump is connected to the motor and console.

6. The patient can be transported to the surgical intensive care unit with the device in place; batteries can each provide 30 minutes of power, and the console can be rolled on a stand or mounted on the patient's bed.

Complications. Complications include vascular or valvular injury, thrombosis, hemolysis, dysrhythmias, bleeding, infection, cardiac injury, failure to wean the patient from the device, and death. Causes of death in patients with the Hemopump are usually irreversible left ventricular failure, multisystem organ failure, and biventricular failure (Rountree and others, 1993).

VENTRICULAR ASSIST DEVICES

More aggressive and sophisticated forms of circulatory assistance are being considered in medical patients with acute MI (Barron, 1989) and in surgical patients whose cardiac function undergoes severe deterioration after termination of CPB despite maximal drug therapy with inotropic agents and vasodilators, and the IABP. Unlike the IABP and Hemopump, which provide pressure assistance to the failing heart by reducing afterload and augmenting existing coronary and systemic circulation, VADs provide volume assistance to the heart by greater decompression of the ventricle and diversion of blood flow from the native ventricle to the artificial pump, which maintains the circulation (Quaal, 1992). Another important difference is that the VAD can function independently of the heart, whereas the IABP and Hemopump can only augment (not replace) existing ventricular function.

The two primary objectives of mechanical assistance are to decrease the workload of the right and/or left ventricle and restore adequate organ perfusion. Determination of VAD placement depends on which side of the heart is affected. Most often VADs are used to support the left ventricle (LVAD), but they may be used for the right ventricle (RVAD) or both pumping chambers (BiVAD).

By taking over cardiac function, VADs enable the heart to rest and recover from reversible injuries. When end-stage cardiomyopathy or irreversible injury preclude recovery, VADs can maintain adequate body perfusion and forestall multisystem organ failure until a donor heart becomes available for transplantation. Although a VAD can support the circulation independently of ventricular function, it cannot replace pulmonary function, which would require an oxygenator to take over the function of the lungs. Patients with cardiac and pulmonary disease may require heart-lung transplantation (see Chapter 18). ECMO (see Chapter 11) has been used when there is a need

---

Box 17-4 Criteria for mechanical circulatory support*

Cardiac index	<2 L/min/m^2
Systolic blood pressure	<90 mm Hg
Left or right atrial pressure	>20 mm Hg
Urinary output	<20 ml/hr (adults)
Systemic vascular resistance	>2100 dynes · sec/cm^{-5}

Exclude patient if:
  Blood urea nitrogen (BUN) >100 mg/dl
  Serum creatinine >5.0 mg/dl
  Chronic lung disease
  Chronic liver disease
  Metastatic cancer
  Sepsis
  Neurologic deficit
  Technically unsatisfactory cardiac operative procedure
  Age >60 years (if bridge to transplant); this may vary

Modified from Richenbacher WE, Pierce WS: Management of complications of mechanical circulatory assistance. In Waldhausen JA, Orringer MB: *Complications of cardiothoracic surgery*, St Louis, 1991, Mosby.

*Criteria may be altered for bridge-to-transplantation candidates depending on the patient's status and the surgeon's judgment.

---

for rapid institution of cardiac and pulmonary support; a thoracic incision is not required (Reedy and others, 1990).

Patient Selection

Patients considered candidates for VADs are usually in one of the following categories (Ley and Hill, 1993; Shiono and others, 1993):

1. Cardiac surgery patients who cannot be weaned from CPB or who have low cardiac output syndrome after surgery
2. Patients who develop cardiogenic shock following MI
3. Patients with end-stage cardiomyopathy awaiting cardiac transplantation

Although similar hemodynamic criteria have been used for all three groups of patients (Box 17-4), they may no longer be directly applicable to bridge-to-transplantation candidates, because myocardial recovery is not anticipated. With a VAD, these patients may be relatively stable, and the goal is maintenance of organ function (versus myocardial recovery) while a donor heart is located. Ironically, hemodynamic stability is often a transplant rejection criterion. Without a VAD, complications (e.g., renal failure, sepsis) can develop that eventually preclude transplantation. Pennington and Swartz (1992) suggest inserting a more sophisticated device to provide a sufficient cardiac output when pharmacologic, respiratory, and

---

Box 17-5 *Exclusion criteria for circulatory support before cardiac transplantation*

Unresolved pulmonary emboli
Chronic renal failure requiring dialysis
Cancer with metastasis
Severe hepatic disease
Irreversible cerebrovascular accident
Unacceptable psychosocial history
Severe bleeding

Modified from Pennington DG, Swartz MT: Assisted circulation and mechanical hearts. In Braunwald E: *Heart disease,* ed 4, Philadelphia, 1991, WB Saunders; and Ruzevich SA, Swartz MT, Pennington DG: Nursing care of the patient with pneumatic ventricular assist device, *Heart Lung* 17(4):399, 1988.

Box 17-6 *Comments on implantation of a ventricular assist device*

O.H. Frazier, MD
Texas Heart Institute
Houston, Texas

For an optimal surgical implant of a ventricular assist device, a knowledgeable team is of the utmost importance. All team members need to be thoroughly informed about the many aspects of the device that is going to be used, such as:

  Indications for use
  Method of insertion
  Proper setup and initiation

  Any time a ventricular assist device is required, it is of an emergent nature, whether the device is approved for general use or is investigational. The physician, OR nurses, and circulatory support team must be able to work quickly and expertly together. Frequently there is little time to "run" for needed supplies.

  A checklist has proved to be beneficial to our team and is used during most implants. From a prepared list, a variety of sutures and equipment are maintained in the operating room to help eliminate any guesswork. For investigational devices, a preimplant checklist is available to ensure adherence to the investigative protocol. The foremost concern to the surgeon is having a well-educated team, working together, to achieve one goal—a good implant—in order to ensure the best possible outcome for the LVAD patient.

IABP support cannot be reduced within 24 to 48 hours. Patients can then receive oral medications, improve their nutritional status, and begin ambulation and muscle-strengthening exercises that offer the potential for rehabilitation and increase the potential for successful transplant outcomes.

Unstable patients requiring immediate mechanical assistance are at even higher risk for developing complications that could exclude them from consideration for transplantation (Box 17-5). Patients do not necessarily have to meet all transplant criteria; acute renal failure and hypoxia that can be reversed should not automatically preclude transplantation (Pennington and Swartz, 1992). When selected to receive a VAD as a bridge to transplantation, patients should have none of the standard contraindications to cardiac transplantation (e.g., severe systemic infection, malignancy, irreversible organ failure) (Vaska, 1991).

Procedural Considerations

In patients who cannot be weaned from CPB, bypass is often reinstituted, with the patient maintained on full bypass for approximately 30 minutes to "rest" the ventricle. During this period surgical team members can assemble necessary VAD supplies and equipment, manage correctable biochemical and hematologic abnormalities, minimize hypothermia, and control dysrhythmias (Golding and others, 1992). Prolonged attempts to wean the patient from CPB are no longer recommended because of the increased risk of aggravating the patient's hemodynamic status. Early institution of mechanical support is favored to avoid further injury both to the myocardium and to major organ systems.

Types of Ventricular Assist Devices

Each type of VAD has its own specific structural characteristics and performance requirements. Perioperative nurses must be familiar with the indications for the device, preparation of its component parts, inser-

tion, and function (Box 17-6). In addition to the regular members of the cardiac team, biomedical engineers are an important resource to ensure that the device functions appropriately.

External Centrifugal and Roller Pumps

Centrifugal pumps (see Chapter 5) are constructed from three smooth rotating blades that are mounted in a cone-shaped housing that is sealed at the bottom with a magnet. The magnet on the cone is connected to a magnet on the console motor. When the motor is activated, the motor magnet and the attached cone magnet revolve, rotating the blades and creating centrifugal force inside the cone. This centrifugal force creates a vortex and supplies kinetic energy to the spinning blood within the lower portion of the cone. Cardiac output is regulated by the number of blade revolutions per minute.

Advantages of the centrifugal pump include widespread availability, relatively low cost, and ease of insertion. Additional advantages include the transference of high volumes of energy at low pressures (thus decreasing blood trauma), reduction of the possibility of air embolus (because air rises to the top of the cone, where it is trapped), and minimal risk of creating excessive outflow pressure (which could lead to disruption of the circuit) (Barden and Lee, 1990).

Another advantage of centrifugal pumps is that they can be used to treat children with postcardiotomy cardiogenic shock. Most other assist devices have limited use because of size constraints. Also, ECMO may not always be feasible because of the intensive labor required and the complications associated with long-term support (Scheinin and others, 1993).

Disadvantages include the need for moderate levels of systemic heparinization when the pump is running at low flow rates and an appreciable degree of hemolysis (although less significant than that seen with roller pumps) (Marchetta and Stennis, 1988). Like roller pumps, centrifugal devices provide nonpulsatile (continuous) flow, which is nonphysiologic (although controversy continues about the relative advantages and disadvantages of pulsatile versus nonpulsatile flow). IABP has been used in conjunction with these devices in an attempt to provide a pulse wave. Two other factors are worth mentioning: one is that frequently the sternum cannot be closed (increasing the risk of infection), and the other is that the patient must remain immobile (with the attendant risks associated with immobility, such as pressure sores, venous stasis, and atelectasis).

Roller pumps, once one of the few assist devices available (Litwak and others, 1976), are used less often for mechanical assistance, primarily because of bleeding from anticoagulation, blood cell injury, and the same disadvantages attributed to centrifugal pumps. Air embolus presents a constant danger, and disconnections between sections of the bypass circuit pose additional risk because of the high pressures that can be generated.

Cannulation techniques for centrifugal and roller pumps are similar. CPB is not necessary, but a sternotomy (or thoracotomy) is required for insertion. Portable roller pumps are used.

Prior to cannulation the surgeon determines whether a patent foramen ovale (or atrial septal defect) exists. Because such a defect could produce interatrial shunting with adverse hemodynamic consequences, the defect is closed primarily or repaired with a patch.

For left ventricular support, a drainage cannula is placed in the left atrium, and the inflow cannula is positioned in the ascending aorta. Right ventricular support is achieved by cannulating the right atrium (outflow) and the pulmonary artery (inflow). When biventricular support is indicated, both right and left ventricular circuits are established.

Operative procedures: cannulation for a centrifugal or roller pump assist device (Joyce, Toninato, and Hansen, 1993; Rose and others, 1993).

Left ventricular support

1. Double concentric pursestring sutures are placed in the left atrium or the atrial appendage (or the right superior pulmonary vein) for outflow and in the ascending aorta for inflow. Teflon pledgets

may be used to buttress the tissue against the cannulas.
2. The atrial appendage is excised, a venous cannula is inserted into the atrium, and the pursestring is tightened.
3. A stab wound is made in the ascending aorta (with or without a partial-occlusion clamp), an arterial cannula is placed in the aorta, and the tourniquet is tightened.
4. Cannulas are connected to tubing that exits through the sternotomy incision or through separate subxiphoid stab wound incisions. As with any arterial cannula-to-tubing connection, precautions are taken to prevent the entry of air into the circuit.
5. The cannulas and tubing are connected to a portable pump, and flow rates are established. Inotropic agents may be used to augment right-sided heart function, and IABP is used for counterpulsation. Hemostasis may be enhanced with the use of fibrin glue around the cannulation exit wounds.
6. The chest is closed cautiously to avoid cardiac compression; in cases where cardiac compression occurs, the skin only is closed. Occasionally the skin cannot be approximated, so the sternal wound is covered with a sterile drape or synthetic material (Rose and others, 1993).

Right ventricular support

Insertion techniques, anticoagulation, and chest closure are similar to those techniques for left ventricular support. The right atrial appendage or the right ventricular apex is cannulated for outflow, and the pulmonary artery is cannulated for inflow.

Postoperative care

Postoperatively, hemodynamic status is monitored, along with renal, pulmonary, and neurologic function. Potential complications include bleeding, renal failure, biventricular failure (after implantation of a univentricular device), low cardiac output, and malfunction of one or more components of the system. Signs and symptoms of hemodynamic deterioration and organ dysfunction are evaluated to determine whether they are due to primary cardiac failure or to hemorrhage or embolism (from air or particulate matter). Patients may be sedated to a greater or lesser degree, but periodically they are allowed to awaken so that their neurologic status can be evaluated (Joyce, Toninato, and Hansen, 1993). Emotional support of the patient and family is important to provide reassurance and to lessen many of the fears and anxieties associated with mechanical assistance.

External Pulsatile Ventricular Assist Devices

Although centrifugal devices have a number of advantages, their disadvantages limit their use in long-term situations, especially in bridge-to-transplantation candidates, who may have to wait weeks or months before a donor heart becomes available. External and internal pulsatile VADs can overcome many of the limitations, making them useful in patients with postcardiotomy shock or end-stage cardiomyopathy (Farrar and others, 1988). Pulsatile flow may result in improved kidney perfusion, decreased peripheral vascular resistance, and enhanced systemic circulation (Barden and Lee, 1990). Other advantages of these VADs are that mobility is less restricted, cardiac output can be adjusted depending on the degree of native cardiac function, and high levels of anticoagulation are not required at normal flow rates.

The pumps are implanted through a median sternotomy incision with the patient under general anesthesia. The devices can provide univentricular or biventricular assistance (BiVAD) for intermediate or long-term support. Although insertion of an LVAD could be performed through a left lateral thoracotomy, this incision is not recommended, because it would limit access to the right ventricle should it fail intraoperatively (and require an RVAD). CPB may not be necessary if the patient is relatively stable and the left ventricle is not going to be cannulated, but CPB should be immediately available. Left ventricular apical cannulation requires a ventriculotomy, necessitating CPB to maintain cardiac output and organ perfusion during insertion of the device. However, the left ventricular apex may be preferred for transplant candidates because apical cannulation provides the largest and most complete pump filling, and because loss of the apex is of less concern in these patients (Ley and Hill, 1993).

Cannulation is similar to that for centrifugal pumps: RVADs cannulate the right atrium and pulmonary artery; LVADs cannulate the left atrium (or left ventricular apex) and the ascending aorta. Typical components of VAD systems are listed in Box 17-7. It is important to remember that when referring to inflow and outflow portions of VAD systems, **inflow** refers to the cannula or conduit bringing blood to the pump, and **outflow** refers to the cannula or conduit ejecting blood from the pump to the body.

Nursing considerations

In addition to being familiar with the technical details of the device and its insertion, the perioperative nurse is responsible for constant assessment of the patient during the perioperative period. Changes in the patient's status may occur suddenly, and thorough preparation prior to the patient's entry into the OR will allow the nurse to focus attention on the patient's needs. When possible, joint meetings between nurses, surgeons, and other members of the surgical team before the operation can reduce uncertainty and confusion, and promote an efficient and successful procedure.

When a device must be inserted on an urgent basis, there may be little time for a preoperative interview, but touching and talking to the patient who has just arrived in the OR can allay some of the fear and anxiety. Families are especially concerned, and an established communication system between designated

---

Box 17-7 *Components of ventricular assist devices*

Cannulas—provide channel between native heart and mechanical pump
 Inflow cannula—cannula bringing blood to VAD pump from body
 Outflow cannula—cannula sending blood out of VAD pump to body
Pump—mechanical ventricle; blood-ejecting device; may be internal or external. Composed of:
 Housing—outer covering of device
 Blood sac—inner chamber into which blood enters and out of which blood is ejected; may be a very smooth lining (e.g., Thoratec, Novacor) or a textured lining (e.g., TCI HeartMate)
 Inflow and outflow valves—maintain unidirectional blood flow; situated at entrance and exit of blood sac, respectively; valves may be mechanical (Thoratec), biologic (Novacor), or constructed from polyurethane (Abiomed)
 Air vent—allows air between housing and blood sac to be removed during device diastole so that blood sac can refill with blood
Drive cable—connects pump to control console; contains monitoring sensing leads, and activating leads
Control console—external device that controls mode of operation; senses level of blood in pump and signals pump to eject; different operating modes include:
 Fixed-rate—nonsynchronized to native heart; commonly used during initiation and weaning of device
 Fill-to-empty—volume mode; asynchronous to heart; blood sac empties as soon as it is full; ejecttion rate depends on blood return to heart from opposite ventricle (preload)
 ECG synchronization—synchronizes VAD to natural heart by detecting R waves of QRS complex; allows VAD ejection to be delayed in order to provide diastolic augmentation
 Manual mode—used in case of power failure and for initial institution of VAD support; may be used to deair pump and to evaluate system function

Modified from Ruzevich SA, Swartz MT, Pennington DG: Nursing care of the patient with pneumatic ventricular assist device, *Heart Lung* 17(4):399, 1988; and Barden C, Lee R: *Update on ventricular assist devices, AACN Clin Issues Crit Care Nurs* 1(1):13, 1990.

---

clinical staff and waiting friends and family members is effective in modifying some of the emotional stress.

Because patients may be debilitated, special caution should be taken to pad dependent areas of the body, as well as hands, elbows, and feet. The patient is at risk for a cardiac arrest during the period of anesthesia induction (May and Adams, 1987), and the nurse should be prepared to institute resuscitative measures quickly. Femoral vein–femoral artery cannulation may be necessary in an emergency, but usually aortocaval (or femoral-caval) CPB is instituted. Table 17-

Table 17-3 ■ *Standards of nursing care for ventricular assist devices*

Nursing diagnosis	Patient outcome	Nursing actions
Powerlessness related to dependence on mechanical device, uncertainty about prognosis, and outcome of treatment	Patient and family understand purpose of treatment and expected outcome so that sense of powerlessness is reduced and coping abilities are enhanced	Discuss questions and concerns about disease and need for cardiac support Identify fears and address specific concerns Allow family interaction with patient to degree possible Address patient/family concerns about critical nature of patient's status/prognosis Keep family informed about patient's status; report changes in condition Support feelings of partnership with health care team
Knowledge deficit about disease, use of VAD, planned surgery, and perioperative events	Patient demonstrates knowledge about physiologic and psychologic responses to disease and VAD	Determine patient's understanding of cardiac disease, need for and purpose of VAD (e.g., bridge to transplantation) Encourage patient and family to ask questions about VAD (right and/or left); explain/teach to patient's and family's level of understanding Determine understanding of VAD complications: stroke, infection, hemorrhage; clarify misconceptions
High risk for infection related to multiple wounds, compromised cardiac function	Patient is free of infection	Prepare VAD components with strict aseptic technique Report deviations in laboratory values (e.g., white blood count) Control room traffic; have necessary supplies and equipment collected in one area Dress all wounds; if sternum is left open, cover incision with sterile dressing; skin and subcutaneous tissue only may be closed
High risk for injury related to: Positioning	Patient is free of injury related to: Positioning	When moving patient, use caution to avoid disrupting lines, cables, cannulas, etc. Avoid bending leg in patient with femoral artery cannula (e.g., IABP)
Physical hazards	Physical hazards	Have available VAD(s), lines, cannulas, connectors, graft material, wrenches, extra vascular clamps, and other implantation supplies; have backup supplies and equipment; avoid scratching or otherwise injuring VAD and VAD components Be familiar with type of VAD (e.g., centrifugal, roller pump, pneumatic, etc.), and how inserted Have VAD drive system in OR; ensure it is functioning properly; have backup power source immediately available Ensure that all connections are tight; avoid kinking of lines Have defibrillator immediately available in anticipation of cardiac arrest Have cannulation supplies appropriate for inflow and outflow sites (e.g., LV apex, aorta, left or right atrium) Prepare prosthetic valve components per manufacturer's instructions (if applicable) Assist with deairing measures to reduce risk of air embolus Ensure that cannula(s) are connected to drive system/power source appropriately Anticipate insertion of hemodialysis catheter, left atrial line; have necessary supplies available Anticipate heparin reversal (in VADs not needing heparinization at standard flow rates); patient may be placed on antiplatelet therapy or heparin therapy depending on type of VAD and physician preference Plan postoperative transport route to minimize delay; ensure transport power source is working (if battery used, ensure it is fully charged before transport)
Electrical hazards	Electrical hazards	Confirm that drive system is working; have backup Avoid contact between VAD and defibrillator paddles, cautery, and pacing wires

Modified from Seifert PC: Cardiac surgery. In Rothrock JC: *Perioperative nursing care planning,* St Louis, 1990, Mosby.

Table 17-3 ■ *Standards of nursing care for ventricular assist devices—cont'd*

Nursing diagnosis	Patient outcome	Nursing actions
High risk for injury related to—cont'd: Foreign objects	Patient is free of injury related to—cont'd: Foreign objects	Account for additional instruments and supplies associated with VAD insertion: wrenches, connectors, etc.; if covers are placed over VAD pump openings to prevent air from entering pump, account for these as well
High risk for altered fluid and electrolyte imbalance	Fluid and electrolyte balance is maintained	Prepare for insertion of hemodialysis catheter (patients often have high potassium levels) Ensure that inotropic drugs are available (per medical order) Check connections and rest of VAD system for bleeding; have hemostatic agents available; avoid puncturing graft components or injuring prosthetic valves Observe chest tubes for excessive drainage; be prepared for mediastinal exploration for excess bleeding

3 lists additional nursing considerations applicable to most patients requiring mechanical assist devices.

Thoratec ventricular assist device

The Thoratec VAD (formerly called the Pierce-Donachy VAD) consists of cannulas connected to a rigid housing that consists of inner and outer compartments separated by a flexible diaphragm (Fig. 17-16). The pumps are powered by compressed air (pneumatic pump), which alternately compress and empty the blood sac to achieve pulsatile flow. Prosthetic (mechanical) valves are incorporated into the inflow and outflow portions of the pump to maintain unidirectional blood flow (Ruzevich, Swartz, and Pennington, 1988). During the filling phase, blood flows from the heart, through the inflow cannula and valve, and into the inner compartment (which is lined with a very smooth polymer to reduce thrombus formation). Pressurized air (between the inner and outer compartment) causes the diaphragm to push against the inner compartment, ejecting blood in pulse waves through the outflow valve and cannula and into the aorta (LVAD) or pulmonary artery (RVAD).

Operative procedure: insertion of an external pulsatile ventricular assist device *(Ley and Hill, 1993; Waldhausen and Pierce, 1985)*

1. After a median sternotomy, the surgeon palpates the atrial septum to ensure closure of the foramen ovale (which, if patent, could cause right-to-left shunting with arterial blood desaturation). If there is an interatrial defect, it is closed with the patient on CPB.
2. In preparation for placement of the inflow and outflow cannulas, tunnels are created from the pericardial space to the skin, just below the costal margin (Fig. 17-17).
3. **LVAD: atrial cannulation:**
   a. The left atrial appendage is exposed by lifting the left ventricular apex and retracting it to the right. (If the right superior pulmonary vein or the left atrial dome is to be cannulated, exposure is achieved by retracting the heart to the left; left ventricular apical cannulation requires elevation of the apex as described in the subsequent section on the TCI HeartMate.)
   b. Double concentric pursestring sutures are placed at the base of the appendage; pledgets may be placed at the beginning and end of each pursestring. The needles are removed, and a tourniquet is applied to each suture.

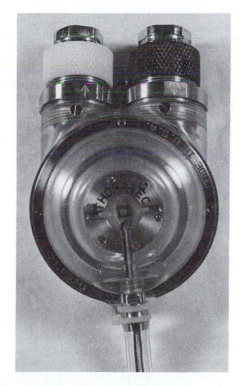

Fig. 17-16 Thoratec ventricular assist device. (Courtesy Thoratec Laboratories Corp., Berkeley, Calif.)

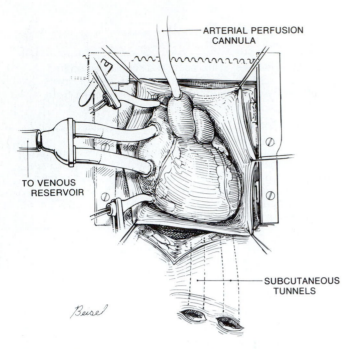

Fig. 17-17 Creation of subcutaneous tunnels for VAD cannulas; the patient is cannulated for CPB. (From Waldhausen JA, Pierce WS: *Johnson's surgery of the chest*, ed 5, St Louis, 1985, Mosby.)

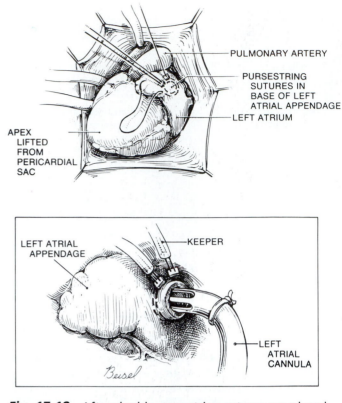

Fig. 17-18 After double pursestring sutures are placed at the base of the left atrial appendage, the atrial cannulas are inserted. (From Waldhausen JA, Pierce WS: *Johnson's surgery of the chest*, ed 5, St Louis, 1985, Mosby.)

   c. The left atrial appendage is incised, and the atrial cannula is inserted (Fig. 17-18). The tourniquet is tightened around the cannula and secured. In addition, a ligature is tied around each tourniquet and cannula.

   d. The cannula is filled with saline and clamped to prevent loss of fluid and the introduction of air into the atrium.

   e. The cannula is passed through the tunnel and brought out through the subcostal incision. The cannula is allowed to fill with atrial blood and is reclamped where it exits the skin (Fig. 17-19). (Or it may be attached to the suction line of the bypass circuit.)

Aortic cannulation:

   f. A partial-occlusion clamp is placed on the ascending aorta, and a small segment of aorta is excised. The Dacron graft end of the arterial cannula is anastomosed to the aortotomy (Fig. 17-20). The cannula is filled with saline, clamped, and tunneled to the medial subcostal incision.

   g. The cannulas are attached to the pump after deairing has been completed (Fig. 17-21). The system is checked, and pumping is initiated.

4. **RVAD** (Fig. 17-22):

Tunnels are prepared as described in step 2.

Atrial cannulation: The right arium is cannulated in a manner similar to step 3, a through e.

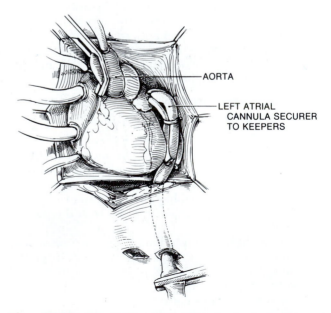

Fig. 17-19 The left atrial cannula is brought out through the subcostal skin incision. (From Waldhausen JA, Pierce WS: *Johnson's surgery of the chest*, ed 5, St Louis, 1985, Mosby.)

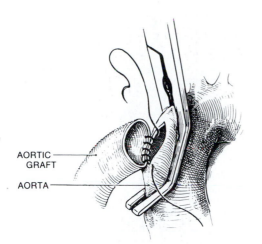

AORTIC
GRAFT

AORTA

Fig. 17-20   **Anastomosis of the graft to the aorta.** (From Waldhausen JA, Pierce WS: *Johnson's surgery of the chest,* ed 5, St Louis, 1985, Mosby.)

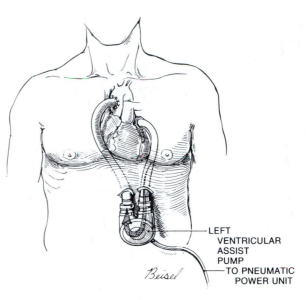

LEFT
VENTRICULAR
ASSIST
PUMP

TO PNEUMATIC
POWER UNIT

Beisel

Fig. 17-21   **Pump attached to cannulas for left ventricular support. The chest has been closed.** (From Waldhausen JA, Pierce WS: *Johnson's surgery of the chest,* ed 5, St Louis, 1985, Mosby.)

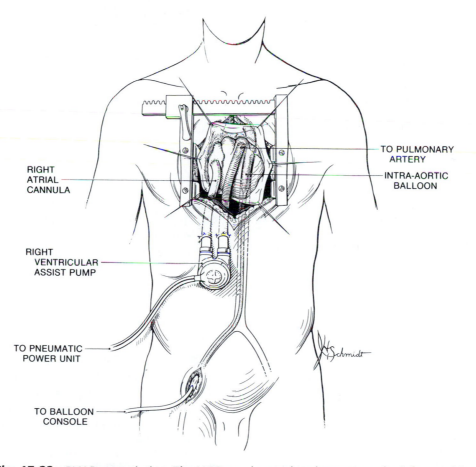

TO PULMONARY
ARTERY

INTRA-AORTIC
BALLOON

RIGHT
ATRIAL
CANNULA

RIGHT
VENTRICULAR
ASSIST PUMP

TO PNEUMATIC
POWER UNIT

TO BALLOON
CONSOLE

Fig. 17-22   **RVAD cannulation. The IABP may be used to decompress the left ventricle and to augment coronary perfusion.** (From Waldhausen JA, Pierce WS: *Johnson's surgery of the chest,* ed 5, St Louis, 1985, Mosby.)

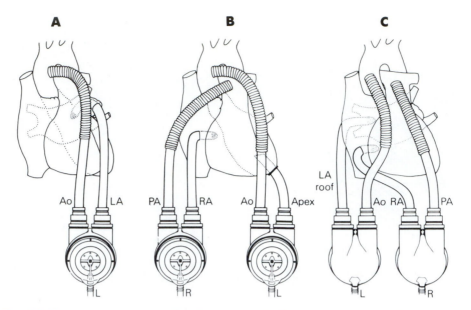

A **B** **C**

Fig. 17-23 **A,** Univentricular (LVAD) support. **B,** Biventricular support (with left ventricular apical cannulation for LVAD inflow to the pump). **C,** Biventricular support (with left atrial roof cannulation for LVAD inflow to the pump). (From Farrar DJ and others: Heterotopic prosthetic ventricles as a bridge to cardiac transplantation: a multicenter study in 29 patients, *N Engl J Med* 318[6]:333, 1988.)

Pulmonary artery cannulation: The pulmonary atery is cannulated in a manner similar to step 3, f. IABP may be used to reduce left atrial pressure and to augment coronary blood flow.

5. **BiVAD**
   Both right and left VADs are inserted. Either the left atrium (left atrial "roof") or the left ventricular apex may be cannulated for LVAD drainage into the pump (Fig. 17-23).
6. CPB is discontinued, and hemostasis is achieved. The chest is closed in the routine manner. Occasionally only subcutaneous tissue and skin are closed (May and Adams, 1987).

Removal of the device

1. The patient is returned to the OR, and the sternotomy is reopened.
2. VAD pumping is discontinued, and the cannulas are clamped.
3. The atrial cannula(s) is removed, and the purse-string sutures are tied.
4. The arterial cannula(s) graft is clamped close to the anastomosis and divided, and the stump is oversewn.
5. The cannulas are removed, and the pericardial ends of the cannula tunnels are oversewn. Chest tubes are inserted, and the sternum is closed.

If the patient is to undergo cardiac transplantation, the donor heart is implanted at this time (see Chapter 18).

Postoperative considerations

Postoperative cardiac arrest can occur; external chest compressions are avoided because they can dislodge the cannulas and otherwise damage cardiac structures.

Treatment consists of pharmacologic and electrical (defibrillation) interventions. Patients who are fibrillating can maintain hemodynamic stability when biventricular support devices are in place.

All VADs are also subject to potential malfunction necessitating replacement of the device. Severe hemolysis, sac rupture, destruction of the outer pump casing, and cannula obstruction have been some of the reasons for replacement. The discussion that follows describes one method for replacing paracorporeal VADs (Lohmann and others, 1992).

The patient is returned to the OR, and general anesthesia is induced. Intravascular lines are inserted for drug infusion and blood pressure monitoring. Antibacterial solution is applied to all exposed VAD structures; all VAD surfaces should be considered contaminated, and they should be separated from the rest of the field as much as possible. Inotropic drugs may be necessary to maintain the circulation; if cardiac function is inadequate to perfuse the body, femoral vein–femoral artery CPB is instituted before the VAD is halted. The exchange procedure can be performed in approximately 30 minutes (Lohmann and others, 1992).

Operative procedure: replacement of a paracorporeal ventricular assist device
(Lohmann and others, 1992).

1. After hemodynamic stability has been achieved, the VAD is halted, and inflow and outflow cannulas are clamped.
2. The old VAD is removed.
3. The new VAD is connected to the VAD inflow cannula. The cannula is slowly unclamped, and the sac is allowed to fill with blood. When the sac is

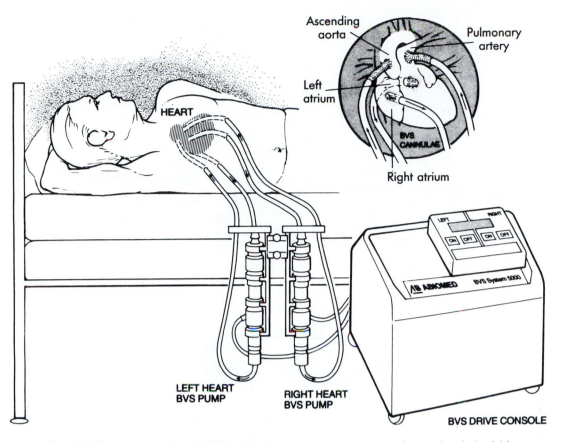

Fig. 17-24 Abiomed BVS 5000 console and blood pumps at the patient's bedside. The inset shows placement of the cannulas. (Courtesy Abiomed, Inc., Danvers, Mass.)

nearly filled with blood and air is evacuated, the inflow cannula is reclamped.

4. The VAD is then partially connected to the VAD outflow cannula. Heparinized normal saline is dripped onto the connection while the outflow cannula is joined to the VAD so that no air remains within the system. The VAD is inspected to ensure that no air remains; the connections are tightened, and VAD function is resumed.

Abiomed BVS 5000 system (external blood pump)

Another external pulsatile device is the Abiomed BVS 5000 system (Fig. 17-24), which can be used for single or biventricular assistance to support patients with postcardiotomy failure (Dixon, Farris, and Jett, 1993; Kaan and others, 1991), or as a bridge to transplantation (Champsaur and others, 1990). The device is disposable, in contrast to most other prosthetic ventricles. It is also the first cardiac assist device to receive Food and Drug Administration (FDA) approval for biventricular support of postcardiotomy heart failure patients (HLB Newsletter, 1992). A disadvantage of the device is that patient mobility is somewhat restricted.

Right atrial–to–pulmonary artery cannulation and left atrial–to–ascending aorta cannulation are used for RVADs and LVADs, respectively. Cannulas and insertion techniques are similar to those in the Thoratec system; femoral vein–femoral artery bypass may be used during device insertion. The distal end of the outflow cannulas have an attached Dacron graft that is anastomosed to the pulmonary artery and/or aorta. Inflow cannulas are inserted directly into the right or left atrium. Trileaflet polyurethane valves are used to maintain unidirectional blood flow (Dixon and others, 1993). The blood pump is composed of two seamless chambers made of polyurethane. The upper chamber is a reservoir that fills passively (like the native atrium). The lower (pumping) chamber contains inflow and outflow valves. When the lower chamber is full, the control console collapses it with a pulse of positive-pressure compressed air (Jett, 1991).

Blood drains by gravity from either atrium into the external blood pumps, which are positioned below the level of the patient's atria (Fig. 17-24). This passive filling prevents the atria from collapsing around the cannulas and minimizes hemolysis from blood trauma. It also prevents air from being suctioned into the system (Dixon and others, 1993). Drainage cannulas must be inserted in a manner that avoids impedance to device filling or obstruction of blood drainage.

Device-related complications are rare and are primarily related to bleeding. The system can be oper-

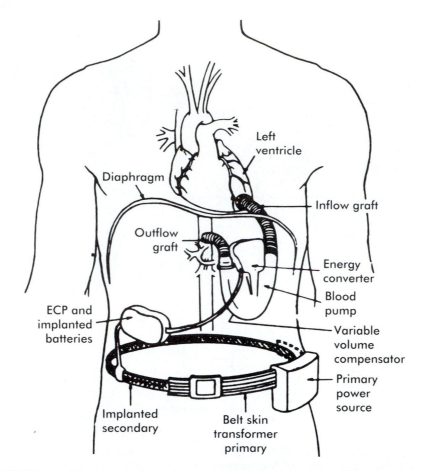

Fig. 17-25 Novacor ventricular assist system (LVAS). A completely implantable version of the Novacor LVAS is shown. The outflow graft is anastomosed to the abdominal aorta rather than to the ascending aorta, as has been frequently done. *ECP,* Electronic control and power unit. (Courtesy Novacor Div., Baxter Healthcare Corp., Oakland, Calif.)

ated by nurses in the critical care unit. Proper function is dependent not only on proper cannula insertion intraoperatively, but also on adequate volume status and appropriate pump height. If the pump is too high, atrial drainage will be inadequate; if it is too low, there will be prolonged filling of the pump, and the heart can become distended (Dixon and others, 1993).

Implantable Left Ventricular Assist Systems

Implantable left ventricular assist systems are investigational devices that represent an important step forward for patients with end-stage cardiac disease because they have the potential for becoming permanent prostheses (Dasse and others, 1992). Although they have been used both for postcardiotomy failure and as a bridge to transplantation, they are less suited for postcardiotomy failure because patients frequently have biventricular failure and the device is designed only for left ventricular support. Another consideration is that implantation requires excision of a portion

of the left ventricular apex, which can hinder left ventricular function on removal of the device and repair of the left ventricular apex. Thus current models are indicated as a bridge to transplantation (Frazier and others, 1992; Shinn and Oyer, 1993).

A major disadvantage of all LVADs is that they require reasonable right ventricular function. Severe right-sided heart failure will lead to inadequate filling of the left side of the heart, and the low preload precludes adequate inflow into the LVAD (Smith, Braunwald, and Kelly, 1992).

Two of these systems—the **Novacor LVAS** (Fig. 17-25) and the Thermo Cardiosystems, Inc. (TCI), **HeartMate** (Fig. 17-26)—are available with electric power sources that free the patient from being constantly tethered to an external power source. (One model of the TCI HeartMate also has an external pneumatic drive system [Fig. 17-27 and 17-28]). As a result, implantable LVADs allow mobility and significantly enhance the quality of life. In the future these devices may become an alternative to cardiac transplantation. However, patient size may be a limiting factor; there must be sufficient room in the left

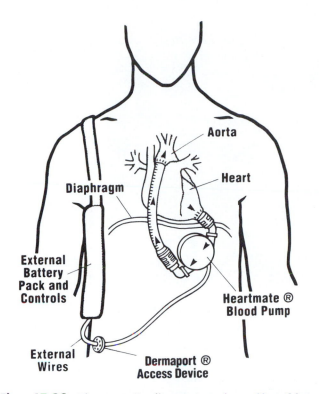

Fig. 17-26 Thermo Cardiosystems, Inc., HeartMate vented electrical system. (Courtesy Thermo Cardiosystems, Inc., Woburn, Mass.)

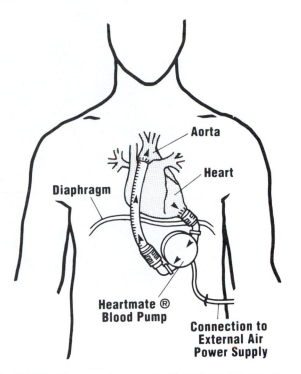

Fig. 17-27   HeartMate pneumatic system. (Courtesy Thermo Cardiosystems, Inc., Woburn, Mass.)

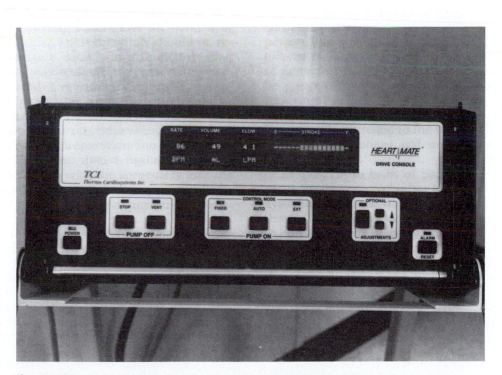

Fig. 17-28   Drive console for the HeartMate pneumatic system. (Courtesy Thermo Cardiosystems, Inc., Woburn, Mass.)

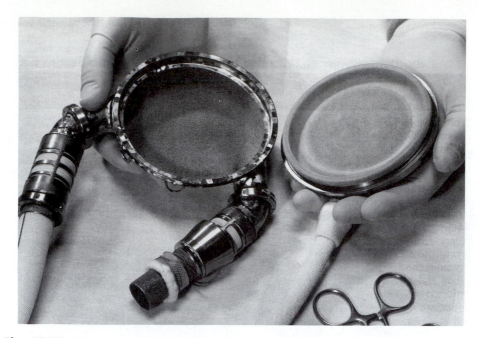

Fig. 17-29 The textured lining of the HeartMate blood sac is designed to facilitate development of a tightly adhering, smooth neointima. (Courtesy Thermo Cardiosystems, Inc., Woburn, Mass.)

upper abdominal quadrant for the pump. Patients who have an adequate body surface area (greater than 1.5 m²), but who are small or short waisted, may be excluded for lack of sufficient space in the abdomen (Shinn and Oyer, 1993).

Both devices are similar in that they withdraw blood from the left ventricular apex into the pump and eject into the ascending aorta. A difference between the Novacor and the TCI HeartMate is that the latter has a textured inner lining within the blood sac (Fig. 17-29) that promotes the development of a neointima and reduces the incidence of thromboembolism (Abou-Awdi and Ragsdale, 1991). This inner layer is made of beaded titanium (the "sintering" process) that stimulates a mild thrombogenesis, leading to the eventual creation of a smooth blood vessel lining (Dasse and others, 1987). In one multicenter series (Frazier and others, 1992), no device-related thromboembolism was observed despite minimal anticoagulation. In contrast the Novacor (and a number of other LVADs) use very smooth linings of polyurethane to reduce clot formation. Neither the smooth nor the textured surface lining has demonstrated proven superiority over the other. Seams and junctions, and areas of blood stasis within all systems still present potential problems. Methods of insertion are similar for both pumps; the operative procedure for one device is described here.

Operative procedure: insertion of the TCI HeartMate ventricular assist device (Abou-Awdi and Frazier, 1993; HeartMate Instructions, 1992)

The drive system should be tested and ready, and the battery power source should be fully charged for use during patient transport postoperatively (see Box 17-8 and Fig. 17-26).

Procedure

1. A median sternotomy is performed, with the excision extended to just above the umbilicus. Thirty milliliters of nonheparinized blood is withdrawn from the patient to be used for preclotting the graft portions of the circuit.

2. While the surgeon is preparing to institute CPB, the VAD pump is prepared and assembled on a separate sterile field prepared for this purpose. The graft conduits are preclotted with the patient's unheparinized blood by dripping the blood over the entire exterior surface of the conduit until clot formation is seen. Clots should not be allowed to enter the interior portion of the conduit. Conduits may be immersed in saline at regular intervals to remove accumulated blood products. The valves within the conduits are rinsed to remove the storage solution per protocol; the valves are evaluated to ensure their integrity. Frequent irrigation with saline prevents drying of the biologic (porcine) valves.

3. After the valve conduits have been preclotted and the valves rinsed, they are attached to the pump in the proper direction (e.g., inflow/outflow).

4. The pump is primed by filling it with saline through the inflow conduit. Tapping and rotating the pump is performed to expel air; the inflow tube is covered with a nonpowdered sterile glove fingertip, and the thread protector is attached to the outflow conduit.

5. CPB is instituted with standard cannulation technique (see Chapter 11).

6. The left ventricular apex is cored with a circular

Box 17-8 *Nursing considerations related to the HeartMate ventricular assist device**

Linda Lewis-Sims, RN, CNOR
Fairfax Hospital
Falls Church, Virginia

Ensure that all necessary consents have been obtained and are documented on chart before VAD insertion; follow established protocols for insertion.

Follow preimplant checklist; confirm that all necessary backup equipment and supplies (e.g., batteries, cables, etc.) are available.

Preparation for pump and Dacron graft:

Remove metal ring with Teflon washer from graft before preclotting graft (according to protocol).

Ensure that ring is replaced in proper position after graft is preclotted so that graft can be attached to pump correctly.

Do not place metal components of graft into any preclotting material (e.g., albumin), since this may prevent their being tightened securely.

Inspect valve conduit for blood in lumen; flush with saline if needed to remove residual blood before implanting device.

Do not use any sharp instruments (e.g., towel clips) on graft to avoid making holes in the material (these will not seal and could cause disastrous bleeding).

Connect drive line to pump before filling pump with saline (if connections are not dry, pump will not work properly); then fill pump to deair it and calibrate system; with electric models, ensure that percutaneous lead does not become wet.

Place a finger cot over outflow conduit (which leads to aorta) and inflow conduit to prevent entry of air into system; be sure that there is no particulate matter or glove powder inside finger cot.

Ensure that all entrapped air is removed before system is activated.

Make sure inflow and outflow valve conduits are placed in correct position to ensure proper direction of blood flow.

Preparation of tissue (bioprosthetic) valves:

Remove storage solution by rinsing in normal saline according to protocol.

Do not allow valves to dry out; keep moistened with saline.

Do not use sharp objects on valve to avoid injury.

Have a piece of Silastic or PTFE (Gore-Tex), depending on surgeon's preference, to cover pump and drive line at time of insertion; after cardiac transplantation, this material helps to facilitate removal of device.

Check and recheck system so that cardiopulmonary bypass time is not unnecessarily increased.

Be familiar with procedure for conversion to air (pneumatic) power if an electrical failure occurs in patient with electric model.

Exteriorized drive line can provide an entry site for infection; strict aseptic practices must be followed.

Communication with patient and family can reduce some of the intense feelings of powerlessness that are often seen in VAD patients.

*Thermo Cardiosystems, Inc.; see Fig. 17-27. Although these considerations describe implantation of the HeartMate, all VAD insertions require similar precautions. Team members should follow a prescribed protocol for implanting the device, ensuring that the system has been deaired, having additional supplies as a backup, checking the power source, and preventing injury to grafts, prosthetic valves, and metal components of the device.

---

cutting knife, and a sewing ring is sutured to the ventriculotomy.

7. An abdominal pocket is created for the pump (prior to systemic heparinization for CPB) just below the left diaphragm, and the pump is placed in the pocket.

8. The inlet conduit is tunneled through an incision in the diaphragm and placed through the left ventricular apical sewing ring. The diaphragm is then closed around the conduit.

9. The outflow graft is placed over the diaphragm and anastomosed to the ascending aorta. The graft is then clamped.

10. The (pneumatic) drive line is brought out of the body through a stab wound in the left lateral abdominal wall above the iliac crest; the exit wound should not be located where it will interfere with clothing (e.g., belt or waistband). The line is connected to the external console.

11. The patient is placed in the Trendelenburg position. A small (19-gauge) needle is inserted into the graft to vent air. CPB flow is reduced to allow the left ventricle to fill. Additional venting maneuvers may be used to remove air from the heart and the outflow graft. The outflow conduit (from the pump) is connected to the outflow graft (anastomosed to the ascending aorta) under dripping saline to prevent entry of air. After air has been removed, pump support is then gradually initiated.

12. Proper pump function is confirmed, and components are secured with nonabsorbable suture.

13. Temporary epicardial pacing wires are attached, CPB is discontinued, and mediastinal drainage tubes are inserted. The chest and abdomen are closed. A small drain may be placed in the abdominal wound.

Internal Orthotopic Pumps

The **Jarvik-7** (see Fig. 17-1) total artificial heart (TAH) has been used to replace the patient's own excised heart (DeVries, 1988). It is implanted in the orthotopic position, in contrast to other prosthetic ventricles that are heterotopically placed externally or within the abdomen. After the initial clinical experiences with TAH implantation, a number of modifications were made to reduce the thromboembolic and hemorrhagic complications that plagued the device. Infection, hemolysis, and device-related malfunctions (Richenbacher and Pierce, 1991b) were additional problems that dimmed the early enthusiasm for orthotopic ventricles.

Although there is no clinical TAH presently in use, experimental models such as the **Utah TAH** (White and others, 1993) are undergoing laboratory investigation with the goal of designing a device that can be used for short-term or long-term support. Given the large number of patients with biventricular failure and the scarcity of cardiac allografts, a permanent TAH would be a valuable treatment option (Davis and others, 1989). Like most other prosthetic assist devices, FDA investigational device exemptions are necessary and require compliance with strict protocols.

Proponents of the TAH cite the advantages of biventricular support, pulsatile flow, and high patient mobility. Disadvantages are related to the need for excision of the native heart, cost, FDA approval, continued thromboembolic and infectious complications, and difficulty of insertion (Jett, 1991). Because biVADs are now available that provide similar advantages and fewer of the disadvantages, interest in TAH research has been limited to a few major centers. However, it should be remembered that the early experiences with the TAH provided valuable contributions to the development of many of the newer, more widely used devices that are currently available.

Complications of Ventricular Assist Devices

Complications may occur during insertion, transport to the postoperative recovery unit, maintenance support, weaning, and removal of the device.

Bleeding

Bleeding from cardiac and vascular suture lines can result in cardiac tamponade and also affect filling of the device (Barker and DeVries, 1993). Devices that require systemic heparinization increase the risk of hemorrhage, as do internal devices that require extensive soft tissue dissection to create a pocket for the pump. Reoperation may be necessary for control of persistent bleeding. The ability to avoid full heparinization during the period of support has reduced bleeding complications significantly. Many devices require only dextran, aspirin, dipyridamole, or low-dose heparin.

Thromboembolism

Thromboembolism has been a persistent, though less frequent, complication. Blood sac linings have been improved, and connections between components of the VAD circuit have been modified to reduce blood trauma. Generally, the risk of thrombus formation is greatest during periods of reduced pump flow such as occurs during weaning. Blood stasis increases the risk of thrombogenesis, and at these times anticoagulation levels are increased.

Infection

Infection is another common complication of circulatory support devices and is often related to preoperative debilitation, invasive lines, and the duration of support. The process is similar to that seen in patients with other prosthetic devices where the foreign body acts as a nidus for infection. Contaminated intravascular lines and urinary drainage catheters can cause bacteremia; the exit sites of cannulas and drive lines are continuously exposed to the patient's skin flora, which can migrate along these lines to invade the mediastinum or skin pockets (Dougherty and Simmons, 1993). Because repeated courses of antibiotics promote the emergence of opportunistic pathogens, specific antibiotic therapy for proven infections is recommended (Pennington and Swartz, 1992). Pressure monitoring lines and drains should be removed when the patient is stable and they are no longer necessary (Shinn and Oyer, 1993).

Other contributing factors, such as multiorgan failure, pneumonia, gastrointestinal bleeding, retained clotted blood, hemolysis, and alterations in host-immune defenses, increase the risk, especially in the presence of catheters and drive lines exiting from multiple skin wounds. Devices that are paracorporeal have more tracts for potential migrating organisms and make the patient more vulnerable to infection as compared with implantable devices that require only one or two percutaneous lines. However, internally placed devices may impinge on the lungs (to cause atelectasis and pneumonia) and other vital organs. Orthotopically placed ventricles (foreign bodies without a tissue-adhering surface) reside in a relatively avascular space; a large area of dead space can accumulate blood and fluid, which can become a source of infection (Hill, 1989).

Hemolysis

Hemolysis is encountered less frequently, in large part because of improvements in the interior portion of the VAD circuit. Seams and connections have been made less traumatic. Increasing experience with insertion techniques has enabled surgeons to implant cannulas in a manner that avoids kinks in the circuit or compression of the conduits.

Biventricular failure

In patients with univentricular support devices, there is a risk of failure of the opposite ventricle. This is of particular concern in patients with LVADs. Maintenance of optimal LVAD support is mandatory so that right ventricular afterload is not increased. Adequate right ventricular function is necessary to provide an adequate left ventricular preload. Venous return cannot be impaired. Inotropic drugs, volume therapy, and afterload reduction are used to maintain filling pressures and to achieve optimal right ventricular performance (Shinn and Oyer, 1993). If right ventricular failure persists, implantation of an RVAD may be required.

Device-related complications

A number of complications are related to the specific design of the support system. Power failures can occur, although they have been rare. Depending on the device, alternative (battery) or additional (extra controller) power sources must be immediately available and capable of being exchanged expeditiously. Device malfunctions are infrequent, but they can be dramatic, as evidenced by the prosthetic valve strut fracture in the TAH; changing to a different mechanical valve has been done to prevent recurrence of this complication.

Abdominally located devices have been associated with wound dehiscence, diaphragmatic hernia, bowel adhesions, and colon perforation (Frazier and others, 1992, Phillips and others, 1992). These complications illustrate some of the physical limitations (e.g., size, shape, and weight) of devices that are positioned internally.

Other complications

Additional potential complications include renal failure, respiratory failure, and stroke. Devices that impair patient mobility may contribute to pressure injuries.

Weaning from Ventricular Assist Devices

Several factors must be considered when attempting to wean a patient with reversible cardiac disease from a VAD. Hemodynamic stability is the primary consideration. Assessment includes cardiac output and cardiac index, pulmonary artery wedge pressure, systemic blood pressure, pharmacologic support required to maintain adequate cellular perfusion, and arterial pulsatility indicating the amount of left ventricular ejection. Hemodynamic monitoring lines and echocardiography can be used to determine hemodynamic function. Other factors to be considered are neurologic, renal, pulmonary, and hematologic status.

Usually the patient's readiness to be weaned is first tested by temporarily slowing or stopping the device to determine the patient's tolerance to the reduction in support. This is done gradually so that the heart can become accustomed to the increased workload. For example, the IABP may be set to augment every second or third heartbeat; Hemopump revolutions per minute may be slowed; centrifugal pump flows are reduced; VAD ejection is decreased to coincide with every other intrinsic cardiac contraction.

Attention to anticoagulation is critical during weaning because diminished flow rates can predispose the patient to thrombus formation. Additional heparin is often required, and clamping of cannulas is generally contraindicated (Ley and Hill, 1993).

DYNAMIC CARDIOMYOPLASTY

The use of skeletal muscle to replace or repair a damaged ventricle was studied experimentally in the 1930s; in the 1960s investigators used the diaphragm as a patch to repair ventricular aneurysms (Chiu, 1991). The first successful clinical dynamic cardiomyoplasty, whereby contracting skeletal muscle was used to augment ventricular function, was performed in 1985 by Carpentier and Chachques (1985, 1991). They applied a left latissimus dorsi muscle pedicle graft to the ventricular surface and stimulated the muscle with a cardiac pacemaker so that it would contract in synchrony with the heart.

To use skeletal muscle, two biologic constraints have to be overcome. The first is the fatigue that develops when skeletal muscle is repeatedly stimulated at a cardiac rate. Studies by Salmons and Sreter (1976) showed that skeletal muscle can be transformed with low-frequency electrical stimulation to a highly fatigue resistant muscle; conditioning for 4 to 6 weeks provides sufficient fatigue resistance to develop to allow indefinite pacing at normal heart rates (Chiu, 1991).

The second biologic problem is related to both structural and functional differences. Skeletal muscle is composed of distinct individual fibers and motor units, in contrast to the myocardium, which is an interconnected system of fibers. Consequently, the heart is capable of responding in an all-or-none manner to a single electrical stimulus that is carried throughout the myocardium to achieve a coordinated contraction. Skeletal muscle response, however, is of short duration and does not affect all of the motor units simultaneously. In addition, the magnitude of contraction can vary depending on the amount of voltage stimulation that is received. To prolong the contraction time, a train of impulses (burst stimulation) delivered with an implantable burst stimulator can be delivered to many motor units at one time to generate a substantially greater force than a single electrical impulse (Koroteyev and others, 1991). Because stimulation must be coordinated with the cardiac cycle so that muscle contraction occurs during systole, sensing electrodes are inserted into the myocardium.

Patient selection

Cardiomyoplasty offers another alternative for patients with severe chronic and medically intractable myocardial failure. Patients in heart failure may not be suitable candidates for transplantation because of associated medical problems, psychosocial contraindications, age, or other exclusion criteria (Jatene and others, 1991). Donor organs are scarce, and patients themselves may refuse transplantation because of concerns about immunosuppression, rejection, and other complications. In addition, mechanical assist devices may be unsuitable or unavailable to some patients in heart failure (although cardiomyoplasty does not necessarily preclude eventual insertion of mechanical assist devices or cardiac transplantation). These considerations have prompted interest in skeletal muscle as a biologic ventricular assist device.

The principal indications for cardiomyoplasty are dilated and ischemic cardiomyopathy (Carpentier and Chachques, 1991; Jatene and others, 1991; Magovern and Benckart, 1991). Hypertrophic cardiomyopathy is usually contraindicated because the latissimus dorsi muscle (LDM) is unable to compress the thickened ventricular wall. Patients with end-stage cardiac disease (who might qualify for transplantation or bridge to transplantation) generally are not candidates for cardiomyoplasty, because there is little hemodynamic benefit from the procedure during the first few postoperative weeks that the muscle pedicle is being conditioned to resist fatigue. Thus patients undergoing the procedure must be able to withstand the stress of the surgery and the immediate postoperative period (Chiu, 1991). Contraindications include significant pulmonary dysfunction, renal failure, or complex ventricular dysrhythmias. Other contraindications include degenerative muscle disease, previous left thoracotomy incision, and preoperative need for inotropic agents and IABP (Magovern and others, 1991). Postoperatively, inotropes and IABP are often used to support the patient until the muscle wrap can begin to function.

Procedural considerations

The left LDM is commonly used because of its proximity to the heart, its large bulk, the presence of a single main blood supply, and a single motor nerve that is suitable for electrode placement and stimulation. In addition, LDM dissection produces little residual functional impairment for the patient (Chiu, 1991; Koroteyev and others, 1991). Other muscles that have been used as pedicle grafts to cover the heart include the right LDM, the pectoralis muscle, and the rectus abdominis muscle. The psoas muscle and the diaphragm have also been used. Concomitant coronary artery bypass grafting and/or left ventricular aneurysmectomy may be performed (see Chapter 12).

Whether the procedure is performed in one or two stages, the muscle is first dissected free (retaining the neurovascular bundle), with the patient lying on the right side for a left LDM and on the left side for a right LDM. Stimulating electrodes are implanted in the muscle and tested (to obtain a response from the skeletal muscle, curariform muscle-paralyzing drugs are omitted). The pedicle is placed in the pleural cavity via a transected second or third rib. A drain is placed, and the wound is closed and dressed. If a two-stage operation is done, the patient is transferred to the postoperative care unit and returned to the operating room a few days later for the second part of the procedure. If the procedure is performed in one stage, after the muscle dissection is completed and the lateral incision is closed, the patient is placed supine, the surgical area is prepared again, and the patient is redraped for the second part of the operation, which is performed via sternotomy (Stewart and others, 1993). Unless concomitant procedures requiring CPB are performed, CPB is not routinely used, although it is available on a standby basis. Patients who are at in-

---

Box 17-9 *Nursing considerations related to cardiomyoplasty*

Gail Kaempf, RN, MSN, CNOR
Presbyterian Medical Center of Philadelphia
Philadelphia, Pennsylvania

Patients usually have end-stage heart failure, so their status is fragile. Try to decrease any stress that the patient is feeling.

Prepare the sterile setup (for a one-stage procedure) in two parts: the first instrument table is used for mobilization of the latissimus dorsi muscle (LDM); the second setup is for muscle wrapping and cardiomyostimulator implantation.*

Be ready to institute cardiopulmonary bypass, although it may not be needed for the cardiomyoplasty procedure alone.*

Insert a urinary drainage catheter and apply sequential compression stockings before prepping and draping.

Supplies and equipment for both lateral and supine positioning are needed because the patient is first placed in the right lateral decubitus position with the arms elevated (for LDM dissection) and then transferred to a dorsal recumbent position, and reprepped and redraped for a median sternotomy (for the cardiac muscle wrap).*

Family members are especially anxious during the intraoperative period; a nurse liaison can help to support the family during this period by providing accurate and up-to-date information about the surgery.*

Although pain relief postoperatively is important to promote lung expansion, placement of an epidural catheter before surgery is not an option because of the location of the muscle dissection. Other methods of pain control are used (e.g., patient-controlled analgesia); the nurse must monitor pain medications closely for adverse effects on the cardiovascular system.*

Expect to see more serosanguineous drainage (50 to 100 ml/hr) from the posterior chest tube immediately after surgery, as compared with that from anterior drainage tubes (because little anterior dissection is performed).*

The procedure may last a long time (up to 6 hours); the perioperative nurse should be rested and have eaten a meal before the start of the procedure.

*Modified from Stewart JV and others: Cardiomyoplasty: treatment of the failing heart using the skeletal muscle wrap, *J Cardiovasc Nurs* 7(2):23, 1993.

---

creased risk and cannot tolerate long procedures may require staged operations.

Perioperative nursing considerations

Because patients are at risk for sudden cardiac decompensation, physiologic and psychologic stress should be minimized. Patients should be kept warm to prevent shivering, which increases myocardial oxygen demand. CPB is not routinely used, but the nurse should be prepared to institute bypass rapidly should

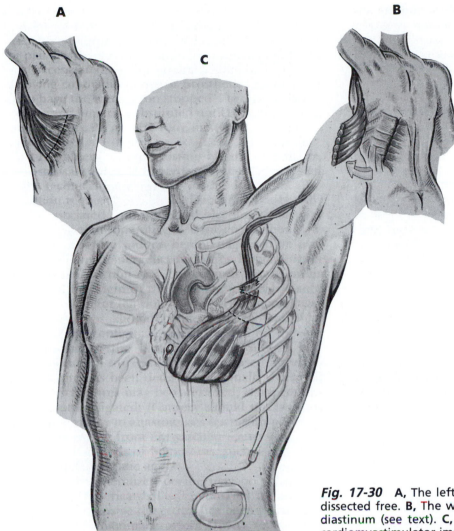

A

B

C

Fig. 17-30 **A,** The left dorsi latissimus muscle (LDM) is dissected free. **B,** The wrap is swung around to the mediastinum (see text). **C,** Completed LDM wrap with the cardiomyostimulator implanted in the abdominal pocket (see text). (From Medtronic, Inc., Minneapolis, Minn.)

the patient require support; usually standard cannulation techniques are used.

Positioning to maximize expansion of the dependent lung is crucial when the patient is in the lateral position and the lung on the side of the muscle pedicle is hypoinflated to improve surgical exposure. Impaired gas exchange causing hypoxemia can produce myocardial ischemia and trigger lethal dysrhythmias (Stewart and others, 1993).

If both the muscle dissection and cardiac wrapping portions of the procedure are to be performed at one time, separate skin preparation and draping supplies, instruments, and other necessary items (including sensing and stimulating electrodes and the cardiac stimulator) for both the thoracotomy and the sternotomy portions of the operation are needed. Additional considerations are described in Box 17-9.

Operative procedure: cardiomyoplasty with the left latissimus dorsi muscle

Part 1: muscle dissection

1. The patient is positioned in a left thoracotomy position with the left arm free and elevated.

2. A longitudinal incision is made from the left axilla to the iliac crest over the lateral border of the LDM.

3. The LDM is dissected and freed from its insertions in the vertebrae, ribs, and iliac crest (Fig. 17-30, *A*). Extreme care is taken to preserve the thoracodorsal neurovascular pedicle. The humeral tendon is cut to prevent possible arm movement during electrostimulation of the LDM (Carpentier and Chachaques, 1991).

4. Two intramuscular pacing electrodes are woven into portions of the muscle. An external stimulator may be used to test electrode function.

5. Approximately 5 cm of the anterior third of the second (or third) rib is removed to create an opening through which the muscle flap and its electrodes can be translocated to the mediastinal space (Fig. 17-30, *B*).

6. A drain is inserted, and the wound is closed; dressings are applied.

Part 2: cardiac wrap

1. The patient is turned to the supine position, and the anterior chest and abdomen are prepared. The

patient is draped to expose the chest and the abdomen, and a midline sternal incision is made. (Some authors have performed this part of the procedure through the initial throacotomy incision, but this has disadvantages, including inadequate exposure and difficulty instituting CPB if it is needed.)

2. The pericardium may be opened in a reversed C shape over the right ventricle in anticipation of the need to supplement the muscle wrap with pericardium should the muscle wrap be too short to surround the heart (Chiu, 1991). The remaining pericardium is widely opened.

3. The LDM muscle is retrieved from the left pleural cavity, and the stimulating electrodes are tested. The LDM is then wrapped around the heart (Fig. 17-30, C). The flap is aligned over the heart, and the tip of the muscle is turned around the apex and approximated to the cardiac anterior and lateral borders with interrupted sutures. The flap may be sutured to the myocardium or to the pericardium, depending on the surgeon's preference.

In patients with large hearts, coverage of the right ventricular outflow tract can be achieved with the pericardial flap anchored to the muscle edge, thus allowing a 360-degree wrap. (Various clockwise and counterclockwise wrapping techniques have been used, but the superiority of one fiber orientation to another has not been clearly established.)

Partial wrapping may be performed to reinforce sites of ventricular aneurysmectomy or tumor excision; the dynamic effectiveness of partial wraps has not been established (Chiu, 1991).

4. A sensing electrode is placed in the epicardium. In patients with ischemic disease involving the left ventricle, the electrode may be placed in the right ventricle; in patients with biventricular dilated cardiomyopathy, the sensing electrode may be placed in the left ventricular wall (Carpentier and Chachaques, 1991). The electrode may also be inserted transvenously into the right ventricular endocardium. It is tested to ensure that it senses the R wave, which will trigger the stimulator.

5. A pocket is formed beneath the rectus abdominis muscle in the upper abdomen, and the sensing electrodes and the muscle-stimulating electrodes are tunneled to the pocket. They are then connected to the burst stimulator/generator. (The stimulator is not activated.)

6. Chest drainage tubes are inserted. All incisions are closed, and dressings are applied. The patient is transferred to the postoperative care unit.

Postoperative period

In the immediate postoperative period, inotropic drugs, IABP, or other assist devices may be needed to support cardiac function. Cardiac tamponade is unusual because both the pericardium and left pleura are incised.

Following the extensive dissection of the LDM, a period of 1 to 2 weeks of rest is required for healing and to restore the collateral blood supply to the pedicle. Immediate stimulation of the muscle is avoided, since it could induce fatigue and lead to possible muscle damage. In addition, stimulation of the mobile muscle against the heart could displace the heart and be detrimental to the circulation (Chiu, 1991).

Once the pedicle has healed and formed adhesions against the heart, a gradual program of stimulation is initiated. A single electrical impulse is applied to the LDM pedicle for every second heartbeat; the number of pulses are increased over the following 4 to 6 weeks until electrical stimuli are delivered as systolic bursts during each cardiac cycle.

The best operative results have been achieved in patients with left ventricular failure but preserved right ventricular function. Patients with biventricular failure derive less benefit from cardiomyoplasty; transplantation may be more appropriate (Magovern and others, 1991).

Skeletal muscle ventricles

Experimental investigations have focused on the use of skeletal muscle to create a separate pumping chamber. Skeletal muscle ventricles (SMVs) may be constructed from LDM, which is wrapped around a conical stent and conditioned with pacing electrodes to achieve fatigue resistance. After conditioning, the muscle is removed from the stent and connected to the cardiovascular system (e.g., the descending thoracic aorta). By stimulating the muscle during diastole, the cardiac wrap augments arterial pressure in a manner similar to that with the IABP. SMVs have also been tested experimentally in the vena cava and the pulmonary artery to augment right ventricular performance (Koroteyev and others, 1991).

ETHICAL CONSIDERATIONS

Ethical considerations are especially pertinent to the topic of mechanical and biologic circulatory assistance. Of all the surgical interventions available for the treatment of cardiac disorders, the use of VADs and other supportive methods have perhaps the most profound impact on the duration and quality of life; the allocation of human, material, and fiscal resources; and the treatment of persons as informed decision makers and consenting research subjects (Katz and Quaal, 1993).

A number of professional, humane, economic, and moral questions are raised by the use of these complex and costly devices (Box 17-10). The questions of when, how, where, and with whom they should be used require careful and compassionate inquiry by patients and families, physicians, nurses, administrators, and legislators (Katz and Quaal, 1993). One can consider costs (nearly $100,000 for some devices) or the quality of life experienced by a patient immobilized by a cumbersome system versus the quality of life experienced

---

Box 17-10 *Questions related to ethical considerations of ventricular assist devices*

Cost

Who should pay if a patient cannot afford a VAD?

Should the selection of a device be based on cost when a more expensive device provides better cardiac support or enhances the quality of life?

Allocation of Resources

Are there sufficient human, material, and fiscal resources to provide devices for those needing them?

What is the impact on donor heart organs for patients supported as a bridge to transplantation?

How should fiscal resources be allocated?

What is the best use of limited resources?

What are acceptable staffing levels for the maintenance of VAD support?

Quality of Life

How is quality of life defined by the:
  Patient?
  Family?
  Surgical team members?
  Society?

Should differences of opinion be arbitrated? By whom? Based on what authority or right?

How is the determination made to terminate VAD support?

Informed Consent

How do patients themselves make an informed decision prior to the use of a VAD?

Should family members have the right to act as surrogate decision makers?

How is the decision made to use a VAD when mechanical support is not anticipated preoperatively?

How are patients' rights as research subjects protected?

Should patients be told not only about the availability of devices and their cost, but also about the level of training and competency that caregivers have in order to operate the devices safely and effectively?

Modified from Katz J, Quaal SJ: Ethical issues associated with a ventricular assist device program. In Quaal SJ, editor: *Cardiac mechanical assistance beyond balloon pumping*, St Louis, 1993, Mosby; and O'Mara RJ: Dilemmas in cardiac surgery: Artificial heart and left ventricular assist device, *Crit Care Nurs Q* 10(2):48, 1987.

---

by a patient with a device that allows ambulation. Also, the question of informed consent is often raised by those who argue that the complexity of the technology precludes a patient's understanding of the options being offered or that obligations to a research protocol may override the obligation to the patient as a person. Katz and Quaal (1993) strongly support the idea that patients and families must be part of the decision process. That decision must be made on an individualized basis and reflect the patient's value system. There is no one standard consent form that can be used for all patients (O'Mara, 1987).

Many of the ethical concerns are due in part to the astounding success of these devices and the demand for their use. The questions and dilemmas being faced today can only become more complicated; and their resolution can only be accomplished by inclusive and open deliberation.

REFERENCES

Abou-Awdi N, Frazier OH: HeartMate ventricular assist system. In Quaal SJ, editor: *Cardiac mechanical assistance beyond balloon pumping*, St Louis, 1993, Mosby.

Abou-Awdi N, Ragsdale D: High-tech help for failing hearts, *RN* 54(5):42, 1991.

Barden C, Lee R: Update on ventricular assist devices, *AACN Clin Issues Crit Care Nurs* 1(1):13, 1990.

Barker LE, DeVries WC: Total artificial heart. In Quaal SJ, editor: *Cardiac mechanical assistance beyond balloon pumping*, St Louis, 1993, Mosby.

Berron K: Role of the ventricular assist device in acute myocardial infarction, *Crit Care Nurs Q* 12(2):25, 1989.

Boncheck L, Olinger G: Direct ascending aortic insertion of the "percutaneous" intra-aortic balloon catheter in the open chest: advantages and precautions, *Ann Thorac Surg* 32:512, 1981.

Braunwald E: The stunned myocardium: newer insights into mechanisms and clinical implications, *J Thorac Cardiovasc Surg* 100(2):310, 1990 (letter to editor).

Braunwald E: Pathophysiology of heart failure. In Braunwald E, editor: *Heart disease*, ed 4, Philadelphia, 1992, WB Saunders.

Braunwald E, Kloner RA: The stunned myocardium: prolonged, postischemic ventricular dysfunction, *Circulation* 66(6):1146, 1982.

Braunwald E, Sobel BE: Coronary blood flow and myocardial ischemia. In Braunwald E, editor: *Heart disease*, ed 4, Philadelphia, 1992, WB Saunders.

Burton NA and others: A reliable bridge to cardiac transplantation: the TCI left ventricular assist device, *Ann Thorac Surg* 55:1425, 1993.

Carpentier A, Chachques JC: Myocardial substitution with a stimulated skeletal muscle: first successful clinical case, *Lancet* 1:1267, 1985.

Carpentier A, Chachques JC: Clinical dynamic cardiomyoplasty: method and outcome, *Semin Thorac Cardiovasc Surg* 3(2):136, 1991.

Champsaur G and others: Use of the Abiomed BVS system 5000 as a bridge to cardiac transplantation, *J Thorac Cardiovasc Surg* 100(1):122, 1990.

Chiu RC: Dynamic cardiomyoplasty: an overview, *PACE* 14(4):577, 1991.

Cooley DA and others: First human implantation of cardiac prosthesis for staged total replacement of the heart, *Trans Am Soc Artif Intern Org* 15:252, 1969.

Dasse KA and others: Clinical experience with textured blood contacting surfaces in ventricular assist devices, *Trans Am Soc Artif Intern Org* 10(3):418, 1987.

Dasse KA and others: Clinical responses to ventricular assistance versus transplantation in a series of bridge to transplant patients, *Trans Am Soc Artif Intern Org* 38(3):M622, 1992.

Davis PK and others: Current status of permanent total artificial hearts, *Ann Thorac Surg* 47:172, 1989.

DeVries WC: The permanent artificial heart: four case reports, *JAMA* 259(6):849, 1988.

Dixon JF, Farris CD, Jett GK: Abiomed BVS 5000 assist device. In Quaal SJ, editor: *Cardiac mechanical assistance beyond balloon pumping*, St Louis, 1993, Mosby.

Dougherty SH, Simmons RL: Infection prophylaxis and treatment. In Quaal SJ, editor: *Cardiac mechanical assistance beyond balloon pumping*, St Louis, 1993, Mosby.

Evans RW and others: Donor availability as the primary determinant of the future of heart transplantation, *JAMA* 255:1892, 1986.

Farrar DJ and others: Heterotopic prosthetic ventricles as a bridge to cardiac transplantation: a multicenter study in 29 patients, *N Engl J Med* 318(6):333, 1988.

Frazier OH, Colon R: Assisted circulation. In Miller TA, editor: *Physiologic basis of modern surgical care*, St Louis, 1988, Mosby.

Frazier OH and others: Multicenter clinical evaluation of the HeartMate 1000 IP left ventricular assist device, *Ann Thorac Surg* 53:1080, 1992.

Gibbon JH: Application of a mechanical heart and lung apparatus to cardiac surgery, *Minn Med* 37:171, 1954.

Golding LA and others: Postcardiotomy centrifugal mechanical ventricular support, *Ann Thorac Surg* 54:1059, 1992.

HeartMate instructions for use, Woburn, Mass, 1992, Thermocardiosystems, Inc..

Hill JD: Bridging to cardiac transplantation, *Ann Thorac Surg* 47:167, 1989.

HLB Newsletter (covering policy development at the National Heart, Lung and Blood Institute, Washington, DC) 8(18):145, 1992.

Holzum D: Intrapulmonary artery balloon pumping after CABG surgery, *Crit Care Nurse* 10(2):48, 1990.

Jatene AD and others: Left ventricular function changes after cardiomyoplasty in patients with dilated cardiomyopathy, *J Thorac Cardiovasc Surg* 102(1):132, 1991.

Jett GK: Left ventricular assist devices: a bridge to the future, *Baylor Univ Med Center Proc* 4(2):27, 1991.

Joyce LD, Toninato C, Hansen JB: Centrifugal ventricular assist devices. In Quaal SJ, editor: *Cardiac mechanical assistance beyond balloon pumping*, St Louis, 1993, Mosby.

Kaan GL and others: Management of postcardiotomy cardiogenic shock with a new pulsatile ventricular assist device: initial clinical results, *Trans Am Soc Artif Int Org* 37(4):1991.

Kantrowitz A: Origins of intraaortic balloon pumping, *Ann Thorac Surg* 50:672, 1990.

Kantrowitz A and others: Initial clinical experience with intra-aortic balloon pumping in cardiogenic shock, *JAMA* 203:113, 1968.

Katz J, Quaal SJ: Ethical issues associated with a ventricular assist device program. In Quaal SJ, editor: *Cardiac mechanical assistance beyond balloon pumping*, St Louis, 1993, Mosby.

Kolff WJ: Total artificial hearts, ventricular assist devices, or nothing? In Quaal SJ, editor: *Cardiac mechanical assistance beyond balloon pumping*, St Louis, 1993, Mosby.

Koroteyev A and others: Skeletal muscle: new techniques for treating heart failure, *AORN J* 53(4):1005, 1991.

Ley SJ, Hill JD: Thoratec ventricular assist device. In Quaal SJ, editor: *Cardiac mechanical assistance beyond balloon pumping*, St Louis, 1993, Mosby.

Litwak RS and others: Use for a left heart assist device after intracardiac surgery: technique and clinical experience, *Ann Thorac Surg* 21:191, 1976.

Lohmann DP and others: Replacement of paracorporeal ventricular assist devices, *Ann Thorac Surg* 54:1226, 1992.

Maccioli GA, Lucas WJ, Norfleet EA: The intra-aortic balloon pump: a review, *J Cardiothorac Anesth* 2(3):365, 1988.

Magovern GJ, Benckart DH: Management of complications related to surgery for ischemic heart disease: ischemic mitral regurgitation, ventricular aneurysm, ventricular septal defect. In Waldhausen JA, Orringer MB: *Complications in cardiothoracic surgery*, St Louis, 1991, Mosby.

Magovern JA and others: Indications and risk analysis for clinical cardiomyoplasty, *Semin Thorac Cardiovasc Surg* 3(2):145, 1991.

Marchetta S, Stennis E: Ventricular assist devices: applications for critical care, *J Cardiovasc Nurs* 2(2):39, 1988.

May DR, Adams MA: Ventricular assist devices: a bridge to cardiac transplantation, *AORN J* 46(4):633, 1987.

Moulopoulos SC and others: Diastolic balloon pumping (with carbon dioxide) in the aorta: a mechanical assistance to the failing circulation, *Am Heart J* 63:669, 1962.

O'Mara RJ: Dilemmas in cardiac surgery: artificial heart and left ventricular assist device, *Crit Care Nurs Q* 10(2):48, 1987.

Packer M: Prolonging life in patients with congestive heart failure: the next frontier, *Circulation* 75(suppl IV):IV-1, 1987.

Pennington DG, Swartz MT: Assisted circulation and mechanical hearts. In Braunwald E, editor: *Heart disease*, ed 4, Philadelphia, 1992, WB Saunders.

Phillips WS and others: Surgical complications in bridging to transplantation: the Thermo Cardiosystems LVAD, *Ann Thorac Surg* 53:482, 1992.

Poirier V: As quoted in Maloney LD: An engineer for the long haul, *Design News*, p 66, Feb 10, 1992.

Quaal SJ: The person with heart failure and cardiogenic shock. In Guzzetta CE, Dossey BM: *Cardiovascular nursing: holistic practice*, St Louis, 1992, Mosby.

Quaal SJ: *Comprehensive intra-aortic balloon pumping*, ed 2, St Louis, 1993, Mosby.

Reedy JE and others: mechanical cardiopulmonary support for refractory cardiogenic shock, *Heart Lung* 19(5):514, 1990.

Richenbacher WE, Pierce WS: Management of complications of intraaortic balloon counterpulsation. In Waldhausen JA, Orringer MB: *Complications in cardiothoracic surgery*, St Louis, 1991a, Mosby.

Richenbacher WE, Pierce WS: Management of complications of mechanical circulatory assistance. In Waldhausen JA, Orringer MB: *Complications in cardiothoracic surgery*, St Louis, 1991b, Mosby.

Rose DM and others: Roller pump ventricular assist device. In Quaal SJ, editor: *Cardiac mechanical assistance beyond balloon pumping*, St Louis, 1993, Mosby.

Rountree WD and others: Johnson & Johnson Hemopump temporary cardiac assist system. In Quaal SJ, editor: *Cardiac mechanical assistance beyond balloon pumping*, St Louis, 1993, Mosby.

Rutan PM, Galvin EA: Adult and pediatric ventricular heart failure. In Quaal SJ, editor: *Cardiac mechanical assistance beyond balloon pumping*, St Louis, 1993, Mosby.

Ruzevich SA, Swartz MT, Pennington DG: Nursing care of the patient with a pneumatic ventricular assist device, *Heart Lung* 17(4):399, 1988.

Salmons S, Sreter FA: Significance of impulse activity in the transformation of skeletal muscle type, *Nature* 263:30, 1976.

Scheinin SA and others: Postcardiotomy LVAD support and transesophageal echocardiography in a child, *Ann Thorac Surg* 55:529, 1993.

Schlant RC, Sonnenblick EH: Pathophysiology of heart failure. In Hurst JW, editor: *The Heart*, ed 7, New York, 1990, McGraw-Hill.

Shinn JA, Oyer PE: Novacor ventricular assist system. In Quaal SJ, editor: *Cardiac mechanical assistance beyond balloon pumping*, St Louis, 1993, Mosby.

Shiono M and others: Overview of ventricular assist devices. In Quaal SJ, editor: *Cardiac mechanical assistance beyond balloon pumping*, St Louis, 1993, Mosby.

Smith TW, Braunwald E, Kelly RA: The management of heart failure. In Braunwald E, editor: *Heart disease*, ed 4, Philadelphia, 1992, WB Saunders.

Stewart JV and others: Cardiomyoplasty: treatment of the failing heart using the skeletal muscle wrap, *J Cardiovasc Nurs* 7(2):23, 1993.

Vaska PL: Biventricular assist devices, *Crit Care Nurse* 11(8):52, 1991.

Waldhausen JA, Pierce WS: *Johnson's surgery of the chest*, ed 5, St Louis, 1985, Mosby.

Wechsler AS: Pharmacologic support of the failing heart. In Waldhausen JA, Orringer MB: *Complications in cardiothoracic surgery*, St Louis, 1991, Mosby.

White RK, Pantalos GM, Olsen DB: Total artificial heart development at the University of Utah. In Quaal SJ: *Cardiac mechanical assistance beyond balloon pumping*, St Louis, 1993, Mosby.

18

Transplantation for Heart and Lung Disease

A new heart will I give you,
A new spirit put within you.
I will remove the heart of stone from your flesh,
And give you a heart that feels.

From the Yom Kippur Morning Service,
"Gates of Repentance"

GENERAL CONSIDERATIONS

Transplantation has become a clinical reality. Programs providing heart, heart-lung, and lung transplantation have proliferated, and acceptance of this treatment option by Medicare has been demonstrated by the decision in 1986 to reimburse institutions for cardiac transplantation (May and Adams, 1992). Other forms of thoracic organ replacement are increasingly being reimbursed by government and third-party payers. Improvements in donor and recipient selection, immunosuppression, methods to diagnose rejection, control of infection, and refined preservation and implantation techniques have improved survival and enhanced the quality of life for patients undergoing transplantation.

Heart Transplantation

The feasibility of performing human transplantation of the heart was described at a meeting in 1960 by Richard Lower (Lower and Shumway, 1960). The only other physician in attendance at the session was Lower's mentor, Norman Shumway, from Stanford University (Cabrol, 1992b). In contrast, almost 1000 participants attended a 1992 meeting of the International Society for Heart and Lung Transplantation (Cabrol, 1992a). The tremendous growth in the popularity of cardiac transplantation during that 32-year interval is due in great part to the work of Lower (who was to continue his work in Richmond, Virginia) and Shumway. They, their colleagues, and other early investigators, such as Alexis Carrel (see Chapter 1), made transplantation a viable intervention for end-stage heart disease. Of historical interest is that Christiaan Barnard (1967), who performed the first human cardiac transplantation in 1967 (see Fig. 1-1), had been impressed by the experimental work of Lower, whose laboratory at the Medical College of Virginia in Richmond had been visited by Barnard in the early 1960s (Cabrol, 1992b).

Although the anastomotic techniques developed by Lower and Shumway gave clinicians a rapid and effective surgical method for performing orthotopic cardiac replacement (e.g., exchanging one person's heart for that of another), rejection of the allograft forced most investigators to abandon transplantation. The problem continued to be studied by Shumway, who was able to improve survival with azathioprine and corticosteroids (e.g., prednisone) for immunosuppression. The addition of cyclosporine led to a triple-drug regimen that has reduced the severity of rejection sequelae, such as intramyocardial edema (Macdonald, 1990). Newer immunosuppressive drugs such as monoclonal antibodies have further enhanced survival and quality of life.

Heart-Lung Transplantation

The development of heart-lung transplantation was stimulated by the studies performed on cardiac replacement. Pulmonary problems such as hypertension and interstitial fibrosis could complicate otherwise successful heart transplants because the right ventricle would be unable to overcome the increased afterload associated with these lung alterations. Thus two organ systems—the heart and the lungs—would fail, necessitating heart-lung transplantation (Ahrens and Powers, 1990). The first long-term survivor of this combined procedure was a patient of Bruce A. Reitz, Shumway, and their associates at Stanford University in 1981 (Reitz, Pennock, and Shumway, 1981).

Lung Transplantation

Lung transplantation—single and double—became clinically feasible as a result of the efforts of Joel D. Cooper (presently at Washington University in St. Louis) and the Toronto Lung Transplant Group (1988). Although numerous lung transplantations had been attempted prior to the first successful experience in Toronto in 1983, respiratory failure, rejection, infection, and dehiscence of the tracheal or bronchial anastomoses made these attempts unsuccessful (Boychuk and Malen, 1990). Use of cyclosporine, avoidance of steroids in the early postoperative period, and methods to protect and revascularize the airway anastomoses enabled Cooper and his associates to demonstrate improved results (Dubois, Chiniere, and Cooper, 1984; Lima and others, 1981).

Availability of Donor Organs

An inadequate supply of donor organs for the growing number of transplant candidates remains a continuing problem. The number of donor organs has actually declined in the past few years, even with ongoing education programs for the public. While there is greater awareness of the need for organs and more frequent family-initiated discussions about organ donation, delays in potential donor identification and insufficient understanding of selection criteria and the recovery process remain problems. In addition, personnel may be hesitant to approach a grieving family, even with required laws that mandate such requests.

Significant increases in organ donation have been demonstrated when the discussion of death and the discussion of donation occur at distinctly separate times—a process known as "decoupling" (Schaeffer, 1993).

EMOTIONAL ASPECTS OF TRANSPLANTATION

Transplantation places great emotional stress on the recipient awaiting transplantation and on the family of the organ donor. It also generates many feelings, sometimes conflicting, among the personnel who participate in the care of "brain-dead" patients prior to removal of organs and among those who are involved in the recovery and implantation procedures.

Transplant Candidate

Patients accepted for organ transplantation worry that they may not survive the waiting period—not an unwarranted fear considering that between 25% and 40% of (heart) transplant candidates may not survive the wait for a donor (Dressler, 1992). Candidates may also be concerned that the new organ, once implanted, will not function. In addition, there may be deep-seated fears about the insertion of another person's body parts into their own. These feelings may be aggravated by symptoms of fatigue, difficulty breathing and sleeping, and generalized weakness (Grady and others, 1992).

Although it is important to educate the patient about the technical and immunologic aspects of organ transplantation, it is also important to provide emotional support. Patients must not only understand the necessity of complying with lifelong immunosuppression therapy, frequent checkups, and endomyocardial biopsies, but must also accept these life-style changes if they are to have a successful outcome. Family support is important to help the candidate cope with the stress of waiting. Often the family's home and social commitments are interrupted so that members can devote their attention to the transplant candidate (Nolan and others, 1992).

Donor Family

Families who are considering organ donation, or who have already consented to donate, undergo a range of emotions that parallel the grieving process described by Kubler-Ross (1969). Nurses, transplant coordinators, surgeons, and others involved with the care of donors can provide support during the period when the family is making or accepting the decision to donate. Emotional assistance before, during, and after donor retrieval is important.

Sammons (1988) has described this process as one that progresses from denial and isolation to anger, bargaining, depression, and acceptance. These stages may not occur in strict sequence; nor are they mutually exclusive—often there is an overlapping of emotions. Feelings of guilt related to the death of the loved one may compound the array of emotions felt by family members.

Although family members at first may deny the diagnosis of brain death and detach themselves emotionally and physically, this does not necessarily imply that they do not wish to talk to someone about the death at a later time. Nurses who are aware of this can be prepared to interact with the family when appropriate; usually the family will initiate this interaction. Nurses and organ recovery coordinators can be especially helpful to families during this period by clarifying the concept of brain death in relation to the artificial maintenance of cardiac and respiratory function. Pelletier's (1993) study showed that unless family members specifically asked questions, most of their information needs went unmet. In addition, confusion over inconsistent terminology, too much information at one time, and too little clarification of brain death contributed to families' concerns.

Once families understand that the patient is dead, they may displace anger toward those around them; such feelings should be allowed to be expressed. Anger does not mean that donation is opposed; in fact, donation can become a way to exert control over a difficult situation. This attempt to control may become a form of bargaining, and families may make specific requests for the allocation of the donor's organs. They may ask that donations be made to a recipient resembling their loved one or that they be allowed to meet the intended recipient. These requests cannot and should not be guaranteed, and this may result in the family's refusal to donate.

As families approach the time that organ recovery would be most feasible, preparatory depression may be evident. This is natural, and families should be allowed to express their sorrow because it will assist them in reaching the stage of acceptance. Families may then be able to accept the fate of their loved one and may no longer be angry. If they have not already done so, families are most likely at this time to make the decision to donate (Sammons, 1988).

Sensitivity to the family's feelings, empathy, and acceptance of the emotions being felt reflect compassionate understanding of this painful experience. This is a critical component in assisting families in viewing organ donation as a humane and honorable act and as a way of attaching meaning to the loss of their loved one (Guinn, 1988). Important needs of families also include receiving information and support, frequent visiting of the loved one, and, for many, consenting to organ donation (Pelletier, 1993).

Caregivers

Transplantation also has an emotional impact on nurses and other caregivers involved in the selection and care of donors, organ recovery, and the transplant procedure. At times staff may be overwhelmed by the reality of death and may demonstrate nervousness, aggression, frustration, boredom, anger, fatigue, and low self-esteem (House and Benitez, 1992).

Kiberd and Kiberd (1992) studied nurses' attitudes toward organ donation, procurement, and transplantation. Operating room (OR) nurses were less likely to consent to donate than were nurses in other units. The authors suggest that this may be related to environmental factors (e.g., participating in the surgery, which was preceived by some respondents to be "mutilating" and "disrespectful"). With respect to organ procurement, they found that only 10% of the operating room nurses in the study felt that they had been supported in their efforts. Comments from these OR nurses included: not enough nursing staff provided; no feedback on the outcome of transplantation; short notice; time consuming; lack of education, psychologic support, and respect from surgeons and physicians; and feelings of discomfort after being left alone with a dead patient after organ retrieval.

Bidagare and Oermann (1991) studied critical care nurses' attitudes toward organ recovery and found that nurses with greater experience in donor care tended to have more positive attitudes toward organ donation. Both Kiberd and Kiberd's (1992) and Bidagare and Oermann's (1991) studies indicate that positive experiences influence attitudes. In addition, the need for support and counsel should be considered for caregivers, as well as for transplant candidates and families of donors.

ORGAN RECOVERY

The current rate of organ procurement from potential donors is only 50% (Darby and others, 1989; MacKensie, Bronsther, and Shackford, 1991). According to Horowitz and colleagues (1992), some of the reasons for the underutilization of potential organs are as follows: inability to obtain family consent, rapid clinical deterioration of the donor, limitations of cardiac ischemic time, economic factors, and logistical problems related to unavailability of personnel and transportation problems.

Initial identification of potential donors is usually made by health care providers who may talk to the family about donation. Members of an organ recovery program may be contacted, and a representative will discuss donation with the family. A patient is not considered a candidate until pronunciation of brain death: total and irreversible absence of all brain and brainstem function. Guidelines for brain death generally include a flat electroencephalogram, absence of reflexes, failure to respond to painful stimuli, and absence of spontaneous respiratory or muscle movement (Smith, Brumm, and Crim, 1991). Inclusion and exclusion criteria for organ donation are used to ensure that the donor's organ(s) will provide optimal function when transplanted. After a donor is identified and accepted, permission is sought from the next-of-kin, and the retrieval process is begun (House and Benitez, 1992). To ensure fair distribution of suitable organs, the United Network of Organ Sharing (UNOS), in collaboration with local procurement organizations, allocates the organs based on a nationwide, computerized waiting list (Smith, Brumm, and Crim, 1991).

Recovery coordinators assist with the donor's medical management, arrange for the arrival of transplant recovery teams (and granting of temporary surgical privileges), collect necessary legal and administrative forms and documents, assist with the procurement procedure, and coordinate donor and recipient teams. Because of the limited supply of donor organs, recovery of a single organ (rather than multiple organ retrieval) is now less common. Coordinators provide an important communication link between the multiple organ recovery teams, which facilitates efficient procurement.

Coordination and communication are essential for successful organ transplantation because extensive preparation with little advance notice is the rule rather than the exception. Multiple organ recovery from a single donor requires a high level of skill and consideration between teams and with the staff from the recovery site (Wiberg and others, 1986). Recovery teams attempt to be as self-sufficient as necessary to avoid delays that could impair organ viability. Cardiac and/or pulmonary teams may bring their own sterile instruments and saws if needed (including cold cardioplegia for donor hearts), although most procurements require commonly used instrumentation. Availability of these items should be confirmed, however.

Table 18-1 ■ *Classification of the cardiomyopathies*

Dilated	Hypertrophic	Restrictive
Causes		
Idiopathic; genetic; alcoholic; pregnancy; viral	Hereditary; possibly result of chronic hypertension	Amyloidosis; postcardiac surgery; postirradiation; endomyocardial fibrosis; idiopathic
Symptoms		
Left or biventricular congestive heart failure	Dyspnea; syncope; chest pain	Dyspnea; fatigue; right-sided congestive heart failure
Chest X-Ray Film		
Enlarged heart; pulmonary congestion	Mild cardiomegaly	Mild to moderate cardiomegaly
Cardiac Catheterization		
Left ventricular dilatation and dysfunction; high diastolic pressures and low cardiac output	Small, hypercontractile left ventricle; diastolic dysfunction	Normal or mildly reduced left ventricular function; high diastolic pressures

Modified from Massie BM, Sokolow M: Heart and great vessels. In Schroeder SA and others, editors: *Current medical diagnosis and treatment*, Norwalk, Conn, 1991, Appleton & Lange.

The transplant coordinator assists this process by discussing requirements with the staff of the donor hospital and providing a list of needed instruments and supplies. The staff can collect these before arrival of the retrieval team (May and Adams, 1992). Often extra tables and round basins are needed, as well, for preparation and packaging of the organs prior to their transport back to the waiting recipient.

Ideally, heart and lung organs will have an ischemic time of less than 4 hours, although lungs may remain undamaged for a few hours longer (Kaiser and Cooper, 1992). To avoid unnecessary delay, which could produce ischemic injury, preparation for implantation of the organs should be completed before the arrival of the donor organ(s).

RECIPIENT PREPARATION

When the recovery team has been notified that a donor is available, the recipient is notified to prepare for surgery. Patients who have been discharged to their homes often carry a beeper so that they can be paged to come to the hospital; on arrival they are admitted and readied for the operation. Patients within the hospital are prepared for transport to the OR suite.

Once the procurement team has confirmed that the donor organ is acceptable, they will contact the recipient team and request transfer of the recipient patient into the OR where the surgery is to be performed. Recipient team members prepare the OR while the patient is being brought to the surgical waiting area. The circulating nurse will greet the patient and family and provide reassurance. Commonly, patients and family members who may be in attendance have mixed feelings—excitement and apprehension—about the upcoming procedure.

Venous and arterial lines will be started. A final review of preoperative protocols and laboratory test results will be performed. Lymphocyte and ABO blood group compatibility of the donor with the recipient will have been determined on testing of the donor organ. The patient may be positioned comfortably, covered with warm blankets, and lightly sedated before anesthesia induction (Sala, 1993).

Patients with ventricular assist devices (VADs) (see Chapter 17) will be transported to the OR with the functioning VAD. Only after confirmation of an acceptable donor organ will the VAD be removed.

HEART TRANSPLANTATION

Cardiac homotransplantation may be orthotopic or, less commonly, heterotopic. In the former the recipient heart is excised and replaced with a donor human heart. Heterotopic transplantation, the so-called piggyback procedure, is the insertion of a donor heart into the right pleural cavity; the donor acts as an auxilliary pump for the remaining native heart (see p. 395).

Xenotransplantation, replacing a human heart with the heart of another species (e.g., a chimpanzee or baboon), has been performed and continues to be investigated as a potential supply of donor organs. Although it caused a sensation, the use of a baboon heart in a neonate by Bailey and associates (1985, 1986, 1989) did demonstrate the technical feasibility of such a procedure and stimulated continuing investigations into the mechanism of rejection.

Approximately half of the patients undergoing cardiac transplantation have dilated cardiomyopathy (Table 18-1; Box 18-1), with generalized left ventricular dysfunction commonly of idiopathic or viral or-

Box 18-1   Comments concerning heart transplantation

Bruce A. Reitz, MD
Stanford University Medical Center
Stanford, California

Heart transplantation is now an accepted therapy that extends the lives of many patients suffering from end-stage heart disease. The procedure is now performed in more than 2000 patients each year in the United States and is limited simply by the number of available organ donors. The current success of heart transplantation in a number of centers has shown that the operative mortality for the procedure can be very low and equivalent to most routine cardiac procedures.

Most patients have a cardiomyopathy that is either due to coronary artery disease or is idiopathic. A number of patients with congenital heart disease, and particularly newborn babies with hypoplastic left heart syndrome,* are now considered good candidates for transplantation.

Since the timing of the procedure depends on the availability of a donor organ, these procedures may be done at any time of the night or day on an urgent basis. The conduct of the operation, including the cannulation, excision of the recipient's old heart, and implantation of the new heart, will be easily accomplished by a nurse with experience in other standard cardiac procedures. The surgeon's goal is to minimize the patient's time on cardiopulmonary bypass and the ischemic time of the donor organ. Furthermore, it is important to maintain strict sterile procedures, especially in handling the donor organ before bringing it to the operative field. Following implantation and cardiopulmonary bypass, meticulous attention to all of the suture lines to ensure hemostasis is essential.

*Hypoplastic left heart syndrome—underdevelopment of all or part of the left side of the heart and associated structures (e.g., left ventricle, aortic arch, aortic valve).

Box 18-2   Selection criteria

End-stage heart disease—prognosis of less than 6 to 12 months
New York Heart Association class III or IV
Unable to be treated by conventional medical or surgical therapy
Age criteria flexible—based on "physiologic age" rather than absolute chronologic age
Psychosocial stability

From Macdonald SN: Heart transplantation, part I. In Smith SL: *Tissue and organ transplantation: implications for professional nursing practice,* St Louis, 1990, Mosby.

igin. About 40% have end-stage heart disease due to coronary artery disease; the remainder have valvular heart disease, congenital disease, or myocarditis (Futterman and Lemberg, 1992; Heck, Shumway, and Kaye, 1989).

Patients frequently have signs of low cardiac output (forward failure), as well as pulmonary and hepatic congestion (backward failure). The ventricles become dilated and unable to eject an adequate right and/or left cardiac output. Although compensatory mechanisms may be adequate to provide a sufficient cardiac output during rest, cardiac output is inadequate during physical exertion or emotional stress. Reduced systemic perfusion can lead eventually to multisystem organ failure and death. Mechanical support devices (see Chapter 17) may be used in these patients to avert organ failure, which may become irreversible.

Selection criteria

Selection criteria (Box 18-2) are becoming more flexible in experienced transplant programs with long-

term success rates (Macdonald, 1990). Careful selection of patients older than 50 years of age—formerly a strict contraindication—has resulted in good outcomes with older recipients. Presently, physiologic, as well as chronologic, age is considered. However, age remains an area of controversy because of ethical considerations related to the scarcity of donor organs, increasing incidence of age-related diseases, and questions concerning extended long-term survival (Macdonald, 1990).

Transplant criteria also apply to patients who have had a VAD inserted as a bridge to transplantation. Although these patients may demonstrate significant improvement in their clinical status, their underlying disease remains an indication for transplantation.

Patient teaching

Patient teaching (Box 18-3) for heart transplant candidates is critical if the chronic immunosuppression and frequent follow-up care regimens are to be successfully integrated into the patient's life-style. Patients may focus on the transplant procedure alone and may not consider their life after transplantation. The ability to concentrate and remember what has been taught may be affected by low cardiac output. These factors make family involvement an important aspect of teaching (Dressler, 1992).

Procedural considerations

Orthotopic transplantation is the most frequent method of cardiac transplantation. As described by Lower and Shumway (1960), the procedure involves excision of the recipient's heart and replacement with a donor heart. Different setups are required for donor organ retrieval and recipient transplantation.

Organ retrieval teams will bring sterile containers for organ transport and any special instruments that may not be available at the organ recovery site. Cold cardioplegia and infusion tubing, along with any other solutions needed, are also transported. To save time, especially after the donor heart has been removed, the recovery team should bring only a minimum number of nondisposable items; this reduces the time that would be needed for cleaning these items before departure.

Implantation procedures are relatively straightforward, but certain considerations are important. The sterile setup should be ready in advance of the arrival of the donor organ. The period of ischemia includes implantation time and ends only after the cross-clamp has been removed and the new heart receives systemic blood flow. Any delay in preparing for surgery can jeopardize the myocardium. Extra-long suture (54 inches) and longer instruments may be useful for deep anastomoses of the left atrium. Immunosuppressive medications given in the OR should be available, along with blood and blood products (Table 18-2).

Operative procedure: orthotopic cardiac transplantation *(Holmquist and Gamberg, 1992; Waldhausen and Pierce, 1985)*

Retrieval of the donor heart

1. A median sternotomy is performed to expose the heart and great vessels.
2. The aorta, pulmonary artery, and venae cavae are dissected. The patient is heparinized.
3. The cavae are occluded, the left atrium is opened to decompress the ventricle, and the heart is rapidly cooled and arrested with cardioplegia solution.
4. The heart is removed by incising the left atrium circumferentially at the level of the pulmonary veins, incising the superior vena cava (SVC) and the inferior vena cava (IVC) (leaving the posterior wall of the right atrium), and severing the aorta and pulmonary artery.
5. The donor heart is placed into two or more sterile bags containing cold saline (or other preservation solution); the bags are placed in a cooler with ice and are immediately transported to the site where the heart will be inserted into the recipient.

Recipient preparation

1. A median sternotomy is performed to expose the heart and great vessels.
2. Bicaval cannulation for cardiopulmonary bypass (CPB) is performed, and a caval tape is placed around each cava. The suitability of the donor organ is confirmed before the procedure is continued.
3. The patient is cooled to the desired temperature, the recipient aorta is cross-clamped, and the caval tapes are tightened.
4. The pulmonary trunk and aorta are transected above their respective semilunar valves. The atria are incised to leave intact posterior portions of the right and left atrial walls, as well as the interatrial septum of the recipient.
5. The recipient heart is then excised.

Implantation of the donor heart

1. The donor heart is removed from the transport container and placed on the back table. The surgeon evaluates the heart and trims the atrial walls and great vessels in preparation for the anastomoses.
2. The donor heart is placed in the pericardial cavity and aligned with the interatrial septum, and the right and left atrial wall remnants of the recipient heart.
3. The donor left atrial wall (Fig. 18-1, *A* and *B*) is anastomosed with a running polypropylene suture. After completion of this anastomosis, cardioplegia solution may be infused retrogradely through the exposed coronary sinus in the right

Table 18-2 ■ *Standards of nursing care for heart and lung transplantation*

Nursing diagnosis	Patient outcome	Nursing actions
Anxiety/fear related to waiting for donor organ, uncertainty about prognosis, function of organ, and outcome of transplant	Recipient and family understand purpose of transplant and expected outcome so that anxiety/fear is reduced and coping abilities are enhanced	Discuss questions and concerns about disease and need for transplant Identify fears and address specific concerns Allow family interaction with patient to provide emotional support Address patient's/family's concerns about critical nature of patient's status/prognosis Keep patient/family informed about patient's status and organ availability
Knowledge deficit about disease, planned transplant surgery/retrieval, and perioperative events	Recipient demonstrates knowledge about physiologic and psychologic responses to disease and transplant	**Recipient:** Determine patient's understanding of cardiac/pulmonary disease, need for, and purpose of transplantation Encourage patient and family to ask questions about transplantation, anticipated life-style changes, need for immunosuppression, need for biopsy/endoscopy, infection, need for close medical supervision; explain/teach to patient's and family's level of understanding Verify recipient's understanding of need to be readily available if a donor is found; devise system to contact recipient at all times (e.g., beeper) Determine understanding of transplant complications: signs/symptoms of infection, rejection, organ failure, related diseases (e.g., CMV, CAD, pulmonary changes)
	Donor family demonstrates understanding of brain death and process of organ recovery	**Donor family:** Clarify "brain death" Explain organ retrieval procedure (as requested) If possible, describe disposition of donor organs
High risk for infection related to immunosuppression, compromised cardiac function	Patient is free of infection	Prepare donor organs with strict aseptic technique; have sterile containers to pack and transport organs Have separate sterile fields for organs Clean outside of transport case before entering recipient OR Have recovery team change into clean scrub clothes before entering recipient OR Control room traffic; have necessary supplies and equipment prepared before implantation procedure
High risk for injury related to: Positioning	Patient is free of injury related to: Positioning	Provide comfort measures (e.g., warm blanket, pillow, head of bed elevated) while awaiting verification from recovery team about organ Determine patient position prior to surgery (e.g., lateral position for single lung transplant, supine position for heart, heart-lung, double lung transplants); have positioning supplies/equipment available When moving patient with a VAD, use caution to avoid disrupting lines, cables, cannulas, etc.
Physical hazards:	Physical hazards:	**Care by donor recovery team:** Be prepared to respond immediately if contacted to retrieve organ(s); have necessary supplies collected and ready to go; collect additional items (such as those requiring refrigeration) Bring only supplies/instruments needed; keep cleaning requirements to minimum to avoid prolonging ischemic time Provide direction and guidance to staff from recovery hospital Provide list of instruments/supplies needed; bring special items unlikely to be found at recovery hospital (e.g., solutions, special staplers for pulmonary procedures) Assist with infusion or cardioplegia solution (heart) and/or lung perfusion, as requested

Modified from Seifert PC: Cardiac surgery. In Rothrock JC: Perioperative nursing care planning, St Louis, 1960, Mosby.
CAD, Coronary artery disease, CMV, cytomegalovirus; CVP, central venous pressure; ETA, estimated time of arrival; ICU, intensive care unit; IJ, internal jugular; LA, left atrium; OR, operating room; PA, pulmonary artery; TAH, total artificial heart; VAD, ventricular assist device.

Table 18-2 ■ *Standards of nursing care for heart and lung transplantation—cont'd*

Nursing diagnosis	Patient outcome	Nursing actions
High risk for injury related to—cont'd: Physical hazards—cont'd:	Patient is free of injury related to—cont'd: Physical hazards—cont'd:	**Care by donor recovery team—cont'd:** If multiple organ recovery is planned, be aware that most other organs are dissected free and the heart is excised first Avoid placing donor organs in direct contact with ice Be prepared to depart donor hospital as soon as possible after donor organ(s) have been excised; notify recipient hospital of ETA If donor and recipient are at same hospital, follow same procedures as above for excision and protection of heart, sterile setups, etc.; transport of organ from OR to OR may be similar to above (per surgeon's request) **Care of donor—staff of recovery hospital:** Prepare OR in advance of recovery team arrival; confirm that consents and other donor documents are in order Place warming blanket on OR bed (to avert cardiac irregularity or standstill from hypothermia) Collect instruments/supplies requested by recovery team; confirm with transplant coordinator or designate Have extra IV poles, portable overhead lights, small tables, basinware, ice, extra suction and cautery, and backup sternal saw and power source Provide brief orientation to recovery team: location of rooms, bathrooms, donor OR, scrub sinks, flash sterilizers, refrigerator (and coffee); familiarize with donor OR—tables, instruments, supplies, etc. Provide assistance with organ recovery **Care of recipient—recipient team:** Prepare patient/OR in advance of arrival of donor organ(s); coordinate with surgeon, anesthesiologist, and recovery team Place warming blanket on bed and activate Anticipate use of CVP (PA line may interfere with surgical site); plan for insertion of PA line after skin closure (as requested) Patient's sternum may be opened before arrival of donor organs (especially if recipient has had previous sternotomy) Cannulation for CPB may or may not be performed, depending on surgeon's preference; be prepared for double atrial cannulation (venous) and ascending aortic cannulation (arterial) for heart transplant; groin cannulation may be used for lung procedures requiring CPB Have long suture for (deep) anastomoses as requested (54-inch suture for example) Anticipate extensive venting procedures; have necessary venting catheters, tubing, etc. Anticipate meticulous hemostasis after each anastomosis; once areas of posterior dissection and anastomosis (e.g., LA) become obscured by anterior anastomoses, hemostasis is more difficult to achieve For lung procedures, have laparotomy instruments for omental pedicle flap(s), staplers, and fiberoptic bronchoscope to inspect lungs, suture lines Notify ICU when donor organ(s) is functioning Be alert for hyperacute rejection in OR; donor heart may have to be removed and replaced by TAH until new heart donor can be found
Foreign objects	Foreign objects	Inspect donor organs for tissue residue from preparation of donor organ (trimmings, etc.)

Continued.

Table 18-2 ■ *Standards of nursing care for heart and lung transplantation—cont'd*

Nursing diagnosis	Patient outcome	Nursing actions
High risk for altered fluid and electrolyte imbalance	Fluid and electrolyte balance is maintained	**Donor:** Have appropriate storage solution/perfusates (patients often have high potassium levels) **Recipient:** Have blood available; communicate with surgeon/blood bank about special orders (e.g., irradiated blood to decrease risk of disease transmission) Ensure that immunosuppressive drugs are available (per order) For single lung procedures, be prepared for CPB Be aware that chest drainage may not accurately reflect amount of blood in pericardium (due to enlarged pericardial cavity of recipient and donor heart smaller than excised native heart)
Risk for ineffective participation in rehabilitation due to not understanding or following prescribed regimens	Patient understands prescribed regimens and verbalizes effects on activities of daily living	Assess patient's/family's understanding of heart biopsy/bronchoscopy to assess organ function, signs of rejection; explain biopsy procedure: right IJ approach, local anesthesia (or anesthesia standby), small specimen excised from right ventricle Explain need for frequent cultures (throat, urine, blood, sputum, bronchial) and blood studies (white blood cell count, platelet count) Describe antibiotic prophylaxis prior to invasive procedures, dental work; need to avoid sick family members and friends; signs and symptoms of infection and/or rejection Elicit patient's/family's understanding of medications, diet, weight control, exercise, cessation of smoking, and other prescribed regimens; refer for cardiopulmonary rehabilitation Provide name(s) of contact persons for follow-up, questions, concerns

atrium (Icenogle, Emery, and Copeland, 1989; Menasche, 1993); or the heart may be kept cold with topical lavage.

4. The right atrial wall is anastomosed (Fig. 18-1, *C*) with a running polypropylene suture. After completion of the right and left atrial anastomoses, the atrial chambers are filled with cold saline to displace air and to maintain hypothermia.

5. The donor and recipient aortas are approximated and joined (Fig. 18-1, *D*), with care being taken not to injure the recipient aortic valve and coronary ostia. Warm cardioplegia solution is infused.

6. The left side of the heart is deaired, and the aortic clamp is removed. Rewarming is begun. The heart usually starts to beat spontaneously.

7. The donor pulmonary artery is occluded with a clamp. The left atrial suture line is inspected for hemostasis before the pulmonary arteries are joined.

8. The pulmonary arteries are anastomosed (Fig. 18-1, *E*), after which the pulmonary artery clamp is removed. (All anastomoses may be performed with the aortic clamp in place.)

9. If the heart is fibrillating, a single direct-current (DC) shock is usually sufficient for defibrillation.

10. Further deairing of the left ventricle is performed with an aortic needle vent and left ventricular apical aspiration. A recuperating period of up to 1 hour may be provided by maintaining CPB and allowing the heart to rest (particularly if ischemic time has been prolonged).

11. When the patient has been rewarmed, CPB is discontinued. Chest drainage tubes and temporary epicardial pacing wires are inserted, and the chest incision is closed. A pulmonary artery pressure catheter may be inserted for postoperative monitoring (Macdonald, 1990).

Heterotopic cardiac transplantation

Heterotopic (piggyback) transplantation is the insertion of a second heart into the right pleural cavity. The donor heart works in tandem with the recipient's native heart. It was originally performed by Carrel and Guthrie (1905), who transplanted a dog heart into the neck of a recipient dog with anastomoses to the recipient's carotid artery and jugular vein.

This type of transplantation has a limited role because the recipient's native heart function continues to deteriorate, producing symptomatic deterioration in the patient. Moreover, chronic anticoagulation, in addition to chronic immunosuppression, is required to prevent thromboembolism from originating in the dysfunctional native heart.

One indication for heterotopic transplantation is the presence of moderately elevated pulmonary vascular resistance in the recipient. Another indication is the size mismatch between a small donor heart and a large recipient. In the case of elevated pulmonary vas-

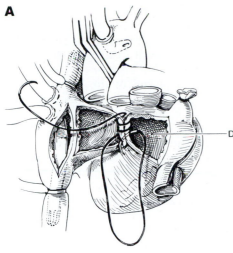

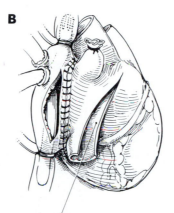

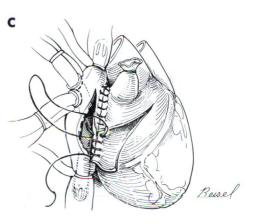

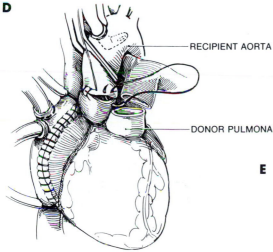

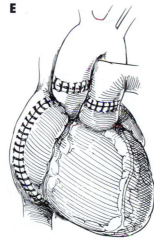

A

DONOR LEFT ATRIUM

B

DONOR RIGHT ATRIUM

C

Bessel

D

RECIPIENT AORTA

DONOR PULMONARY ARTERY

E

Fig. 18-1   Orthotopic cardiac transplantation. **A** and **B,** Anastomosis of the left atrial wall. **C,** Right atrial anastomosis. **D,** Aortic anastomosis. **E,** The pulmonary artery has been attached. (From Waldhausen JA, Pierce WS: *Johnson's surgery of the chest,* ed 5, St Louis, 1985, Mosby.)

cular pressure with a hypertrophied right ventricle, another procedure may be preferable to the heterotopic operation: the "domino" donor procedure whereby a heart-lung donor's organs are given to a patient with pulmonary disease and mild right ventricular hypertrophy (with no other abnormalities) secondary to the pulmonary hypertension. The excised heart from the heart-lung recipient is in turn implanted into a patient with elevated pulmonary vascular resistance requiring a cardiac transplant. The rationale is that implanting a heart with a normal right ventricular wall into a patient with elevated pulmonary pressures will cause the transplanted heart to fail before it can compensate by hypertrophy (Baumgartner, 1992).

Relative or absolute contraindications to heterotopic transplantation may include preoperative angina, a prosthetic valve, major ventricular dysrhythmias, and a previous cardiac operation. Fixed high pulmonary vascular resistance is an absolute contraindication to heterotopic transplantation. If pharmacologic reversal of pulmonary vascular resistance can be demonstrated, orthotopic transplantation may be considered (Baumgartner, 1992; Yacoub, Mankad, and Ledingham, 1990).

Donor recovery

Donor recovery is similar to that for orthotopic heart recovery, except that more tissue (e.g., SVC) is taken during recovery. A prosthetic graft is used to bridge the gap between one or both great vessels of the donor and recipient. Nursing considerations are similar to those for orthotopic transplantation.

Preparation of the heterotopic donor heart
(Novitsky, Cooper, and Barnard, 1983)

1. After excision of the arrested donor heart, the orifices of both right pulmonary veins and the IVC are closed with a continuous suture technique or a heavy tie (Fig. 18-2, *A*). Care is taken to avoid occluding the coronary sinus.
2. The bridge of tissue between the left superior and inferior pulmonary veins is excised to make a single opening into the left atrium.

Preparation of the recipient heart

1. After a median sternotomy and longitudinal opening of the pericardium, a right-sided pleuropericardial flap is created by dividing the pleura inferiorly and superiorly, taking care to avoid the phrenic nerve.
2. The patient is heparinized and cannulated for CPB. Venous cannulas are inserted into the IVC through a low atrial incision and into the SVC through the right atrial appendage in order to preserve the SVC for later anastomoses (Fig. 18-2, *A*).
3. CPB is instituted, and a left ventricular apical vent is introduced. The recipient heart is arrested with cardioplegia.

Implantation of the heterotopic heart
Left atrial anastomosis:
1. The recipient left atrium is incised longitudinally, posterior to the interatrial groove (as for mitral valve procedures).
2. The donor heart is placed in the right thoracic cavity anterior to the collapsed right lung and alongside the native heart.
3. The donor and recipient left atria are anastomosed with a continuous suture; this results in a common atrium from which blood can enter either the donor or recipient left ventricle (Fig. 18-2, *A* and *B*).
4. A second left ventricular venting catheter is inserted into the donor left ventricle.
5. If there is myocardial activity, cardioplegia can be infused through the donor ascending aorta.

Right atrial anastomosis:
6. Caval clamps or tourniquets are placed around the IVC and SVC.
7A. The donor SVC is anastomosed end-to-side (Fig. 18-2, *C*) to the recipient SVC (Waldhausen and Pierce, 1985), or
7B. An incision is made in the recipient SVC and right atrium, and the opening is widely anastomosed to the donor right atrium (Novitzky, Cooper, and Barnard, 1983).

Aortic anastomosis:
8. The lungs are temporarily inflated to determine the appropriate donor aorta length, and the donor vessel is trimmed to the desired length.
9. A partial-occlusion clamp is placed on the right side of the recipient aorta, and the donor aorta is anastomosed end-to-side to the recipient aorta (Fig. 18-2, *C*). Some surgeons may interpose a section of low-porosity graft material between aortas (Baumgartner, 1992). The previously placed aortic vent is activated, and the caval tapes are released.
10. The partial-occlusion clamp is released, and the donor heart is allowed to receive blood from the heart-lung machine.
11. A suction catheter can be placed in the donor pulmonary artery to aspirate blood.
12. Rewarming is begun.

Pulmonary artery anastomosis:
13. Because the donor pulmonary artery is usually not sufficiently long to reach the recipient artery without undue tension, a conduit (preclotted woven graft or allograft) is inserted.
14. The graft is anastomosed end-to-side to the recipient pulmonary artery and end-to-end to the donor pulmonary artery (Fig. 18-2, *C*).
15. As rewarming continues, both hearts are deaired. The donor heart may begin to beat spontaneously; if it fibrillates, one DC shock is usually sufficient to resume normal contractions.
16. Chest tubes and pacing wires are inserted, CPB is terminated, and hemostasis is achieved. Closure is similar to that for orthotopic transplantation.

A

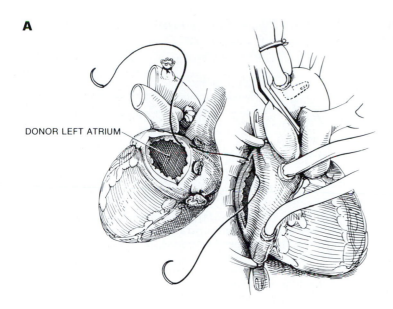

DONOR LEFT ATRIUM

B

C

Beisel

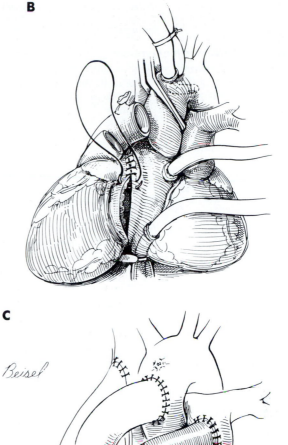

Fig. 18-2 Heterotopic cardiac transplantation. **A** and **B,** Left atrial anastomosis. **C,** A remnant of the donor SVC is anastomosed to the side of the recipient SVC. The donor ascending aorta and pulmonary artery are anastomosed end-to-side to their respective counterparts. A graft may be interposed between donor and recipient pulmonary arteries to provide additional length. (From Waldhausen JA, Pierce WS: *Johnson's surgery of the chest,* ed 5, St Louis, 1985, Mosby.)

Once cardiac activity resumes, blood flows preferentially into the heart with the least resistance (e.g., the chamber with the greater compliance). Ejection is asynchronous and depends on different heart rates. Electrocardiographic (ECG) complexes may be confusing because complexes from both hearts are superimposed on each other. It is important to determine the origin of dysrhythmias or ECG changes because, for example, premature ventricular beats may be expected in the diseased native heart but not in the donor heart, and ECG evidence of ischemia related to atherosclerotic changes in the donor heart (considered a form of chronic rejection) should be differentiated from that associated with the native organ. Supraventricular dysrhythmias are expected in the donor heart, and ventricular dysrhythmias are expected in the recipient heart. To distinguish between the two organs, separate telemetry systems are used for each heart (and the display screen is labeled according to the heart being monitored). The leads for the donor heart are positioned over the right chest wall to correspond with the location of the right and left donor ventricles, and the leads for the native heart are placed over the left chest wall (Rafalowski, 1991).

Postoperative care

Postoperatively the patient is taken to a private room in the surgical intensive care unit (ICU). Isolation practices vary, but strict isolation procedures have not been shown to be more beneficial than modified pro-

Table 18-3 ■ *Effects of denervation on the heart*

Normal	Denervation
Loss of Sympathetic Innervation	
Sympathetic fibers release norepinephrine and acetylcholine, leading to:	Without direct stimulation, response to stress and exercise depends on other mechanisms
Increased conduction through sinoatrial and atrioventricular nodes	Muscle activity increases venous return to heart, increasing cardiac output
Increased heart rate	Later, heart rate and cardiac output increase from circulating catecholamines
Increased stroke volume	There is delayed response to exercise
Immediate response to exercise	When preload is decreased, orthostatic hypotension occurs, resulting from a lack of compensatory increase in heart rate
Loss of Parasympathetic Innervation	
Parasympathetic fibers (including vagus nerve) inhibit conduction through atrioventricular node	Faster resting heart rate (usually 90 to 100 beats per minute) occurs
	Valsalva maneuver, carotid massage, and atropine have no effect on heart rate
Loss of Pain Receptors	
Angina is present during cardiac ischemia	There is no angina

From Dressler DK: The patient undergoing cardiac transplant surgery. In Guzzetta CE, Dossey BM: *Cardiovascular nursing: holistic practice*, St Louis, 1992, Mosby.

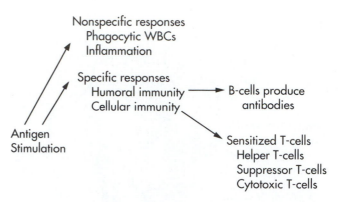

Fig. 18-3 Overview of the immune response. When confronted with a foreign substance, the immune system may respond through specific or nonspecific responses. Cellular immunity with the stimulation of small sensitized T-cells is thought to be the most important response in relation to transplant rejection. (From Dressler DK: The patient undergoing cardiac transplant surgery. In Guzzetta CE, Dossey BM: *Cardiovascular nursing: holistic practice*, St Louis, 1992, Mosby.)

tective isolation procedures consisting of gowns, masks, and careful handwashing (Dressler, 1992; Gamberg, Miller, and Lough, 1987). Centers for Disease Control (CDC) (1983) guidelines recommend private rooms, hand washing with antiseptic soap prior to patient contact, and the wearing of masks by persons with upper respiratory tract infections (Vaska, 1993).

Although a healthy donor heart is tolerant of ischemia, postoperative cardiac dysfunction is a common occurrence. Patients often require a combination of inotropic drugs and vasodilators for a few hours or days after surgery. Isoproterenol may be used to support the right ventricle of the donor heart. Heart failure may be aggravated by pulmonary hypertension due to pretransplant pulmonary dysfunction in the recipient, increased cardiac output ejected by the donor, reperfusion injury, and/or the adverse effects of CPB (see Chapter 11) during the transplant procedure. Drug therapy, adequate ventilation, and monitoring of blood gasses are all important considerations during postoperative care (Bahnson and others, 1991).

Another factor is the effect of severing the neural connections to the heart. Because sympathetic (e.g., adrenergic) and parasympathetic (e.g., vagus) nerves

are interrupted, the denervated heart (Table 18-3) must rely on noncardiac mediators to augment heart rate and contractility, to increase the cardiac output. Manipulation of volume (preload) and inotropic medications, as well as atrial pacing, may be necessary to maintain adequate stroke volume. Circulating, noncardiac catecholamines provide another means of increasing heart rate and contractility.

Chest pain receptors are also cut, resulting in an inability to feel angina pectoris. Studies (Stark, McGinn, and Wilson, 1991) have shown, however, that sensory afferent reinnervation of the donor heart can occur months after transplantation and is thought to be related to the reestablishment of sympathetic fibers and myocardial norepinephrine stores. These findings are significant because patients are at risk for accelerated coronary atherosclerosis, and anginal symptoms are an important warning signal.

Because right atrial tissue from both donor and recipient is present, the electrocardiogram (ECG) will show two P waves. Only the P wave of the donor heart will be conducted to the rest of the heart, because the impulse from the recipient's native atrial tissue is unable to cross the suture line (Augustine, 1990). Bradycardia and other dysrhythmias are not unusual after surgery and may be related to immunosuppression therapy, as well as to altered conduction pathways (Little and others, 1989). A number of patients may require a permanent pacemaker.

Bleeding may be another problem encountered postoperatively. Because the recipient pericardium is often enlarged, secondary to cardiomegaly, there is additional space between the pericardium and the smaller donor heart in which blood can accumulate without detection. Moreover, many patients are taking anticoagulants preoperatively (e.g., warfarin) to protect them from thromboembolism related to left ventricular dilatation and atrial fibrillation. Adhesions

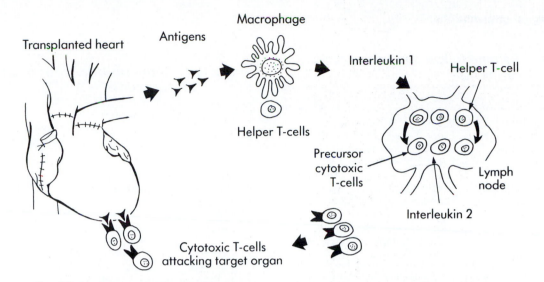

Fig. 18-4 Acute rejection process. Antigens on the transplanted cells are recognized as foreign by macrophages and precursors of helper T-cells. The interaction between these cells results in the release of IL-1, which causes helper T-cells to mature. The helper T-cells then interact with precursors of cytotoxic T-cells. Another hormone, IL-2, is released and promotes proliferation and maturation of the cytotoxic T-cells. These cells then circulate to the transplanted heart, combine with the antigens on the transplanted cells, and attempt to destroy the transplanted cells. (From Dressler DK: The patient undergoing cardiac transplant surgery. In Guzzetta CE, Dossey BM: *Cardiovascular nursing: holistic practice*, St Louis, 1992, Mosby.)

from previous surgery may cause increased bleeding, and liver dysfunction (from preoperative right-sided congestion) may impair coagulation processes. Homologous blood transfusions are avoided, when possible, to reduce the risk of disease transmission; autotransfusion is used whenever possible (Bahnson and others, 1991).

Rejection

Rejection of the transplanted heart remains a major threat to long-term survival. The basic problem is the specific and nonspecific responses of the recipient's immune system to foreign antigens (Fig. 18-3) (Futterman and Lemberg, 1992). The immunologic process that affects the donor heart can be hyperacute, acute, or chronic.

Hyperacute rejection occurs immediately after transplantation and becomes apparent in the OR. It is caused by a humoral response related to ABO incompatibility and a reactive lymphocyte crossmatch between recipient and donor. Platelet thrombi are deposited throughout the coronary arteries, and endothelial damage and interstitial hemorrhage are manifested. This produces global myocardial ischemia and cardiac failure (Macdonald, 1990). When hyperacute rejection occurs, the donor heart must be removed and replaced with a total artificial heart until another cardiac organ becomes available for transplantation.

Acute rejection (Fig. 18-4) commonly occurs within the first 3 months after transplant. It is activated by T-lymphocytes producing interstitial and perivascular mononuclear cell infiltration. If untreated, it progresses to cellular death (Macdonald, 1990).

Transvenous endomyocardial biopsy (Fig. 18-5) is performed to study the histologic changes character-

istic of acute rejection. Results should be correlated to the clinical picture because sampling errors can occur (e.g., tissue from scarred regions, tissue taken from an area free of rejection but surrounded or adjacent to an area of rejection) (Wingate, 1991).

Rejection is categorized as mild, moderate, severe, or resolving (or resolved). During the first few months postoperatively, biopsies may be performed weekly; after 3 to 6 months they may be done every 2 to 3

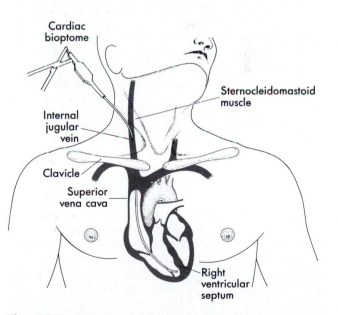

Fig. 18-5 Technique of endomyocardial biopsy. The bioptome is inserted through the right internal jugular vein. (From Macdonald SN, Naucke NA: Heart transplantation. In Smith SL: *Tissue and organ transplantation*, St Louis, 1990, Mosby.)

Table 18-4 ■ *Routine follow-up care for heart recipients*

Test	Frequency
Endomyocardial biopsy (more difficult with heterotopic trans- plantation)	Weekly for 4 weeks Every 2 weeks for 1 month Monthly for 3 months Every 3 months until 1 year Every 4 to 6 months indefinitely
Coronary angiography	Yearly
Complete blood count, chemistry panel	Monthly with clinic visits
Cyclosporine level	Monthly with clinic visits
Echocardiogram	Every 6 months
Chest x-ray study	Every 6 months

From Dressler DK: The patient undergoing cardiac transplant surgery. In Guzzetta CE, Dossey BM: *Cardiovascular nursing: holistic practice*, St Louis, 1992, Mosby.

months, and then quarterly after that. Clinical signs and symptoms of rejection warrant prompt biopsy. Noninvasive methods such as radionuclide testing and transesophageal and transsternal echocardiography are among the routine tests performed in patients (Table 18-4).

Immunosuppression and infection

Immunosuppression therapy is used to prevent or minimize rejection, but it increases the risk of opportunistic pathogens normally controlled by the body's immune system. Infection can occur anywhere, but the most common site is the lungs. Bacterial, viral, fungal, and parasitic organisms may be responsible (Vaska, 1993; Box 18-4).

Prevention is the best protection. Preoperatively donors are screened for transmissible diseases. Recipients are extubated within the first 24 hours if possible, and invasive lines and catheters are discontinued as soon as permissible (Box 18-5). Patients are also encouraged to ambulate soon after surgery to prevent pulmonary complications. Strict infection control practices, especially frequent hand washing, are important. Perioperative antibiotic treatment is standard; long-term prophylaxis may be used, but generally organism-specific drugs are preferred (Dressler, 1992).

Patient discharge teaching

Discharge planning (Box 18-6) focuses on assisting patients and families in coping with the short- and long-term effects of transplantation. A large amount of information is provided that requires repetition and reinforcement. New information should build on what is already known (Cifani and Vargo, 1990) and should take into consideration the psychologic makeup of the patient (Wingate, 1991). It is especially important that patients know about rejection, infection, drug complications, expected quality of life, and life-style recommendations (Dressler, 1992); this can be facilitated by making them part of an OR transplant "care team" (Lefrak, 1993).

Box 18-4 **Common infections in cardiac recipients**

Bacterial Infections
Early
Escherichia coli
Enterococci
Klebsiella organisms
Pseudomonas organisms
Serratia organisms
Staphylococcus organisms
Streptococcus organisms

Late
Legionella organisms
Listeria organisms
Mycobacterium organisms
Nocardia organisms
Salmonella organisms

Viral Infections
CMV, (cytomegalovirus)
Herpes simplex
Epstein-Barr virus
Varicella zoster virus

Fungal Infections
Aspergillus organisms
Cryptococcus organisms
Histoplasmosis
Coccidioidomycosis
Blastomycosis
Candida organisms

Parasitic Infections
Pneumocystis organisms
Toxoplasmosis

From Dressler DK: The patient undergoing cardiac transplant surgery. In Guzzetta CE, Dossey BM: *Cardiovascular nursing: holistic practice*, St Louis, 1992, Mosby.

HEART-LUNG TRANSPLANTATION

Patients with end-stage lung disease associated with severe right ventricular failure are candidates for heart-lung procedures (Box 18-7). The most common indications are primary pulmonary hypertension or Eisenmenger's syndrome. The latter is a condition in patients with atrial or ventricular septal defects who have pulmonary overloading, which leads to hypertension; eventually this causes reversal of the shunt from one that is left-to-right to one that is right-to-left, producing cyanosis (Bolman, 1991). Closure of the defect does not result in improvement when a severely elevated pulmonary vascular resistance poses too high an afterload for the right ventricle to overcome; heart-lung replacement is the only therapeutic option (Jamieson and others, 1984a).

With the development of improved lung transplantation techniques, a number of these patients may

Box 18-5 Infection

Assessment

Defining Characteristics

Presence of etiologic risk factors increasing patient's susceptibility to infection

Subjective
- Lethargy
- Weakness
- Chills
- Dyspnea
- Pain
- History of fevers

Objective
- Shortness of breath
- Cough/sputum production
- Crackles or wheezes
- Fever
- Abnormal laboratory values—elevated WBC, leukopenia
- Positive culture results
- Presence of lesions, invasive lines or tubes

Assessment Techniques

Assess wounds and line/tube insertion sites for signs or symptoms of infection: redness, swelling, drainage.

Obtain vital signs every 4 hours, particularly temperature.

Auscultate lungs for crackles/wheezes every 4 hours.

Obtain chest x-ray studies daily.

Monitor laboratory abnormalities.

Obtain cultures per order.

Interventions

Administer antimicrobial therapy as prescribed.

Institute protective isolation precautions.

Use good handwashing technique.

Discontinue invasive lines and tubes as soon as possible.

Maintain aseptic wound and invasive line care.

Report infection around wounds or lines.

Limit unnecessary procedures.

Report temperature elevations above 38° C or per specified parameters.

Employ aggressive pulmonary therapy as ordered.

Report laboratory abnormalities.

Report positive culture results.

Restrict visitors and health professionals with known infection or exposure to communicable disease.

Maintain optimal nutrition and hydration.

Teach patient and significant others: prevention, transmission, signs and symptoms of infection.

From Macdonald SN: Heart transplantation, part I. In Smith SL: *Tissue and organ transplantation: implications for professional nursing practice*, St Louis, 1990, Mosby.

Box 18-6 Discharge teaching plan for heart transplant patient

Prior to discharge the patient and family will:

Demonstrate accuracy related to self-administration of medications:
- Cyclosporine
- Azathioprine
- Prednisone
- Other prescribed medications

Verbalize information related to immunosuppressive drugs:
- Common side effects
- Timing of doses
- Laboratory measurement of cyclosporine levels
- Adequate supply of medication

Verbalize strategies to prevent infection:
- Avoidance of people with infection
- Careful dietary choices

Verbalize signs and symptoms of infection and when to call physician:
- Fever above 100° F
- Respiratory symptoms (e.g., cough and sore throat)
- Gastrointestinal symptoms
- Cutaneous lesions

Verbalize strategies to prevent rejection:
- Taking medication exactly as directed
- Notifying transplant team of change in medications
- Avoiding alcohol and over-the-counter drugs

Verbalize possible signs and symptoms of rejection:
- Hypotension
- Dysrhythmias
- Symptoms of congestive heart failure

Accurately record vital signs and weight daily:
- Record keeping
- Knowledge of acceptable parameters

Maintain body weight within normal parameters:
- Verbalize guidelines for low-cholesterol, no-added-salt diet
- Balance intake with activity

Demonstrate compliance with activity and exercise recommendations:
- Progressive cardiac rehabilitation
- Expectations regarding return to work and normal activities

Demonstrate an understanding of routine follow-up care:
- Laboratory work and office visits
- Endomyocardial biopsy schedule
- Yearly heart catheterization

Verbalize satisfaction with life-style after transplant:
- Management of emotional problems
- Daily stress management such as relaxation, music therapy, and imagery

From Dressler DK: The patient undergoing cardiac transplant surgery. In Guzzetta CE, Dossey BM: *Cardiovascular nursing: holistic practice*, St Louis, 1992, Mosby.

Box 18-7 *Comments regarding heart-lung transplantation*

Bruce A. Reitz, MD
Stanford University Medical Center
Stanford, California

Combined heart and lung transplantation was first successfully accomplished in 1981. Since that time more than 1000 patients worldwide have undergone the procedure. This demonstration of successful transplantation of lung tissue led to the ability to transplant single lungs and bilateral lung grafts. All of these procedures were made possible by the availability of better immunosuppression and monitoring techniques.

The goals of the surgeon in heart-lung transplantation are to minimize potential bleeding complications because of the extensive dissection required, to minimize pulmonary injury following transplant (through gentle handling of the lung and heart graft), and to minimize the ischemic time of the graft. Since the trachea of the donor and the trachea of the recipient are open during portions of the procedure, careful attention must be given to minimizing contamination from this potentially contaminated source.

With currently available preservation techniques and careful attention to surgical detail, the operative mortality after heart-lung transplantation has been significantly reduced and is now in the range of 5% to 10%. The ultimate success in patients is related more to the later control of rejection in the lung and to the prevention of chronic rejection changes such as obliterative bronchiolitis. Heart-lung transplantation has resulted in significant improvement in the quality and length of life in a number of otherwise desperately ill patients.

Box 18-8 *Specific donor criteria for heart-lung transplants*

No thoracic trauma (penetrating chest injury or lung contusion)
No history of pulmonary or cardiac disease (ECG normal)
No evidence of pulmonary or systemic infection
Insignificant smoking history
PaO_2 more than 90 mm Hg with FiO_2 0.40 and PEEP <5 cm H_2O
PaO_2 more than 350 mm Hg with FiO_2 1.0 and PEEP 0
Peak inspiratory pressure <20 cm H_2O with tidal volume 15 ml/kg and normal blood gases
Sputum negative for Gram stain and culture
Fiberoptic bronchoscopy (optional)
Chest measurements compatible with potential recipient
    Sternal notch to xiphoid
    Sternal notch to acromial process
    Chest circumference at fourth intercostal space (expiration)
    Chest circumference in maximum arch (expiration)
    Axilla to costal arch in midaxillary line
    Clavicle to costal arch in midclavicular line

From Ahrens TS, Powers C: Heart-lung transplantation. In Smith SL: *Tissue and organ transplantation: implications for professional nursing practice*, St Louis, 1990, Mosby.

---

benefit from single or double lung transplantation (see following section), especially if it is performed before irreversible right ventricular decompensation occurs. This technique allows distribution of organs to more candidates because the donor heart can be used in another patient requiring cardiac transplantation.

Donor criteria (Box 18-8) requiring both the heart and the lungs to be normal or satisfactory significantly impacts organ availability. The weight, height, and size of the chest should be similar for both the donor and the recipient; height tends to be a more reliable indicator of lung size than is weight (Bolman, 1991). Size matching is especially important between the donor lungs and recipient thorax, because lungs that are too large could produce cardiac tamponade when the sternum is closed; when this occurs, sternal closure may have to be delayed for a few days to allow reduction in the amount of pulmonary edema (Reichart, Vosloo, and Holl, 1990). Careful fluid management helps to prevent pulmonary overload and possible damage to the lungs.

Avoiding pulmonary infection related to endotra-

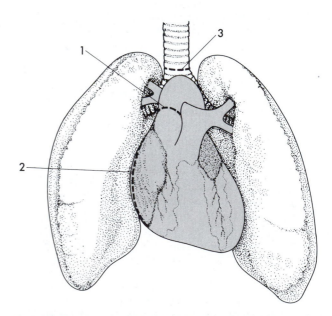

Fig. 18-6 Anastomotic sites in heart-lung transplantation. *1*, Aorta; *2*, right atrium; *3*, trachea. (From Ahrens TS, Powers C: Heart-lung transplantation. In Smith SL: *Tissue and organ transplantation*, St Louis, 1990, Mosby.)

cheal intubation preoperatively in the donor, or to spillage from the trachea during either retrieval or transplantation procedures, is another consideration in heart-lung procedures (Baldwin and Shumway, 1986). Often, trachial or bronchial stumps are closed with disposable stapling devices to prevent cross-contamination.

Recipient preparation varies from cardiac transplantation in that in addition to removal of the heart, removal of the diseased native lungs and insertion of the donor lungs must be done in such a way that the phrenic, vagus, and recurrent laryngeal nerves are not injured during dissection. Transection of the right and/or left phrenic nerves can cause unilateral or bilateral paralysis of the diaphragm; recurrent laryngeal nerve injury affects laryngeal motor function; and vagal interruption can cause, among other problems, severe gastrointestinal dysfunction and persistent diarrhea.

A three-anastomosis technique (Fig. 18-6) is used to ensure preservation of the donor's sinus node and the recipient's nerves. Additional supplies include staplers (TA30, TA55, TA90, depending on the surgeon's preference) for the bronchus/trachea. Instruments used to transect the airway are considered contaminated after use and should be passed off the field.

Operative procedure: heart-lung transplantation (Casale and Reitz, 1991; Holmquist and Gamberg, 1992; Jamieson and others, 1986b).

Organ retrieval

Excision of the donor organ is done only after careful inspection of the organs. Retrieval of the heart and lungs is accomplished through a median sternotomy, and the organs are usually removed separately (e.g., the heart is excised, and then each lung is separately removed).

Procedure
1. A median sternotomy is performed, and the heart is inspected; the pleural spaces are opened, and the lungs are inspected.
2. The anterior pericardium is excised.
3. The aorta is encircled with an umbilical tape and tagged with a hemostat.
4. The SVC, IVC, and innominate artery are dissected free. The azygos vein is doubly ligated and divided.
5. The trachea is encircled with a tape.
6. Heparin is administered via the right atrial appendage after the timing is coordinated with the other organ retrieval teams present.
7. Prostaglandin E_1 (a pulmonary dilator that enhances lung perfusion with preservative solutions) is administered prior to aortic cross-clamping.
8. The IVC is unclamped. The SVC is doubly ligated and divided, and the blood is allowed to empty from the head and upper body.
9. The aortic cross-clamp is applied, and cold cardioplegia solution is infused through the aortic root.
10. Lung preservation solution is infused through the pulmonary artery. The left atrial appendage is amputated to allow the returning pulmonary fluid to drain into the pericardium (rather than flow into the left ventricle, which could produce ventricular distension). Coronary drainage exists from the coronary sinus into the opened right atrium.
11. Topical hypothermic solutions are used to irrigate the heart and lungs.
12. After infusions are complete, the aorta is divided at the level of the innominate artery.
13. The heart and lungs are removed by dividing the posterior pleural reflections at the pulmonary ligament.
14. The trachea is clamped at least five rings above the carina while the lungs are kept inflated. The trachea is stapled (TA55) and excised above the staple line.
15. The heart and lungs are placed in a sterile basin on a separate table prepared with a sterile bag (or container) containing cold physiologic solution. This bag is placed in another container and prepared for transport as described under cardiac transplantation.

Recipient operation

Large bronchial collateral vessels in many recipients (especially those with Eisenmenger's syndrome), in association with the problem of providing adequate exposure to revise or repair completed anastomoses during implantation, make meticulous hemostasis a crucial factor in the recipient operation (Casale and Reitz, 1991).

Procedure.
1. A median sternotomy is performed, and the pleural cavities are entered by incising each pleura anterior to the pericardium. (Incising the pleura laterally could injure the phrenic nerves running along the lateral borders of the pericardium.)
2. The lungs are inspected and palpated. Existing adhesions are divided prior to the administration of heparin (to reduce bleeding).
3. The prepericardial fat and thymic remnants are excised. The pericardium is incised, and the great vessels are exposed. Tapes with tourniquets are placed around the IVC and SVC.
4. Heparin is administered.
5. A high aortic cannulation is performed to retain a sufficient collar for the aortic anastomosis to the donor heart. The SVC and the IVC are cannulated via the right atrium. The caval tapes are tightened to prevent entry of air (Fig. 18-7, *A*).
6. CPB is instituted, and the patient is cooled to 28° C (82.4° F).
7. The aorta is cross-clamped.

Heart:
8. The heart is removed in the manner described previously for cardiac transplantation.

Left lung:
9. The anterior left pericardium is excised longitudinally, leaving intact the pericardium containing the phrenic nerve.

A

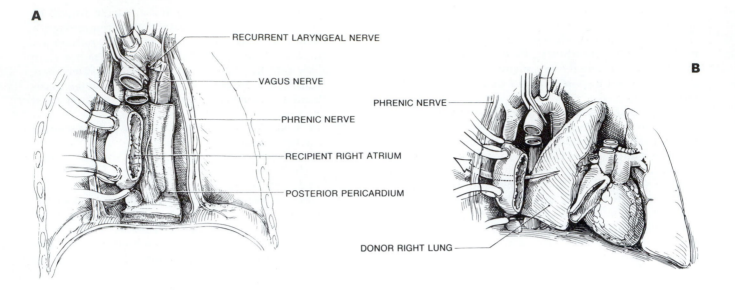

RECURRENT LARYNGEAL NERVE

VAGUS NERVE

PHRENIC NERVE

RECIPIENT RIGHT ATRIUM

POSTERIOR PERICARDIUM

B

PHRENIC NERVE

DONOR RIGHT LUNG

C

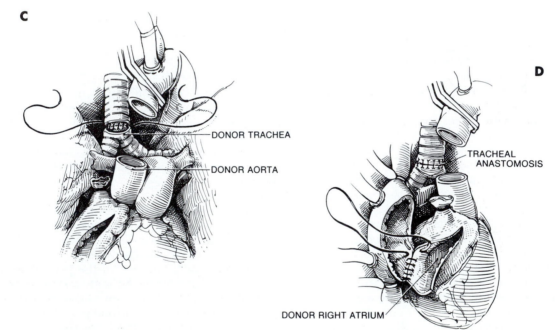

DONOR TRACHEA

DONOR AORTA

D

TRACHEAL ANASTOMOSIS

DONOR RIGHT ATRIUM

E

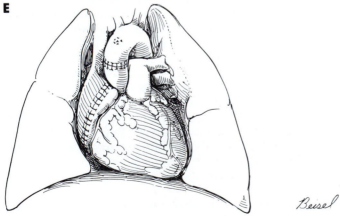

Beisel

Fig. 18-7 Heart-lung transplantation. **A,** The recipient heart and lungs have been excised, exposing the posterior pericardium. Note the location of the phrenic, vagus, and recurrent laryngeal nerves and the right and left phrenic nerve pedicles. **B,** The recipient heart and lungs are brought onto the field; the right lung is passed beneath the recipient atriocaval remnant and right phrenic nerve to lie in the right pleura; the left lung will be placed beneath the left phrenic nerve and positioned in the left pleural space. **C,** The tracheal anastomosis is performed, followed by **D,** the right atrial anastomosis, and finally, **E,** the aortic anastomosis. (From Waldhausen JA, Pierce WS: *Johnson's surgery of the chest,* ed 5, St Louis, 1985, Mosby.)

10. The left pericardium posterior to the left phrenic nerve is incised longitudinally anterior to the pulmonary veins and from the left pulmonary artery down to the diaphragm (Fig. 18-7, *A*).
11. The pulmonary veins and the right pulmonary artery are divided carefully to prevent injury to the vagus nerve situated in the posterior mediastinum and to the recurrent laryngeal nerve around the ductus ligament between the aorta and the pulmonary artery (Fig. 18-7, *A*).
12. The left main bronchus is exposed and transected with a stapler. Instruments used on the bronchus are passed off the field. Large bronchial arteries and collateral vessels may be found in this area; they are clipped or ligated.
13. The left lung is removed and placed in a basin off the sterile field.

Right lung:

14. A right phrenic nerve pedicle is created in a manner similar to the one for the left lung (see steps 9 and 10).
15. The right atrium is dissected free; the right pulmonary ligament is divided.
16. The right pulmonary artery is divided.
17. The right mainstem bronchus is transected with another stapler. The right lung is removed from the field, along with bronchus instruments.
18. After the recipient's native heart and lungs are removed, the posterior mediastinum and surrounding tissue are inspected carefully for bleeding sites, which are ligated, clipped, or cauterized.
19. The tracheobronchial junction (carina) is resected, leaving the surrounding tracheal blood supply intact to promote healing of the anastomosis.
20. The trachea is cut between two and four rings above the carina.

Implantation of the donor organs:

21. The donor heart and lungs are brought to the field, and the donor trachea is divided two rings above the carina.
22. The donor trachea is gently suctioned and cultured.
23. The organs are positioned by passing the right lung underneath the right phrenic pedicle, and the left lung under the left phrenic pedicle (Fig. 18-7, *B*).
24. The trachea may be further trimmed, and the anastomosis (Fig. 18-7, *C*) to the donor is performed first with a running 3-0 polypropylene suture (Jamieson and others, 1984a, 1984b). The heart and lungs may be protected with a continuous lavage of cold physiologic solution.
25. A venting catheter is placed in the left atrial appendage to remove air from the left side of the heart.
26. The right atrial anastomosis (Fig. 18-7, *D*) is also performed with a continuous 3-0 polypropylene suture.
27. The donor and recipient aortas (Fig. 18-7, *E*) are anastomosed end-to-end with a continuous 4-0 polypropylene suture. Topical lavage is discontinued, and rewarming is begun. Air is removed from the aorta and left side of the heart, and the cross-clamp is removed.
28. Caval tourniquets are removed, and ventilation is started. Venting catheters are taken out of the heart, and the entry sites are oversewn. CPB is terminated.
29. Temporary pacing wires and chest tubes are placed; hemostasis is achieved, and the sternum is closed.

Postoperative period

In addition to the problems associated with cardiac transplantation discussed previously, heart-lung recipients are also at risk for developing complications relating to the lung transplant (see following section). Perioperative complications include injury to major nerves, pulmonary edema, and tracheal or bronchial anastomotic dehiscence. The major late complication is bronchiolitis obliterans, a syndrome producing small airway obstruction. Chronic pulmonary rejection is thought to be the cause, but this has not yet been confirmed (Casale and Reitz, 1991).

LUNG TRANSPLANTATION

Experimental lung transplants were performed in the 1940s and 1950s, and the first human lung transplant was accomplished in 1963 by James Hardy in Mississippi (Runyon, 1990). Early poor results were attributed not only to poor patient selection, but also to ischemia and deterioration of the bronchial airway, rejection, and sepsis. Bronchovascular or bronchopleural fistulas developed, and the use of immunosuppressive therapy with prednisone and azathioprine was found to further retard healing of the bronchial anastomoses (Dickey, 1992).

With the substitution of cyclosporine for the steroids and the use of a circumferential omental pedicle flap to revascularize the bronchial anastomosis and prevent the formation of fistulas, survival improved significantly for investigators from the University of Toronto. They performed the first successful long-term single lung transplant in 1983 on a patient with end-stage pulmonary fibrosis (Toronto Lung Transplant Group, 1988).

Bilateral, en bloc lung transplantation was performed a few years later in a patient with end-stage emphysema caused by alpha$_1$-antitrypsin deficiency (Moberly, Trapp-Jackson, and Girard, 1992). Bilateral single lung transplantation with one lung from one donor and a second lung from another donor is also performed and is preferred to the double lung, en bloc procedure. Single lung transplantation can be performed without CPB and is currently favored over the technically more difficult double lung procedure; single lungs also provide another organ for another patient requiring transplantation (Egan, Kaiser, and Cooper, 1989). Selection criteria and evaluation of

> **Box 18-9 *Selection criteria for lung transplant recipients***
>
> I. End-stage lung disease with evidence of progression of disease and life expectancy < 12–18 months
> II. No other systemic disease
> III. No significant coronary artery disease
> IV. Demonstrated compliance with medical regimens
> V. No contraindication to immunosuppression
> VI. Psychologically stable; no history of alcohol or drug abuse
> VII. Must be ambulatory with O_2 as required
> VIII. Must *not* be on systemic steroids
> IX. Single lung transplant
>   A. Age ≤ 60 years
>   B. No chronic infectious lung disease such as chronic bronchitis, bronchiectasis, or cystic fibrosis
> X. Bilateral lung transplant
>   A. Age < 50 years
>
> From Kaiser LR, Cooper JD: The current status of lung transplantation. In Cameron J and others, editors: *Advances in surgery*, vol 25, St Louis, 1992, Mosby.

> **Box 18-10 *Lung transplantation inpatient evaluation***
>
> I. Pulmonary assessment
>   A. Pulmonary function tests
>   B. Ventilation: perfusion scan
>   C. Computed tomographic scan, when indicated
> II. Cardiac assessment
>   A. Radionuclide ventriculogram
>   B. Two-dimensional echocardiogram
>   C. Right heart catheterization, when indicated
>   D. Coronary angiography
>   1. All patients over 40 years of age
>   2. All bilateral lung candidates over 30 years of age
> III. Evaluation by social worker, psychologist
> IV. Assessment by physical therapist
>   A. Define exercise tolerance with O_2 saturation monitoring
>   1. 6-minute walk
>   2. Treadmill
>   3. Stair climbing
> V. Assessment by pulmonary rehabilitation
> VI. Assessment by dietitian
>
> From Kaiser LR, Cooper JD: The current status of lung transplantation. In Cameron J and others, editors: *Advances in surgery*, vol 25, St Louis, 1992, Mosby.

potential recipients are outlined in Boxes 18-9 and 18-10.

Present indications for the type of lung transplantation in patients with end-stage pulmonary disease depend on the predominant physiologic impairment. These can be classified as restrictive, obstructive, infective, or related mainly to increased pulmonary vascular resistance. Idiopathic pulmonary fibrosis is the most common restrictive disorder; obstructive lung disease is due mainly to chronic bronchitis and emphysema from smoking or alpha₁-antitrypsin deficiency. (The latter is an inherited deficiency in antitrypsin, which inhibits proteolytic enzymes from damaging and destroying alveoli and pulmonary parenchyma; increased circulating levels of the destructive enzymes create emphysematous changes that eventually impair gas exchange. Patients undergoing double lung transplantation often have obstructive disease, but single lung procedures have been performed successfully [Kaiser and Cooper, 1992]).

Infectious lung disease requiring transplantation is often related to cystic fibrosis, which fosters frequent episodes of infection and leads to destruction of lung tissue. Single lung transplantation is contraindicated because of widespread bacterial colonization of the airways. Heart-lung transplantation has been performed in these patients, even if the recipient's heart is functioning adequately. Yacoub, Mankad, and Ledingham (1990) and Cavarocchi and Badellino (1988) have used the "domino procedure" whereby the cystic fibrosis patient receives the heart-lung and donates his or her heart to another. Patients with shunts producing volume overloading (Eisenmenger's syn-

drome) may have heart-lung transplants but may also be considered for single lung transplants and correction of the defect producing the shunt.

Another form of domino replacement has been applied to patients requiring pulmonary transplantation. In a case described by Shumway (1992), a 46-year-old mother donated her right upper lobe to her 12-year-old daughter, whose right lung had been pneumonectomized as a result of bronchopulmonary dysplasia secondary to prolonged oxygen ventilation in the neonatal period. This use of living, related donors of pulmonary organs may widen the potential donor pool. Individual lobes can be dissected free relatively easily (as compared with the liver), and success with renal grafts from living, related donors has supported the concept.

Procedural considerations

For both single and bilateral lung transplants, the retrieval team reviews the chest x-ray films to determine the size and condition of the lungs. Evidence of infiltrates, aspiration, or consolidation would make a donor unacceptable (Box 18-11). Adequate gas exchange is confirmed by arterial blood gas analysis. If the arterial oxygen saturation declines over time, the donor lung may not be suitable. A flexible fiberoptic bronchoscopy is performed, and specimens are taken for culture and Gram stain. (Gram stain results can be used to guide antibiotic therapy in the recipient.) The final assessment of the donor lungs is direct inspection after both pleural spaces have been opened (Kaiser and Cooper, 1992).

Patients with head injuries due to motor vehicle trauma provide a significant number of potential donors, but associated blunt chest trauma causing pulmonary contusion can contraindicate use of the lungs. Ideally, retrieval time is no more than 4 to 6 hours; when multiple organ procurement is performed or retrieval sites are a great distance, close coordination is mandatory to maintain an ischemic time of less than 6 hours. Flying time (one way) may be limited to under 2½ hours (Kaiser and Cooper, 1992).

For single lung transplants, CPB is available on a standby basis; the groin is prepared and draped for cannulation if needed (Sala, 1993). If CPB is not used, heparinization can be avoided. In certain patient populations (e.g., those with pulmonary fibrosis) receiving a single lung, 25% of the recipients required CPB (Low and Cooper, 1991). Strict aseptic technique is used for endotracheal intubation and nasogastric tube insertion. For bilateral lung transplants, CPB is routinely used.

If an omental pedicle flap is used, abdominal instruments will be required. This flap will be brought up to the chest and wrapped around the airway anastomoses. Staplers are used to close and transect the airways (e.g., trachea, bronchi). A fiberoptic bronchoscope may be needed for examining the airways and lungs (Kaiser and Cooper, 1992; Moberly, Trapp-Jackson, and Girard, 1992).

Operative procedure: lung organ retrieval
(Calhoon and others, 1991; Kaiser and Cooper, 1992; Low and Cooper, 1991)

If the donor heart is to be used for transplantation, cardiectomy is performed before the lung(s) is removed.

Procedure
1. A left atrial incision is made, leaving an adequate cuff for both the heart and the lung(s) (Fig. 18-8).
2. Prostaglandin E_1 is injected intravenously, and cold electrolyte solution is flushed through the inflated lungs via the pulmonary artery. Cold lavage may be used in the pleural spaces.
3. The left atrial appendage is amputated or cannulated to allow returning flush solution to exit the heart (the rationale for this is the same as it is for heart-lung procedures, described previously). The right side of the heart is vented by transecting the IVC. The aorta is then clamped (and cardioplegia solution is infused).

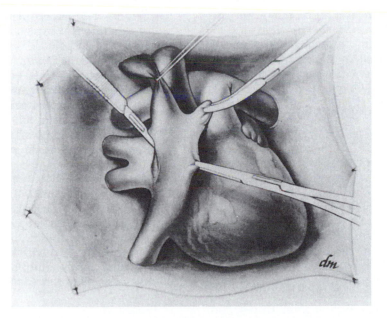

Fig. 18-8 Development of the interatrial groove provides sufficient atrial cuff for both cardiac and pulmonary transplantation. (From Egan TM, Kaiser LR, Cooper JD: Lung transplantation, *Curr Probl Surg* 25:680, 1989.)

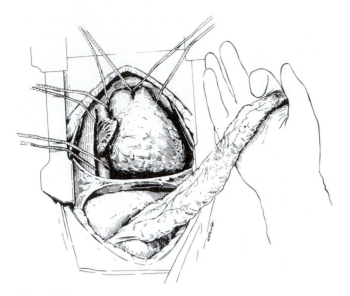

Fig. 18-9 The omentum is mobilized after the sternotomy incision has been extended. Creation of the omental pedicle may also be performed through a small laparotomy prior to median sternotomy or lateral thoracotomy. Umbilical tapes have been passed around the IVC, SVC, aorta, and pulmonary artery. (From Egan TM, Kaiser LR, Cooper JD: *Lung transplantation, Curr Probl Surg* 25:680, 1989.)

4. After flushing has been completed, the pulmonary artery is divided at the bifurcation.
5. The bronchus is dissected and divided between staple lines. (Stapling the bronchus prevents flooding of the lungs by the transport solution and reduces the risk of infectious matter spilling into the lungs.)
6. One lung (or both lungs) is removed; it remains connected by the left atrial cuff and the pulmonary artery.
7. The organ is immersed in cold solution and packed for transport. The lung(s) can be used either for single lung transplant(s) or for bilateral or sequential lung procedures.

Operative procedure: single lung transplantation

Recipient preparation:

1. Approximately 1 hour before arrival of the donor lung, arterial and pulmonary pressure lines are inserted, and the patient is anesthetized and intubated with a double-lumen tube.
2. For single lung transplants, the patient is positioned laterally with the affected side up; the position is maintained for the entire procedure.
3. The chest, abdomen, and both groins are prepared and draped (usually the contralateral groin is used if CPB is necessary).
4. When the omentum is used, a small upper midline laparotomy is made to mobilize the pedicle (Fig. 18-9), which is tunneled beneath the sternum or subxiphoid region for subsequent re-

trieval. If there is time before arrival of the donor lung, the laparotomy incision may be closed.

5. A lateral thoracotomy incision is made, and the recipient pulmonary artery, veins, and mainstem bronchus are dissected free. The pericardium is opened around the pulmonary veins.
6. To determine if the patient can withstand lung transplantation without CPB, the pulmonary artery is occluded for about 5 minutes to test the patient's response. If CPB is deemed necessary, it is instituted after arrival of the donor organ.
7. Once the donor lung has arrived and is found to be acceptable, the recipient lung is excised.
8. The recipient pulmonary artery is occluded and transected just beyond the first bifurcation.
9. A long-handled, partial-occlusion clamp (e.g., a Statinsky clamp) is placed on the left atrium adjacent to the pulmonary veins. The tissue between the venous orifices is removed to form one larger opening.
10. The bronchus is transected just before its bifurcation. The endotracheal tube to the affected bronchus is used to occlude the bronchial orifice.
11. The bronchial arteries are cauterized.

Implantation of the donor lung:

12. The donor lung is brought to the field and oriented into the chest. The pulmonary vein cuff of the left atrium is anastomosed to the native left atrial cuff with a continuous suture of 4-0 polypropylene (Fig. 18-10).
13. The bronchi are anastomosed end-to-end with a running polypropylene suture technique. The omental pedicle is placed around the bronchial anastomosis and loosely secured (Fig. 18-11). It should be noted that many surgeons do not use the omentum technique.
14. The pulmonary artery is connected with a continuous 4-0 polypropylene suture. Just before the suture line is completed, the left atrium and pulmonary veins are deaired with a small-gauge (18-gauge) needle. The pulmonary artery is reaired, and the suture line is completed.
15. The lung is inflated and placed on 10 cm of water positive end-expiratory pressure (PEEP) to prevent severe pulmonary edema secondary to inflammatory changes that can occur on reperfusion of the revascularized lung.

Operative procedure: bilateral lung transplantation (Kaiser and Cooper, 1992)

Donor retrieval is similar to that for single lung recovery. Each lung is removed from the donor after left atrial incision and transection of the pulmonary arteries and the bronchi. The en bloc procedure is infrequently performed; bilateral single lung transplants or sequential single lung transplants are more common.

Procedure

1. A median sternotomy is made, and pleuropericardial windows are created in a manner that protects the recipient's phrenic nerves (Figs. 18-12

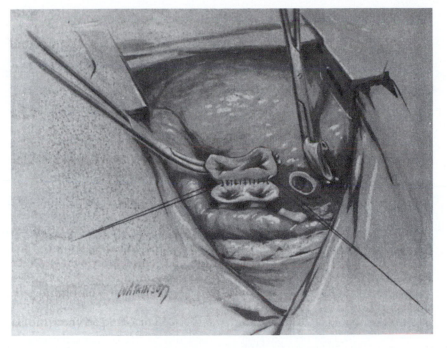

Fig. 18-10   Anastomosis of donor and recipient left atria; the bronchus is occluded with an inflated balloon. (From Egan TM, Kaiser LR, Cooper JD: Lung transplantation, Curr Probl Surg 25:680, 1989.)

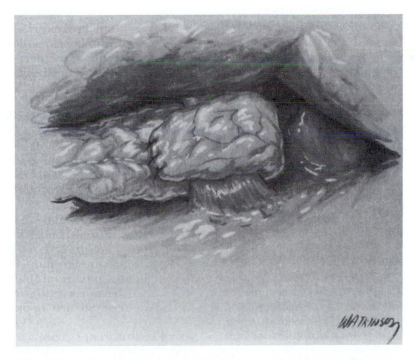

Fig. 18-11   After completion of the bronchial anastomosis, the omental pedicle is wrapped around the anastomosis and secured loosely. (From Egan TM, Kaiser LR, Cooper JD: Lung transplantation, *Curr Probl Surg* 25:680, 1989.)

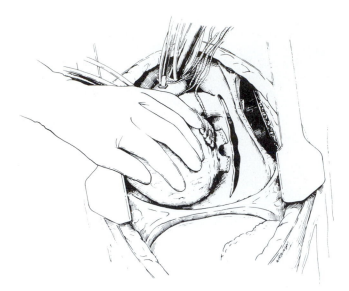

Fig. 18-12 A left pleuropericardial window is created posterior to the phrenic nerve and exposes the pulmonary veins. (From Egan TM, Kaiser LR, Cooper JD: Lung transplantation, *Curr Probl Surg* 25:680, 1989.)

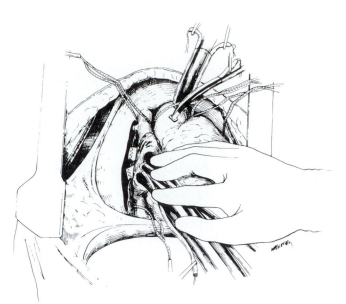

Fig. 18-13 The right pleuropericardial window is created posterior to the right phrenic nerve and near the exit site of the right pulmonary veins. The azygous vein is divided to enlarge the window. (From Egan TM, Kaiser LR, Cooper JD: Lung transplantation, *Curr Probl Surg* 25:680, 1989.)

and 18-13). The patient is prepared for CPB.
2. CPB is initiated.
3. The pulmonary veins are stapled closed to prevent air from entering the left side of the heart and systemically embolizing. The recipient lungs are excised.
4. The donor lungs are passed into their respective pleural cavity through the pleuropericardial opening.
5. The donor bronchi are positioned in the posterior mediastinum and anastomosed to the recipient bronchi.
6. On completion of the anastomoses, the aorta is cross-clamped, cardioplegia solution is infused retrogradely (or antegradely), and the heart is arrested.
7. The left atrial and pulmonary artery anastomoses are completed. The left atrium and ventricle are deaired, and the cross-clamp is removed to perfuse the heart.

Completion of the procedures

After the skin incision(s) is closed, the double-lumen endotracheal tube is removed and replaced with a single-lumen tube. Immunosuppression (methylprednisolone) begins in the operating room (Calhoon and others, 1991). Cyclosporine will be started after gastrointestinal function returns. After dressings are applied, the patient is covered with a warm blanket (Dickey, 1992).

Postoperative period

The transplanted lung is susceptible to fluid overload. This may be due to a number of causes. Reperfusion

edema may be the result of hypothermia and CPB (if used), as well as intraoperative ischemia; it may be affected by the disruption of pulmonary lymphatics and increased extravascular water accompanying implantation. In patients who have undergone CPB, bleeding may be a problem; and suboptimal myocardial preservation may cause postoperative left ventricular dysfunction. Oximetry and arterial and pulmonary pressures are monitored continuously; cardiac output and mixed venous saturation are measured intermittently (Kaiser and Cooper, 1992; Todd, 1990). Continuous cardiac output may be used.

Patients are sedated and ventilated for approximately 48 hours and then extubated when the lung(s) is working well. Patients may have a prolonged ileus, necessitating nasogastric tube suctioning and intravenous total parenteral nutrition. Chest physiotherapy is started while the patient is intubated. Ambulation is started as early as possible.

Immunosuppression consists of cyclosporine, azathioprine, and prednisone. Monoclonal antibodies (OKT-3), successfully used for heart transplant patients, have not shown a benefit in lung transplant patients and are associated with development of cytomegalovirus (CMV) infections (Calhoon and others, 1991). Bacterial infections are common but are generally not lethal (Maurer, 1990).

Methylprednisone is used to treat episodes of rejection. Acute rejection is common, with two or three episodes often occurring within the first month. Rejection is manifested by temperature elevation (which may be slight), deterioration of gas exchange as evidenced by decreased exercise tolerance, and infiltrates (seen on chest x-ray films).

Obliterative bronchiolitis is a complication in lung transplant patients, as well as heart-lung recipients. The incidence of airway necrosis has decreased, and bronchial stenosis may require insertion of Silastic stents. Infectious complications, especially those related to CMV, continue to be a problem (Low and Cooper, 1991).

Follow-up care includes frequent blood tests to monitor immunosuppression levels and blood counts. Exercise testing, pulmonary function studies, and arterial blood gases are also used, especially in anticipation of the onset of bronchiolitis obliterans. "Colds" or other illnesses persisting for more than a few days warrant prompt investigation. Cardiac and pulmonary function are evaluated every 3 months (or more) the first year, and every 6 months after that (Maurer, 1990).

CONCLUSION

Despite the advances made in all forms of transplantation, donor organ shortages have limited the widespread use of transplantation techniques. Methods to optimize the efficient utilization of available organs is reflected in the variety of combinations used for heart-lung, single lung, and bilateral lung replacement procedures. Nurses and other health care professionals can help these efforts by engaging in educational activities for the community and professional colleagues, and by participating in the identification of potential donors. Future efforts will be aimed at overcoming problems associated with xenotransplantation, refining immunosuppression therapy, and gaining greater insights into the mechanisms of rejection.

REFERENCES

Ahrens TS, Powers C: Heart-lung transplantation. In Smith SL: *AACN tissue and organ transplantation: implications for professional nursing practice,* St Louis, 1990, Mosby.

Augustine SM: Nursing care of the heart and heart-lung transplant patient. In Baumgartner WA, Reitz BA, Achuff SC, editors: *Heart and heart-lung transplantation,* Philadelphia, 1990, WB Saunders.

Bahnson HT and others: Management of complications related to cardiac transplantations. In Waldhausen JA, Orringer MB: *Complications in cardiothoracic surgery,* St Louis, 1991, Mosby.

Bailey LL and others: Baboon-to-human cardiac zenotransplantation in a neonate, *JAMA* 254:3321, 1985.

Bailey LL and others: Method of heart transplantation for treatment of hypoplastic left heart syndrome, *J Thorac Cardiovasc Surg* 92(1):1, 1986.

Bailey NA, Lay P, Loma Linda University Infant Heart Transplant Group: New horizons: infant cardiac transplantation, *Heart Lung* 18(2):172, 1989.

Baldwin JC, Shumway N: Cardiac and cardiopulmonary homotransplants. In Sabiston DC, editor: *Textbook of surgery,* ed 13, Philadelphia, 1986, WB Saunders.

Barnard CN: A human cardiac transplant: an interim report of a successful operation performed at Groote Schuur Hospital, Cape Town, *S Afr Med J* 41:1271, 1967.

Baumgartner WA: Heterotopic transplantation: is it a viable alternative? *Ann Thorac Surg* 54:401, 1992.

Bidagare SA, Oermann MH: Attitudes and knowledge of nurses regarding organ procurement, *Heart Lung* 20(1):20, 1991.

Bolman RM: Cardiac and cardiopulmonary homotransplants. In Sabiston DC, editor: *Textbook of surgery,* ed 14, Philadelphia, 1991, WB Saunders.

Boychuk JE, Malen JF: Lung transplantation. In Smith SL: *AACN tissue and organ transplantation: implications for professional nursing practice,* St Louis, 1990, Mosby.

Cabrol C: Presidential address, *J Heart Lung Transplant* 11(4, pt 1):595, 1992a.

Cabrol C: Special recognition award to Richard Lower, *J Heart Lung Transplant* 11(4, pt 1):597, 1992b.

Calhoon JH and others: Single lung transplantation: alternative indications and technique, *J Thorac Cardiovasc Surg* 101:816, 1991.

Carrel A, Guthrie CC: The transplantation of veins and organs, *Am Med* 10:1101, 1905.

Casale AS, Reitz BA: Management of complications in transplantation: heart-lung. In Waldhausen JA, Orringer MB: *Complications in cardiothoracic surgery,* St Louis, 1991, Mosby.

Cavarocchi NC, Badellino M: Heart/heart-lung transplantation: the domino procedure, *Ann Thorac Surg* 48:130, 1988.

Centers for Disease Control (CDC): Guidelines, section 4. Modification of isolation precautions, *Infect Control* 4:155, 1983.

Cifani L, Vargo R: Research review: teaching strategies for the transplant recipient: a review and future directions, *Focus Crit Care* 17(6):476, 1990.

Darby JM and others: Approach to management of the heart-beating brain-dead organ donor, *JAMA* 261:2222, 1989.

Dickey D: Transplantation for end-stage lung disease: a nurse's perspective, *Todays OR Nurse* 14(2):6, 1992.

Dressler DK: The patient undergoing cardiac transplant surgery. In Guzzetta CE, Dossey BM: *Cardiovascular nursing: holistic practice,* St Louis, 1992, Mosby.

Dubois P, Chiniere L, Cooper JD: Bronchial omentopexy in canine lung allotransplantation, *Ann Thorac Surg* 38:11, 1984.

Egan TM, Kaiser LR, Cooper JD: Lung transplantation, *Curr Probl Surg* 26(10):680, 1989.

Futterman LG, Lemberg L: Cardiac transplantation: update, *Am J Crit Care* 1(2):118, 1992.

Gamberg P, Miller JL, Lough ME: Impact of protective isolation on the incidence of infection after heart transplantation, *J Heart Transplant* 6(3):147, 1987.

Grady KL and others: Symptom distress in cardiac transplant patients, *Heart Lung* 21(5):434, 1992.

Guinn NJ: Organ procurement in the community hospital, *Todays OR Nurse* 10(2):10, 1988.

Heck CF, Shumway SJ, Kaye MP: Sixth Official Report: The Registry of the International Society for Heart Transplantation—1989, *J Heart Transplant* 8(4):272, 1989.

Holmquist T, Gamberg PL: Heart and heart-lung transplantation, *Todays OR Nurse* 14(2):12, 1992.

Horowitz MD and others: Donor cardiectomy for other transplant centers, *J Heart Lung Transplant* 11(4, pt 1):683, 1992.

House MA, Benitez N: Multiple organ retrieval: impact on staff and institutions, *Semin Periop Nurs* 1(1):51, 1992.

Icenogle TB, Emery RW, Copeland JG: Donor operation—myocardial protection: current and future practice. In Wallwork J, editor: *Heart and heart-lung transplantation,* Philadelphia, 1989, WB Saunders.

Jamieson SW and others: Heart and lung transplantation for pulmonary hypertension, *Am J Surg* 147:740, 1984a.

Jamieson SW and others: Operative technique for heart-lung transplantation, *J Thorac Cardiovasc Surg* 87(6):930, 1984b.

Kaiser LR, Cooper JD: The current status of lung transplantation, *Adv Surg* 25:259, 1992.

Kiberd MC, Kiberd BA: Nursing attitudes towards organ donation, procurement, and transplantation, *Heart Lung* 21(2):106, 1992.

Kirklin JW, Barratt-Boyes BG: *Cardiac surgery,* ed 2, New York, 1993, Churchill Livingston.

Kubler-Ross E: *On death and dying*, New York, 1969, Macmillan.

Lefrak EA: Personal communication, 1993.

Lima O and others: Effects of methylprednisone and azothioprine on bronchial healing following lung autotransplantation, *J Thorac Cardiovasc Surg* 82(2):211, 1981.

Little RE and others: Arrhythmias after orthotopic cardiac transplantation, *Circulation* 80(5, suppl III):111-140, 1989.

Low DE, Cooper JD: Lung transplantation. In Sabiston DC, editor: *Textbook of surgery*, ed 14, Philadelphia, 1991, WB Saunders.

Lower RR, Shumway NE: Studies on orthotopic homotransplantation of the canine heart, *Surg Forum* 11:18, 1960.

Macdonald SN: Heart transplantation. In Smith SL: *Tissue and organ transplantation: implications for professional nursing practice*, St Louis, 1990, Mosby.

Mackensie RC, Bronsther OL, Shackford SR: Organ procurement in patients with fatal head injuries, *Ann Surg* 213:143, 1991.

Maurer JR: Therapeutic challenges following lung transplantation, *Clin Chest Med* 11(2):279, 1990.

May D, Adams RH: Management and administration of the operating room during transplantation, *Semin Periop Nurs* 1(1):3, 1992.

Menasche P: Coronary sinus retroperfusion for myocardial protection: pragmatic observations and caveats based on a large experience. In Karp RB, editor: *Advances in cardiac surgery*, vol 4, St Louis, 1993, Mosby.

Moberly DL, Trapp-Jackson K, Girard NJ: Single-lung transplantation for alpha 1-antitrypsin deficiency, *Semin Periop Nurs* 1(1):25, 1992.

Nolan MT and others: Perceived stress and coping strategies among families of cardiac transplant candidates during the organ waiting period, *Heart Lung* 21(6):540, 1992.

Novitsky D, Cooper DKC, Barnard CN: The surgical technique of heterotopic heart transplantation, *Ann Thorac Surg* 36(4):476, 1983.

Pelletier ML: The needs of family members of organ and tissue donors, *Heart Lung* 22(2):151, 1993.

Rafalowski M: The heterotopic heart transplant patient: cardiac monitoring challenges, *Crit Care Nurse* 11(2):28, 1991.

Reichart B, Vosloo S, Holl J: Surgical management of heart-lung transplantation, *Ann Thorac Surg* 49:333, 1990.

Reitz BA, Pennock JL, Shumway NE: Simplified operative method of heart and lung transplantation, *J Surg Res* 31:3, 1981.

Runyon VD: Single lung transplantation: new treatment for end-stage pulmonary disease, *AORN J* 51(3):694, 1990.

Sala P: Simultaneous transplantation, *Todays OR Nurse* 15(2):23, 1993.

Sammons BH: Opinion: organ recovery coordinators can help family work through the grieving process, *AORN J* 48(6):1181, 1988.

Schaeffer P: "Decoupling" improves organ donation rates, *Kardia* 4:7, fall 1993.

Shumway NE: *Transplantation of the heart and heart-lungs*. Paper presented at the Fifth Annual Symposium, Cardiac Surgery: 1993, St Thomas, US Virgin Islands, Nov 14, 1992.

Smith SE, Brumm J, Crim BJ: A donation to life: organ procurement, *Todays OR Nurse* 13(12):2, 1991.

Stark RP, McGinn AL, Wilson RF: Chest pain in cardiac-transplant recipients: evidence of sensory reinnervation after cardiac transplantation, *N Engl J Med* 324(25):1791, 1991.

Todd TRJ: Early postoperative management following lung transplantation, *Clin Chest Med* 11(2):259, 1990.

Toronto Lung Transplant Group: Experience with single-lung transplantation for pulmonary fibrosis, *JAMA* 259:2258, 1988.

Waldhausen JA, Pierce WA: *Johnson's surgery of the chest*, ed 5, St Louis, 1985, Mosby.

Wiberg CA and others: Multiorgan donor procurement, *AORN J* 44(6):936, 1986.

Wingate S: Cardiac transplantation. In Wingate S, editor: *Cardiac nursing: a clinical management and patient care resource*, Gaithersburg, Md, 1991, Aspen.

Yacoub M, Mankad P, Ledingham S: Donor procurement and surgical techniques for cardiac transplantation, *Semin Thorac Cardiovasc Surg* 2(2):153, 1990.

Vaska PL: Common infections in heart transplant patients, *Am J Crit Care* 2(2):145, 1993.

19

Surgery for Cardiac Dysrhythmias

The heart is always marching, unless it misses signals from its conductor.

John Stone, MD, 1990

Disorders affecting the electrical activity of the heart produce changes in the rate or rhythm of cardiac impulses. These disorders are commonly divided into those affecting impulse formation, those affecting impulse conduction, or a combination of the two (Zipes, 1992). Originally, treatment for these disturbances was transvenous or open thoracotomy insertion of pacemakers in patients with symptomatic, excessively slow heart rates (bradycardia). These early pacemakers generated an electrical stimulus at a fixed number of impulses per minute in order to increase the heart rate and improve cardiac output. In the late 1960s operations involving conduction tissue and surrounding structures were devised.

Corrective surgery on the heart itself for underlying dysrhythmias was introduced in 1968 when Sealy and his associates (Cobb and others, 1968) surgically divided an abnormal conduction pathway that was producing an excessively fast heart rate (tachycardia) in a patient with Wolff-Parkinson-White (WPW) syndrome. Since then, greater understanding of the anatomic and electrophysiologic principles of the conduction system, combined with the development of electrophysiologic diagnostic capabilities, has led to the creation of sophisticated devices and procedures to modulate the heart rate, terminate dysrhythmias, or remove (or isolate) the origin of the dysrhythmia.

CONDUCTION SYSTEM

The action of contraction and relaxation reflects the heart's conversion of electrical stimulation into mechanical work. The resulting pumping activity is performed in a regular pattern and at a sufficient rate to optimize cardiac output for the individual's hemodynamic needs (Hoops-Nast, 1986). Disturbances in the initiation, rate, rhythm, or conduction of the electrical impulses that stimulate the myocardium can alter contractility, making the pumping action of the heart less efficient and tissue perfusion inadequate (Feeney, 1992). Ventricular fibrillation, for example, is considered a lethal dysrhythmia because the uncoordinated impulses being discharged in the ventricle produce an unorganized ventricular contraction that is ineffectual in ejecting blood (Berne and Levy, 1992). However, minor rhythm disturbances are common, and those that do not interfere with cardiac output and are not life-threatening may not require treatment (Spittle, 1991). The severity of the dysrhythmia is determined by its effect on cardiac output and the clinical status of the patient.

Automatic and rhythmic beating of the heart begins early in embryonic life. During cardiogenesis two types of cardiac tissue develop: contractile cells of the myocardium that can respond to a stimulus and pacemaker cells capable of spontaneously initiating an electrical impulse that will stimulate myocardial cells to contract (Hoops-Nast, 1986). Although all normal cardiac tissue is excitable (able to respond to an electrical stimulus), only pacemaker cells are capable normally of initiating the impulse without an outside stimulus (automaticity). When a cardiac impulse (also known as the action potential) is generated, the heart's inherent conductivity allows it to be transmitted to other areas of the heart (Marriott and Conover, 1989) (Box 19-1).

To understand why and how surgery and other invasive techniques are used to treat dysrhythmias, it is helpful to review how electrical impulses are normally generated and transmitted from the atria to the ventricles through the network of cells and fibers that make up the conduction system.

CONDUCTION OF ELECTRICAL IMPULSES

The conduction system comprises the sinoatrial (SA) node, internodal pathways, the atrioventricular (AV) junction, the bundle of His and its right and left

Box 19-1 *Glossary of terms*

Aberrancy   Temporary, abnormal intraventricular conduction of a supraventricular impulse (e.g., a premature atrial beat conducted to the ventricle).

Accessory pathway   Extramuscular tract between the atrium and the ventricle, outside the normal conduction tract, that is capable of conducting an impulse, either antegrade or retrograde; seen in Wolff-Parkinson-White (WPW) syndrome.

Action potential   Generation and transmission of an electrical impulse through the cell. It is a precise and rapid sequence of changes in the movement of transmembrane ionic currents (mainly sodium, calcium, and potassium) that represents the electrical cardiac cycle. It consists of five phases: phases 0 to 3 make up electrical systole, and phase 4 makes up electrical diastole.

Phase 0   Depolarization; the electrical gradient changes rapidly from -90 mV to $+20$ mV as sodium rapidly enters the cell (fast sodium channels). Because it is a significant change, it appears on the electrocardiogram (ECG).

Phase 1   Initial rapid repolarization of the cell caused by an exodus of potassium from the cell.

Phase 2   Plateau of the action potential; results from the influx of calcium and sodium (slow channels).

Phase 3   Terminal rapid repolarization phase that begins with closing of the slow channels. It is completed by the passive movement of potassium out of the cell and the active transport of sodium out of the cell by the sodium pump. During this phase, the electrical gradient (transmembrane potential) is returned to -90 mV. Because this is a major electrical change, it is evident on the ECG. Activation can be initiated during this phase with a lessor stimulus than is required at maximal repolarization.

Phase 4   Electrical diastole; the resting phase of the electrical cardiac cycle; the interval between action potentials.

Fast-response action potential   Action potential produced when all of the fast sodium channels are available for depolarization. This results in rapid upstroke velocity, maximal amplitude for phase 0, and consequent optimal conduction velocity.

Slow-response action potential   Action potential produced when none of the fast sodium channels is available for depolarization and only slow sodium-calcium channels are available to depolarize the fiber; the action potential has a slow upstroke velocity, low amplitude, and consequent slow conduction.

Automaticity   Capability of a cell to depolarize spontaneously, reach threshold potential, and initiate an action potential. Characteristic of pacemaker cells.

Altered automaticity   Ability of cells, not normally possessing the property of automaticity, to depolarize automatically.

Enhanced normal automaticity   Rapid automatic activity caused by steepening of phase 4 depolarization in pacemaker cells; can occur with excess catecholamines, especially in the presence of ischemia.

Circus movement tachycardia   Any reentry tachycardia; generally reserved for atrioventricular (AV) reentry using an accessory pathway and the AV node.

Conductivity   Ability of cardiac cells to receive an electrical stimulus and transmit it to other cells.

Depolarization   Reduction of a membrane potential to a less negative value.

Ectopy   Cardiac dysrhythmia caused by initiation of an excitation impulse at a site other than the sinus node; may occur in healthy and diseased hearts at a site of irritated myocardium.

Excitability   Ability of a cardiac cell to respond to an electrical stimulus; irritability.

Preexcitation   Activation of part of the ventricular myocardium earlier than would be expected if the activating impulses traveled only down the normal routes.

Reentry   Reactivation of a tissue for the second or subsequent time by the same impulse.

Refractory period   Period during which the cell (or fiber) is unable to respond normally to a stimulus because it has been too recently activated by a previous stimulus. During the *effective* refractory period, no stimulus can evoke a response; during the *relative* refractory period, a strong stimulus can evoke a response, but conduction velocity may be reduced through the AV node.

Repolarization   Restoration of the cell's resting membrane potential; occurs between phase 1 and the end of phase 3 of the action potential.

Resting membrane potential   Electrical gradient that exists between the inside and the outside of a myocardial cell at rest.

Rhythmicity   Ability of the heart to contract with regularity.

Threshold potential   Transmembrane potential (electrical gradient) that must be achieved before an action potential can be initiated.

Triggered activity   Rhythmic activity that results when a series of after-depolarizations reach threshold potential; can be induced by digitalis.

Modified from Marriott HJL, Conover MB: *Advanced concepts in arrhythmias*, ed 2, St Louis, 1989, Mosby.

branches, and the Purkinje fibers (Goldenbeger, 1990). In the healthy heart these impulses travel from right to left and from head to toe (Thelan, Davie, and Urden, 1990). The electrocardiogram (ECG) provides a pictorial record of this electrical activity by registering potential changes in the electrical field of the heart (Fig. 19-1). The ECG does not record this electrical activity directly (that would require the placement of

an electrode into the cell itself), nor does it represent the mechanical activity of the heart.

Sinoatrial Node

Impulses originate in the SA node (see Chapter 4 on anatomy and physiology), a mass of neuromuscular tissue lying between the entrance of the superior vena

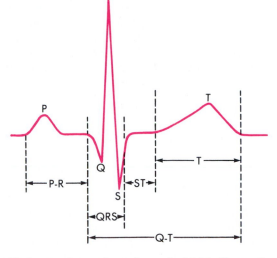

Fig. 19-1 Configuration of a typical ECG, illustrating important deflections and intervals. (From Berne RM, Levy MN: *Cardiovascular physiology,* ed 6, St Louis, 1992, Mosby.)

cava and the right atrium in the sulcus terminalis. The SA node receives its blood supply from the sinus node artery arising from the right coronary artery or, less commonly, from the left coronary artery. (Ischemic injury due to obstructive lesions in the coronary artery supplying the SA node can cause nodal dysfunction.)

Electrophysiologic mapping of the right atrium has demonstrated a number of sites within the area of the SA node that can initiate impulses spontaneously. Collectively, these sites serve as an atrial pacemaker complex (Berne and Levy, 1992). Two types of cells have been identified. P-cells within the center of a pacemaker site initiate the action potential, and surrounding T-cells conduct the impulse to atrial tissue. Because the SA node generates impulses at a faster rate (approximately 60 to 100 times per minute) than other neuromuscular tissues of the heart, it excites other potential pacemakers before they can reach the threshold necessary to spontaneously depolarize themselves and initiate an impulse (Mandel, 1987). As a result, the SA node suppresses the automatic generation of impulses by other (potential) pacemaker sites, such as the AV junction (which has an intrinsic rate of approximately 40 to 60 impulses per minute) and the ventricular fibers (approximately 20 to 40 impulses per minute). Because of the higher rate of impulse formation, the normal SA node acts as the primary pacemaker of the heart and the main controller of the heart rate (Berne and Levy, 1992). Conversely, when the sinus node does not generate impulses at a sufficiently rapid rate, it does not suppress latent pacemakers. One or more of these may reach threshold and depolarize to take over the function of primary pacemaker.

From the atrial pacemaker complex the impulse is conducted to the AV junction. There is some controversy as to whether these impulses travel through his-

tologically discrete pathways or through plain atrial myocardium whose fiber orientation, size, and chamber geometry promote rapid conduction (Zipes, 1992). For example, impulses traveling down fibers parallel to the long axis of the heart (the normal direction of the impulse) have a greater velocity than impulses moving through fibers running perpendicular to the direction of the impulse. (The effect of fiber orientation on impulse conduction is termed anistrophy.)

Anatomic studies have been interpreted to show that there are preferential pathways that consist of three neuromuscular bands forming specific conduction tracts: the anterior, middle, and posterior internodal pathways (Goldenberger, 1990). A branch of the anterior pathway, Bachmann's bundle, is thought to transmit the impulse to the left atrium. According to this theory, the greatest conduction velocity between the sinus node and the AV junction occurs along the posterior internodal tract. However, autonomic nervous system stimuli, along with those factors just described, may contribute to the speed with which the impulse is transmitted to the AV junction.

Atrioventricular Junction

The AV node, situated between the atria and the ventricles, is now understood to comprise three regions: (1) the atrionodal (AN) region, located between the atrium and the anatomic AV node; (2) the nodal (N) region (corresponding to the AV node), located posteriorly on the right side of the interatrial septum near the coronary sinus; and (3) the nodal-His (NH) region, situated between the N region and the bundle of His. Collectively these three regions, along with the bundle of His, are called the AV junction. Cardiac rhythms formerly classified as "nodal" are now more appropriately considered "junctional." Blood flow to the AV junction is received from the right coronary artery in most persons (Goldenberger, 1990).

Recent investigations have shown that the N region does not contain true pacemaker cells from which junctional rhythms arise. Rather, impulses originate from the AN or NH region, or from the bundle of His. When the sinus node fails to act as the primary pacemaker, pacemaker cells within the AN or NH region take over this function, but at the slower rate of 40 to 60 impulses per minute.

What is physiologically and clinically significant about the AV node itself is the reduction in the velocity of the impulse that occurs in this area. This is due to the fibrotic nature of the tissue, which, unlike faster conducting myocardial cells, impedes the speed of the impulse. (Conduction is also delayed in the AN region, but this is attributed to the longer distance of this region rather than to an actual slowing of velocity such as that occurring in the N region.) This delay (seen on the ECG between the P wave and the QRS complex) allows the atria to contract and the ventricles to fill. This delay also protects the ventricle when there are excessively rapid atrial impulses. Without the delay, too many of these impulses would be conducted to the ventricles, producing excessive contractions and limiting ventricular filling. In the normal heart, the AV node allows only one third to one half of these excessive, rapid atrial impulses to traverse the junctional region (Berne and Levy, 1992).

Accessory pathways

In most persons AV junctional tissue and the bundle of His provide the only pathway for impulses traveling from the atrium to the ventricles. In some persons alternative routes (accessory pathways) exist between the atria and the ventricles that can allow impulses to travel not only in a forward normal (antegrade) fashion, but also in a backward (retrograde) or circular direction. These accessory pathways are thought to be the result of a developmental failure to interrupt the AV myocardial continuity present in the primitive heart and are related to gestational development.

During the early stages of development there is a discrete ring of muscle fibers surrounding the AV junction. This ring becomes fibrotic, thereby slowing conduction velocity between the upper and lower cardiac chambers. When the continuity of some fibers fails to be divided, one or more pathways remain, in addition to the AV node and bundle of His, through which an impulse can pass from atria to ventricles. Often these conduct faster than the AV node because they are made up of working myocardium, which offers less resistance to the impulse than AV nodal tissue. These accessory pathways may be responsible for conducting impulses that can prematurely excite the ventricles (preexcitation) and produce lethal dysrhythmias. Some impulses may be delayed in one of the pathways and reenter the circuit, thereby self-perpetuating the impulse (see subsequent section on reentry). Catheter ablation using direct electrical current or radiofrequency waves, cryosurgery, or direct severing of these accessory pathways can be performed. Patients with the WPW syndrome, the most common form of preexcitation, frequently benefit from these interventions (Marriott and Conover, 1989).

Ventricular Conduction

Cells in the NH region gradually merge with the bundle of His, which forms the upper portion of the ventricular conduction system. The bundle is situated along the right side and the top of the ventricular septum (near the septal leaflet of the tricupsid valve). It then divides into a right bundle and a left bundle. The right bundle follows the right side of the septum. The left bundle penetrates the septum and further divides into an anterior and a posterior division, or fascicle; there may be a third fascicle supplying the midseptum (Marriott and Conover, 1989). Right or left bundle-branch block occurs when transmission is delayed or interrupted in the respective main bundle branch; left anterior or left posterior hemiblock refers to conduction blocks within the respective left bundle branches (fascicles).

The right bundle branch and the left bundle branches subdivide into the Purkinje fibers, which penetrate the subendocardium of each ventricle. Conduction is most rapid through the Purkinje system, allowing rapid activation of the ventricles. The Purkinje system also plays a protective role in limiting the number of atrial impulses that can stimulate ventricular contraction. It can accomplish this because the Purkinje fibers have a long refractory period during which they will not respond to further excitation. Consequently, they will not normally allow premature contractions of the ventricles. When there are accessory pathways or other AV connections that bypass the AV node, rapidly firing impulses can be transmitted to the ventricles, producing ventricular tachycardia. Transmission of the impulses over the ventricles begins with the right and left endocardial surface of the interventricular septum (except the basal portion) and the papillary muscles. (Early papillary muscle contraction helps to tether the mitral and tricuspid valve leaflets so that they do not evert into their respective atria during ventricular systole.)

The impulse rapidly spreads along the endocardial surface of both ventricles. It spreads less rapidly from endocardiucm to epicardium, especially in a hypertrophied left ventricular wall. The basal epicardial and septal regions are activated last (Berne and Levy, 1992).

Factors Influencing the Initiation or Conduction of Impulses

In addition to intrinsic disturbances of cardiac tissue, electrical events can be modified by chamber geometry (such as left ventricular hypertrophy or atrial septal defect), autonomic nervous system influences, hemodynamics, and blood flow, wall motion changes, electrolyte abnormalities, drugs, surgical trauma and edema, and ischemic heart disease.

Both sympathetic (adrenergic) and parasympathetic fibers of the autonomic system can modify the generation and transmission of impulses. The sympathetic system directly affects both atria and ventricles by stimulating an increase in the rate and conduction of impulse and augmenting the force of atrial and ventricular contractions. It also increases the excitability of the heart. The parasympathetic system has little control over the ventricles, but the vagus branches do influence the sinus node and the AV junction by causing a reduction in the rate of discharge from the SA node, decreasing the excitability of the AV junctional fibers, and further slowing conduction through the AV node (Gary and Guzzetta, 1991). Increased heart rates are usually the result of decreased vagus tone (e.g., as can be produced pharmacologically with atropine) rather than increased sympathetic activity (Goldenberger, 1990).

It is likely that the autonomic nervous system may have competitive effects on cardiac rhythm. For example, sympathetic stimuli may be antidysrhythmic by improving contractility and coronary blood flow in a failing heart; however, the increase in myocardial oxygen demand accompanying increased contractility in a heart with ischemic coronary artery disease may promote the development of cardiac dysrhythmias. The effects of sympathetic stimulation may explain why anxiety and psychologic stress can be significant factors in the onset of ventricular fibrillation (Zipes, 1989). An awareness of this interaction provides an important rationale for providing emotional support and comfort measures in the anxious patient.

The electrophysiologic effects of coronary ischemia can be especially deleterious because inadequate blood flow alters regional myocardial pH, potassium and other electrolyte levels, and the concentration of metabolic end-products. Infarction or ischemic injury to conducting tissue alters the ability to generate or conduct impulses and is responsible for a number of supraventricular and ventricular dysrhythmias. Surgical interruption or pharmacologic blockade of efferent sympathetic responses can be used to control the dysrhythmias.

Surgery can produce direct trauma or tissue injury (such as edema) leading to temporary (or permanent) conduction blocks. Surgery on the tricuspid valve, repairs of congenital anomalies involving the atrial septum, and other operations in areas containing conduction tissue pose a risk of injury. The surgical division of accessory pathways may also produce conduction blocks.

Although the nervous system does affect heart rate and contractility, intact nervous pathways are not required for the heart to function, as cardiac transplant patients with denervated hearts have demonstrated. This is because the heart is capable of initiating its own impulse, responding to that impulse, and doing so with regularity. These reflect, respectively, the characteristics of automaticity, excitability, and rhythmicity (see Box 19-1).

CATEGORIZING DYSRHYTHMIAS

Categorizing rhythm disturbances is complicated by the variety of classification systems available: major dysrhythmias (that require treatment) and minor dysrhythmias (that may not); bradydysrhythmias (slow heart rates) and tachydysrhythmias (fast heart rates); and disorders of impulse formation and impulse conduction. Or, dysrhythmias may be classified according to the sites from which they originate (Goldenberger, 1990). Regardless of the system used, abnormal electrophysiologic mechanisms, such as altered automaticity, triggering, and reentry (see Box 19-1), are often responsible for many dysrhythmias.

Altered Automaticity

Altered automaticity is caused either by enhancement of normal automaticity or by the development of abnormal automaticity in both pacemaker cells and nonpacemaker cells as a result of certain disease states (Conover, 1992). Enhanced automaticity may develop in the sinus node or His-Purkinje fibers. For example,

sympathetic nervous system activity with increased catecholamine release can alter sinus node automaticity to produce sinus tachycardia. Such stimulation can be related to strong emotions, such as fear or anxiety, or to emotional tension. Additional factors include exercise, fever, anemia, hyperthyroidism, myocardial disease, or anoxia. Medications such as atropine, isoproterenol, or epinephrine may also enhance automaticity (Gary and Guzzetta, 1992). Excessive vagal tone may depress automaticity and produce sinus bradycardia. Depressed sinus function can also allow lower centers, such as the bundle of His, to fire impulses faster and thereby usurp the sinus node as the primary pacemaker (Marriott, 1991).

Abnormal automaticity producing dysrhythmias occurs in working atrial or ventricular myocardium, as well as pacemaker, cells. A declining membrane potential enables the cell membrane to reach threshold prematurely, resulting in a spontaneous depolarization. Often this is related to disease or metabolic derangements such as ischemia, infarction, cardiomyopathy, hypokalemia, or hypocalcemia (Conover, 1992).

Triggered Activity

Triggered activity is another disorder of impulse formation producing dysrhythmias. Triggered impulses are those that are repetitively fired during or after the repolarization phase of an ectopic cell. If the cell reaches threshold potential during the period when the calcium or sodium channels are activated, it can be "triggered" to depolarize (again) spontaneously. Excess digitalis or catecholamines are often the cause of this mechanism; other factors include ischemia, increased ventricular wall tension (e.g., from the pressure overload of aortic stenosis), and heart failure (Conover, 1992).

Reentry

The reentry mechanism (Fig. 19-2) is responsible for sustaining the majority of ventricular dysrhythmias, such as ventricular tachycardia, and supraventricular dysrhythmias, such as supraventricular tachycardia, atrial flutter, and atrial fibrillation (Kutalek and Michelson, 1991a). Reentry occurs when a cardiac impulse restimulates a portion of the heart that has already been stimulated. Three conditions are necessary: an additional circuit (e.g., an accessory pathway), unequal responsiveness in the limbs of the circuit, and slow conduction (Marriott, 1991). For example, a descending impulse enters two limbs of a circuit: the normal AV route and an accessory pathway. When one limb has recovered while the other remains refractory, the refractory limb prevents passage of the impulse when it first approaches; the wave front will travel only down the responsive limb. (If both limbs were still refractory, the impulse would be arrested; if both limbs had recovered, the impulse would have continued. In either case, reentry could not occur.)

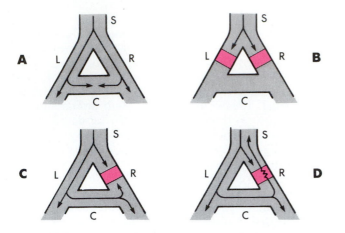

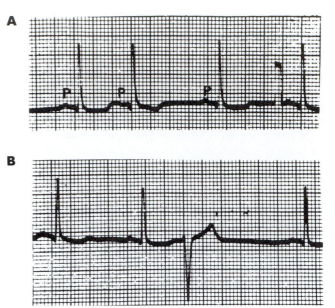

Fig. 19-2 Reentry and the role of unidirectional block. **A,** An excitation wave traveling down a single bundle *(S)* of fibers continues down the left *(L)* and right *(R)* branches. The depolarization wave enters the connecting branch *(C)* from both ends and is extinguished at the zone of collision. **B,** The wave is blocked in branches *L* and *R*. **C,** Bidirectional block exists in branch *R*. **D,** Unidirectional block exists in branch *R*. The antegrade impulse is blocked, but the retrograde impulse is conducted through and reenters bundle *S* (see text). (From Berne RM, Levy MN: *Cardiovascular physiology*, ed 6, St Louis, 1992, Mosby.)

Fig. 19-3 **A,** Premature atrial depolarization and **B,** premature ventricular depolarization. The premature atrial depolarization (the second beat in the top tracing) is characterized by an inverted P wave and normal QRS and T waves. The interval following the premature depolarization is not much longer than the usual interval between beats. The brief rectangular deflection just before the last depolarization is a standardization signal. The premature ventricular depolarization, **B,** is characterized by bizarre QRS and T waves and is followed by a compensatory pause. (From Berne RM, Levy MN: *Cardiovascular physiology*, ed 6, St Louis, 1992, Mosby.)

When the wave front reaches the distal end of the refractory limb and that region has had time to recover, the impulse is transmitted backward through the previously refractory portion and arrives at the original forking point. The two pathways available to the impulse have by now also recovered and accept the impulse. It is as though a new impulse has originated from the forking point, but actually it is still the sinus impulse starting a second wave front. This mechanism creates a reciprocal rhythm that produces a circulating wave, or "circus movement" (Marriott, 1991).

Surgical Considerations

From a surgical perspective a practical way to categorize disturbances of rhythm and conduction is to divide them into bradydysrhythmias and tachydysrhythmias, that are supraventricular or ventricular. Determination of their origin is important because prognosis and treatment differ. Supraventricular dysrhythmias (such as sinus tachycardia, atrial fibrillation, or premature atrial complexes) originate in the atrium or AV junction. Electrophysiologically, these are generally characterized by normal (narrow) QRS complexes. Ventricular dysrhythmias (such as ventricular tachycardia or fibrillation, or premature ventricular complexes) commonly produce a bizarre (wide) QRST complex that has a prolonged QRS interval (Kutalek and Michelson, 1991b; Marriott, 1991). Fig. 19-3 illustrates this difference by comparing premature atrial complexes and premature ventricular complexes; Fig. 19-4 demonstrates differences between

supraventricular tachycardia and ventricular tachycardia. The tachydysrhythmias are of special concern because they can result in life-threatening symptoms such as hypotension, syncope, or pulmonary edema (Ross and Mandel, 1987). Persistent ventricular tachycardia can degenerate into ventricular fibrillation, causing sudden death. These dysrhythmias, usually caused by abnormal mechanisms (e.g., altered automaticity, triggered activity, and reentry), may be evaluated with a number of diagnostic tests.

DIAGNOSTIC EVALUATION OF DYSRHYTHMIAS

In addition to the diagnostic tests commonly performed to assess and plan treatment for ischemic, valvular, and other forms of acquired or congenital heart disease, special ECG and electrophysiologic (EP) studies of the conduction system may be required to determine the site and mechanism of the dysrhythmia.

Noninvasive studies include the 12-lead ECG and ambulatory monitoring devices. These are often among the first diagnostic methods to be used. More specific information can be obtained with atrial electrograms and signal-averaged ECGs.

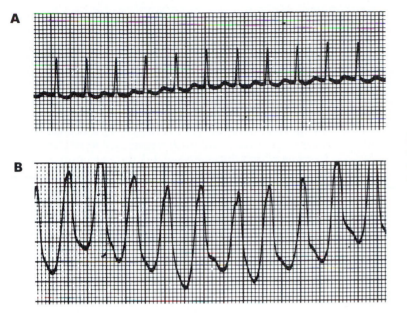

Fig. *19-4* Paroxysmal tachycardias. **A,** Supraventricular tachycardia. **B,** Ventricular tachycardia. (From Berne RM, Levy MN: *Cardiovascular physiology,* ed 6, St Louis, 1992, Mosby.)

Atrial ECGs can be performed with the temporary epicardial pacing wires implanted in cardiac sugery patients. Disturbances of rate and rhythm are common postoperatively, and atrial ECGs can be used to diagnose and plan treatment for sinus abnormalities, atrial fibrillation or flutter, and sinus or junctional tachycardias. For differentiating the origin of rapid heart rates, atrial ECGs are especially valuable because they enable the clinician to select the most appropriate therapy (Lombness, 1992).

Signal-Averaged Electrocardiography

Signal-averaged ECG is another diagnostic technique widely used for patients at risk for sudden cardiac death from ventricular dysrhythmias. Signal averaging enables detection of low-amplitude waveforms in the ECG that are normally masked by muscle movement, and electronic "noise" from amplifiers and electrodes (Schactman and Greene, 1991). These low-amplitude signals are called "late potentials," occurring at the end of or just after the QRS complex. They are thought to originate from damaged (e.g., infarcted) areas of myocardium, which conduct more slowly than normal tissue. The resulting delayed conduction provides one of the requirements for reentry ventricular tachycardia, which can lead to sudden death (Lansdowne, 1990).

A computer-based technique is used to combine hundreds of QRS complexes. Noise is canceled, and a high-resolution signal is created and amplified to detect late potentials (Schactman and Greene, 1991).

Electrophysiologic Studies

EP testing is an invasive method that can be used to both diagnose and select treatment modalities for dys-

rhythmias. Therapeutic interventions can also be performed with EP testing techniques. The most common indication for EP studies is assessing tachycardias, diagnosing the dysrhythmia, and determining the mechanism and site of the disturbance (Prystowsky and Noble, 1992).

Although bradydysrhythmias and conduction blocks can often be diagnosed by the ECG, invasive EP studies may be indicated for these disorders when a diagnosis cannot be determined by conventional methods or when the patient is asymptomatic. For example, EP testing may be required to distinguish between an intrinsic conduction abnormality of the sinus node and an autonomic nervous system dysfunction (such as excessive vagal tone producing a bradycardia) (Ross and Mandel, 1987).

EP testing can be performed at the bedside, in the EP laboratory, or in the operating room (ACC/AHA, 1989). EP studies commonly use programmed electrical stimulation and have both diagnostic and therapeutic applications. Preoperative studies are used to assess sinus node function, AV conduction, and bundle of His function, and the mechanisms of atrial and ventricular bradydysrhythmias and tachydysrhythmias. The electrophysiologist attempts to reproduce the clinical dysrhythmia in an effort to uncover the causes of the disturbance and to institute treatment (Kowey and Friehling, 1986).

Studies are also useful for predicting the efficacy of pharmacologic and nonpharmacologic therapy and for evaluating the patient's prognosis. When surgery is indicated, intraoperative EP studies are used to confirm the preoperative findings and to define more precisely the site and the characteristics of the dysrhythmia. Testing of implantable cardioverter defibrillator (ICD) devices, for example, may be done intraoperatively. Postoperative studies are routinely performed to evaluate the effectiveness of therapeutic interventions.

Preoperative electrophysiologic studies

Preoperative EP studies use multichannel recorders that can simultaneously display multiple-surface ECG leads and intracardiac leads, as well as intravascular pressures. Before the initial study, antidysrhythmic therapy is discontinued, if possible, and the patient is placed on NPO status. Lidocaine is used to anesthetize the catheter insertion site, but excessive amounts of lidocaine should be avoided so that test results are not subject to being affected by systemic absorption of the drug.

Intracardiac stimulators are used to deliver single or multiple impulses through the percutaneously inserted catheter in an attempt to induce or reproduce the clinical dysrhythmia. Pacing capability is also available to enable the electrophysiologist to suppress or overdrive the dysrhythmia. A monitor-defibrillator with external defibrillator patches applied to the patient should be prepared prior to testing.

Patient safety considerations mandate that defibrillation capability has been verified. Backup equipment should be available, and personnel directly involved with patient care should be thoroughly familiar with the use of both external defibrillator adhesive pads and external defibrillator paddles. When applying patches (or paddles), the nurse should ensure that they are applied in such a way that the defibrillation current can cross the left ventricle. Patch placement may be the right shoulder–left ventricular apex (near the left midclavicular line), anteroposterior to the left ventricle, or some other configuration that allows current to reach the left ventricle (Barbiere and Liberatore, 1992). (During surgery, when patches may interfere with the sterile field, sterile external paddles can be used.)

Emergency drugs and supplies for assisted ventilation should also be available, along with oxygen and suction. The procedure is performed under strict sterile technique with the patient prepared and draped to expose the catheter entry sites. This is usually both femoral veins and arteries, but internal jugular and subclavian sites can be used at the discretion of the electrophysiologist (Bierman and Wong, 1987). Arterial pressure is measured with a catheter in the femoral artery; the femoral veins are used for the electrode catheters.

Baseline measurements are taken of the conduction times between sections of the conduction pathway. Usually two to five multipolar electrode catheters are inserted into the femoral veins to permit stimulation and recording from each catheter. Each electrode is connected to recorders and to the stimulator. Catheter electrodes are positioned in the high right atrium, low right atrium, coronary sinus, and right ventricular apex, and along the bundle of His. The electrodes can simultaneously stimulate, pace, and record activities at these various sites to produce an EP map of the heart. Programmed stimulation may be used to induce

a variety of dysrhythmias and to define their underlying electrical basis.

Bundle of His recordings (Fig. 19-5) have provided valuable information in differentiating supraventricular causes of ventricular disturbances from ventricular ones. Impulses originating in the atrium will be reflected in recordings of bundle of His activity, whereas ectopic ventricular foci will not produce bundle of His activation (Marriott, 1991). Because treatment depends on the underlying problem, bundle of His recordings have enhanced the selection and effectiveness of antidysrhythmic drugs and have provided valuable information for determining nonpharmacologic treatments.

Patient stress. Patients undergoing EP studies have identified a number of stressors. Anxiety is common among these patients, as is fear of dying, losing control, and undergoing cardioversion (Menza, Stern, and Cassem, 1988). Connelly (1992) found that illness-related stressors were important (e.g., concern about diagnosis/treatment, being away from home, requiring cardioversion, pain, discomfort, death). Patients need clear, accurate information about the procedure and the treatment options available. Emotional support can also reduce some of the fears and concerns of these patients (DeBasio and Rodenhausen, 1984).

Intraoperative electrophysiologic studies

Intraoperative EP studies can reproduce and confirm the preoperative findings. Intraoperative mapping can also provide additional information about specific dysrhythmias, such as reentrant ventricular tachycardias, that are located on the epicardial portion of the ventricle.

A hand-held probe electrode is moved over various sites along the epicardium and the exposed endocardium to locate critical portions of the dysrhythmic circuit. Because transvenous catheter electrodes (used during the preoperative study) are of limited use in mapping the epicardium, direct probing of the surface of the heart intraoperatively is used to locate these critical epicardial circuits when they exist (Waldo, Biblo, and Carlson, 1991). Another testing method is to apply a "sock" over the heart; the sock is covered with electrodes for mapping.

Drawbacks of intraoperative mapping include the length of time required to perform sequential mapping of multiple sites, the relative imprecision of the technique, and frequent prolonged cardiopulmonary bypass (CPB) times that can increase operative morbidity (Waldo, Biblo, and Carlson, 1991).

THERAPY FOR DYSRHYTHMIAS
Pharmacologic Therapy

Antidysrhythmia drugs are selected according to their mechanism of action (Table 19-1) and may be used for either ventricular or supraventricular rhythm disturbances (Karb, 1992). All have side effects of varying severity. Some may be "proarrhythmic;" that is, their

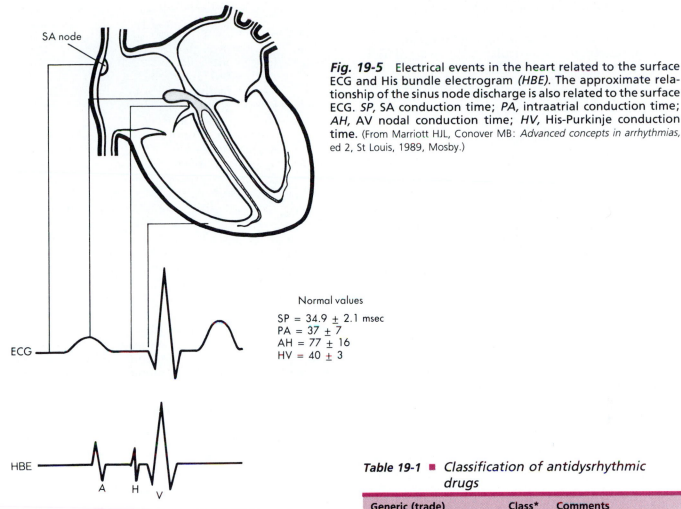

Fig. 19-5 Electrical events in the heart related to the surface ECG and His bundle electrogram *(HBE)*. The approximate relationship of the sinus node discharge is also related to the surface ECG. *SP*, SA conduction time; *PA*, intraatrial conduction time; *AH*, AV nodal conduction time; *HV*, His-Purkinje conduction time. (From Marriott HJL, Conover MB: *Advanced concepts in arrhythmias,* ed 2, St Louis, 1989, Mosby.)

Normal values

SP = 34.9 ± 2.1 msec
PA = 37 ± 7
AH = 77 ± 16
HV = 40 ± 3

use creates a new or more serious form of ventricular dysrhythmia as a result of drug toxicity.

In patients with sustained or symptomatic ventricular dysrhythmias, amiodarone therapy may be used. Amiodarone is a drug that slows SA nodal firing and AV nodal conduction time, and prolongs the refractory period in the AV node, the atria, and the ventricles. It is used to treat refractory supraventricular and ventricular dysrhythmias. Because it has a number of serious side effects and a long half-life, it is not considered a first-line antidysrhythmic; it is used when other drugs are ineffective or intolerable. The drug is generally not used in patients with asymptomatic ventricular tachycardia of short duration. Side effects include SA node blockade, bradycardia, myocardial depression, pulmonary toxicity, and hypotension. Other effects include headache, depression, tremor, hallucinations, nausea, anorexia, and constipation. Photosensitivity, impaired vision, and bluish discoloration of the skin (from crystal deposition) may occur with long-term use (Karb, 1992).

Patients scheduled for EP testing related to insertion of an ICD will have the drug discontinued whenever possible because it makes the heart more refractory to defibrillation. (Also, because of its long half-

Table 19-1 ■ *Classification of antidysrhythmic drugs*

Generic (trade)	Class*	Comments
Quinidine (Quinidex, others)	IA	
Procainamide (Procan, Pronestyl, others)	IA	
Disopyramide (Norpace)	IA	
Lidocaine (Xylocaine)	IB	
Mexiletine (Mexitil)	IB	
Tocainide (Tonocard)	IB	
Flecainide (Tambocor)	IC	
Propafenone (Rythmol)	IC	
Propranolol (Inderal)	II	Other β-adrenergic blockers would also be included in this class
Bretylium (Bretylol)	III	
Amiodarone (Cordarone)	III	
Verapamil (Calan)	IV	Other calcium channel blockers would also be included in this class

From Karb VB: Selected cardiovascular drugs. In Guzzetta CE, Dossey BM: *Cardiovascular nursing: holistic practice,* St Louis, 1992, Mosby.
*Class I drugs change the sodium ion influx that allows cells to depolarize. Class IA drugs slow conduction and prolong refractoriness. Class IB drugs shorten the refractory period. Class IC drugs slow conduction without changing refractoriness. Class II drugs are adrenergic blockers. Class III drugs prolong refractoriness. Class IV drugs block calcium influx.

life, it may be uncertain if the drug's effects are still present.)

One of the newer drugs being used for paroxysmal (sudden-onset) supraventricular tachycardia (PSVT) is adenosine (Owens and Zellers-Jacobs, 1992; Severson and Meyer, 1992). It's very rapid onset of action, short half-life, and minimal side effects have made it a first-line treatment for PSVT.

Because it is not within the scope of this book to provide a more thorough discussion of pharmacologic treatment, the reader is referred to the extensive nursing and medical literature available.

Nonpharmacologic Therapy

Because of the serious complications of many dysrhythmic drugs and their inefficacy in some patients, nonpharmacologic therapy has gained increasing attention as an alternative or adjunctive form of therapy (Zipes, 1992). Among the various forms of treatment are ablative therapy; surgical interruption, isolation, or excision of dysrhythmogenic myocardial tissue; and implantable defibrillation-pacing devices.

Ablation therapy

Endocardial catheter ablation may be performed with direct-current (DC) shock, radiofrequency energy, lasers, and cryogenic devices. These techniques are most often performed in patients with AV reentry tachycardias (e.g., WPW syndrome) and ventricular tachycardia (Zipes, Klein, and Miles, 1991). The precise location of the dysrhythmogenic focus is identified by EP testing. If multiple foci exist, there is less likelihood of successful catheter abaltion (Kinney and Craft, 1992).

Ablation may be performed percutaneously in the EP laboratory (Klein and others, 1992; Moulton and others, 1993; Valle and Lemberg, 1990) or in the operating room (Cox and others, 1990; Regas, Hill, and Schmidt, 1986). Prior to ablation, EP testing is again performed to confirm the location of the site(s) to be destroyed. The ablation catheter is maneuvered into position, and the energy source is activated to ablate the selected tissue (Cox and others, 1990) (Figs. 19-6 through 19-8). If AV junctional ablation is performed, complete AV block may develop, necessitating permanent pacemaker insertion. Other complications include ventricular tachycardia and fibrillation, thromboembolism, hemopericardium with tamponade, and transient hypotension (Zipes, Klein, and Miles, 1991).

SUPRAVENTRICULAR DYSRHYTHMIAS

Bradydysrhythmias

Pacemakers

Traditionally, temporary and permanent pacemakers have been used for patients with compromised cardiac output due to profound bradycardia. Early pacemakers fired at a fixed rate; they did not have the ability

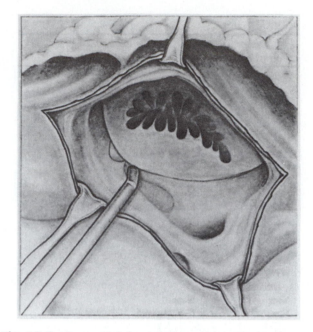

Fig. 19-6 Opened right atrium and identification of the bundle of His with a hand-held electrode. The patient's head is to the left, and a right atriotomy has been performed to expose the atrial septum. The bundle of His can usually be identified just posterior to the junction of the membranous portion of the intraatrial septum and the tricuspid valve annulus, as shown in the diagram. (From Cox JL and others: Perinodal cryosurgery for atrioventricular node reentry tachycardia in 23 patients, *J Thorac Cardiovasc Surg* 99(3):440, 1990.)

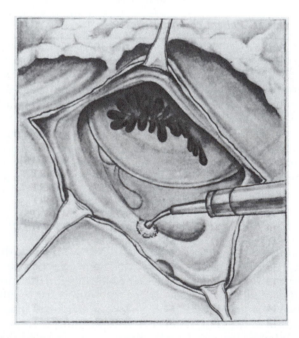

Fig. 19-7 Placement of the first 3 mm cryolesion in relation to the location of the AV node and bundle of His. (From Cox JL and others: Perinodal cryosurgery for atrioventricular node reentry tachycardia in 23 patients, *J Thorac Cardiovasc Surg* 99(3):440, 1990.)

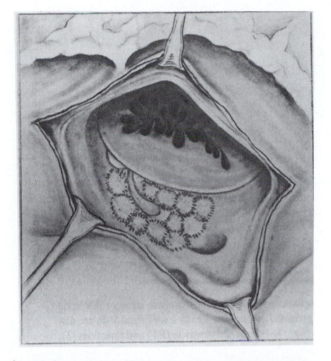

Fig. 19-8 Diagrammatic representation of the overlapping 3 mm cryolesions that are placed around and within the borders of the triangle of Koch (defined by the tendon of Todaro, the orifice of the coronary sinus, and the tricuspid annulus—see Fig. 19-16). The objective of the perinodal cryosurgical procedure is to ablate as much atrial septal tissue within the triangle of Koch as possible without causing permanent heart block. (From Cox JL and others: Perinodal cryosurgery for atrioventricular node reentry tachycardia in 23 patients, *J Thorac Cardiovasc Surg* 99(3):440, 1990.)

maker competing with the intrinsic heartbeat (and potentially creating a ventricular dysrhythmia) and prolonged the battery life of the generator (Stafford and Kleinschmidt, 1991).

Pacemakers have evolved from devices that were capable of stimulating a single chamber to those able to sense and stimulate both atrial and ventricular chambers; adjust rates to physiologic demands; provide telemetric information, and autoprogram and reprogram functions; and provide antitachycardia functions (Futterman and Lemberg, 1992). The ability to program pacemakers has led to greater flexibility in adapting to changing metabolic requirements and underlying rhythm derangements. Newer systems are capable of modulating the rate of impulse generation (the rate-responsive mode), as well as modifying the amount of energy (the output) required to stimulate an impulse. Dysrhythmia detection is also available in the latest systems. Pacemakers can be used in combination with antidysrhythmic drugs to control reentrant tachydysrhythmias. They can also be used to treat tachycardias by sensing a rapid ventricular rate and instituting a faster (overdrive) pacing stimulus to terminate the tachydysrhythmia (Kutalek and Michelson, 1991a). These newer functions have been included in the descriptive code established by the Inter-Society Commission on Heart Disease Resources (Table 19-2). Patients likely to benefit from these newer devices are those with a clinical tachycardia that can be reliably initiated and terminated in the EP laboratory (Friehling, Marinchak, and Kowey, 1988). Patients at risk for ventricular fibrillation due to ventricular tachydysrhythmias originating from multiple sites may be treated more appropriately with an internal defibrillator.

Temporary pacemakers. Temporary pacing may be used as an emergency measure to stabilize a patient with deteriorating hemodynamic function due to sudden heart block related to acute ischemia or electrolyte disturbances (Futterman and Lemberg, 1992). A permanent pacemaker can be implanted later, once the patient is stabilized. Temporary pacemaker leads (contained within a pacing Swan-Ganz catheter) may be

to sense the patient's native heartbeat. With the introduction of sensing capabilities, pacemakers could determine the intrinsic heart rate and generate an electrical impulse whenever the heart did not initiate a beat on its own within a preset period of time. With an adequate underlying rate, the pacemaker impulse is inhibited. This shift from continuous pacing to continuous sensing eliminated the hazard of the pace-

Table 19-2 ■ *Pacemaker function identification codes*

Position 1: chamber paced	Position 2: chamber sensed	Position 3: response	Position 4: programmable functions	Position 5: antitachyarrhythmia functions
A, Atrium *V,* Ventricle *D,* Dual (atrium and ventricle) *0,* None *S,* Single chamber	*A,* Atrium *V,* Ventricle *D,* Dual (atrium and ventricle)	*I,* Inhibited *T,* Triggered *D,* Dual (inhibited and triggered) *0,* None	*P,* Programmable rate and/or output *M,* Multiprogrammable (rate, output, mode, sensitivity, etc.) *T,* Antitachyarrhythmia mode *R,* Rate response *0,* None	*P,* Pacing *S,* Shock *D,* Dual (pacing and shock)

Modified from Kutalek SP, Michelson EL: Cardiac pacing and antiarrhythmic devices: newer modes of antiarrhythmia pacing, *Mod Concepts Cardiovasc Dis* 60(6):31, 1991; and Stafford MJ, Kleinschmidt KM: Physiological cardiac pacing: the DDD pacemaker system and rate-responsive modes, *Cardiovasc Nurs* 27(3):13, 1991.

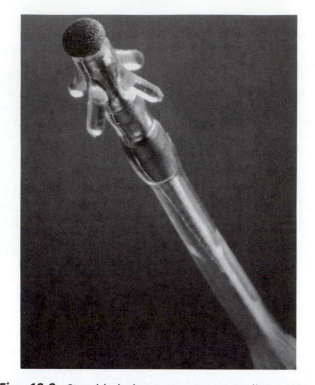

Fig. 19-9 Steroid-eluting transvenous cardiac pacing lead with tined tip. Treating the lead with a steroid reduces inflammation of the myocardium and can extend the battery life by allowing effective stimulation with electrical impulses of less intensity. (Courtesy Medtronic, Inc., Minneapolis, Minn.)

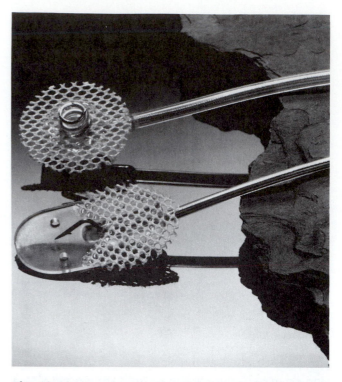

Fig. 19-10 Permanent epicardial screw-in *(top)* and stab *(bottom)* pacemaker leads. (Courtesy Medtronic, Inc., Minneapolis, Minn.)

inserted transvenously with a percutaneous method, or leads can be applied externally in the form of adhesive patches. Epicardial leads are commonly used in postoperative cardiac surgery patients to control transient postoperative rhythm disturbances (see Chapter 9).

Permanent pacemakers. Permanent pacing systems are indicated for patients with chronic or recurrent severe bradycardia due to AV block or sinus node malfunction. They may also be used for overdrive pacing in patients with ventricular tachycardia or tachycardia-bradycardia syndromes (Barbiere and Liberatore, 1993). Transvenous atrial leads often have a screw configuration; ventricular lead tips may have a tined tip (Fig. 19-9).

When concomitant cardiac procedures are performed, epicardial leads (see Chapter 9) can be permanently affixed to the heart. The permanent epicardial atrial lead usually has a fishhook configuration. The ventricular lead has a pigtail design that screws into the muscle; manufacturer's instructions should be reviewed to determine the number of rotations required for the screw-in leads (Fig. 19-10). The leads are tunneled to a subcutaneous pocket created for the generator in a manner similar to that described later for transvenous insertion.

Pacemaker system

A cardiac pacemaker can be thought of as a system consisting of a power supply, housing, leads, and an electronic circuit. These components are necessary for both temporary and permanent pacemakers.

Power supply. Implantable (permanent) pacemaker generators most often contain lithium batteries, whose longevity is determined by battery size and capacity, current settings, rate and mode of stimulation, and lead design (Harthorne, 1989). Dual-chamber pulse generators (having two sensing and stimulating channels) have a shorter life span than single-chamber pacemakers—typically 4 to 8 years for dual-chamber models versus 6 to 12 years for single-chamber devices. Rate-responsive pacers have an even shorter operating life (Futterman and Lemberg, 1993). Alternative power sources continue to be investigated.

Temporary generators (see Chapter 9) are powered by alkaline batteries. They are never line-powered (attached to a wall outlet) because of the danger of current leaks into the myocardium.

Housing. The power supply and the electronic circuitry of the generator are separately enclosed within an inert metal container (Fig. 19-11). The box is hermetically sealed to prevent moisture and tissue from injuring the internal components of the device and to prevent the surrounding tissue from being harmed (Sager, 1992).

Lead. The lead acts as the conductor of the pacing

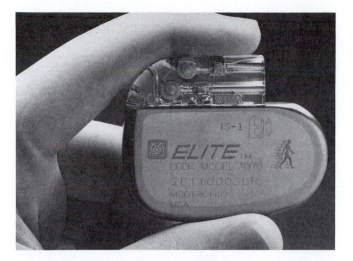

Fig. 19-11 Dual-chamber cardiac pacemaker. This model offers synchronized rate-responsive pacing in both chambers of the heart. It is capable of counting and recording electrical events, and this information can be retrieved to enhance pacer function. (Courtesy Medtronic, Inc., Minneapolis, Minn.)

stimulus to the myocardium and as the sensor of P waves or QRS complexes (depending on whether the atrium or the ventricle, respectively, is sensed). Rubber or plastic is used to insulate all but the distal tip of the lead that directly contacts the myocardium. The contacting portion of the lead is known as the **electrode.**

Electronic circuit. The electronic circuit modifies the energy available in the power supply in order to create the appropriate duration and amplitude of an impulse. A timing element within the circuit determines the frequency of stimulation. The stimulus is applied to the atrium or to the ventricle, or to both chambers sequentially, depending on the type of pacemaker device inserted. When two chambers are paced, two output and timing circuits are required, along with two sensing components; a separate timing mechanism is used to create an AV delay (Harthorne, 1989). Additional circuitry is necessary for other pacing/anti-tachycardia functions.

Patient teaching considerations

Pacemaker insertion is a commonplace procedure and may be perceived as a "routine" operation by clinicians. Assumptions about the relative simplicity of insertion and the positive effects that these devices have on the clinical status of the patient should not be generalized to patients' psychologic perceptions about the impact that a pacemaker has on their lives. Dependence on a machine that the patient cannot control may have a profound emotional effect. Wingate (1986) has demonstrated that patients' acceptance levels vary depending on demographic variables such as support systems, environment, and socioeconomic status. These considerations should be integrated into the educational programs designed for patients and families.

Patient teaching addresses the reason for pacemaker insertion, the system components, the surgical procedure (usually local anesthesia is used), and postoperative considerations related to the pacemaker and to functional activities (Table 19-3). The perioperative nurse can show the patient a pacemaker similar to the one being implanted. Many patients may not be aware that pacemaker generators are relatively small (1¾ by 1½ by ¼ inches) and lightweight (a little more than 1 ounce). The patient can be shown the pacing leads (transvenous or epicardial) and how they are implanted into the heart distally and attached to the generator proximally. Photographs of the small scar and the slight skin pocket bulge can help the patient to prepare for his or her postoperative appearance. The location of the pocket should be discussed, with preferences (if any) for chest or abdominal placement elicited. These teaching sessions also provide the patient with an opportunity to ask questions and clarify misconceptions (Dugan, 1991).

Patient preparation for transvenous insertion in the operating room (or cardiac catheterization laboratory) focuses on what can be expected during the procedure. Including sensory stimuli (color, temperature, size or room; sounds, conversations; number and roles of personnel, etc.) enables the patient to anticipate and mentally plan for the experience. If the patient wears a hearing aid, it is helpful to allow the patient to keep it in place so that questions asked of the patient during surgery will be heard. The patient should be aware that local anesthesia will reduce the discomfort from the incision, that sedation is usually available, and that a drape will separate his or her face from the periclavicular incision site. The procedure lasts approximately 1 hour, and that information can be relayed to the patient and waiting family; efforts to make the patient as comfortable as possible will enhance the smoothness of the procedure. Additional teaching is performed during the postoperative period.

Procedural considerations

When the patient is not undergoing open sternotomy, the transvenous route is the most common, although epicardial leads are sometimes inserted via a left anterior thoracotomy. Insertion of a permanent transvenous pacemaker system usually is performed with local anesthesia and fluoroscopy. Location of the generator pocket is important. A unit that is too close to the axilla may be painful and interferes with arm movement. It may also lead to skin breakdown and infection. A generator that is too close to the clavicle may be painful during arm motion and when the patient is supine (Waldhausen and Pierce, 1985). (Excessive arm movement during the early postoperative period may also cause the leads to become dislodged.)

The perioperative nurse will coordinate efforts with the OR control desk and the radiology department to

Table 19-3 ■ *Standards of nursing care for pacemakers and implantable cardioverter defibrillators*

Nursing diagnosis	Patient outcome	Nursing actions
Anxiety related to dysrhythmia surgery/pacemaker insertion, postoperative events	Patient demonstrates acceptable level of anxiety that promotes effectiveness of pacemaker/ICD treatment	Elicit questions and concerns about dysrhythmia and proposed treatment Identify and reinforce effective coping mechanisms; respect some denial; expect concern about relying on a "machine" Provide comfort measures; identify perceived needs and expectations

Knowledge deficit related to inadequate knowledge of planned surgery and function of devices	Patient demonstrates knowledge of physiologic and psychologic responses to device insertion	Determine patient's understanding of dysrhythmia, conduction disturbance
		Determine patient's/family's understanding of surgical procedure; briefly describe perioperative events; if local anesthesia is used, tell patient what to expect; reinforce or clarify what patient (and family) has been told by surgeon; elicit expected outcome of surgery
		
		Pacer:
		  Elicit patient's preference (if any) for location of generator pocket
		  Allow patient to keep hearing aid if local anesthesia is used; provide comfort measures (e.g., pillow, drapes off face)
		ICD:
		  If generator placement is to be performed with patient under local anesthesia, prepare for sensation of fibrillation/defibrillation (usually sedation used); provide emotional support and comfort measures

High risk for infection related to surgery	Patient is free of infection related to aseptic technique	Protect sterility of test cables, guidewires, etc. Confine and contain instruments and supplies used to excise infected tissue Keep instruments and guidewires free of blood and debris Document lot and serial numbers of implants
High risk for altered skin integrity	Patient's skin integrity is maintained	In thin, malnourished, or very elderly patients with poor skin turgor, use additional padding to protect skin, joints, and bony prominences

High risk for injury related to:
  Retained foreign objects
	Patient is free of injury related to:
	  Retained foreign objects
		Account for screwdrivers, electrode caps, and other small accessory items
		Check generator pockets for retained sponges

Physical hazards	Physical hazards	Have available appropriate equipment/supplies such as leads, generators, testing devices, and accessory items; confer with technical representative and surgeon to ensure that all necessary items are available If fluoroscopy is used, provide lead shields, aprons for personnel and patient Monitor ECG for severe bradycardia or ventricular ectopy, tachycardia, and/or fibrillation When transvenous leads are inserted (pacer or ICD), be alert for signs of pneumothorax or hemothorax: SOB, absent or diminished breath sounds, cyanosis, restlessness, tachypnea, decreased oxygen saturation, hypotension For ICD insertion, be prepared to open chest; institute CPB if patient does not defibrillate Use magnets with caution and in consultation with physician when activating/deactivating devices Keep instruments, device components clean; wash powder off gloves
Electrical hazards	Electrical hazards	Minimize use of electrocautery; avoid near generator or leads, and with active ICD Confirm defibrillator settings with surgeon when testing ICD (e.g., 10-20 J for internal defibrillation; 350 J or more for external shock)

Modified from Seifert PC: Cardiac surgery. In Rothrock JC: *Perioperative nursing care planning*, St Louis, 1990, Mosby.
CPB, Cardiopulmonary bypass; *CPR*, cardiopulmonary resuscitation; *ECG*, electrocardiogram; *ICD*, implantable cardioverter defibrillator; *J*, joule; *MRI*, magnetic resonance imaging; *SOB*, shortness of breath.

Table 19-3 ■ *Standards of nursing care for pacemakers and implantable cardioverter defibrillators—cont'd*

Nursing diagnosis	Patient outcome	Nursing actions
Electrical hazards— cont'd	Electrical haz- ards—cont'd	Apply appropriate conducting gel with external defibrillator paddles Defibrillate on verbal command of surgeon When testing (fibrillating) patient, have defibrillator charged and ready to shock
Thermal injury	Thermal injury	Avoid pouring ice slush or ice chips directly on phrenic nerve (in lateral pericardium)

High risk for self-care def- icit related to inade- quate knowledge of device function	Patient demonstrates knowledge of de- vice as it relates to self-care abilities	Assess patient's knowledge of signs/symptoms of pacer/ICD function
		Assess patient's understanding of signs/symptoms of infec- tion: redness, swelling, warmth, pain, fever
		Use patient education material provided by manufacturer
		Complete documentation and submit forms as indicated for follow-up and patient ID card; stress importance of keeping ID card on person at all times (may be required for security clearance at airport because devices can set off security alarms)
		Provide information for obtaining medical alert ID bracelet/ necklace; provide name of person to contact in emergen- cies (or dial 911)
		Pacer:
		  Discuss safety issues:
		    Limit use of electric razors, hairdryers, and other electrical devices over generator site
		    Do not lean directly over running engines
		    Inform physician before undergoing diagnostic proce- dures that use magnetic fields or intense radiation
		  Provide instruction related to:
		    Taking own pulse and maintaining record
		    Reporting prolonged hiccoughing or chest twitching
		    Battery failure; note change in heart rate (5 beats more or less than set rate), dizziness or fainting, weakness or fatigue, chest pain, swelling in extremities; failure is gradual
		    Telephonic testing procedure
		ICD:
		  Discuss possible personal concerns:
		    Driving restrictions
		    Appearance of generator pocket
		    Dependence on ICD, fear of shocks and/or malfunction, sensation of shock
		  Instruct patient to report:
		    ICD shocks; keep diary
		    Rapid heart rate, dizziness, fainting
		  Instruct patient that precautions are required for (Moser, Crawford, and Thomas, 1993):
		    Arc welders, large transformers
		    Security systems (e.g., airport)
		    MRI, diathermy, lithotripsy, nerve stimulators, electrocau- tery, radiation therapy
		  Instruct patient that precautions are not required for (Moser, Crawford, and Thomas, 1993):
		    Small hand tools
		    Microwave ovens, satellite dish
		    Ultrasound, lasers, diagnostic radiation
		  Address family concerns (Arato, 1992):
		    ICD discharge, notification of physician
		    Activities of daily living, travel, driving
		    Signs and symptoms of malfunction
		    Need for CPR if device fails or has already delivered full sequence of shocks
		    Making contact with person receiving a shock (produces "buzzing" or tingling)

Box 19-2 *Surgery for dysrhythmias: procedural considerations*

Instrumentation

Basic sternotomy setup for open chest procedure and all ICD procedures

Mitral valve retractors if mitral valve exposure is necessary for dysrhythmia surgery

Minor set for transvenous insertion of pacemaker leads

Supplies*

Sterile drapes for fluoroscopy unit

Sterile sleeves for "wands" and other testing devices that cannot be sterilized

Sterile magnet

Leads and/or patches

Generators

Guidewires, introducers, stylets

Alligator test cables, probes, ECG cables

Device programmers/analyzers

External defibrillator patches

EP "socks," belts for intraoperative EP testing

Service kits (e.g., screwdrivers, sterile caps, etc.)

Adaptor kits and connectors

Culture tubes (e.g., if revising pacer or ICD pocket)

Equipment

Defibrillator (and backups); internal and external defibrillation capability; external defibrillation patch system may also be requested

Fibrillator (for induction of dysrhythmia during testing)

Testing equipment appropriate for device inserted (EP machines, computer programmers, analyzers)

Fluoroscopy machine (if transvenous route is used)

Positioning

Supine

Modified thoracotomy may be used for some ICD procedures

Skin Preparation

Chin to groin, side to side

Draping

Anterior and lateral chest and abdomen, right and left sternoclavicular areas (over subclavian vein) exposed

Anesthesia screen placed over head to keep drapes off face

Special Infection Control Measures

Confine and contain tissue and instruments from infected tissue

Secure leads, testing devices, etc., that are passed off field

Culture tissue and other items as requested by surgeon

Keep guidewires, leads, etc., free of blood and debris

Special Safety Measures

Label syringes and containers holding medications and solutions:
  Antibiotic solution
  Heparinized saline
  Lidocaine topical anesthetic

Documentation/Report to Postoperative Care Unit†

Procedure: type of device, manufacturer, lot and serial numbers of all implanted components

Preoperative diagnosis (e.g., complete heart block, ventricular tachycardia, sudden death)

Pacemaker: rate settings; type and location of leads, generator; pacer function (e.g., DDD—both atrium and ventricle paced and sensed, and capable of either triggering or inhibiting a response)

ICD: location of patches (and tranvenous electrode if used), generator; ICD function (e.g., defibrillation with bradycardia pacing; status—active, inactive)

Patient problems, concerns related to dysrhythmia, surgery, function of device

Documentation required for investigational devices

ECG, Electrocardiogram; *EP,* electrophysiologic; *ICD,* implantable cardioverter defibrillator.

*As applicable to procedure.

†In addition to standard documentation/postoperative report; see Chapter 9.

---

have the appropriate x-ray equipment ready and tested prior to the start of the procedure. Pacing leads, generators, testing devices, and other necessary supplies to insert and test the system should be available (Boxes 19-2 and 19-3).

In patients with existing pacemaker generators, special precautions should be taken with the use of electrosurgical units. Excessive currents near the vicinity of the generator may cause dysrhythmias or myocardial burns from transmission of the current down the electrode (Waldhausen and Pierce, 1985). Patients with exteriorized wires are also susceptible to electrical shock hazards.

Operative procedure: insertion of a transvenous pacemaker system

1. The patient is in the supine position with both subclavian vein areas of the upper chest and shoulders exposed.

2. Local anesthetic (1% lidocaine [Xylocaine]) is infiltrated into the skin over the area where the subclavian vein is to be punctured; this may be the same site as the pocket for the generator (Fig. 19-12).

   The patient is placed in the Trendelenburg position (to engorge the vein). The patient's head is turned to the opposite side.

> **Box 19-3** *Pacemakers and implantable cardioverter defibrillators: special considerations*
>
> Kimberly L. Hill, RN
> Arrhythmia Associates
> Fairfax, Virginia
>
> ### Implantable Cardioverter Defibrillator
>
> Nonsterile personnel should wear gloves to reduce risk of shock when patient receives shock during ICD testing.
>
> Always have external defibrillator capability, preferably sterile external paddles on field (for nonthoracotomy procedures).
>
> If external defibrillator (R-2) pads are applied, ensure that their position will provide an adequate flow of current across ventricles (see Fig. 19-20).
>
> Be prepared to open chest (and possibly institute CPB) if patient cannot be defibrillated.
>
> Do not use electrocautery without first checking with electrophysiologist (may cause dysrhythmia or burn injury; may harm device).
>
> Have available sterile covers for wands and programmer heads used on sterile field.
>
> Be aware that presence of previously placed ICD ventricular patches (in patient returning to OR for ICD testing) may affect ability to externally defibrillate (patches create impedance to current flow).
>
> Have clear understanding of sequence of defibrillation methods to be used for patient rescue when fibrillation is induced; for example:
>
> If open chest: (1) ICD testing device, then (2) internal paddles (10 to 20 joules; may require higher setting on occasion)
>
> If closed chest: (1) ICD testing device, (2) external defibrillation patches, then (3) external paddles (up to 360 joules or higher if necessary)
>
> Before inducing VT/VF, determine whether shock should be synchronized to R wave if patient has VT, so that shock does not occur on T wave and cause VF; if patient has VF, shock must be nonsynchronized.
>
> ### Pacemaker and/or Implantable Cardioverter Defibrillator
>
> Patients should be aware that there is a possibility of sternotomy or thoracotomy; anticipate need for patient resuscitation and be able to institute promptly.
>
> Always prepare area over both subclavian veins (in case surgeon cannot enter one side and needs to use contralateral side).
>
> Wash powder off gloves when handling devices/wires.
>
> Always have extra defibrillator available.
>
> Make sure all cables (alligators, etc.) are sterile before start of procedure.
>
> Protect sterile devices, patches, and leads from falling off field; contamination can be very costly.
>
> Never place internal or external defibrillator paddles over pacer or ICD generator.
>
> Keep guidewires free of blood when passing transvenous ICD or pacemaker leads (accumulated blood can impede passage of wire and leads).
>
> When passing leads to abdomen, pass through chest tube to avoid breaking or fracturing lead (see text).
>
> Anticipate need for atropine (to prevent vagus nerve–induced bradycardia) when passing any leads.
>
> Make sure device is deactivated while handling on field.
>
> Never allow magnets to be in contact with or within 12 inches of pacer or ICD unless requested to do so (this also includes heads of programmers).
>
> Verify that there are no retained sponges in pacer/ICD pocket(s).
>
> Know type, brand, and manufacturer of device implanted; document all model, lot, and serial numbers; use stickers supplied by manufacturer.
>
> Have appropriate consents; have regulatory agency approval for investigational devices.
>
> Document all personnel involved in procedure: nurses, physicians (including electrophysiologists), sales representatives, technical representatives, investigational associates.
>
> Include settings and operational status (e.g., activated, deactivated) of devices when reporting to patient recovery unit.
>
> *ICD*, Implantable cardioverter defibrillator; *OR*, operating room; *VF*, ventricular fibrillation; *VT*, ventricular tachycardia.

3. A cutdown is performed to isolate the (right or left) subclavian vein, and the vessel is encircled with heavy sutures or umbilical tapes.

4. The vein is punctured with a needle through which a guidewire is introduced (Fig. 19-13).

5. A dilator-sheath is advanced over the guidewire to enlarge surrounding tissue; the dilator is removed. The lead is introduced over the guidewire, and the sheath is peeled away (Fig. 19-14). The guidewire is removed.

6A. If a single ventricular lead (e.g., VVI) is to be inserted, it is threaded through the right atrium and tricuspid valve, and into the right ventricle under fluoroscopy. Stylets inserted through the electrode can be used to manipulate the lead into position within the right ventricle.

Alligator cables are attached: one prong of each cable is connected to the lead, and the second prong is clipped to the subcutaneous tissue as a ground. The proximal ends of the cables are passed off the field and inserted into the pacing analyzer system. Thresholds and other conduc-

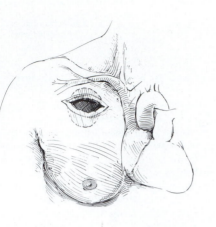

Fig. 19-12 An incision is made where the pocket is to be formed. (From Waldhausen JA, Pierce WS: *Johnson's surgery of the chest,* ed 5, St Louis, 1985, Mosby.)

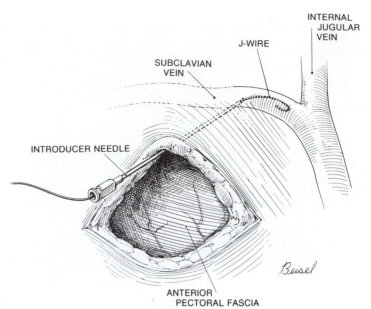

Fig. 19-13 With the patient in the Trendelenburg position and the head turned to the opposite side, the subclavian vein is punctured through the upper margin of the wound. The guidewire is introduced. (From Waldhausen JA, Pierce WS: *Johnsons's surgery of the chest,* ed 5, St Louis, 1985, Mosby.)

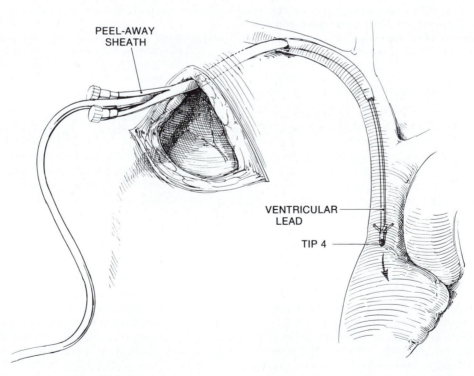

Fig. 19-14 The dilator-sheath is advanced over the guidewire; the wire and dilator are then removed, and the pacer lead is introduced into the sheath. The electrode lead is advanced into the right atrium. (From Waldhausen JA, Pierce WS: *Johnson's surgery of the chest,* ed 5, St Louis, 1985, Mosby.)

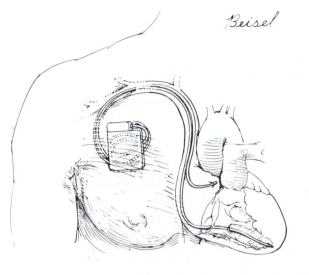

Beisel

Fig. 19-15 Both atrial and ventricular leads have been inserted and tunneled to the pacer pocket, where they are connected to the generator. (One pocket may be used for the leads and the generator.) Excess electrode is coiled and placed behind the generator, which is put into the pocket. (From Waldhausen JA, Pierce WS: *Johnson's surgery of the chest*, ed 5, St Louis, 1985, Mosby.)

tion parameters are tested to confirm that the lead will function appropriately.

6B. If dual-chamber pacing is used, a second electrode is placed in the right atrium and the position is checked by fluoroscopy. Leads may have a tined tip or a screw-in tip to foster a secure attachment in the right atrium; a stylet may be used to position the lead within the atrial trabeculations. Testing is performed (see step 6A).

7. The incision site is enlarged, if necessary, to become a pocket for the pacer generator; or a pocket is formed near the venous insertion site, and the leads are tunneled to the pocket.

8. The leads are connected to the generator, which is placed into the pocket. Excess lead is coiled and placed behind the generator (Fig. 19-15). Incisions may be irrigated with antibiotic solution.

9. Subcutaneous tissue and skin are closed with absorbable suture, and dressings are applied.

The generator may be affixed to the pectoral fascia in patients who may be considered at risk for the generator to migrate (e.g., those with poor wound healing). (Sewing the generator to the pectoral fascia is done more commonly with heavier devices, such as internal defibrillators, and is described in the procedure for inserting an ICD.)

Postoperative period

In the immediate postoperative period, pacemaker function will be assessed, and additional teaching will be performed. The patient is taught to take an apical pulse and to inspect the incisional area for signs of infection. Signs of pacemaker malfunction are reviewed, and the telephone number of a person to

contact should be available for reporting occurrences. An identification card will be given to the patient, who should carry it at all times. The card includes information such as the name of the pacemaker manufacturer; model, lot, and serial numbers; implantation date; and name and telephone number of the physician. If problems arise, this information is vital for troubleshooting and, if necessary, for reprogramming the generator. Complications and malfunctions are outlined in Table 19-4.

Transtelephonic monitoring is used for periodic assessment of pacemaker function. ECG rhythm strips are transmitted to the physician's office and reviewed. These rhythm strips can also detect when a generator battery change is needed.

Battery/lead changes. When the power source or a transvenous lead must be replaced (or reprogrammed), the procedure can be performed on an outpatient basis (Huffman, 1988). The skin pocket is reopened, and the generator is exposed and removed along with the attached leads. The leads are disconnected, and a new generator is connected to the leads and tested. It is then replaced in the skin pocket, and the incision is closed.

Transvenous lead replacement may be necessary. Generally, the existing leads have become embedded in the atrial and/or ventricular endocardium. If they cannot be dislodged and removed with gentle traction, they are left in place to avoid possible injury during an attempted extraction. New leads are inserted percutaneously into the contralateral side and positioned in the heart under fluoroscopy. The existing generator is disengaged from the malfunctioning leads, attached to the new leads, and implanted into a new skin pocket. The old leads are capped so that there are no exposed wires remaining (Luck and Pae, 1991).

Tachydysrhythmias

There are two goals in the surgical treatment of supraventricular tachydysrhythmias. The first is to localize the initiating focus or abnormal conduction pathway, and the second is to excise, divide, or in some way ablate the arrhythmogenic site. Preoperative EP tesing is done to identify the ectopic focus or the abnormal pathway, and intraoperative studies are done to confirm the data. Two conduction disturbances that may be amenable to surgical intervention are WPW syndrome and atrial fibrillation. Some of the anatomic landmarks used during surgery are shown in Fig. 19-16.

Surgery for Wolff-Parkinson-White syndrome

Dysrhythmias in patients with WPW syndrome is related to the existence of one or more accessory pathways (also known as Kent bundles) producing early activation (preexcitation) of a part or all of the ventricle by an impulse originating in the sinus node or

Table 19-4 ■ *Complications and malfunctions of permanent pacemakers*

Complication or malfunction	Causes	Diagnosis	Treatment
Failure to pace with artifact present (loss of capture)	Lead displacement (can occur up to 2 to 3 months after implant)	Diagnosis is assumed with loss of capture in early postoperative period; x-ray film is of little help unless displacement is gross	Replace lead using active fixation type
	High threshold (exit block) resulting from fibrosis or ischemia at lead tip	Diagnosis is assumed if loss of capture occurs in late postoperative phase, or there is AMI; invasive lead threshold studies can make definitive diagnosis	Programming: increase pacemaker output (and/or pulse width); if programming is unsuccessful and problem appears to be permanent, replace lead and/or use high-output pulse generator; for repeated episodes use epicardial leads.
Failure to pace with artifact absent Intermittent	Electromagnetic interference from sources within and outside body	Isometric exercise test demonstrates muscle inhibition in patient with chest wall implant; patient may have history of symptoms when near potential source of electromagnetic interference	Programming: decrease pacemaker sensitivity; if possible, change to bipolar or use triggered mode (VVT or AAT) Replace pulse generator and lead with bipolar system Tell patient to avoid source of outside interference if possible During electrocautery, program pacemaker to VOO, AOO, or DOO
	Incomplete lead fracture	Lead resistance is increased and R or P wave size decreased on electrogram; x-ray study confirms diagnosis	Replace or repair lead
	T wave sensing	Characteristic ECG with pauses in output equal to escape interval from T wave to next pacing artifact is seen	Programming: decrease sensitivity to level in which oversensing is eliminated
Continuous	Complete lead fracture	There is high lead resistance, flat electrogram, and fracture seen on x-ray film	Replace or repair lead
	Broken or loose connection between lead and pulse generator	Diagnosis is assumed if there is no activation of pulse generator with use of magnet	Repair connection or pulse generator, depending on type of damage
	Pulse generator battery failure	Diagnosis is assumed if there is no activation of pacemaker on ECG with use of magnet; battery condition indicators from interactive programmer (battery impedance and output) will be low	Replace pulse generator
Undersensing	Reduced size of intrinsic R or P wave sensed from lead tip, less than millivolt-sensitivity capability of pacemaker	On ECG, there is no recycling of pacemaker by intrinsic beats; on electrogram R or P wave measurements are less than the millivolt-sensitivity capability of pulse generator	Programming: increase sensitivity: increase rate to override non-sensed intrinsic beats; if ectopy is present, treat pharmacologically to suppress; reposition lead to obtain larger R or P wave on electrogram, or use pacemaker with greater sensitivity according to size of R or P wave on electrogram

From Sager DP: The person with an artificial cardiac pacemaker. In Guzzetta CE, Dossey BM: Cardiovascular nursing: holistic practice, St. Louis, 1992, Mosby.

Table 19-4 ■ *Complications and malfunctions of permanent pacemakers—cont'd*

Complication or malfunction	Causes	Diagnosis	Treatment
Oversensing of T wave, QRS complex, or afterpotential	Short refractory period or excessively high sensing capability of pulse generator	There are pauses in output or a continuous slowing of set rate of pacemaker; distance from oversensed wave or complex to next pacemaker artifact is equal to normal escape interval	Programming: decrease sensitivity or increase refractory period
Pacemaker-mediated tachycardia	In DDD pacemaker, retrograde conduction sensed by atrial channel; after AV delay another impulse is fired into ventricle, and cycle repeats at a rate limited by upper rate limit of system	ECG shows rapid rate equal to upper rate limit; magnet over pulse generator terminates tachycardia and puts pacemaker into DDD mode	Reprogram postventricular atrial refractory period to a time greater than that needed for conduction to atrium; if it takes 300 msec for retrograde impulse to produce a P wave, program to 325 msec
Diaphragmatic or phrenic nerve pacing	Tip of a ventricular lead placed too close to diaphragmatic portion of right ventricle Tip of atrial lead too close to phrenic nerve Pulse generator output too high Perforation of lead tip through myocardium to close proximity with diaphragm or phrenic nerve	Diaphragmatic contractions at pacemaker rate are occurring, with pacemaker artifact Fluoroscopy will show diaphragm contracting with pacemaker output If perforation has occurred into pericardial sac, there may be a friction rub and positive echocardiogram	Programming: decrease pacemaker output until contractions cease but capture is maintained, or decrease paced rate if patient has adequate intrinsic rhythm; if these measures fail and patient is uncomfortable, reposition lead
Chest or abdominal muscle stimulation around pulse generator in unipolar pacing systems (muscle twitch)	High pacemaker output or high current density	Reducing pacemaker output with programming may stop twitching	Programming: reduce pacemaker output and pulse width to level above that needed to maintain capture; change polarity to bipolar; reduce paced rate if patient has adequate intrinsic cardiac rhythm
	Lead fracture or break in lead insulation (current leaks out of lead into muscle)	X-ray film may show lead fracture; patient may complain of pinprick sensation	Replace or repair fractured lead
	Flipped pulse generator (in unipolar pacemakers with posterior covering on anodal metal case)	On x-ray film, pacemaker identification letters appear backward	Reposition pulse generator in pocket, and use two-point sutured fixation of pulse generator to chest or abdominal wall muscle; instruct patient not to "twiddle" pacemaker
	Low threshold to muscle pacing	Inappropriate muscle pacing occurs at low pacemaker output in absence of any of preceding problems	Use bipolar pacing system in sensitive patients or commercially prepared boot for unipolar pulse generator metal case to insulate electrically active anode from underlying muscle
Pacemaker syndrome (symptomatic reduction in cardiac output)	Loss of AV synchrony in VVI or VVT pacing, reducing cardiac output	Symptoms are weakness, decreased exercise tolerance, and persistent unmanageable congestive heart failure	Programming: increase paced rate if there is no intrinsic rhythm; decrease paced rate if there is adequate intrinsic cardiac sinus rhythm; if programming is unsuccessful, replace pacing system with physiologic one
Runaway pacemaker	Component failure	Paced rate will accelerate to upper rate limit of pulse generator, usually 140 to 150 bpm; this may be intermittent; patient may report dizziness or syncope and sensation of rapid heart rate	Replace pulse generator

Continued.

Table 19-4 ■ *Complications and malfunctions of permanent pacemakers—cont'd*

Complication or malfunction	Causes	Diagnosis	Treatment
Change in rate or other parameter	Incorrect programming	Reprogramming with new programmer returns pacemaker to normal function	If necessary replace pulse generator if reprogramming is unsuccessful
	Phantom or inadvertent programming by electromagnetic interference	Same as above	Same as above
	Spontaneous self-reprogramming (rare)	Same as above	Same as above
	Programmer malfunction such as power failure	Same as above	Same as above
	Pacemaker circuitry failure	Attempts at reprogramming fail	Replace pulse generator
	Reed switch malfunction	Pacemaker fails to sense intrinsic beats or remains in magnet rate after removal of magnet	Replace pulse generator
	Pacemaker battery exhaustion	Battery information (impedance and current) from interactive programmer is abnormal	Replace pulse generator
Muscle inhibition	Myopotentials inhibiting pacemaker output	Pectoral muscle isometric test is positive; patient may report dizziness during activities requiring use of arms such as lifting windows or pushing up in bed	Reprogram to lower sensitivity if possible (e.g., from 0.5 mV to 2 mV) Reprogram to triggered mode if pulse generator is capable (only with single-chamber pacing systems) Reprogram to bipolar mode if possible Instruct patient to avoid activities that produce symptoms Replace system with bipolar or triggered one if problem is severe and not remedied by any of preceding steps

the atrium. The most common rhythm disturbance is "circus movement" reentry tachycardia (ACC/AHA, 1989).

During circus movement tachycardia, the impulse travels in a circuit: atrium—AV node—bundle of His—bundle branch—ventricle—accessory pathway—atrium. In this situation the impulse travels antegradely from the atrium to the ventricle (AV) through the normal (AV node–bundle of His) pathway and then reenters the atrium retrogradely from the ventricle through the accessory pathway. Retrograde conduction through the accessory pathway does not produce ventricular preexcitation (Cox, Gallagher, and Cain, 1985).

Alternatively, antegrade AV conduction can occur over the accessory pathway (causing preexcitation of the ventricle), and retrograde ventricular atrial (VA) conduction can occur through the bundle of His—AV node pathway. For circus movement to occur, the car-

diac impulse travels a loop of cardiac fibers and reenters previously excited tissue (see Fig. 19-2). To achieve this, the impulse must be conducted slowly around the loop, and one of the two AV pathways must be blocked in one direction in order to allow the impulse to reenter the circuit (Berne and Levy, 1992). When atrial fibrillation occurs in patients with WPW syndrome, the accessory pathways may provide a relatively unimpeded route for the rapid atrial impulses to reach the ventricle and thereby stimulate ventricular fibrillation.

Patients with life-threatening dysrhythmias will have had preoperative EP testing to identify the general area of the accessory pathway (ACC/AHA, 1989), which is commonly in one of four areas: the left free wall, posterior septal wall, anterior septal wall, and right free wall (Fig. 19-17). Some patients (e.g., those with Ebstein's anomaly) may have accessory pathways in more than one region (Cox, Gallagher, and Cain, 1985).

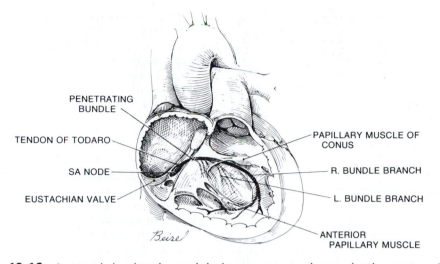

PENETRATING BUNDLE

TENDON OF TODARO

SA NODE

EUSTACHIAN VALVE

PAPILLARY MUSCLE OF CONUS

R. BUNDLE BRANCH

L. BUNDLE BRANCH

ANTERIOR PAPILLARY MUSCLE

Beise

Fig. 19-16 Anatomic landmarks used during surgery on the conduction system. The AV node lies at the apex of the triangle of Koch, which is formed by the tendon of Todaro, the tricuspid valve annulus, and the coronary sinus (the base of the triangle). The penetrating bundle of His passes through the central fibrous body into the septum, staying at the inferior border of the membranous septum on the left side. The branching portion gives off the fasciculi of the posterior radiation of the left bundle branch. At its bifurcation it then divides into the right bundle and the anterior radiation of the left bundle branch. The right bundle branch passes to the right side of the septum and goes to the anterolateral papillary muscle (moderator band). Conduction tissue does not extend beyond the papillary muscle of the conus (medial papillary muscle). (From Waldhausen JA, Pierce WS: *Johnson's surgery of the chest,* ed 5, St Louis, 1985, Mosby.)

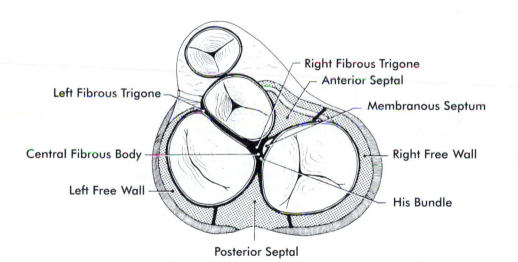

Left Fibrous Trigone

Central Fibrous Body

Left Free Wall

Right Fibrous Trigone

Anterior Septal

Membranous Septum

Right Free Wall

His Bundle

Posterior Septal

Fig. 19-17 Diagram of the superior view of the heart with the atria cut away, demonstrating the boundaries of each of the four anatomic areas where accessory pathways can occur in Wolff-Parkinson-White (WPW) syndrome. The boundaries of the **left free wall space** are the mitral valve annulus and the ventricular epicardial reflection extending from the left fibrous trigone to the posterior septum. The boundaries of the **posterior septal space** are the tricuspid valve annulus, the mitral valve annulus, the posterior superior process of the left ventricle, and the ventricular epicardial reflection. The boundaries of the **right free wall space** are the tricuspid valve annulus and the epicardial reflection extending from the posterior septum to the anterior septum. The boundaries of the **anterior septal space** are the tricuspid valve annulus, the membranous portion of the interatrial septum, and the ventricular epicardial reflection. All accessory connections must insert into the ventricle somewhere within these anatomic **boundaries.** (From Cox JL, Gallagher JJ, Cain ME: Experience with 118 consecutive patients undergoing operation for the Wolff-Parkinson-White syndrome, *J Thorac Cardiovasc Surg* 90(4):490, 1985.)

Intraoperative EP mapping may be performed; ideally this is performed prior to cannulation (which can interfere with EP mapping) and initiation of CPB. This may not be possible if the patient becomes hemodynamically unstable. A band (or finger ring) or sock of sensing electrodes is used for testing (Edmunds, Norwood, and Low, 1990; Gay, 1990).

The band is moved over the heart to map the accessory pathway(s). Mapping of additional pathways can be done after initiation of CPB.

When the accessory pathway has been located (most often the left free wall), cannulation for bypass is performed, and bypass is initiated.

Operative procedure

1. A median sternotomy is performed.
2. EP studies are performed, and the accessory pathway is located. Cannulation is performed for CPB, and bypass is instituted.
3. The left atrium is opened. Left free wall division of the accessory pathway (Cox, Gallagher, and Cain, 1985) is performed by exposing the mitral valve to access the left posterior free wall.
4. Dissection of the space is completed, exposing the entire mitral valve annulus, the left fibrous trigone (Fig. 19-17), and the posterior ventricular septum. The identified accessory pathway is transected with a sharp nerve hook, cryoablation, or other method selected by the surgeon.
5. Additional, potential accessory pathways are transected.
6. The left atrial incision is closed, and the chest tubes and temporary pacing wires are inserted. The patient is weaned from CPB, hemostasis is achieved, and all incisions are closed.

Postoperatively, conduction abnormalities requiring insertion of a permanent pacemaker may occur, but this is not common. Surgical mortality of 5% has been reported (Cox, Gallagher, and Cain, 1985).

Surgery for atrial fibrillation

Atrial fibrillation is the most commonly occurring sustained cardiac dysrhythmia, affecting up to 1% of the general population, 8% to 17% of patients over 60 years of age, and up to 79% of patients with mitral valve disease (Cox and others, 1991c). Medical and surgical therapy has been largely unsuccessful in treating the detrimental sequelae of the disorder: (1) an irregularly irregular ventricular response to the chaotic atrial impulses, (2) hemodynamic compromise resulting from loss of an atrial kick and decreased ventricular filling time, and (3) increased vulnerability to thromboembolism due to loss of effective atrial contraction and stasis of blood in the atrium (Cox and others, 1991a, 1991c).

Although many patients can adapt to the irregular heartbeat and the altered hemodynamics, thromboembolism remains a serious risk. The prevalence of thromboembolism associated with atrial fibrillation is approximately 33%, and the majority of these events involve the brain, leading to death or permanent severe neurologic deficit (Cox, Schuessler, and Boineau, 1991; Cox and others, 1991c).

Early surgical procedures attempted to blunt the sequelae of atrial fibrillation by ablating the bundle of His or by creating an isolated strip of muscle to direct impulses from the SA node to the AV node/bundle of His and from there to the ventricles (the "corridor procedure"). Unfortunately, the first procedure could not reestablish sinus rhythm and therefore could not provide an atrial kick; the risk of thromboembolism also remained. The corridor procedure could correct the irregular ventricular rhythm produced by atrial fibrillation, but right and left AV synchrony could not be reestablished, and the atrial kick remained absent (Cox and others, 1991a).

Another operation, called the "maze procedure" and developed by Cox and associates (1991a), is an attempt to reroute the multiple wave fronts, nonuniform conduction, bidirectional block, and large reentrant circuits occurring during atrial fibrillation. These results are achieved by making multiple incisions so that the impulses (which are unable to cross suture lines) are routed from the SA node to the AV node. (This inability of the impulse to cross suture lines is also seen in the cardiac transplant patient whose native SA node impulses cannot cross the anastomosis to the transplanted heart.) Based on the findings of EP mapping (Cox and others, 1991b), a maze is created (Fig. 19-18) whereby there is one entrance point (the SA node) and one exit site (the AV node). In cases with smaller reentrant circuits between suture lines and a short refractory period allowing impulses to escape, adjunctive drug therapy may be used to prolong the atrial refractory period so that fewer impulses can propagate (Cox and others; 1991a).

Operative procedure: the maze procedure (Cox, 1991a)

Excellent surgical exposure is critical. The patient is placed in the supine position.

Procedure

1. A median sternotomy is performed.
2. The superior vena cava (SVC) is mobilized from the azygos vein to the right atrium. The anatomic groove between the right pulmonary artery and the right superior pulmonary vein is developed, and the posterior left atrium is freed from the pericardium.
3. The aorta and the pulmonary artery are retracted to the left.
4. The interatrial groove is developed as for mitral valve surgery (see Chapter 13), except that the dissection is completed as much as possible inferiorly and superiorly.
5. The aorta is dissected from the pulmonary artery and encircled with an umbilical tape.
6. The SVC and inferior vena cava (IVC) are encircled with caval tapes and cannulated; the aorta is cannulated, and a cardioplegia vent needle is inserted into the ascending aorta.
7. A pulmonary artery vent is placed just beyond the

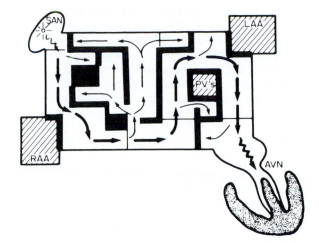

Fig. 19-18 The maze procedure for atrial fibrillation. Because atrial fibrillation is characterized by the presence of multiple macroreentrant circuits that are fleeting in nature and can occur anywhere in the atria, a surgical procedure based on the principle of the maze was developed. Both atrial appendages are excised, and the pulmonary veins are isolated. Appropriately placed atrial incisions not only interrupt the conduction routes of the most common reentrant circuits, but also direct the sinus impulse from the SA node to the AV node along a specified route. The entire atrial myocardium (except for the atrial appendages and pulmonary veins) is electrically activated by providing for multiple blind alleys off the main conduction route between the SA node and the AV node, thereby preserving atrial transport function postoperatively. *SAN*, Sinoatrial node; *RAA*, right atrial appendage; *LAA*, left atrial appendage; *PV's*, pulmonary veins; *AVN*, atrioventricular node. (From Cox JL and others: The surgical treatment of atrial fibrillation. III. Development of a definitive surgical procedure, *J Thorac Cardiovasc Surg* 101(4):569, 1991.)

pulmonary valve and connected to the aortic vent line.

8. CPB is instituted, the caval tapes are tightened, and the patient is systemically cooled.
9. The right atrial appendage is excised.
10. Two intersecting slits are made in the atrial free wall.
11. The aorta is cross-clamped, and the heart is arrested with hyperkalemic cardioplegia.
12. A stab wound is made in the left atrium and extended to connect with the right atriotomy.
13. A standard left atriotomy is performed in the interatrial groove.
14. Retractors are inserted.
15. After adequate exposure is achieved, incisions are made to create an electrical maze of the atrium (Fig. 19-19). The incisions are closed with a 3-0 (nonpledgeted) monofilament. Cryoablation is also performed on additional fibers. Patch closure of the SVC and anterior right atriotomy (with a piece of pericardium) may be performed to prevent narrowing of the SVC.
16. Atrial and ventricular pacing wires are attached: two wires on the right atrium, one wire on the left atrium, and two wires on the right ventricle. CPB is discontinued.
17. Hemostasis is obtained, and chest tubes are inserted. The incisions are closed.

Postoperative complications

Complications specifically related to the surgical treatment for dysrhythmias include heart block and injury to cardiac structures within the surgical field (e.g., coronary sinus, coronary arteries, tricuspid and mitral valves). Other complications that are associated with

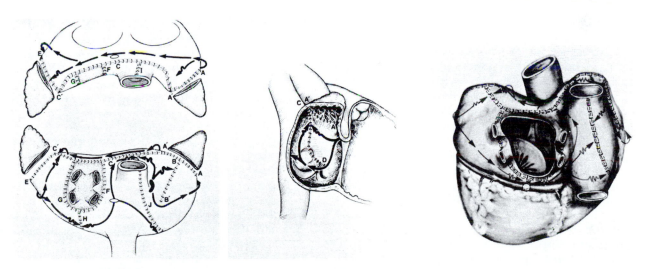

Fig. 19-19 Two-dimensional *(left and middle)* and three-dimensional *(right)* depiction of the incisions used for the maze procedure. (From Cox JL and others: The surgical treatment of atrial fibrillation. III. Development of a definitive surgical procedure, *J Thorac Cardiovasc Surg* 101(4):569, 1991.)

most open heart procedures include stroke, coagulopathy, hemorrhage, infection, pulmonary embolism, ventricular dysfunction, and chylopericardium (abnormal lymphatic drainage into the pericardium) (Ferguson and Cox, 1991).

VENTRICULAR DYSRHYTHMIAS
Bradydysrhythmias

Ventricular bradycardias may be seen in patients with chronic conduction delay due to bundle-branch or fascicular block. Complete trifascicular block is rare, and the rate of progression is slow when there are no intervening causes (such as ischemia, drugs, or electrolyte imbalances). EP studies may be indicated in symptomatic patients whose bundle-branch block is suspected of causing symptoms (e.g., syncope or near-syncope) or in whom knowledge of the site of the block, the severity of the conduction delay, or the response to drug therapy requires further investigation (ACC/AHA, 1989). Pacemaker implantation (discussed earlier) is the therapy of choice.

Tachydysrhythmias

The most serious of the ventricular rhythm disturbances are the tachydysrhythmias that may deteriorate into ventricular fibrillation because of a primary electrical instability or hemodynamic compromise associated with the rapid heart rate.

Unlike many patients with supraventricular dysrhythmias, patients undergoing surgical therapy for ventricular rhythm disturbances often have left ventricular dysfunction related to ischemic heart disease. Ischemic ventricular tachycardias are commonly due to reentrant circuits located in the border region between a myocardial infarction or left ventricular aneurysm and the surrounding normal myocardium (Cox, 1991b). The type of surgery performed will be influenced by the etiology of the underlying cardiac disease (Zipes, 1992); the surgical approach may be direct or indirect.

Nonischemic forms of ventricular tachydysrhythmias exist, but these occur less often and are most often due to cardiomyopathy or congenital ventricular dysplasia. Occasionally the tachydysrhythmia is idiopathic, without macroscopic or microscopic evidence of primary cardiac disease (Cox, 1991a, 1991b). Surgical resection or ablative techniques have not demonstrated long-term success. A cardioverter defibrillator may be implanted to reduce the risk of sudden death in these patients (Ferguson and Cox, 1991).

Indirect procedures

Indirect procedures such as coronary artery bypass grafting and valve repair or replacement can be useful in improving myocardial blood flow and cardiac hemodynamics, but they do not destroy or excise the tissue responsible for the dysrhythmia. In patients with a previous myocardial infarction, there may be extensive scarring of the left ventricle and, in some cases, a well-defined ventricular aneurysm (Gay, 1990). Left ventricular aneurysmectomy has been performed to excise myocardium from which the dysrhythmias were thought to originate. If the dysrhythmogenic site is contained within the resected portion of the aneurysm, then aneurysmectomy could be expected to be curative. Unfortunately, this procedure is rarely effective, because typically there are multiple dysrhythmogenic sites outside, as well as inside, the borders of the aneurysm or the infarct (Cox, 1991a, 1991b; Zipes, Klein, and Miles, 1991).

Direct procedures

Direct surgical procedures to remove the dysrhythmogenic focus or foci fall into two categories: resection and ablation. When these procedures fail to correct the disturbance, termination of the dysrhythmia is achieved with an internal defibrillator.

Indications for surgery

The major indications for surgery are drug resistance to symptomatic, recurrent ventricular tachydysrhythmias; drug intolerance; or unwillingness of the patient to adhere to medication regimens. Surgical resection or ablation may be contraindicated in patients with severe left ventricular dysfunction. In these patients implantation of an ICD may be the preferred treatment (Cox, 1991b; Zipes, 1989).

Operative procedure: mapping and resection of endocardium for ventricular tachycardia

These operations require EP mapping of the heart to determine the point or location of the dysrhythmogenic focus so that it can be excised, isolated, or ablated.

Procedure

1. A median sternotomy is performed. Cannulation for CPB is performed, but bypass is not initiated until intraoperative EP studies are performed. The vena cavae may be cannulated directly to provide maximal epicardial surface area on the atrium for the application of EP electrodes (Cox, 1991b).

   Normothermia is maintained during the mapping procedure to enhance the accuracy of the EP measurements.
2. An expandable sock with multiple electrodes is placed over the heart with the open end at the level of the AV groove. The sock may have a dark seam corresponding to the left anterior coronary artery (used for reference purposes).
3. Additional electrodes are sutured to the tip of the left atrial appendage and on the left or right ventricle (through the sock material). The ventricular electrode is for pacing and sensing. The electrodes are passed off the field and attached to EP equipment.
4. Ventricular tachycardia is induced, and the ec-

topic focus is localized. This may require multiple tests to locate the correct site(s).

5. The sock is removed, leaving the ventricular electrode.

6. Normothermic CPB is initiated, and a left ventriculotomy is made. (If a resectable aneurysm is present, the incision is made through the aneurysmal wall.)

7. Ventricular tachycardia is again induced through the ventricular electrode. A finger ring electrode is applied to different points along the septum and endocardial surface of the left ventricle to further localize the activation site. Once this has been achieved, hypothermia is induced.

8. The endocardium containing the tachyarrhythmic focus is excised. If a ventricular septal defect is created from the resection, it is repaired (see Chapter 12).

9. The ventriculotomy is closed with felt-buttressed sutures. Ventricular aneurysms may be repaired according to the location and extent of the lesion.

10. Temporary atrial and ventricular pacing wires are attached.

11. Several attempts are made to induce ventricular tachycardia in order to determine if the dysrhythmogenic site has been ablated and to uncover any additional foci.

12. If internal defibrillator patches are to be placed, they are applied at this time.

Implantable cardioverter defibrillator (ICD)

Sudden cardiac death (SCD), affecting more than 450,000 people per year, represents a major health problem. SCD is thought to result from ventricular fibrillation or from sustained ventricular tachycardia that deteriorates into ventricular fibrillation; less often it is due to myocardial infarction. In patients at high risk for SCD, antidysrhythmic drugs may not provide adequate protection; implantable defibrillators are used to terminate the dysrhythmia (Mason and McPherson, 1992).

The difficulties of managing ventricular tachydysrhythmias are related to the fact that electrical countershock is the only treatment for ventricular fibrillation. Realizing that patients often died of ventricular tachycardia/fibrillation because the necessary equipment and personnel to defibrillate patients were unavailable, Mirowski (1983) and his associates conceived of an implantable device that could sense the dysrhythmia and deliver a countershock to terminate the life-threatening disorder. The first device of this kind was implanted clinically at the Johns Hopkins Hospital in Baltimore, in 1980. The first defibrillators were used to treat ventricular fibrillation; by 1982 modifications allowed the Mirowski defibrillator to treat both ventricular fibrillation and ventricular tachycardia (Arato, 1992).

Defibrillator patches are placed on the ventricle and connected to an internal defibrillator that is activated when it senses ventricular tachycardia or fibrillation.

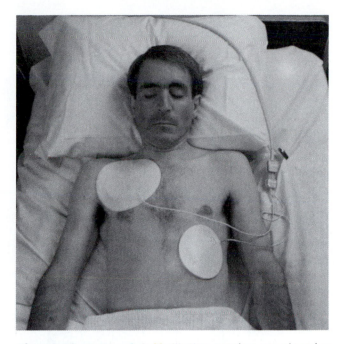

Fig. 19-20 External defibrillation patches are placed so that current can cross the heart. (Courtesy R-2 Medical Systems, Inc., Niles, Ill.)

Up to four or five shocks can be delivered per episode of dysrhythmias (Prinkey, 1992).

The ICD is prescribed for patients at risk for spontaneous ventricular fibrillation or ventricular tachycardia unresponsive to pharmacologic therapy, or when a specific dysrhythmogenic site cannot be located and resected, or when additional irritable foci are present (which would make more extensive resection of the ventricle unfeasible). Some internal defibrillators bear the proprietary name A.I.C.D. (automatic implantable cardiovertor defibrillator, manufactured by Cardiac Pacemakers, Inc.); ICD is the generic name for the device.

Extensive preoperative testing is done in the EP laboratory to determine the need for ICD insertion. Generally, these patients are unresponsive to drug therapy or are unable to tolerate pharmacologic treatment. Patients taking antidysrhthmics preoperatively may have the drug(s) discontinued to reduce their interference with defibrillation during intraoperative ICD testing (Arato, 1992). Because testing requires induction of ventricular fibrillation or tachycardia, external defibrillation capability is necessary. Defibrillation may be achieved with external hand-held paddles (see Chapter 5) or adhesive patches (Fig. 19-20).

Surgical implantation is performed alone or in conjunction with other procedures (most commonly, myocardial revascularization). When performed with other cardiac procedures, implantation is done through the median sternotomy (see Table 19-3 and Boxes 19-2 and 19-3). Anterior left thoracotomy or subxiphoid incisions are often used when the proce-

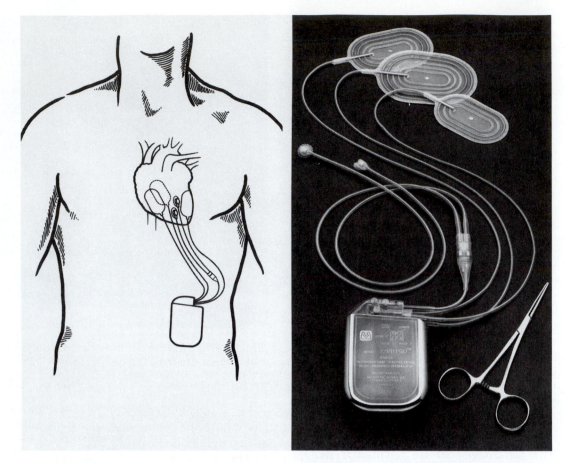

Fig. 19-21 Pacemaker-cardiac-defibrillator is designed to control tachydysrhythmias, as well as the bradycardia that often occurs after defibrillation with the device. *Left:* The device shown in the typical position with two sensing leads and three possible patch positions. The pulse generator (in the abdominal pocket) receives information from the sensing leads and delivers precisely programmed electrical impulses to the heart through the patch leads. The sensing and patch leads are attached during cardiac surgery. This system provides tiered therapy whereby the generator can be programmed to pace at increasing levels of intensity to treat ventricular tachycardia or, if necessary, provide sufficient energy to defibrillate ventricular fibrillation. *Right:* Small, medium, and large patches *(top):* sensing leads *(middle):* and generator *(bottom, with hemostat for comparison).* (Courtesy Medtronic, Inc., Minneapolis, Minn.)

dure consists of defibrillator implantation only. A variety of electrode configurations are possible. The most common is an anterior patch and a posterior patch. If this configuration does not provide adequate defibrillation, a third patch may be attached to the heart. However, only two patches can be used to defibrillate (the remaining third patch would be inactive).

An alternative is to introduce a transvenous sensing/defibrillation lead. This would be programmed to function in conjunction with one of the three patches. (The remaining two patches would then be inactive.) ICD generators are at least twice the size of most pacemaker generators; an abdominal pocket is more suitable than a chest pocket (where there is less room for the generator).

Operative procedure: insertion of an implantable cardioverter defibrillator

1. A median sternotomy, anterior left thoracotomy, or subxiphoid incision is performed.
2. The pericardium is opened and retracted with sutures.
3. The posterior defibrillator patch (Fig. 19-21) is placed behind the heart on the posterolateral surface of the left ventricle. The patch is anchored to the myocardium with two or three sutures.

   Occasionally the patch is attached to the pericardial surface so that the ventricle is in contact with the patch. The patch is positioned so that the side containing the electrodes makes contact with the ventricular surface.
4. The anterior patch is attached to the right ven-

tricular surface opposite the posterior patch. When adhesions from previous surgery are present, the patch can be placed on the outside of the pericardium over the appropriate area of the right ventricle (Edmunds, Norwood, and Low, 1990).

Having the anterior and posterior patches opposite each other will allow most of the defibrillator current to pass through the ventricular septum.

5. Two sensing electrodes (corkscrew) are placed on a free area of the right or left ventricular epicardium. The sensing leads and patch leads are attached to sterile cables that are connected to sensing and defibrillation equipment. Ventricular tachycardia/fibrillation is induced, and the patches are activated to test the necessary cardioversion/defibrillation threshold (acceptable threshold levels are generally between 10 and 25 joules). During testing, internal defibrillator paddles should be immediately available for rescue if the testing device cannot defibrillate the patient.

6. A subcutaneous pocket for the defibrillator generator is made in the left upper abdominal wall.

7. When testing of the sensing electrodes and patches is completed, the distal ends of the leads can be transferred to the abdominal pocket. This is accomplished by inserting the distal ends of the patch and sensing leads into one end of a chest tube that has been tunneled from the abdominal pocket to the pericardium. The leads (two sensing and two patch) are inserted into the pericardial end of the chest tube, which is then pulled out through the abdominal incision, carrying the leads with it.

8. The leads are connected to the defibrillator generator. The generator is tested, after which it is placed in the subcutaneous pocket. All incisons are closed.

The device is often deactivated after insertion and testing because myocardial irritability and discontinuation of antidysrhythmia medications can trigger tachydysrhythmias. Standard resuscitative measures are instituted if sustained ventricular tachycardia or fibrillation occurs. External defibrillation can be used, but the paddles should not be placed directly over the generator (Arato, 1992). Occasionally, external defibrillation is hampered by the insulating effects of the ICD patches; higher energy levels may be required to cardiovert the patient.

Postoperatively the patient will undergo EP studies to ensure that the system is working properly. Antidysrhythmic medications may be added or restarted (Prinkey, 1992). Regular checkups are recommended; generator changes can be done with the patient under local anesthesia. Additional teaching considerations are listed in Table 19-3.

REFERENCES

ACC/AHA Task Force Report: Guidelines for clinical intracardiac electrophysiologic studies, *J Am Coll Cardiol* 14(7):1827, 1989.

Arato A: Elderly care: automatic implantable cardioverter defibrillators, *J Gerontol Nurs* 18(12):15, 1992.

Barbiere CC, Liberatore K: Automated external defibrillators: an update of additions to the ACLS algorithms, *Crit Care Nurse* 12(5):17, 1992.

Barbiere CC, Liberatore K: From emergent transvenous pacemaker to permanent implant and follow-up, *Crit Care Nurse* 13(2):39, 1993.

Berne RM, Levy MN: *Cardiovascular physiology,* ed 6, St Louis, 1992, Mosby.

Bierman PQ, Wong ES: Prospective evaluation of infections associated with pacing catheters for electrophysiologic testing, *Heart Lung* 16(4):350, 1987.

Cobb FR and others: Successful surgical interruption of the bundle of Kent in a patient with Wolff-Parkinson-White syndrome, *Circulation* 38:1018, 1968.

Connelly AG: An examination of stressors in the patient undergoing cardiac electrophysiologic studies, *Heart Lung* 21(4):335, 1992.

Conover MB: *Understanding electrocardiography,* ed 6, St Louis, 1992, Mosby.

Cox JL: The surgical treatment of atrial fibrillation. IV. Surgical technique, *J Thorac Cardiovasc Surg* 101(4):584, 1991a.

Cox JL: Surgical treatment of cardiac arrhythmias. In Sabiston DC, editor: *Textbook of surgery,* ed 14, Philadelphia, 1991b, WB Saunders.

Cox JL, Gallagher JJ, Cain ME: Experience with 118 consecutive patients undergoing operation for the Wolff-Parkinson-White syndrome, *J Thorac Cardiovasc Surg* 90(4):490, 1985.

Cox JL, Schuessler RB, Boineau JP: The surgical treatment of atrial fibrillation. I. Summary of the current concepts of the mechanisms of atrial flutter and atrial fibrillation, *J Thorac Cardiovasc Surg* 101(3):402, 1991.

Cox JL and others: Perinodal cryosurgery for atrioventricular node reentry tachycardia in 23 patients, *J Thorac Cardiovasc Surg* 99(3):440, 1990.

Cox JL and others: Successful surgical treatment of atrial fibrillation: review and clinical update, *JAMA* 266(14):1976, 1991a.

Cox JL and others: The surgical treatment of atrial fibrillation. II. Intraoperative electrophysiologic mapping and description of the electrophysiologic basis of atrial flutter and atrial fibrillation, *J Thorac Cardiovasc Surg* 101(3):406, 1991b.

Cox JL and others: The surgical treatment of atrial fibrillation. III. Development of a definitive surgical procedure, *J Thorac Cardiovasc Surg* 101(4):569, 1991c.

DeBasio N, Rodenhausen N: The group experience: meeting the psychological needs of patients with ventricular tachycardia, *Heart Lung* 13(6):597, 1984.

Dugan L: What you need to know about permanent pacemakers, *Nursing 91,* p. 46, June, 1991.

Edmunds LH, Norwood WI, Low DW: *Atlas of cardiothoracic surgery,* Philadelphia, 1990, Lea & Febiger.

Feeney MK: Dysrhythmias. In Guzzetta CE, Dossey BM: *Cardiovascular nursing: holistic practice,* St Louis, 1992, Mosby.

Ferguson TB, Cox JL: Complications related to the surgical treatment of supraventricular and ventricular cardiac arrhythmias. In Walhausen JA, Orringer MB: *Complications in cardiothoracic surgery,* St Louis, 1991, Mosby.

Friehling TD, Marinchak RA, Kowey PR: Role of permanent pacemakers in the pharmacologic therapy of patients with reentrant tachyarrhythmias, *PACE* 11:83, 1988.

Futterman LG, Lemberg L: Pacemaker update: 1992. I. General remarks and electrocardiographic assessment of pacemaker function, *Am J Crit Care* 1(3):118, 1992.

Futterman LG, Lemberg L: Pacemaker update. II. Atrioventricular synchronous and rate-modulated pacemakers, *Am J Crit Care* 2(1):96, 1993.

Gary LC, Guzzetta CE: Cardiac monitoring and dysrhythmias. In Dossey BM, Guzzetta CE, Kenner CV: *Critical care nursing: body—mind—spirit*, Philadelphia, 1992, JB Lippincott.

Gay WA: *Atlas of adult cardiac surgery*, New York, 1990, Churchill Livingstone.

Goldenberger E: *Treatment of cardiac emergencies*, ed 5, St Louis, 1990, Mosby.

Harthorne JW: Cardiac pacing. In Grillo HC and others, editors: *Current therapy in cardiothoracic surgery*, Philadelphia, 1989, BC Decker.

Hoops-Nast EJ: Cardiac electrophysiology. In Weeks LC, editor: *Advanced cardiovascular nursing*, Boston, 1986, Blackwell Scientific Publications.

Huffman M: Pacemaker battery change: an outpatient procedure, *AORN J* 48(4):733, 1988.

Karb VB: Selected cardiovascular drugs. In Guzzetta CE, Dossey BM: *Cardiovascular nursing: holistic practice*, St Louis, 1992, Mosby.

Kinney MR, Craft MS: The person undergoing cardiac surgery. In Guzzetta CE, Dossey BM: *Cardiovascular nursing: holistic practice*, St Louis, 1992, Mosby.

Klein LS and others: Radiofrequency catheter ablation of ventricular tachycardia in patients without structural heart disease, *Circulation* 85(5):1666, 1992.

Kowey PR and Friehling TD: Uses and limitations of electrophysiology studies for the selection of antiarrhythmia therapy, *PACE* 9:231, 1986.

Kutalek SP, Michelson EL: Cardiac pacing and antiarrhythmic devices: antitachycardia and antifibrillatory devices. I. Arrhythmia detection and antitachycardia pacing, *Mod Concepts Cardiovasc Dis* 60(2):7, 1991a.

Kutalek SP, Michelson EL: Cardiac pacing and antiarrhythmic devices: antitachycardia and antifibrillatory devices. II. Electrical cardioversion and defibrillation, *Mod Concepts Cardiovasc Dis* 60(3):13, 1991b.

Lansdowne LM: Signal-averaged electrocardiograms, *Heart Lung* 19(4):329, 1990.

Lombness PM: Taking the mystery out of rhythm interpretation: atrial electrograms, *Heart Lung* 21(5):415, 1992.

Luck JC, Pae WE: Pacemaker complications. In Waldhausen JA, Orringer MB: *Complications in cardiothoracic surgery*, St. Louis, 1991, Mosby.

Mandel WJ: *Cardiac arrhythmias: their mechanisms, diagnosis and management*, ed 2, Philadelphia, 1987, JB Lippincott.

Marriott HJ: *Practical electrocardiography*, ed 8, Baltimore, 1991, Williams & Wilkins.

Marriott HJL, Conover MB: *Advanced concepts in arrhythmias*, ed 2, St Louis, 1989, Mosby.

Mason P, McPherson C: Implantable cardioverter defibrillator: a review, *Heart Lung* 21(2):141, 1992.

Menza MA, Stern TA, Cassem NH: Treatment of anxiety associated with electrophysiologic studies, *Heart Lung* 17(5):555, 1988.

Mirowski M: Management of malignant ventricular tachyarrhythmias with automatic implanted cardioverter-defibrillators, *Mod Concepts Cardiovasc Dis* 52(8):41, 1983.

Moser SA, Crawford D, Thomas A: Updated care guidelines for patients with automatic implantable cardioverter defibrillators, *Crit Care Nurse* 13(2):62, 1993.

Moulton L and others: Radiofrequency catheter ablation for supraventricular tachycardia, *Heart Lung* 22(1):3, 1993.

Owens M, Zellers-Jacobs L: Adenosine: the newest drug for PSVT, *RN* 55(12):38, 1992.

Prinkey LA: Defibrillation, cardioversion, and the automatic implantable cardioverter-defibrillator. In Guzzetta CE, Dossey BM: *Cardiovascular nursing: holistic practice*, St Louis, 1992, Mosby.

Prystowsky EN, Noble RJ: Electrophysiological studies: who to refer, *Heart Dis Stroke* 1:188, 1992.

Regas ML, Hill SB, Schmidt CV: Wolff-Parkinson-White syndrome: cryosurgical ablation of accessory pathways, *AORN J* 44(5):742, 1986.

Ross TF, Mandel WJ: Invasive cardiac electrophysiologic testing. In Mandel WJ: *Cardiac arrhythmias: their mechanisms, diagnosis and management*, ed 2, Philadelphia, 1987, JB Lippincott.

Sager DP: The person with an artificial cardiac pacemaker. In Guzzetta CE, Dossey BM: *Cardiovascular nursing: holistic practice*, St Louis, 1992, Mosby.

Schactman M, Greene JS: Signal-averaged electrocardiography: a new technique for determining which patients may be at risk for sudden cardiac death, *Focus Crit Care* 18(3):202, 1991.

Severson AL, Meyer LT: Treatment of paroxysmal supraventricular tachycardia with adenosine: implications for nursing, *Heart Lung* 21(4):350, 1992.

Spittle L: Dysrhythmias. In Wingate S, editor: *Cardiac nursing: a clinical management and patient care resource*, Gaithersburg, Md, 1991, Aspen.

Stafford MJ, Kleinschmidt KM: Physiological cardiac pacing: the DDD pacemaker system and rate-responsive modes, *Cardiovasc Nurs* 27(3):13, 1991.

Stone J: *In the country of hearts: journeys in the art of medicine*, New York, 1990, Delacourt Press, p 127.

Thelan LA, Davie JK, Urden LD: *Textbook of critical care nursing: diagnosis and management*, St Louis, 1990, Mosby.

Valle BK, Lemberg L: Wolff-Parkinson-White syndrome, *Heart Lung* 19(6):690, 1990.

Waldhausen JA, Pierce WS: *Johnsons's surgery of the chest*, ed 5, St Louis, 1985, Mosby.

Waldo AL, Biblo LA, Carlson MD: New directions in intraoperative mapping and surgical treatment of ventricular tachycardia, *Circulation* 83(5):1824, 1991.

Wingate S: Levels of pacemaker acceptance by patients, *Heart Lung* 15(1):93, 1986.

Zipes DP: Cardiac electrophysiology: promises and contributions, *J Am Coll Cardiol* 13(6):1329, 1989.

Zipes DP: Management of cardiac arrhythmias: pharmacological, electrical, and surgical techniques. In Braunwald E: *Heart disease*, ed 4, Philadelphia, 1992, WB Saunders.

Zipes DP, Klein LS, Miles WM: Nonpharmacologic therapy: can it replace antiarrhythmic drug therapy? *J Cardiovasc Electrophysiol* 2(suppl):S255, 1991.

SUGGESTED READINGS

Guzzetta CE, Dossey BM: Cardiovascular assessment. In Dossey BM, Guzzetta CE, Kenner CV: *Essentials of critical care nursing*, Philadelphia, 1990, JB Lippincott.

Lamb LS, Judson EB: Maximal rate response in a permanent pacemaker during chest physiotherapy, *Heart Lung* 21(4):390, 1992.

Lowe JE: Cardiac pacemakers. In Sabiston DC, editor: *Textbook of surgery*, ed 14, Philadelphia, 1991, WB Saunders.

Scheinman MM: Catheter and surgical treatment of cardiac arrhythmias, *JAMA* 263(1):79, 1990.

Scheinman MM: Catheter ablation: present role and projected impact on health care for patients with cardiac arrhythmias, *Circulation* 83(5):1489, 1991.

Stevens LL, Redd RM: Bedside electrophysiology study, *Crit Care Nurse* 7(4):36, 1987.

20

Surgery for Adult Congenital Heart Disease

The complications arising from the persistence of a patent ductus arteriosus would seem to make surgical ligation of this anomalous vessel a rational procedure, if such a procedure could be completed with promise of a low operative mortality.

Robert E. Gross, MD, and John P. Hubbard, MD, 1939

The successful ligation in 1939 by Gross (Gross and Hubbard, 1939) of a persistent ductal shunt between the aorta and the pulmonary artery in a 7-year-old girl is often considered the beginning of surgical treatment for congenital malformations of the heart (Taussig, 1982). This achievement also focused on the importance of collaborative efforts between surgeons and their pediatric cardiologic associates and stimulated the development of procedures to palliate and/or repair a number of congenital deformities (Rashkind, 1982).

Catheter therapy has greatly expanded the treatment options for congenital anomalies. Balloon angioplasty techniques can be used to dilate stenotic valves or vascular strictures (Radtke and Lock, 1990). Occlusive devices inserted to close anomalous intracardiac or extracardiac communications have also been used, but these have undergone reappraisal by the Food and Drug Administration.

Before the introduction of extracorporeal circulatory support, surgical treatment of congenital anomalies was primarily limited to extracardiac lesions (such as patent ductus arteriosus [PDA] and coarctation of the aorta) (Table 20-1) that could be operated on without the necessity of arresting the heart. Surgery for intracardiac malformations, such as the tetralogy of Fallot, consisted of the creation of palliative extracardiac shunts (e.g., the Blalock-Taussig subclavian artery–to–pulmonary artery shunt). Total repair of this and other complex intracardiac lesions had to await cardiopulmonary bypass (CPB) capability and the development of diagnostic methods that were more sophisticated than the stethoscope, three-lead electrocardiogram (ECG), and chest radiograph, which were the only tools available to Gross in 1939 (Engle, 1989).

Improvements in early diagnosis and perinatal management of congenital disorders has resulted in enhanced survival for many of these patients. As a result, the number of adults with congenital heart disease is increasing and encompasses those who have never undergone palliative or reparative procedures in childhood, but who require correction in adulthood (Box 20-1), those who have had palliation with or without anticipation of repair, and those who have had surgery and require no further operation (Perloff, 1992). These patients are also susceptible to acquired cardiac disease and may require surgery for coronary artery disease and valvular dysfunction. Thus perioperative nurses specializing in acquired cardiac disorders are increasingly likely to see patients with congenital heart disease.

Although this chapter is limited to the congenital deformities most likely to await repair in adulthood, it is helpful to be familiar with the congenital anomalies commonly requiring correction in childhood, because the perioperative nurse may encounter these patients when they require surgery for acquired disorders. Nurses can plan care better knowing that there may be sternal (or thoracic) adhesions from prior surgery, altered anatomy without the familiar landmarks, prostheses (e.g., conduits, occlusive devices, intracardiac or extracardiac patches) that should not be disturbed, and other alterations that will affect the performance of surgery.

Among the congenital disorders discussed in this chapter are PDA, atrial septal defect (ASD), and coarctation of the aorta. This chapter also includes a discussion of closure of a PDA in the infant. PDA, a frequently occurring extracardiac congenital disorder, does not require CPB in the infant (unless it is associated with other complex malformations) and is rel-

Table 20-1 ■ *Selected congenital cardiac lesions*

Lesion	Description
Anomalous pulmonary venous return	Pulmonary venous return enters systemic venous system rather than left atrium; may be partial or total return of pulmonary venous blood flow; usually produces increased pulmonary blood flow, variable cyanosis
ASD	Communication between right and left atria; there are three common types: **Sinus venosus:** Area of entry is superior vena cava into atrium; commonly associated with partial anomalous pulmonary venous return **Ostium secundum:** Area of fossa ovalis (formerly fetal foramen ovale); midportion of septum; most common **Ostium primum:** Area inferior to fossa ovalis; associated with cleft anterior leaflet of mitral valve; least common ASDs usually occur as isolated lesions; produce volume overloading of right side of heart and pulmonary circulation
Coarctation of aorta	Aortic constriction caused by both external narrowing and intraluminal membrane **Postductal** (adult): Coarctation located distal to left subclavian artery and PDA, near or at aortic isthmus; produces systolic and diastolic hypertension in proximal aorta, increases left ventricular workload, and stimulates fetal and postnatal development of large collateral vessels to perfuse organs distal to coarctation **Preductal** (Infant): Coarctation located proximal to PDA; lower body perfusion dependent on patent ductus; may produce cyanosis of lower extremities; collateral circulation not formed; less common than adult form
PDA	Persistent, patent fetal shunt between aorta and pulmonary artery; produces increased pulmonary blood flow
Pulmonary atresia	Absence of pulmonary valve causing decreased pulmonary blood flow; blood flows from right and left ventricles into aorta; pulmonary blood flow depends on PDA or collateral circulation; produces cyanosis
Tetralogy of Fallot	Consists of four anatomic abnormalities: VSD, pulmonary stenosis, aorta that overrides VSD, and right ventricular hypertrophy; results in decreased pulmonary blood flow, causing hypoxia and cyanosis
TGA	Aorta arises from right ventricle, and pulmonary artery arises from left ventricle, creating two independent circulations; for survival, there must be some anatomic communication (e.g., ASD, PDA, or VSD) to allow for mixing of blood; associated with multiple problems such as hypoxia (seen as cyanosis), pulmonary overloading, congestive heart failure
Tricuspid atresia	Absence of tricuspid valve causing decreased pulmonary blood flow; requires ASD to relieve systemic venous engorgement and VSD to allow blood to enter lungs; produces cyanosis; if large VSD is present, pulmonary overloading may develop
VSD	Communication between right and left ventricles; may occur beneath aortic valve in membranous septum, in infundibular (perimembranous) septum, beneath septal leaflet of tricuspid valve, or in muscular septum; produces volume overloading of right ventricle and pulmonary circulation

ASD, Atrial septal defect; *PDA,* patent ductus arteriosus; *TGA,* transposition of the great arteries; *VSD,* ventricular septal defect.

atively easy to repair. Perioperative cardiac nurses may be presented with such a patient, especially when there are no pediatric centers in the near vicinity.

Other congenital deformities and syndromes already discussed in previous chapters include:

When adult patients appear with a congenital lesion more commonly seen in the pediatric population, perioperative nurses can apply principles of surgical management for acquired disorders to these congenital malformations. Although the etiology is different, there are similarities that the perioperative nurse can consider in preparing for these unusual cases. (It is also helpful if a nurse in this situation consults a colleague familiar with congenital cardiac disorders.) For example, patients with tetralogy of Fallot (see Table 20-1) require closure of the ventricular septal defect (VSD), relief of the pulmonary stenosis, and enlargement of the right ventricular outflow tract (often with a synthetic patch). Repair of a congenital VSD would include techniques similar to those used for repair of a postmyocardial infarction VSD (see Chapter 12). Pulmonary stenosis at the valvular level could be repaired by incision of the stenotic pulmonary valve (see Chapter 15) or insertion of a pulmonary allograft (see Chapter 14); subvalvular stenosis may require excision

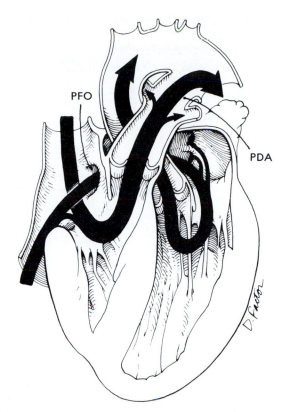

Fig. 20-1 Intracardiac fetal circulation depicting the normal fetal shunts: the patent foramen ovale *(PFO)* and the patent ductus arteriosus *(PDA)*. Most inferior vena cava (IVC) blood passes across the PFO into the left atrium. The superior vena cava (SVC) return is directed predominantly across the PDA, which is large and nonrestrictive. Note that relatively little blood enters or exits the lungs. Persistent postnatal shunting of blood through the PFO and PDA creates hemodynamic disturbances that may require surgical correction. (From Bove EL: Congenital heart lesions. In Miller TA, editor: *Physiologic basis of modern surgical care*, St Louis, 1988, Mosby.)

of a portion of the hypertrophied right ventricular outflow tract. Patch closure of the right ventriculotomy may be required: the patch material, suture, and felt pledgets, as well as the surgical technique, may be similar to those used for a standard repair of a left ventricular apical aneurysm (see Chapter 12).

INTRAUTERINE CIRCULATION

The fetal lungs do not oxygenate blood; the lungs are nonaerated and filled with fluid, which produces a high pulmonary vascular resistance. Both oxygen and nutrients are provided by the mother, whose blood is circulated to the placenta, where oxygen and other metabolic substrates are exchanged for the metabolic waste products of the fetus. Enriched blood is carried to the fetus through the umbilical vein, passes through the liver, and enters the inferior vena cava (IVC) and right atrium. Most of this blood passes preferentially across the patent foramen ovale (bypassing the high-pressure pulmonary vascular bed) into the left atrium, left ventricle, and ascending aorta to perfuse the brain and coronary circulation (Fig. 20-1).

Blood returning to the superior vena cava (SVC) enters the right atrium and passes through the tricuspid valve into the right ventricle and the pulmonary artery. Much of this blood passes across the nonrestrictive, widely patent ductus arteriosus into the descending aorta rather than into the high-pressure pulmonary system. Because the right and left ventricles face similar resistances, both ventricles function essentially as one unit (Bove, 1988). Blood in the aorta returns to the placenta via the umbilical arteries.

POSTNATAL CIRCULATORY CHANGES

At birth, closure of the normal fetal shunts—the foramen ovale and the ductus arteriosus—is necessary to achieve separation of the pulmonary and systemic circulations. Elimination of the placenta (which in utero creates a low systemic vascular resistance) results in an abrupt increase in systemic vascular resistance. Aeration of the lungs gradually decreases pulmonary vascular resistance, promoting greater blood flow to the lungs (Rudolph and Nadas, 1962).

Increased pulmonary venous return to the left atrium elevates left atrial pressure. This causes the septum primum (a flap of tissue on the left atrial wall) to seal closed the foramen ovale (which becomes the fossa ovalis). Increased arterial oxygen tension causes constriction of the smooth muscle in the wall of the ductus arteriosus (which becomes the ligamentum ar-

Table 20-2 ■ *Congenital malformations seen in the adult*

Malformation	Example
Defects: Absent tissue in cardiac septa (walls), causing shunts	Atrial septal defect
Obstructions: Excess tissue at or near level of cardiac valves or major arteries	Coarctation of aorta; idiopathic hypertrophic subaortic stenosis
Anomalous connections: Abnormal communications between arteries and veins or between vessels and cardiac chambers	Anomalous pulmonary venous return (e.g., into right atrium)
Improperly formed tissue: Having normal function at birth and during adolescence but later causing cardiac dysfunction	Bicuspid aortic valve
Combinations of the above	Tetralogy of Fallot

Modified from Roberts WC: Congenital cardiovascular abnormalities usually "silent" until adulthood. In Roberts WC: *Adult congenital heart disease*, Philadelphia, 1987, FA Davis.

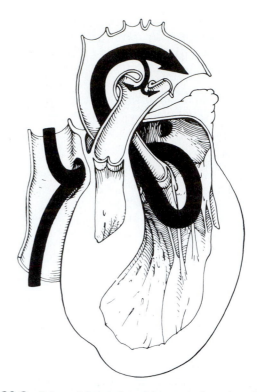

Fig. 20-2   Tricuspid atresia with normally related great vessels and without a ventricular septal defect (VSD). Pulmonary blood flow depends on an atrial septal defect (ASD) to shunt blood to the left atrium, from where it enters the left ventricle. From there, blood enters the aorta and enters the lungs via a patent ductus arteriosus. When a VSD is also present, blood can cross to the right ventricle and enter the lungs. (From Bove EL: Congenital heart lesions. In Miller TA, editor: *Physiologic basis of modern surgical care*, St Louis, 1988, Mosby.)

teriosum). When either the ductus arteriosus or the foramen ovale fails to close, mixing of oxygenated and unoxygenated blood persists. The higher pressure in the systemic circulation (as compared with the pulmonary circulation) leads to shunting of blood into the pulmonary system that, if severe enough, eventually results in congestive heart failure.

CONGENITAL MALFORMATIONS

Unlike acquired cardiac disease, which imposes pathologic anatomic and physiologic changes in previously "normal" structures, the major problems associated with congenital disorders of the heart and great vessels are the disturbed hemodynamics, and in some lesions the hypoxemia, that result from abnormal morphology, intracardiac shunting, and altered pulmonary blood flow (Hickey and Wessel, 1987).

Why some congenital malformations do not require intervention until later childhood or adulthood is related to the nature of the lesion (Table 20-2), the altered volume and pressure loads affecting cardiac function in the neonatal period, and the degree of oxygen saturation of the blood supplying the tissues. Lesions are often categorized as **acyanotic** (those that do not produce systemic arterial desaturation) or **cyanotic** (those that produce a bluish discoloration from venous blood entering the arterial circulation and causing arterial oxygen desaturation). Cyanotic lesions can be due to right-to-left shunts within the heart or aorta, or to transposition of the pulmonary artery and the aorta (Hazinski, 1992).

Also important are the status of the lungs, which can be affected by increased pulmonary blood flow; the type and size of the malformation or defect; the

resistance to flow through the abnormal, as well as the normal, vascular pathways; and the direction and magnitude of the shunts. For example, an abnormal opening in the ventricular septum produces shunting of blood from the area of higher pressure (usually the left ventricle) to the area of lower pressure (e.g., the right ventricle). An isolated, small VSD will have fewer adverse hemodynamic consequences than a large VSD or multiple VSDs, both of which would substantially increase the left-to-right shunting of blood into the pulmonary vasculature, eventually resulting in increased pulmonary vascular resistance. If, however, the VSD is associated with a severe obstruction to right ventricular outflow (such as a tightly stenotic pulmonary valve), then there is likely to be higher pressure in the right ventricle as it tries to overcome the resistance to ejection, and this can cause blood to be shunted to the (relatively lower pressure) left ventricle.

Other developmental cardiac abnormalities may be present. Valves may be absent (e.g., tricuspid atresia; Fig. 20-2); chambers may be underdeveloped (e.g., hypoplastic left heart syndrome); systemic and pulmonary arteries may be attached to the "wrong" ven-

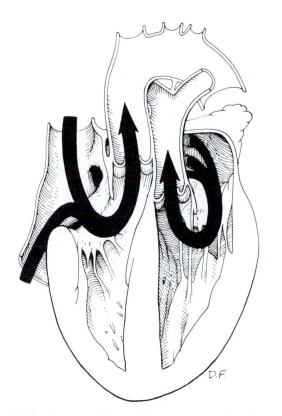

Fig. 20-3 Transposition of the great arteries. The aorta arises from the right ventricle, and the pulmonary artery arises from the left ventricle, producing severe hypoxemia. For survival, an intracardiac shunt is needed to allow oxygen-saturated blood to enter the aorta and the systemic circulation. (From Bove EL: Congenital heart lesions. In Miller TA, editor: *Physiologic basis of modern surgical care*, St Louis, 1988, Mosby.)

tricle (e.g., transposition of the great arteries; Fig. 20-3). Combinations of malformations (e.g., in tetralogy of Fallot) are not uncommon and may not be evident during the initial diagnostic workup. Because of the possibility of finding additional anomalies at operation, a surgeon will explore cardiac and related anatomy meticulously during surgery.

The frequency of congenital lesions seen in the adult is a reflection not only of their rate of occurrence, but also of the mortality in childhood. The more serious lesions are not seen in later life because they are more likely to cause death in infancy (Cooley, Hallman, and Hammam, 1966).

DIAGNOSTIC EVALUATION OF CONGENITAL HEART DISEASE

A complete history and physical examination incorporates the extent of the cardiopulmonary impairment and other, extracardiac congenital anomalies that are frequently associated with congenital heart disease. Pulmonary infections are common in lungs that are chronically volume overloaded, and the pres-

ence, severity, and duration of hypoxemia should be investigated (Hickey and Wessel, 1987). Bacterial endocarditis is also seen in these patients and is related to the endothelial trauma that can occur from altered circulatory patterns.

Electrocardiogram

The ECG provides information about cardiac rhythm, the adverse effects of volume and pressure overload on the ventricles, conduction abnormalities such as bundle-branch blocks, and signs of ventricular hypertrophy (Liebman and Plonsey, 1989). Interpretation of the ECG should take into consideration the effects of diuresis on electrolyte levels. The classic histologic studies of the conduction system by Lev (1958, 1959, 1960) have been valuable in interpreting ECG patterns, as well as in guiding the surgeon during intraoperative repairs of congenital cardiac anomalies.

Chest Radiography

Posteroanterior and lateral chest radiographs illustrate cardiac size and configuration, the pattern of pulmonary blood flow, the position of the aortic arch, and skeletal abnormalities (such as rib notching, seen in patients with coarctation of the aorta). In adults who have had previous surgery for palliation of congenital malformations, the chest x-ray film may show rib deformity from thoracotomy or the extent of adhesions from sternotomy, conduits or shunts, or postoperative complications (Gross and Steiner, 1991). Currently, contrast angiography is infrequently used, but it may be required for some complicated lesions.

Echocardiography

Two-dimensional echocardiography with color flow Doppler is practically indispensable for the diagnosis of congenital (and acquired) cardiac disorders. Its use may obviate the need for cardiac catheterization, which can be risky in the neonate. Uncomplicated ASD, PDA, and coarctation of the aorta may be diagnosed with precision in many cases. For more complex defects of the atrial or ventricular septum or for small-lumen PDAs, echocardiography has limitations, and diagnosis may require more invasive techniques (Meyer, 1989). Doppler technology provides information about the movement of blood (direction and velocity), pressure gradients across valves and obstructions, and the valve area (Goldberg, 1989). In addition to its noninvasiveness, echocardiography avoids ionizing radiation and is relatively inexpensive (Gross and Steiner, 1991).

Cardiac Catheterization

Cardiac catheterization with cineangiocardiography remains an important diagnostic technique for assessing congenital malformations, although echocardiography is becoming increasingly useful for initial diagnosis. Because adults with congenital lesions are also at risk for developing acquired heart disease, cardiac catheterization is routinely done to determine the existence and extent of obstructive atherosclerotic lesions and other acquired disorders and to assess left ventricular function. It is also used to study the direction, magnitude, and approximate location of intracardiac shunts. Intracardiac and intravascular pressures, pressure gradients, and blood oxygen saturations can be measured. For example, the patient whose arterial blood is fully saturated in the aorta can be safely assumed to have no significant right-to-left shunt, whereas documentation of hypoxemia in the aorta indicates shunting of desaturated blood into the systemic circulation (Hickey and Wessel, 1987).

Other Diagnostic Techniques

Computed tomography (CT) is helpful for diagnosing a number of congenital disorders. CT scans may be especially useful in anomalies associated with the great vessels.

Magnetic resonance imaging (MRI) and positron emission tomography can provide information about morphology and altered hemodynamics; they are also being used to study cardiac metabolism noninvasively by measuring the phosphorus found in high-energy phosphates (e.g., adenosine triphosphate [ATP]) and other biologically important atomic nuclei used in metabolic processes. MRI is useful for visualizing coarctation of the aorta and is especially valuable in the older patient whose aortic isthmus may not be easily assessed with ultrasonic techniques. (Echocardiography is superior, however, for evaluating flow velocity through shunts and defects.) Ventricular septal defects are not as easily demonstrated with MRI (Jacobstein, 1989).

Radionuclide techniques can be used to quantify left-to-right shunting and systolic ventricular performance, and there is great potential for measuring ventricular volumes and diastolic function (Hurwitz and Treves, 1989).

PATENT DUCTUS ARTERIOSUS

PDA is the most common cause of left-to-right shunting at the level of the great arteries (see Fig. 20-1). Because aortic pressure is higher than pulmonary artery pressure throughout the cardiac cycle, shunting occurs in both systole and diastole. This produces a continuous murmur, often described as "machinery like." In addition, the low-resistance pulmonary circulation allows a significant amount of aortic diastolic runoff, resulting in a wide pulse pressure and a bounding arterial pulse. A large PDA will produce a substantial increase in pulmonary blood flow, leading to pulmonary overloading and eventual heart failure (Bove, 1988). A smaller PDA, producing less left-to-right shunting, may not be clinically significant for many years.

Infant Patent Ductus Arteriosus

Pharmacologic closure with indomethacin (a prostaglandin inhibitor) may be attempted in small babies with a physiologically significant shunt. (Conversely, in babies with congenital lesions that severely limit pulmonary blood flow, such as a stenotic or absent tricuspid valve, a PDA may be necessary for survival until surgery can be performed. In such cases prostaglandin may be used to maintain the patency of the ductus.) Nonsurgical methods to close the ductus have included the insertion of occlusive devices under fluoroscopy in the cardiac catheterization laboratory.

Procedural considerations

Surgical closure of a PDA is indicated when the patient is at risk for or has congestive heart failure. The procedure can be performed in the operating room (OR) or in the neonatal intensive care unit (NICU). Where surgery is performed is based on the ability of the infant to withstand the stress of transport to and from the nursery, the availability of infant carrier systems, the creation of a suitable operative environment, the availability and skill of personnel, and surgeon preference (Huddleston, 1991; Taylor and others, 1986). For infants who are critically unstable and require high-frequency ventilation or extracorporeal membrane oxygenation (ECMO) (see Chapter 11), PDA ligation in the NICU may be preferred in order to avoid the risks of transport.

When PDA ligation is performed in the NICU, the primary concern is maintenance of sterility (Huddleston, 1991) to protect the infant from infection. Sterile instruments and supplies required for surgery are often brought to the unit. Other items may be present in the unit or may be transported from the OR as needed (Box 20-2).

Closure of the ductus can be performed in a number of ways. Gross (Gross and Hubbard, 1939) originally ligated the ductus of a 7-year-old girl with No. 8 braided silk. Current ligation techniques may use double ligature of heavy silk (e.g., No. 1) or a pursestring ligature of polypropylene. The ligated ductus may or may not be divided.

Division and oversewing of the cut ductal ends and double application of metal vascular clips with or without division are other methods of ligation. The use of vascular clips has gained some popularity; its proponents maintain that the technique minimizes the risk of tearing friable ductal tissue (especially in the posterior wall of the ductus) in infants, as well as in adults. Prior to application of the clips, the applier must be checked for easy release of the clip and for correct apposition of the clip applier jaws (Taylor and others, 1986).

In neonates an important consideration is distinguishing between the various vascular structures: the PDA, aorta, pulmonary artery, and left subclavian artery (Box 20-3). A careful evaluation is necessary to avoid ligating the wrong vessel, because in neonates the PDA may be quite large and resemble the aorta.

Box 20-2 Instruments and supplies for ligation of a patent ductus arteriosus outside of the operating room

Instruments*

Knife handles
Vascular forceps
Adson tissue forceps with teeth
Fine dissecting scissors
Suture scissors
Towel clips
Mosquito clamps
Hemostats
Kelly clamps
Right-angle clamps
Vascular clip appliers (assorted sizes)
Needle holders
Vascular clamps (straight and angled)
Suction tip(s)
Sponge sticks
Ribbon retractors
Brain retractors
Vein retractors
Army-Navy retractors
Senn retractors
Eyelid retractors
Rib spreader

Sterile Supplies

Gowns, gloves, drapes
Peanut (Kittner) sponges
Suture (heavy silk ties, vascular suture, closing suture)
Mineral oil
Electrocautery pencil
Suction tubing
Chest catheter (standard chest tube for older patient or red rubber catheter for infant)
Vascular ligating clips (assorted sizes)
Skin preparation materials
Hand scrub brushes

Nonsterile Supplies and Equipment

Electrosurgical unit
Electrosurgical dispersive pad
Spotlight
Radiant warmer (infants)
Surgeon headlights and magnifying loupes
Privacy screens
Surgical hats and masks
Positioning supplies
Physiologic monitoring devices
(Blood and blood products should be available at the start of surgery)

Modified from Huddleston KR: Patent ductus arteriosus ligation: performing surgery outside the operating room, *AORN J* 53(1):69, 1991.

*Size of instruments is dependent on size and weight of patient; type of instruments is dependent on surgeon's preference.

Box 20-3 Special considerations for patients with congenital heart disease

JoAnn Desilets, RN (JD)
Children's Hospital of Philadelphia
Philadelphia, Pennsylvania

Jill Montgomery, RN (JM)
Children's Hospital Medical Center
Boston, Massachusetts

General Considerations

Participate in preoperative evaluation; include parents and significant others (JM).

Develop instrument sets that can be used for most patients within a particular size range (e.g., under 15 kg, 15 to 30 kg, over 30 kg); add longer instruments if needed for deep cavities (JD).

In patients with prior palliative surgery (e.g., creation of a shunt), consider type, location, and purpose of shunt: central shunts (e.g., aorta to main pulmonary artery) may be directly under sternum and may pose a risk of laceration during sternotomy (JD).

Occasionally, when patient has not undergone cardiac catheterization for diagnosis, other (undetected) anomalies or defects may be found at surgery: always plan, and be prepared, for a more complex lesion than originally anticipated; unexpected findings are not uncommon in patients with congenital cardiac anomalies (JM).

Have blood (and blood products) immediately available in OR (JM).

Know where lesion is situated (e.g., does aorta arch to the right or to the left?) (JM).

Patent Ductus Arteriosus (PDA) Repair

There is always the potential risk of ligating the wrong vessels during closure of a PDA; anticipate a thorough assessment of vascular structures within operative field before ligating ductus (JD).

Double check that there is no malocclusion of jaws of vascular clamps; nonfunctioning clamps can cause vascular rupture with severe hemorrhage, which is very poorly tolerated in neonates with (relatively) low circulating blood volume (JM).

Pay special attention to positioning to avoid brachial plexus injury (JM).

Local anesthetic may be injected in area of thoracotomy incision to reduce postoperative incisional pain and to facilitate breathing and recovery; have (preferred) medication on field (JM).

If occlusion is to be performed in cardiac catheterization laboratory, maintain communication and obtain patient data (e.g., age, weight, availability of blood) in the event that patient needs to come to operating room for emergency surgery; have a plan that can be implemented quickly (JM).

Continued.

Box 20-3   *Special considerations for patients with congenital heart disease—cont'd*

Atrial Septal Defect (ASD)

Plan for bicaval venous cannulation (but may use cardiotomy suction to drain venous return in very small patients with simple lesions) (JD); very complex lesions may require hypothermic circulatory arrest (JM).

Have temporary and permanent epicardial pacemaker leads and generator available (JM).

Anticipate insertion of right atrial and/or left atrial pressure monitoring lines (JM).

ASD: Secundum

Anticipate patch repair or suture closure, depending on lesion (JD); patch material includes pericardium, knitted Dacron, PTFE (JM).

ASD: Primum

Be aware that surgeon will look for VSD and other anomalies in addition to evaluating ASD (JD).

Surgeon will assess mitral valve for cleft leaflet or evidence of more severe mitral regurgitation; depending on degree of mitral valve dysfunction, valvuloplasty, suture reconstruction, or valve replacement may be performed (JD).

ASD: Sinus Venosus

Anticipate presence of anomalous pulmonary venous return into right atrium (JM).

May use right-angle venous cannulas to provide better operative visualization (JM).

Ventricular Septal Defect (VSD)

Determination of surgical incision (e.g., right or left ventriculotomy) depends on location and type of defect: multiple muscular VSDs may be approached via left ventriculotomy; membranous VSD may be best approached through right ventriculotomy (JD).

Have atrioventricular (AV) sequential pacemaker available following repair (JM).

Coarctation of the Aorta

Anticipate use of bilateral (arm) blood pressure monitoring (JM).

Have a selection of aortic vascular clamps in different sizes and angles for total or partial occlusion of aorta (type of clamp depends on repair intended); be prepared for anything (JM).

Have selection of tube grafts (JD, JM).

Because paralysis due to prolonged ischemia is a dreaded complication, be especially attentive to preventing unnecessary aortic cross-clamp time (JM).

The PDA may seem to be in continuity with the descending aorta, whereas the aortic isthmus and aortic arch are smaller (Walhausen and Pierce, 1985).

Operative procedure: ligation of a patent ductus arteriosus in the infant

The patient is placed in the lateral position with the left side up. Positioning supplies (e.g., axillary rolls, padding between the knees) are the same as those used for any lateral position (see Chapter 11). Small axillary rolls can be made from a rolled cloth diaper, Webril, or a washcloth. Pressure areas are padded, and a dispersive electrode pad is placed around the buttocks. Adhesive tape across the hips may be used to stabilize the patient, although in neonates this may be unnecessary.

Routine monitoring includes ECG, pulse oximetry, and monitoring of blood pressure, temperature, and end-tidal carbon dioxide (when possible). Head coverings are used to reduce heat loss from the head; radiant warmers may be used to provide additional warmth. Very small infants present special needs. Finding sufficient space for ECG electrodes and dispersive pads may be a challenge. However, dispersive pads should not be trimmed down, because this could cause inadequate dispersion of electrical currents and result in skin burns.

Procedure

1. A thoracotomy incision is made in the third or fourth intercostal space (Fig. 20-4).

2. The ribs are spread with hand-held retractors for initial dissection. A Finochietto rib spreader is then inserted.

   The lungs are carefully retracted downward and forward, taking care to protect the phrenic, recurrent laryngeal, and main vagus nerves (Fig. 20-5).

3. The mediastinal pleura is opened over the aortic isthmus (the portion of the aorta over the PDA, between the left subclavian artery and the descending aorta); the incision is extended to expose the subclavian artery, the ductus, and the pulmonary artery.

4. The vascular structures are inspected and identified, and the determination is made as to which occlusion technique to use. Retraction sutures

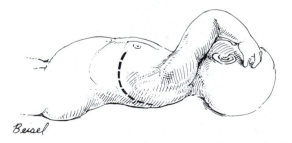

Fig. 20-4   Incision for repair of a PDA. (From Waldhausen JA, Pierce WS: *Johnson's surgery of the chest*, ed 5, St Louis, 1985, Mosby.)

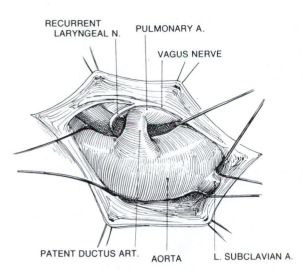

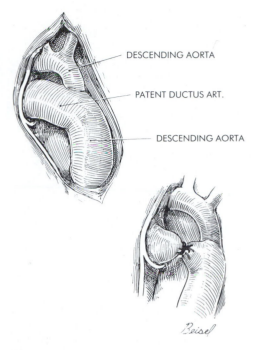

Fig. 20-5 Surgical exposure for closure of a PDA. Note the relationships between the PDA, aorta, left subclavian artery, and pulmonary artery, and the location of the vagus nerve and its branch, the recurrent laryngeal nerve. (From Waldhausen JA, Pierce WS: *Johnson's surgery of the chest,* ed 5, St Louis, 1985, Mosby.)

Fig. 20-7 In the neonate the ductus arteriosus may be quite large and difficult to distinguish from the aorta. (From Waldhausen JA, Pierce WS: *Johnson's surgery of the chest,* ed 5, St Louis, 1985, Mosby.)

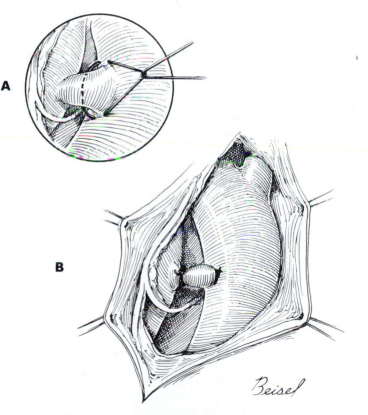

Fig. 20-6 **A,** A pursestring ligature of a PDA may be preferred to passing a ligature around the ductus with a ligature carrier, which requires more extensive dissection and increases the risk of hemorrhage from the posterior wall of the ductus. **B,** Completed, double suture ligation. (From Waldhausen, JA, Pierce WS: *Johnson's surgery of the chest,* ed 5, St Louis, 1985, Mosby.)

may be placed around the aorta proximally and distally, and around the subclavian artery.

5A. **Suture ligation:** A heavy (No. 1) silk suture may be placed around the ductus and tied (Fig. 20-6, *A*); a second ligature may be placed around the ductus (Fig. 20-6, *B*). Coating the ligature with sterile mineral oil may facilitate its passage around the ductus.

In some neonates the ductus may be very large, and it must be distinguished from the aorta (Fig. 20-7).

5B. **Vascular clip:** A medium to medium-large vascular clip may be placed across the ductus. This technique minimizes the risk of hemorrhage associated with dissection of the posterior wall of the ductus. (Retraction sutures may not be required.)

5C. **Division and oversewing:** The ductus may be clamped proximally and distally and divided, and the ends may be oversewn (Fig. 20-8).

5D. **Pursestring ligation:** A pursestring ligature may be sewn on the aortic side, and another one may be sewn on the pulmonary side; these are tied, occluding the PDA.

6. If the pleura has been entered, air can be removed with the chest tube. In neonates a red rubber catheter can be placed into the pleura through the partially closed incision and then gradually withdrawn while the lungs are inflated and the pneumothorax is evacuated. Once the catheter is removed, the incision is completely closed.

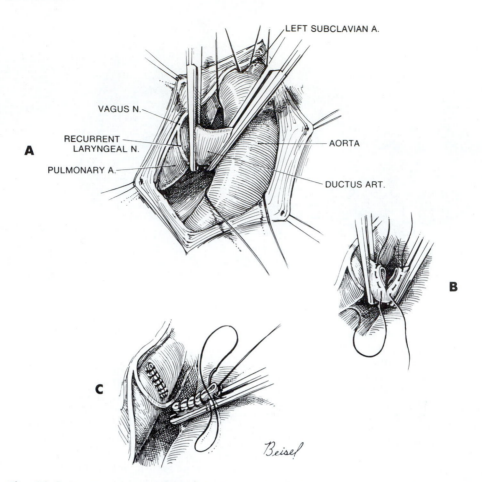

LEFT SUBCLAVIAN A.

VAGUS N.

A

RECURRENT
LARYNGEAL N.

PULMONARY A.

AORTA

DUCTUS ART.

B

C

Beisel

Fig. 20-8 **A,** Clamps are applied to the aortic and pulmonary sides of the ductus arteriosus. **B,** The ductus arteriosus may be divided halfway through and partially sutured as a precaution in the event that a clamp slips. **C,** Division of the ductus is completed, and an over-and-over technique is used to close each end of the ductus.
(From Waldhausen JA, Pierce WS: *Johnson's surgery of the chest,* ed 5, St Louis, 1985, Mosby.)

7. The skin closure is completed, and dressings are applied.

Postoperative period

In the absence of other problems, the postoperative course after PDA closure is usually uneventful. Occasionally a ligated ductus becomes patent again; if the reopened ductus is hemodynamically significant, reoperation is performed to divide and oversew the vessel. Even when a reopened ductus has little clinical impact, closure is advised to reduce the susceptibility to endarteritis (Myers and Waldhausen, 1991).

Adult Patent Ductus Arteriosus

A ductus that does not close spontaneously within 2 months of birth usually remains persistently patent. It is also more commonly an isolated anomaly. Dyspnea and recurrent respiratory infections are typical presenting symptoms. The presence and severity of symptoms in adults is determined by the size of the PDA, the presence of pulmonary hypertension, and the direction of the shunt. Congestive heart failure is a significant cause of death in adult patients with PDA. With improved diagnostic techniques and selective antibiotic prophylaxis, the incidence of infective endarteritis has been greatly decreased (McManus, 1987). Because progressive pulmonary vascular disease may lead to rapid and irreversible cardiac failure, it is recommended that adults with PDA undergo surgical closure (Wright and Newman, 1978).

In adults the ductus may be calcified, sclerotic, and aneurysmal, increasing the risk of rupture. Double ligation (similar to that used in infants) is effective in the uncomplicated adult ductus. In more complicated cases where the ductus is broad and fragile, felt-buttressed sutures or patch closure of the ductal opening inside the aorta may be performed. Bypass shunts or CPB (occasionally with hypothermia) may be used for the difficult ductus (Johnson and Kron, 1988). In patients with marked elevation of pulmonary vascular resistance, operative closure may not significantly reduce pulmonary hypertension, and outcomes may be less favorable (Borow and Braunwald, 1988).

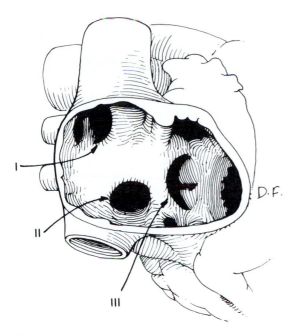

Fig. 20-9 Location of the three types of ASD. The sinus venosus defect *(I)* is shown with anomalous drainage of the right upper pulmonary vein. The ostium secundum defect *(II)* is in the midportion of the septum in the area of the fossa ovalis. The ostium primum defect *(III)* is located in the base of the septum, with its inferior edge formed by the continuity of the tricuspid and mitral valves. There is often a cleftlike anomaly in the anterior leaflet of the mitral valve visible through the defect. (From Bove EL: Congenital heart lesions. In Miller TA, editor: *Physiologic basis of modern surgical care*, St Louis, 1988, Mosby.)

ATRIAL SEPTAL DEFECT

ASDs are among the most common of the congenital malformations seen in adulthood. The defect can occur in three forms (Fig. 20-9): the ostium secundum (the most common), the sinus venosus, and the ostium primum (least common). A common associated lesion in the sinus venosus ASD is partial anomalous pulmonary venous return into the right atrium.

Although blood being shunted from the left atrium to the right atrium increases pulmonary blood flow, the right atrium and the lungs are generally able to tolerate this increased volume for many years. This is due to the distensibility of the atrial wall and the pulmonary vasculature, as well as to the low pressures found within the right side of the heart. Eventually, pulmonary overloading can produce pulmonary hypertension and elevated pulmonary vascular resistance. Pulmonary arterial pressure may begin to approximate systemic arterial pressure, which in turn can lead to a balanced (bidirectional) shunt or to reversal of the shunt whereby higher right-sided pressures create a right-to-left shunt, producing systemic arterial desaturation (e.g., cyanosis). With advancing age, patients can also develop cardiomegaly, atrial dysrhythmias, right ventricular hypertrophy, and right

ventricular failure (cor pulmonale) (Hamilton and others, 1987; Schaff and Danielson, 1987).

The ECG usually demonstrates incomplete right bundle-branch block and a clockwise shift of the heart. Posteroanterior and lateral chest radiographs demonstrate an enlarged right atrium and right ventricle, reflecting the increased ratio of pulmonary blood flow to systemic blood flow (see later discussion). The pulmonary artery shadow is also enlarged. Echocardiography is almost always diagnostic, with transesophageal echocardiography (TEE) widely used to differentiate between the forms of ASD. Atrioventricular valve regurgitation can be demonstrated as well (Cleveland, 1993).

Although bacterial endocarditis is often a risk in patients with congenital heart disease, it is unusual in a patient with an ASD because the relatively large septal defect does not produce a "jet" lesion (the forceful squirting of blood against endocardium or endothelium—as occurs with PDA), which would traumatize the inside of the heart and create a potential site for infection (Seifert and Lefrak, 1984).

Symptoms are usually exertional dyspnea and fatigue. Initially these complaints may be attributed to coronary artery disease or rheumatic valvular problems rather than to an ASD. Incomplete right bundle-branch block or atrial fibrillation may also be present, particularly in adults (Schaff and Danielson, 1987).

Diagnosis can usually be made with modern echocardiographic techniques, but cardiac catheterization may be performed in adults to determine the presence of coronary or valvular heart disease. Cardiac catheterization techniques have also been extensively used to measure pulmonary and systemic pressures, to determine the oxygen saturation of the cardiac chambers and major vessels, and to compute the ratio of pulmonary blood flow to systemic blood flow (Qp/Qs). In the normal heart the stroke volume of the right ventricle equals that of the left ventricle. In the presence of an ASD, which shunts some of the left ventricular preload into the right side of the heart, the pulmonary circulation receives more blood than the systemic circulation. Thus the ratio of pulmonary blood flow to systemic blood flow is higher than the normal Qp/Qs of 1:1. The patient also has an increased oxygen saturation of the right atrial blood (normal is 75%). This is due to the shunting of freshly oxygenated blood to the right atrium (the increase in venous oxygen saturation is referred to as a "step-up"). Blood samples can be taken from a number of locations between the SVC and the IVC in order to determine the site of the defect and whether there is anomalous pulmonary venous return to the right atrium (which would be reflected in higher oxygen saturation of the blood near the SVC as compared with that near the IVC). Table 20-3 lists cardiac catheterization data of a patient with a secundum ASD.

Procedural considerations

Monitoring lines consist of arterial and central venous pressure lines; a pulmonary artery pressure catheter

Table 20-3 ■ *Cardiac catheterization laboratory results of a patient with ostium secundum atrial septal defect*

Measurement	Defect	Normal
Pressures:		
Right atrium	Mean = 1 mm Hg	Less than 5 mm Hg
Right ventricle	46/0-3 mm Hg	25/0-5 mm Hg
Pulmonary artery	46/18 (mean 26) mm Hg	25/12 (mean 16) mm Hg
Pulmonary artery wedge pressure	Mean = 4	4-12 mean
Left atrium	Mean = 4	8-12 mean
Left ventricle	140/0-6	100-140/0-5
Aorta	140/68	100-140/60-80
Oxygen saturations:		
Superior vena cava	76%	75%
Inferior vena cava	81%	75%
High right atrium	82%	75%
Mid right atrium	84%	75%
Low right atrium	85%	75%
Right ventricle inflow	85%	75%
Right ventricle outflow	85%	75%
Left atrium	98%	95%
Left-to-right shunt (ratio of pulmonary blood flow to systemic blood flow)	1.9 : 1	1 : 1
Systemic vascular resistance	25 Wood units	Less than 20 Wood units
Total pulmonary resistance	3.4 Wood units	Less than 3.5 Wood units
Pulmonary vascular resistance	2.9 Wood units	Less than 2 Wood units
Angiography: Normal contraction of left ventricle without evidence of mitral regurgitation or mitral valve prolapse		
Coronary angiography: Normal coronary arteries		

Modified from Seifert PC, Lefrak EA: Atrial septal defect: the adult patient, *AORN J* 39(4):617, 1984.

hampers exposure of the right atrial surgical site (insertion may also be complicated by the presence of large defects through which the catheter could travel). If left ventricular function requires monitoring, a left atrial line can be inserted during surgery, or a pulmonary artery catheter can be introduced after completion of the operation. Nurses should be aware that air in venous lines can pass through the defect and embolize into the systemic circulation. Therefore great caution should be taken to remove any air from peripheral or central venous lines (Weller and others, 1984). TEE is commonly used during surgery for ASD in the adult.

Bicaval cannulation is used for venous return so that systemic blood does not obscure the field. A right-angle SVC cannula may be needed if the ASD is high in the right atrium (e.g., sinus venosus ASD). Mild hypothermia (32° C [90° F]) is usually sufficient for simple defects. Cardioplegia solution is given antegradely; cardioplegia solution given retrogradely through the coronary sinus is cumbersome with the right atrium opened, but some surgeons do give intermittent retroplegia infusions with a hand-held catheter.

A median sternotomy is routinely performed, but a modified right thoracotomy approach can also be used if there are no other suspected anomalies. The cosmetic results of such an anterolateral (submammary) incision have been excellent (Rosengart and Stark, 1993).

Instrumentation that is used for mitral valve surgery (Chapter 13) can also be used for ASD repair.

Knitted patch material is preferred for closing the defect because it is easier to handle and frays less than woven material; autogenous pericardium may also be inserted. Primary closure is generally avoided in adults with large defects in order to avoid distortion of the atrium or excessive tension on the suture line.

Surgery is associated with some risk to the atrioventricular node, which is situated near the coronary sinus and the septal leaflet of the tricuspid valve (Bharati, Lev, and Kirklin, 1983) (Fig. 20-10). Permanent epicardial pacemaker leads should be available in the event that heart block is created (see Box 20-3).

Operative procedure: repair of an atrial septal defect

1. A median sternotomy is made, and bicaval cannulation for CPB is performed. A cardioplegia infusion line/venting catheter is placed in the anterior aorta. If pericardium is to be used for closure of the defect, a piece of sufficient size is excised and kept moist and pliable in normal saline until it is needed.

2. After bypass is initiated, the heart is arrested and the right atrium is opened (see Fig. 20-10). Retractors are inserted to expose the atrial septum.

3. The right atrium is carefully inspected to locate the defect and to determine its size and configuration. Surrounding tissue is inspected for other anomalies. If a prosthetic patch is to be used, sterile patch material is delivered to the field and cut to the appropriate size and shape.

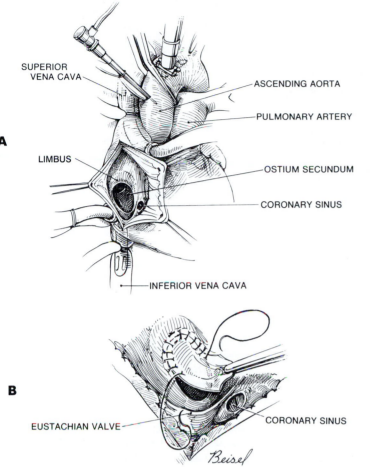

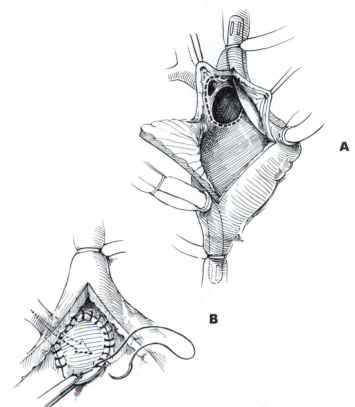

Fig. 20-11 Exposure of a sinus venous ASD with partial anomalous pulmonary venous return (the smaller opening next to the defect). (From Waldhausen JA, Pierce WS: *Johnson's surgery of the chest*, ed 5, St Louis, 1985, Mosby.)

Fig. 20-10 **A,** The right atrium is opened to expose the secundum ASD. Occasionally a very small defect may be closed primarily. **B,** Patch repair. (From Waldhausen JA, Pierce WS: *Johnson's surgery of the chest*, ed 5, St Louis, 1985, Mosby.)

4A. **Repair of secundum ASD:** Suturing of the patch to the edges of the defect is started at the superior margin and proceeds along one side and then the other. Excess material may be further trimmed, and the inferior repair is then completed (Fig. 20-11). Just before patch closure is completed, air within the left atrium and left ventricle is allowed to escape through the opened portion of the patch.

4B. **Repair of sinus venosus ASD:** Repair is similar to that described in 4A. If there is pulmonary venous drainage into the right atrium (Fig. 20-11, *A*), the patch is placed in such a way that it redirects pulmonary venous drainage into the left atrium through the defect but does not impede systemic venous return from the SVC into the right atrium (Fig. 20-11, *B*).

5. Closure of the right atrium is performed so that narrowing of the SVC is avoided. The right atrium is partially closed with 4-0 polypropylene. Air is removed from the right atrium and the pulmonary artery, and closure of the atrium is completed. The aortic vent needle is turned on to remove residual air from the left side of the heart.

6. The cross-clamp is removed, and the heart is defibrillated if it does not resume contraction spontaneously. The ECG is monitored for signs of conduction blocks or dysrhythmias. TEE is used to test the repair and to detect the presence of intracardiac air.

7. Temporary atrial and ventricular pacing wires are inserted. A left atrial pressure line may be inserted to monitor left ventricular response to the increased volume and pressure load resulting from closure of the defect.

8. Chest tubes are placed, and the patient is weaned from bypass.

9. After hemostasis has been achieved, the chest and skin are closed.

Postoperative period

Closure of ASDs in adults increases longevity and provides significant improvement in clinical symptoms. The operative risk is low; increased risk is due primarily to associated problems (e.g., coronary artery

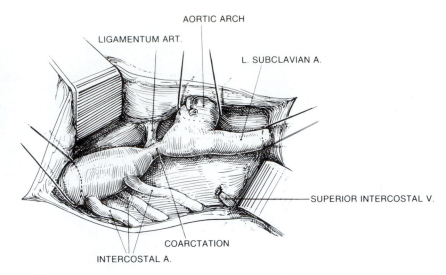

LIGAMENTUM ART.

AORTIC ARCH

L. SUBCLAVIAN A.

SUPERIOR INTERCOSTAL V.

COARCTATION

INTERCOSTAL A.

Fig. 20-12 Exposure of coarctation of the aorta. Note the relationships between the various structures. The superior intercostal vein has been ligated and divided to facilitate exposure. It is common to find greatly enlarged intercostal arteries, which provide collateral circulation to the distal aorta. The ligamentum arteriosum is the former PDA. (From Waldhausen JA, Pierce WS: *Johnson's surgery of the chest,* ed 5, St Louis, 1985, Mosby.)

disease, valvular dysfunction, dysrhythmias). Although it may require a number of months, there is often a decrease in the size of the heart and a reduction in elevated pulmonary pressures. Cardiac rhythm and atrioventricular conduction often remain unchanged (Hamilton and others, 1987; Stewart and Bender, 1991).

COARCTATION OF THE AORTA

Coarctation of the aorta is characterized by a localized narrowing of the aortic wall (Fig. 20-12; see also Table 20-1). Abnormally thick medial tissue (Fig. 20-13) projects into the lumen of the aorta, forming a shelf, which creates an obstruction to left ventricular outflow. Blood pressure proximal to the coarctation is elevated (promoting left ventricular hypertrophy), whereas blood pressure distal to the lesion is decreased. Upper-body hypertension and absent or diminished femoral or pedal pulses may be detected on physical examination. There may be a murmur at the left sternal border caused by blood flow through the narrowed aorta. Left-sided rib notching from the extensive collateral circulation and enlarged intercostal vessels pressing against the thorax is often seen on the chest radiograph. These clinical findings suggest coarctation, which is often confirmed by MRI (which is rapidly becoming the gold standard diagnostic test for coarctation). Cardiac catheterization is usually necessary only if MRI cannot demonstrate the lesion (Cleveland, 1993). The most common associated congenital malformation is a bicuspid aortic valve (see Chapter 14). Other anomalies include VSD, PDA, and mitral valve abnormalities.

In adults (Fig. 20-14, *A*) the coarctation is often found at the junction of the aortic arch and the de-scending aorta distal to the left subclavian artery and the ligamentum arteriosum (formerly the PDA). This postductal form of coarctation, in contrast to the preductal (infant) type of constriction (Fig. 20-14, *B*), is the more common form of coarctation and is also more likely to allow survival into adulthood. This is due to the extensive collateral circulation, which provides blood flow to the kidneys and lower extremities. Collaterals develop in utero and continue after birth in response to the resistance to blood flow through

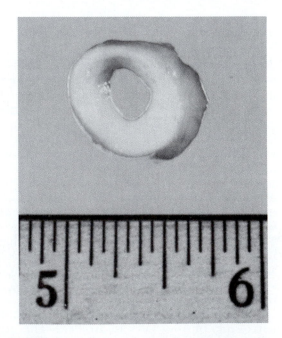

Fig. 20-13 Excised coarcted segment of the aorta. (Courtesy Nevin M. Katz, MD.)

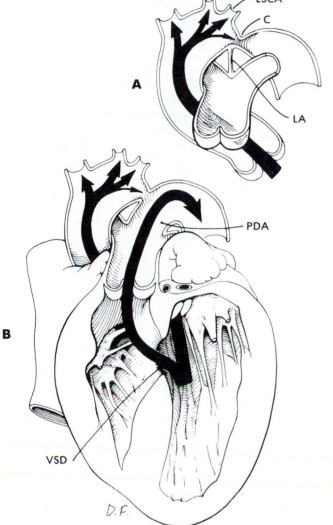

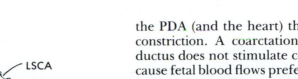

Fig. 20-14 Hemodynamic abnormalities in coarctation of the aorta. **A,** Pathophysiology in the older child or adult. The coarctation *(C)* is distal to the former patent ductus arteriosus *(PDA)*—the ligamentum arteriosum *(LA)*—and the left subclavian artery *(LSCA)*. With this postductal form of coarctation, because there is resistance to flow even in utero, the development of collateral circulation is stimulated and provides a means of perfusing the lower body. **B,** In preductal coarctation, there is little stimulus to develop collateral circulation, because in the fetus blood flow through the ductus is unimpeded. It is only at birth, when the heart must eject against a greatly increased afterload, and perfusion to the lower body is severely compromised, that the effects of the coarctation manifest themselves. Without a ventricular septal defect *(VSD)* to allow blood to pass through into the pulmonary artery and cross the PDA into the distal aorta, severe hypoxemia develops. (From Bove EL: Congenital heart lesions. In Miller TA, editor: *Physiologic basis of modern surgical care*, St Louis, 1988, Mosby.)

the PDA (and the heart) that is created by the aortic constriction. A coarctation located proximal to the ductus does not stimulate collateral development, because fetal blood flows preferentially through the PDA into the descending aorta (with little blood flow traveling through the aorta proximal to the ductus). Although blood flow in utero is relatively unimpeded with preductal coarctations, at birth this changes dramatically as the ductus closes and the heart must eject the full cardiac output into the constricted aorta. Without collateral circulation a PDA becomes an important conduit for distal blood flow. As the ductus begins to close, heart failure will occur if the coarctation is severe (Hazinski, 1992).

Procedural considerations

In the adult, longstanding collateral circulation to the distal aorta will have enlarged the left subclavian artery and the arteries in the muscles and intercostal spaces. These arterial walls tend to be very thin, and hemorrhage from them may be troublesome (Waldhausen and Pierce, 1985). A PDA may be found near the most constricted portion of the coarctation; the PDA may be ligated or clipped as previously described.

Positioning, skin preparation, draping, and instrumentation are similar to those used for descending thoracic aortic aneurysms (see Chapter 16). Different sizes of tube grafts should be available. If preclotting is required, preparations should be made sufficiently in advance; unnecessary prolongation of aortic cross-clamp time creates a risk for spinal ischemia and paralysis (see Box 20-3).

Resection of a short coarctation with end-to-end anastomosis of the aorta can be performed in infants, whose tissue may be easily reapproximated. Because recoarctation can occur after the initial operation, a subclavian flap procedure has been devised whereby the left subclavian artery is divided, brought down, and anastomosed to the aorta to create an adequately enlarged lumen. A reverse subclavian flap may be used to enlarge a coarcted aortic arch; the artery is divided, swung around to the proximal portion of the aorta, and anastomosed to the aortic arch. Because ligation of the subclavian artery restricts blood flow to the affected arm, this technique is usually reserved for very young patients who may be able to develop collateral circulation to perfuse the arm. In children with longer coarctations, or in older patients with less elastic tissue or a sclerotic aorta, patch repair or resection with interposition of a tube graft may be necessary to prevent excessive tension on the suture line. Occasionally the coarctation is left in place and a bypass graft (tube graft) is anastomosed to the aorta proximal and distal to the coarctation (Hallman, Cooley, and Gutgesell, 1987).

Operative procedure: resection of a coarctation of the aorta *(Walhausen and Pierce, 1985)*

1. The patient is placed in the lateral position with the left side up, and a thoracotomy incision is made in the fourth intercostal space.

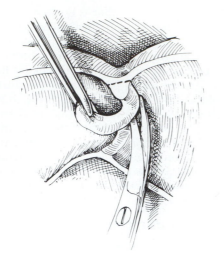

Fig. 20-15 Excision of the coarctation "shelf". (From Waldhausen JA, Pierce WS: *Johnson's surgery of the chest*, ed 5, St Louis, 1985, Mosby.)

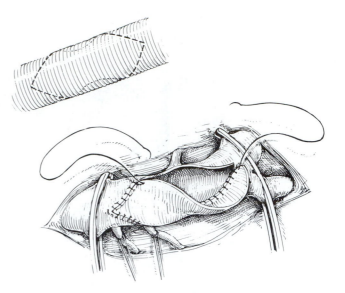

Fig. 20-16 The diamond-shaped patch is anastomosed to the aorta with a continuous suture technique. (From Waldhausen JA, Pierce WS: *Johnson's surgery of the chest*, ed 5, St Louis, 1985, Mosby.)

2. The pleura is opened over the coarctation and aortic isthmus, and the lungs are retracted anteriorly and inferiorly.
3. The area of the coarctation, including the transverse aortic arch, the distal aorta, and the left subclavian artery, is dissected as much as possible, using caution to avoid injury to the recurrent laryngeal, vagus, and phrenic nerves. Distally the aorta may be freed almost to the diaphragm.
4. Heavy silk ligatures or umbilical tapes may be placed around the left subclavian artery, the vertebral artery, and the aorta.
5. Vascular occluding clamps are placed on the aorta above and below the coarctation. Intercostal arteries may be occluded temporarily to control bleeding during the repair.
6. The aorta is opened, and the coarctation shelf is excised (Fig. 20-15).
7A. **Patch repair:** Patch material is cut into an oval or diamond shape and sewn to the aorta with 3-0 or 4-0 polypropylene (Fig. 20-16).
7B. **Resection with graft replacement:** The appropriate-size graft is delivered to the field and anastomosed end-to-end proximally and distally to the aorta. Because the distal aorta tends to be larger than the proximal aorta (related to poststenotic dilatation), the graft can be beveled to approximate the proper lumen size. This technique is similar to that used for resection of a descending thoracic aortic aneurysm (see Chapter 16).
7C. **Subclavian flap repair:** The left subclavian artery is ligated at the origin of the vertebral artery, which is also ligated. The subclavian artery is divided and swung down onto the aorta, where it is sutured (Fig. 20-17).
8. After completion of the anastomoses, the distal clamp is removed first. The proximal clamp is then removed slowly to prevent a sudden increase in the arterial pressure.

9. Hemostasis is achieved, a chest tube is inserted, and the pleura is closed with absorbable suture. The chest is closed, and dressings are applied.

Postoperative period

Complications that may require reoperation in the early postoperative period include hemothorax (usually from a branch of an intercostal artery) and chylothorax (from injury to the thoracic duct, which allows lymph to drain into the chest). Patients may complain of abdominal pain after surgery; this is thought to be related to the sudden and unaccustomed strong blood flow to the mesentery after repair. In severe cases, bowel infarction may result. Recurrent coarctation is a late complication that may require surgery, although this is most likely to occur in infants who have undergone resection and anastomosis of the resected aorta (Hallman, Cooley, and Gutgesell, 1987).

Although resection of an aortic coarctation results in significant reduction in systemic blood pressure in most adults, persistent and unexplained systemic hypertension can be seen in up to 50% of patients (Maron, 1987). Although it is unclear why there is continuing hypertension (in the absence of a residual coarctation), it has been suggested that it is related to the period of time that hypertension existed preoperatively (Clarkson and others, 1983). Thus resection performed in young patients is less likely to result in persistent hypertension; however, the incidence of recoarctation is higher in this group (Kappetein, 1993). Other possible factors are reduced distensibility of the proximal aorta, renovascular abnormalities involving the renin angiotensin system, and essential hypertension (Maron, 1987).

Unfortunately, other cardiovascular complications are not uncommon and may shorten life expectancy.

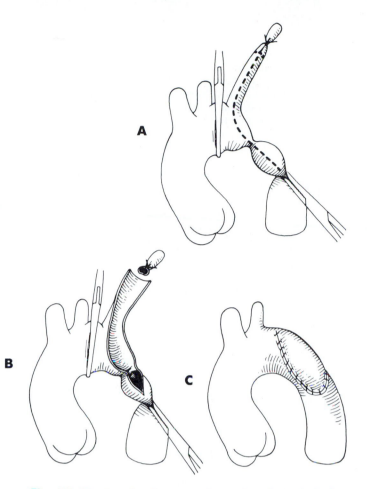

Fig. 20-17 Repair of coarctation using the subclavian flap procedure. **A,** The left subclavian artery is mobilized and divided distally. **B,** A longitudinal incision is made through the artery and the adjacent aorta; the incision must extend distally beyond the coarctation to normal aorta. **C,** The subclavian flap is brought down onto the aorta and anastomosed. (From Bove EL: Congenital heart lesions. In Miller TA, editor: *Physiologic basis of modern surgical care,* St Louis, 1988, Mosby.)

These include unexplained congestive heart failure, aortic or cerebral vascular rupture, and problems associated with the aortic or mitral valve. Because of the high incidence of abnormal valves associated with coarctation, antibiotic prophylaxis is recommended before invasive procedures are done (Smith, 1984).

CONCLUSION

Congenital malformations are not uncommon in the adult. Future trends in congenital heart disease will depend not only on the number of infants born with malformations (often reported as 8 in 1000 live births), but also on the impact of early surgical repair and the effects of survivors having children of their own. Although there is variance in the reported incidence of survivors of congenital heart disease having children with cardiac deformities, the American College of Cardiology (Schlant and others, 1988) has predicted a definite increase. Perioperative nurses are likely to encounter an increasing number of adult patients with lesions ranging from the simple secundum ASD to the more complex tetralogy of Fallot.

REFERENCES

Bharati S, Lev M, Kirklin JW: *Cardiac surgery and the conduction system,* New York, 1983, John Wiley & Sons.

Borow KM, Braunwald E: *Congenital heart disease in the adult.* In Braunwald E, editor: Heart disease, ed 3, Philadelphia, 1988, WB Saunders.

Bove EL: *Congenital heart lesions.* In Miller TA, editor: *Physiologic basis of modern surgical care,* St Louis, 1988, Mosby.

Clarkson PM and others: Results after repair of coarctation of the aorta beyond infancy: a 10 to 28 year follow-up with particular reference to late systemic hypertension, *Am J Cardiol* 51:1481, 1983.

Cleveland DC: Personal communication, 1993.

Cooley DA, Hallman GL, Hammam AS: Congenital cardiovascular anomalies in adults: results of surgical treatment in 167 patients over age 35, *Am J Cardiol* 17(3):303, 1966.

Engle MA: Growth and development of state of the art care for people with congenital heart disease, *J Am Coll Cardiol* 13(7):1453, 1989.

Goldberg SJ: Noninvasive diagnostic methods. III. Doppler echocardiography. In Adams FH, Emmanouilides GC, Riemenschneider TA, editors: *Moss' heart disease in infants, children, and adolescents,* ed 4, Baltimore, 1989, Williams & Wilkins.

Gross RE, Hubbard JP: Surgical ligation of a patent ductus arteriosus, *JAMA* 112:729, 1939.

Gross GW, Steiner RM: Radiographic manifestations of congenital heart disease in the adult patient, *Radiol Clin North Am* 29(2):293, 1991.

Hallman GL, Cooley DA, Gutgesell HP: *Surgical treatment of congenital heart disease,* ed 3, Philadelphia, 1987, Lea & Febiger.

Hamilton WT and others: Atrial septal defect secundum: clinical profile with physiologic correlates. In Roberts WC: *Adult congenital heart disease,* Philadelphia, 1987, FA Davis.

Hazinski MF: Congenital heart disease. III: Obstructive heart lesions, *Life Support Nurs,* p 15, Dec 1982.

Hazinski MF: *Nursing care of the critically ill child,* ed 2, St Louis, 1992, Mosby.

Hickey PR, Wessel DL: Anesthesia for treatment of congenital heart disease. In Kaplan JA, editor: *Cardiac anesthesia,* ed 2, Philadelphia, 1987, WB Saunders.

Huddleston KR: Patent ductus arteriosus ligation: performing surgery outside the operating room, *AORN J* 53(1):69, 1991.

Hurwitz RA, Treves ST: Nuclear cardiology. In Adams FH, Emmanouilides GC, Riemenschneider TA, editors: *Moss' heart disease in infants, children, and adolescents,* ed 4, Baltimore, 1989, Williams & Wilkins.

Jacobstein MD: Magnetic resonance imaging and positron emission tomography. In Adams FH, Emmanouilides GC, Riemenschneider TA, editors: *Moss' heart disease in infants, children, and adolescents,* ed 4, Baltimore, 1989, Williams & Wilkins.

Johnson AM, Kron IL: Closure of the calcified patent ductus in the elderly: avoidance of ductal clamps and shunts, *Ann Thorac Surg* 45:572, 1988.

Kappetein PA and others: Noninvasive long-term follow-up after coarctation repair, *Ann Thorac Surg* 55:1153, 1993.

Lev M: The architecture of the conduction system in congenital heart disease. I. Common atrioventricular orifice, *AMA Arch Pathol* 65:174, 1958.

Lev M: The architecture of the conduction system in congenital heart disease. II. Tetralogy of Fallot, *AMA Arch Pathol* 67:572, 1959.

Lev M: The architecture of the conduction system in congenital heart disease. III. Ventricular septal defect, *AMA Arch Pathol* 70:529, 1960.

Liebman J, Plonsey R: Noninvasive diagnostic methods. I. Electrocardiography. In Adams FH, Emmanouilides GC, Riemenschneider TA, editors: *Moss' heart disease in infants, children, and adolescents,* ed 4, Baltimore, 1989, Williams & Wilkins.

Maron BJ: Aortic isthmic coarctation. In Roberts WC: *Adult congenital heart disease,* Philadelphia, 1987, FA Davis.

McManus BM: Patent ductus arteriosus. In Roberts WC: *Adult congenital heart disease,* Philadelphia, 1987, FA Davis.

Meyer RA: Noninvasive diagnostic methods. I. Echocardiography. In Adams FH, Emmanouilides GC, Riemenschneider TA, editors: *Moss' heart disease in infants, children, and adolescents,* ed 4, Baltimore, 1989, Williams & Wilkins.

Meyers JL, Waldhausen JA: Management of complications following repair of coarctation of the aorta, patent ductus arteriosus, interrupted aortic arch, and vascular rings. In Waldhausen JA, Orringer MB: *Complications in cardiothoracic surgery,* St Louis, 1991, Mosby.

Perloff JK: Congenital heart disease in adults. In Braunwald E, editor: *Heart disease,* ed 4, Philadelphia, 1992, WB Saunders.

Radtke W, Lock J: Balloon dilation, *Pediatr Clin North Am* 37(1):193, 1990.

Rashkind WJ: Historical aspects of surgery for congenital heart disease, *J Thorac Cardiovasc Surg* 84(4):619, 1982.

Roberts WC: Congenital cardiovascular abnormalities usually silent until adulthood. In Roberts WC: Adult congenital heart disease, Philadelphia, 1987, FA Davis.

Rosengart TK, Stark JF: Repair of atrial septal defect through a right thoracotomy, *Ann Thorac Surg* 55:1138, 1993.

Rudolph AM, Nadas AS: The pulmonary circulation and congenital heart disease, *N Engl J Med* 267:968, 1962.

Schaff HV, Danielson GK: Advances in surgical management of congenital heart disease in adults, *Cardiovasc Clin* 17:221, 1987.

Schlant RC and others: Trends in the practice of adult cardiology: implications for manpower, *J Am Coll Cardiol* 12(3):822, 1988.

Seifert PC, Lefrak EA: Atrial septal defect: the adult patient, *AORN J* 39(4):617, 1984.

Smith EF: Acyanotic obstructive lesions: coarctation of the aorta and congenital aortic stenosis, *Nurs Clin North Am* 19(3):471, 1984.

Stewart JR, Bender HW: Management of complications of surgery for septal defects. In Waldhausen JA, Orringer MB: *Complications in cardiothoracic surgery,* St Louis, 1991, Mosby.

Taussig HB: World survey of the common cardiac malformations: developmental error or genetic variant? *Am J Cardiol* 50:544, 1982.

Taylor RL and others: Operative closure of patent ductus arteriosus in premature infants in the neonatal intensive care unit, *Am J Surg* 152:704, 1986.

Waldhausen JA, Pierce WS: *Johnson's surgery of the chest,* ed 5, St Louis, 1985, Mosby.

Weller D and others: Atrial septal defect: a nursing care plan, *AORN J* 39(4):634, 1984.

Wright JS, Newman DC: Ligation of the patent ductus, *J Thorac Cardiovasc Surg* 75:695, 1978.

21

Cardiac Trauma and Emergency Surgery

Luck plays a role in outcome.

Malcolm M. Fisher, MD, 1990

Chance favors the prepared mind.

Louis Pasteur*

Emergency situations are not unusual for perioperative cardiac nurses, many of whom have a "disaster mentality" that enables them to anticipate and prepare for unusual or unexpected events. Cardiac perioperative nurses are aware that "routine" cardiac procedures have the potential for turning into emergencies, given the underlying instability of many patients. When the patient's clinical status deteriorates suddenly outside of the operating room (OR), such as can occur with failed percutaneous transluminal coronary angioplasties (PTCAs), acute rupture of an ischemic mitral papillary muscle, and postmyocardial infarction ventricular septal defects (VSDs), prompt surgical intervention is needed. Efficient and experienced cardiac perioperative nurses are able to respond quickly in these situations and implement the most appropriate treatment. Predetermined protocols, jointly developed by nurse and physician members of the surgical team and confirmed or reviewed as warranted by the patient's clinical status, are invaluable for expeditiously transferring the patient to the OR, opening the chest, instituting cardiopulmonary bypass (CPB), and performing the appropriate repair.

Occasionally patients are too unstable to transport to the OR, and surgery must be performed wherever the patient is located (e.g., the cardiac catheterization laboratory, emergency/trauma department, or critical care unit). When these areas do not have OR capability, portable systems incorporating CPB systems, instruments, and supplies enable the surgical team to perform lifesaving procedures in these and other settings within the hospital.

Factors that facilitate prompt intervention include an awareness of the pathophysiology and the intended goal of therapy, familiarity with the roles and responsibilities of various team members, and coordination of efforts. Emergency situations, whether due to trauma, complications of surgery, or accidents, depend on close cooperation and communication.

This chapter describes some of these emergency situations. Many of the principles involved in trauma care, for example, are similar to those applied when life-threatening alterations occur during any cardiac procedure.

TRAUMA

Trauma is the most common cause of death in individuals less than 44 years of age (Rice and McKenzie, 1989), with automobile and motorcycle crashes constituting the major cause of death. Alcohol is frequently a contributing factor. In the very young and the elderly, falls are a leading cause of death (Kidd, 1993). Only cardiovascular disease, cancer, and cerebrovascular accidents cause more deaths than trauma (Trauma Nursing Coalition, 1992).

The earliest trauma patients were soldiers injured during war. Not surprisingly, the heart was the assailant's preferred target (Unkle, 1988). Military surgeons were instrumental in developing not only methods of vascular and myocardial repair, but also endotracheal intubation, mechanical ventilation, management of pulmonary injuries, and chest drainage systems. Especially notable is Harkin's (1946) accomplishment during World War II (see Chapter 1). He operated on 134 patients with shell fragments and other missiles in or near the heart with no deaths in the series (Symbas and Justicz, 1993).

In addition to improved surgical techniques and

---

*As quoted in Vallery-Radot R: *The life of Pasteur*, 1927. From Beck EM, editor: *Bartlett's familiar quotations*, ed 14, Boston, 1968, Little, Brown.

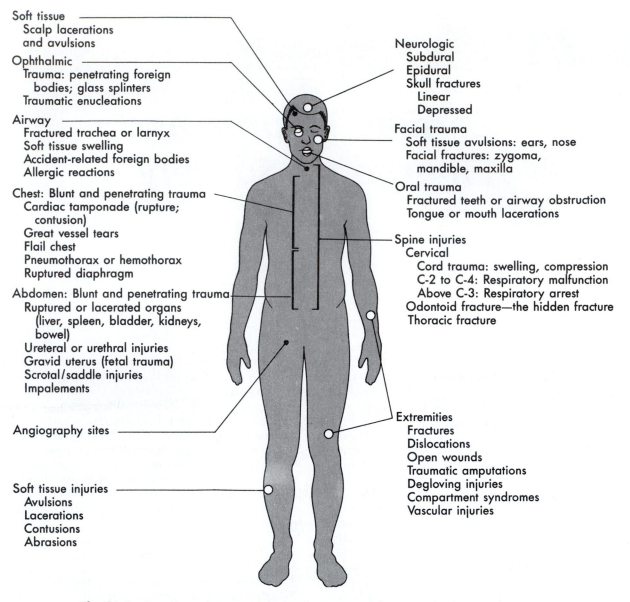

Soft tissue
Scalp lacerations
and avulsions

Ophthalmic
Trauma: penetrating foreign
bodies; glass splinters
Traumatic enucleations

Airway
Fractured trachea or larnyx
Soft tissue swelling
Accident-related foreign bodies
Allergic reactions

Chest: Blunt and penetrating trauma
Cardiac tamponade (rupture;
contusion)
Great vessel tears
Flail chest
Pneumothorax or hemothorax
Ruptured diaphragm

Abdomen: Blunt and penetrating trauma
Ruptured or lacerated organs
(liver, spleen, bladder, kidneys,
bowel)
Ureteral or urethral injuries
Gravid uterus (fetal trauma)
Scrotal/saddle injuries
Impalements

Angiography sites

Soft tissue injuries
Avulsions
Lacerations
Contusions
Abrasions

Neurologic
Subdural
Epidural
Skull fractures
Linear
Depressed

Facial trauma
Soft tissue avulsions: ears, nose
Facial fractures: zygoma,
mandible, maxilla

Oral trauma
Fractured teeth or airway obstruction
Tongue or mouth lacerations

Spine injuries
Cervical
Cord trauma: swelling, compression
C-2 to C-4: Respiratory malfunction
Above C-3: Respiratory arrest
Odontoid fracture—the hidden fracture
Thoracic fracture

Extremities
Fractures
Dislocations
Open wounds
Traumatic amputations
Degloving injuries
Compartment syndromes
Vascular injuries

Fig. 21-1 Overview of trauma injuries that may require operative intervention. (From Foss J, Feistritzer N: Perioperative care of the trauma patient. In Neff JA, Kidd PS: *Trauma nursing: the art and science,* St Louis, 1993, Mosby.)

multidisciplinary teamwork, rapid transport systems, trauma facilities designed for early resuscitation and stabilization, and prompt surgical intervention have contributed to the success of civilian trauma systems (Morgan and others, 1986; O'Connel, 1992).

Mechanism of Injury

Although many improvements in the surgical treatment of trauma patients have been made as a result of battle experiences, war injuries are not always comparable to civilian injuries (Hood, 1990). The mechanism of injury is usually different. Battle injuries are commonly due to high-velocity gunshot wounds and missile fragments that produce severe, lethal hemorrhage at the site of injury, whereas civilian trauma

involves many motor vehicle accidents and knife wounds or low-velocity missile injuries that produce less severe hemorrhage. These factors may allow the victim to reach a health care facility for prompt treatment. Unfortunately, increased use of high-velocity weapons has resulted in a greater number of deaths at the site of injury.

Traumatic injury is related to the kinds of forces impacting the body and the type of energy dissipated. Thermal or chemical energy, for example, may cause burns; kinetic energy can cause lacerations, avulsion, amputation, puncture wound, or contusion (Huggins, 1990) (Fig. 21-1). Injuries produced by kinetic energy can be further subdivided into two categories: **blunt trauma** and **penetrating trauma.**

The mechanism of injury is related to three com-

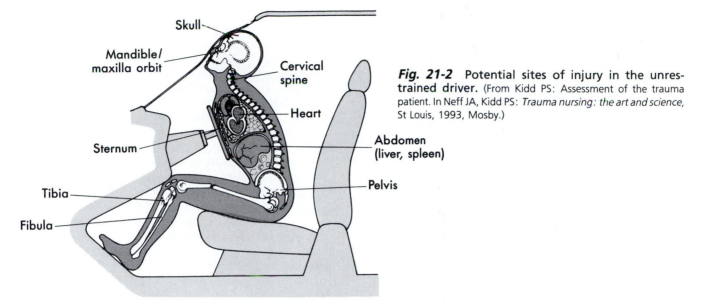

Fig. 21-2 Potential sites of injury in the unrestrained driver. (From Kidd PS: Assessment of the trauma patient. In Neff JA, Kidd PS: *Trauma nursing: the art and science,* St Louis, 1993, Mosby.)

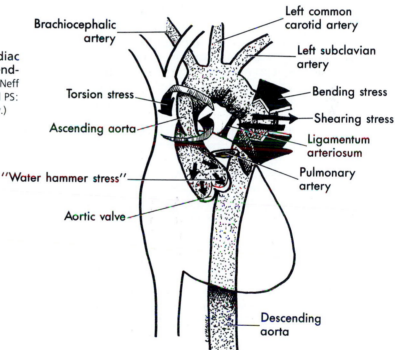

Fig. 21-3 Diagrammatic representation of cardiac and great vessel anatomy, and sites of torsion, bending, shearing, and "water hammer" stress. (From Neff JA: Perfusion: cardiac and vascular injuries. In Neff JA, Kidd PS: *Trauma nursing: the art and science,* St Louis, 1993, Mosby.)

ponents of biomechanics: compression, stretch, and stress. **Compression** occurs as the tissues at the point of impact are pushed together. **Stretch** occurs as the tissues are pulled apart; extreme stretch tears the moving tissue free from the nonmoving component. **Stress** is a specific point where nonmoving tissue is in contact with moving tissue (McSwain, 1991).

As accurate and complete a description as possible of the type of trauma incurred is important for anticipating the types of injuries that have occurred. For example, in blunt injuries caused by motor vehicle frontal collisions (Fig. 21-2), compression, stretch, and stress (Fig. 21-3) are all present in varying degrees.

The occupant of the car continues to move in a forward direction until some object (e.g., the steering wheel or dashboard) is impacted. If the chest hits an object, the vertebral column may continue to move forward and compress the heart between the vertebrae and the sternum, producing myocardial contusion or rupture. Death can also be caused by dysrhythmias.

Such impacts also raise suspicion of aortic injuries. Although the aortic arch and the heart are relatively freely suspended in the mediastinum, the descending aorta is attached at the ligamentum arteriosum (the remnant fetal ductus arteriosus). If the posterior tho-

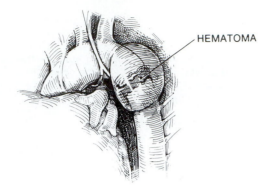

Fig. 21-4 Hematoma contained within the adventitial layer of a descending thoracic aorta creating a pseudo-aneurysm. (From Waldhausen JA, Pierce WS: *Johnson's surgery of the chest,* ed 5, St Louis, 1985, Mosby.)

racic wall and the vertebral column stop, so does the descending aorta. The aortic arch and heart, however, continue to swing forward. This action can result in shear forces sufficiently strong enough to partially or completely lacerate the aorta circumferentially. If all three layers of the aortic wall (intima, media, and adventitia) are torn, exsanguination is practically immediate. If only the intima and media are torn, the adventitia may encapsulate the hematoma and tamponade the bleeding. The resulting pseudoaneurysm (Fig. 21-4) may remain intact long enough for the victim to receive emergency treatment.

Lateral impacts may fracture the ribs and produce flail chest and pulmonary contusion. Penetrating injuries caused by knife or gunshot wounds depend on the original energy of the penetrating object and the number of tissue particles it impacts (Hood, 1990).

Nursing Considerations

Nursing care focuses on the identification and treatment of the patient's response to injury. Factors that affect a patient's response include the type of injury, age and developmental level, previous and current health problems, family and social support systems, economic status, level of education, and psychosocial impact of the injury on the victim and family. Appropriate material resources should be selected without duplication. Inadequate or inappropriate instrumentation delays prompt intervention and can foster confusion, increase the level of stress, and possibly incur litigation (Trauma Nursing Coalition, 1992).

The perioperative nurse's role as a patient advocate is especially critical in a setting where the patient enters the system severely wounded, often unconscious and intubated, and incapable of communication and self-protection. The legal rights of patients must be protected; advance directives such as those relating to organ donation should be honored, and safety considerations outlined in institutional policies and procedures should be followed. Minimal standards relating to basic aseptic technique, counts, and documen-

tation are adhered to in all but the most critical situations; exceptions should be covered by written policies (e.g., taking an x-ray film postoperatively when sponge or needle counts cannot be performed) (Trauma Nursing Coalition, 1992).

Families and significant others must also cope with the stress that traumatic injuries impose. Because of the suddenness with which such injuries occur, families have little time to prepare for these events and often feel helpless to cope with the situation. Nurses can have a positive impact by engendering a sense of hope and providing information about the patient's condition and the care being received (Reeder, 1991).

Diagnostic Evaluation

The initial diagnosis and treatment are provided in the field and in the emergency facility. Primary assessment and treatment focus on a patent airway, breathing, and circulation (i.e., the ABCs of resuscitation). After ensuring adequate ventilation, administering oxygen, and protecting the spine, the emergency/trauma team assess the victim for other potentially lethal injuries (Hefti, 1991). Vital signs are monitored frequently, and arterial blood gasses and electrolyte levels are determined.

Severe bleeding of the heart or great vessels requires immediate surgical intervention, and there may be little time for diagnostic radiography or arteriography. In thoracic vascular injuries, the surgeon must achieve rapid proximal and distal control of the vessel under unfavorable conditions in an anatomically complex area. In patients who are relatively stable on arrival to the emergency department, electrocardiograms (ECGs), chest radiographs, and echocardiograms are frequently performed. Cardiac enzyme levels may be tested in patients suspected of having myocardial contusion.

Computed tomographic (CT) scanning may be performed, but the time delay often limits its usefulness, and precise imaging of the injury is not always possible. Thoracoscopy is being used for some chest injuries (Moore, 1992).

Blunt (Nonpenetrating) Injury

Blunt cardiovascular injuries result from external physical forces that create pressure waves on the body tissues (Hammond, 1990; Turner, 1990). A blast, blunt force, or deceleration may produce injuries such as rib fracture, flail chest, pneumothorax, hemothorax with or without cardiac tamponade, pulmonary or myocardial contusion, or rupture of cardiac chambers or great vessels. Automobile collisions (see Fig. 21-2) are the most common cause of blunt trauma; falls and blunt objects striking the victim also produce injuries.

Because blunt injuries do not break the skin, external evidence of internal injury may be limited to bruises and discoloration of the skin. Injury may result from the direct impact of a force against the skin, deceleration, compression against the chest, upward displacement of blood and abdominal contents, and/

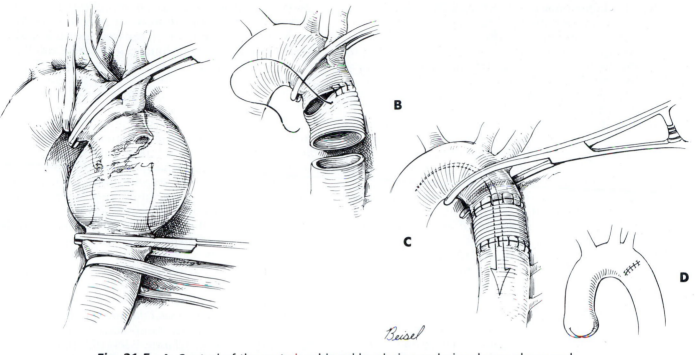

Fig. 21-5 **A,** Control of the aorta is achieved by placing occlusive clamps above and below the lacerated aorta. Occasionally the proximal clamp is placed across the aorta between the left carotid and the left subclavian arteries, and a separate clamp is applied to the subclavian artery. **B,** The proximal anastomosis is performed with a continuous suture technique (the distal aortic clamp is not shown). **C,** The completed repair. After the distal clamp is removed, the proximal clamp is released slowly. **D,** Primary closure of a small aortic tear. (From Waldhausen JA, Pierce WS: *Johnson's surgery of the chest,* ed 5, St Louis, 1985, Mosby.)

or concussion that interferes with cardiac rhythm (Turner, 1990). Having this information allows the clinician to anticipate the kinds of injuries that are likely to be found.

Rupture of the interventricular septum produces an acute left-to-right shunt that is poorly tolerated. Surgical treatment (e.g., patch closure) is similar to that for postmyocardial infarction VSD (see Chapter 12). Valvular injuries (e.g., ruptured chordae tendineae or papillary muscles of the tricuspid or mitral valves, or leaflet tears in any of the cardiac valves) often require valve replacement, although reparative techniques are preferred when feasible (see previous chapters for discussion of valve surgery). Repair of the thoracic aorta is described below.

Surgery for injury to the thoracic aorta

Deceleration injuries may cause a tear in the aorta at the isthmus, just distal to the subclavian artery. Creation of a pseudoaneurysm may temporarily tamponade the bleeding. The mechanism of injury and radiographic evidence provide information about the extent of the injury. Superior mediastinal widening, depression of the left main bronchus, and deviation of the esophagus to the right are significant and warrant aortography, when feasible, for confirmation (Cohn and Braunwald, 1992).

If the hematoma (e.g., surrounding the lacerated descending thoracic aorta) is not massive or expanding

rapidly (on repeat chest x-ray films), diagnostic arteriography may be performed. Preoperative imaging of the aorta and surrounding vessels is beneficial because it documents the presence or absence of other vascular injuries and localizes the site of the tear. This information is especially useful if there are other injuries requiring surgery, and it helps in planning the appropriate incision and operative procedure (Waldhausen and Pierce, 1985).

In preparation for surgery, perioperative nurses will have instrumentation, supplies, and positioning equipment for a left thoracotomy. The procedure is similar to that for a descending thoracic aneurysm (see Chapter 16). Synthetic tube grafts should be available for resection and repair of the aorta. Autotransfusion capability, as well as an adequate supply of bank blood, is necessary. CPB is generally avoided because of the risk of hemorrhage from systemic heparinization.

Operative procedure: repair of a transected aorta

1. After skin preparation and draping for a left lateral thoracotomy, an incision is made in the fifth intercostal space. The lungs are retracted anteriorly and inferiorly.
2. The hematoma is located, and the aorta above and below is partially dissected to allow placement of occlusive clamps (Fig. 21-5, *A*).

3. The hematoma is incised, and the edges of the aortic wall are trimmed in preparation for insertion of a prosthetic graft.
4. An appropriately sized tube graft is delivered to the field, and the proximal anastomosis is performed (Fig. 21-5, *B*).
5. The distal anastomosis is then performed (Fig. 21-5, *C*).
6. The distal clamp is removed first, and the anastomoses are checked for bleeding. Additional sutures are placed as necessary. The surgical site is assessed for other injuries or areas of bleeding; these are repaired.
7. After hemostasis is achieved, the proximal clamp is slowly removed.
8. Free blood and clotted blood are removed, and the pleural space is irrigated.
9. A chest tube is inserted, and the incision is closed.
10. In rare instances there is a small tear in the aorta that can be repaired primarily with a running suture (Fig. 21-5, *D*).

Pharmacologic control of the aortic blood pressure (with nitroprusside), expeditious surgery, and early reexpansion of the lung are important considerations. Postoperatively, pulmonary impairment, empyema, and sepsis may complicate recovery. Ischemic injury to the spinal cord or kidneys is less likely to occur with cross-clamping times of less than 30 minutes (Turney and others, 1976).

Penetrating Injury

Penetrating cardiac injuries are caused by bullets, knives, ice picks, and other objects that can pierce the skin and underlying structures. The amount of injury is related to the velocity, size, and internal movement of the object and the tissue being penetrated. Gunshot wounds are generally more lethal than stab wounds because of the higher velocity and the larger area of tissue destroyed. Because of its accessibility, the anterior surface of the heart (primarily the right ventricle) is the most frequent site of injury. Acute hemorrhage or tamponade severely compromises hemodynamic status, leading to shock and acidosis, and the victim often dies before reaching a health care facility (Smith and Fitzpatrick, 1993).

When patients do survive long enough to receive treatment, an ECG, chest radiograph, and echocardiography are often performed for diagnosis. Serial enzymes may provide evidence of the extent of the myocardial injury. Some patients may undergo coronary arteriography and ventriculography. In patients with suspected hemothorax, thoracentesis or chest tube insertion can decompress the chest and confirm the diagnosis (Smith and Fitzpatrick, 1993), although performance of these procedures should not delay definitive treatment.

Iatrogenic injury constitutes another category of penetrating trauma. Cardiopulmonary resuscitation (CPR) may fracture ribs and puncture the heart and abdominal organs. Cardiac catheterization and angiographic procedures can be complicated by laceration or dissection of the heart or major vessels from guidewires and catheters. Transvenous leads and intravascular monitoring lines can produce similar injuries (Markovchick and Duffens, 1992; Turner, 1990).

Cardiac Tamponade

Acute tamponade is the most common cardiac emergency seen in patients with penetrating injuries to the heart and pericardium (Fig. 21-6); the condition is seen less often in patients with blunt trauma to the chest. Because the pericardium is a relatively nondistensible sac encasing the heart, accumulated blood from the injured heart muscle or coronary arteries can cause compression of the myocardium. If the pericardial opening is obliterated by blood clot, lung tissue, or a flap of pericardial tissue, blood within the pericardial sac cannot escape. This in turn prevents adequate filling of the ventricles, resulting in a reduction of cardiac output (Hammond, 1990).

The classic signs of tamponade, referred to as "Beck's triad" (after Claude Beck who described the condition in 1937), consist of hypotension, distended neck veins, and distant (muffled) heart sounds. It may be difficult to demonstrate clinically the complete triad, especially during major resuscitation efforts when heart sounds are difficult to hear or when patients are uncooperative or combative. The most reliable signs include elevated central venous pressure (CVP) in association with hypotension and tachycardia (Markovchick and Duffens, 1992).

If the pericardium has been lacerated or ruptured (and the opening in the sac has not been obliterated by clot or adjacent tissue), blood can enter the pleural cavities or mediastinum, and cardiac tamponade may not develop, at least initially. Presenting signs and symptoms will be those of hemorrhage (e.g., hypotension, tachycardia, low CVP) or hemothorax (e.g., dyspnea; radiographic or echocardiographic evidence of blood in the chest) (Cohn and Braunwald, 1992; Markovchick and Duffens, 1992). In extremely critical patients, diagnostic studies may be omitted in order to avoid delaying treatment.

There has been considerable debate over the effectiveness of thoracotomy in the emergency department. The earlier popularity of this technique waned as it became apparent that this procedure did not produce the expected increase in survival. Although in patients brought in without signs of life, thoracotomy with release of tamponade and control of hemorrhage is the only chance for survival (Buchman, Phillips, and Menker, 1992), mortality is high. With the increase in violent trauma and the number of published studies describing resuscitative efforts, indications for emergency thoracotomy have been modified. This reappraisal has also been influenced by the increasing risk of viral infection to health care personnel during resuscitation (Millham and Grindlinger, 1993). At present, patients demonstrating either hemody-

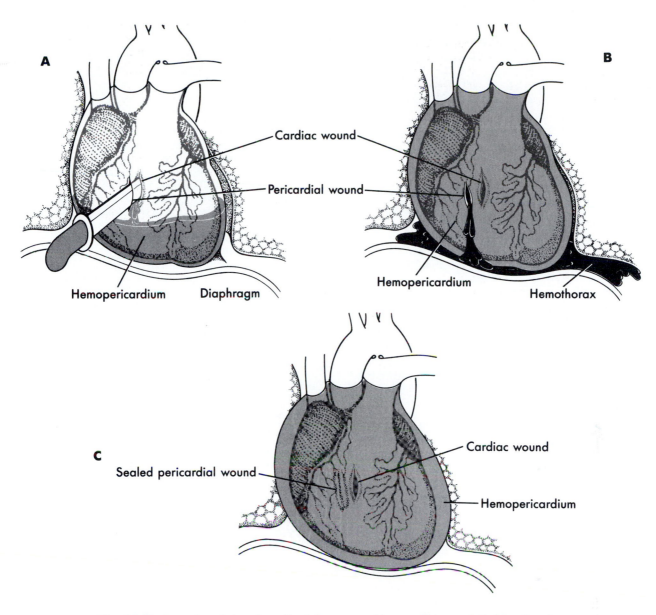

Fig. 21-6 **A,** Pericardial and cardiac injury caused by a stab wound. **B,** Bleeding from the heart through the pericardial tear into the pleural space. Tamponade may not occur if blood can exit the pericardium. **C,** If the pericardial wound is sealed, blood collects within the pericardial sac and produces cardiac tamponade. (From Neff JA: Perfusion: cardiac and vascular injuries. In Neff JA, Kidd PS: *Trauma nursing: the art and science,* St Louis, 1993, Mosby.)

namic or neurologic activity at some time between the initial encounter in the field and admission to the emergency department have a better chance of survival with thoracotomy. Patients who respond appropriately to resuscitation and are relatively stable can be transported to the OR for mediastinal exploration under controlled conditions (Crawford, 1991). Patients without signs of life (e.g., no evidence of mentation; absent blood pressure or pulse) are unlikely to benefit from emergency thoracotomy (Buchman, Phillips, and Menker, 1992; Millham and Grindlinger, 1993).

Perioperative considerations

Institutions with trauma centers often have perioperative nurse team members functioning within the trauma unit or on call from the OR. Roles vary from institution to institution. Some perioperative nurses function in a separate trauma OR; some act as a liaison between the OR and the emergency/trauma department; and others participate in transporting and treating patients in a designated OR within the surgical suite. The degree of interdepartmental interaction may differ, but a system of communication and planning for rapid intervention is essential to avoid a cha-

Box 21-1 *Nursing considerations in thoracic trauma*

Cecil A. King, RN, CNOR
Maryland Institute for Emergency
Medical Services Systems
Baltimore, Maryland

Thoracic trauma, when presenting in the level I trauma center, whether blunt or penetrating, often requires a thoracotomy for definitive management. Blunt trauma is most common in the unbelted driver as the chest is thrown forward into the steering column on impact. Penetrating trauma occurs in the gunshot wound (GSW) or stabbing victim and may or may not involve vital structures of the thoracic cavity. These injuries may disrupt vascular integrity and/or actually penetrate the heart muscle itself. Angiography may have to be omitted in locating the internal injuries secondary to the patient's instability.

With penetrating trauma, it is important to note the entrance and exit wounds in reference to internal structures in order to anticipate potential disruption and plan the surgical course. Close communication with the resuscitation nurse will enable the perioperative nurse to prepare the OR for emergency exploration and repair. The patient requiring "stat" perioperative intervention will show widening mediastinum on the (true) upright chest x-ray film and/or profound hemodynamic instability.

When the patient arrives in the OR, be ready to open the chest and cross-clamp.

Key Points

1. Never deflate or remove the pneumatic antishock garment (PASG) or MAST trousers; this may be the only means of maintaining a blood pressure and perfusion of vital organs. The perioperative nurse is now also a resuscitative nurse.
2. Be prepared for massive hemorrhage on opening the chest cavity; frequently a tamponade may have somewhat stabilized the patient; do not be fooled by this

pseudostability. This type of hemorrhage can be "heard" and is described as the sound of a waterfall. Have blood products ready, such as universal type O, Rh-negative packed red blood cells (PRBCs), and plan to keep 10 units ahead of needs; also have available crystalloids, such as Plasma-Lyte A, which is compatible with blood products and contains no calcium or lactate.
3. These patients will require a rapid infusion system (RIS) to maintain blood pressure.
4. As you position and prepare these patients, check all pulses and continue to palpate pulses frequently throughout the procedure. Many a blood pressure has been maintained in the pulseless patient by RIS alone.
5. Have the crash cart in the OR and ready to use. These patients will frequently require internal defibrillation.

Secondary Considerations

Get the patient off the backboard as he or she arrives in the OR and is moved to the OR table. Have available aortic occlusion instrumentation, vascular grafts, and appropriate suture materials. This issue can best be addressed before the "stat" thoracic case by having the OR closest to the resuscitative area set up and equipped to handle this population. Have general surgery, chest, and vascular instrumentation in your emergency OR at all times.

The family of these patients (and the nursing staff) must be cognizant of the fact that the trauma patient with the need for emergency thoracotomy many times has a bleak prognosis; rarely does this patient have single-system trauma, and this increases morbidity.

---

otic situation that can adversely affect patient outcomes (Foss and Feistritzer, 1993).

Case carts prepared in advance can be especially helpful in avoiding delays. Carts (or other portable units) containing items specific to the type of injury (e.g., thoracic, abdominal, extremity) include instruments and supplies likely to be required. Separate carts can also facilitate performing simultaneous procedures for two or more life-threatening injuries. And because they are portable, these carts can be taken to the emergency department (or other area) if the patient is too unstable to transport to the OR.

When the patient arrives in the OR, positioning, application of dispersive pads, and skin preparation are performed expeditiously. Prior communication with the liaison in the emergency department will assist the perioperative staff in having ready the most appropriate supplies and instruments for the intended procedure. If pneumatic antishock garments (PASG) or MAST trousers are in place, they should

not be removed unless specifically requested by the surgeon or anesthesiologist; these garments may be necessary to maintain a blood pressure (Box 21-1). Perioperative standards of care for the trauma patient are shown in Table 21-1.

Other considerations in patients with cardiac tamponade relate to anesthetic management and the type of incision. Positive-pressure ventilation may increase intrathoracic pressure and further compromise cardiac filling. It may be preferable to anesthetize the patient with a mask, open the chest, and relieve the tamponade before tracheal intubation and forced positive-pressure breathing is initiated (Mattox, 1989).

The type of incision depends on the location of the injury. Anterolateral thoracotomy through the fourth or fifth interspace provides excellent cardiac exposure and can be extended across the sternum if necessary. This incision has the advantage of keeping the abdominal cavity separate from the thorax and is an important consideration when there are concomitant

Table 21-1 ■ Perioperative care of the trauma patient

Nursing diagnosis	Nursing intervention	Evaluative criteria
High risk for ineffective airway clearance and impaired gas exchange Related to obstruction, local trauma, aspiration, loss of jaw position, effects of anesthetic, procedure, position	**Maintain clear airway** Ensure patent airway, and maintain cervical spine precautions Provide high-flow oxygen Ensure patent nasogastric tube, and empty stomach Administer histamine receptor antagonists as ordered Monitor airway and respirations during extubation, and transport to postanesthesia care unit, using pulse oximetry Suction Use artificial airway to maintain jaw position	PaO_2 will be greater than 80 mm Hg on room air, and $PaCO_2$ will be between 35 and 45 mm Hg; pH will be 7.35-7.45 A patent airway will be maintained for the patient Respiratory rate, rhythm, and depth will be in the patient's normal range No aspiration will occur
High risk for fluid volume deficit Related to hemorrhage, shock, previous illness	**Maintain normovolemia** Administer IV fluids and/or blood as needed to maintain blood pressure via large-bore needle or catheter Consider PASG application Insert urinary catheter, and monitor intraoperative output	The patient will have a systolic blood pressure of greater than 100 mm Hg Capillary refill will be 2 seconds or less Urinary output will be 30 ml or more per hour
High risk for electrolyte disturbance Related to the nature of the injury, medication, choice of resuscitative fluid	**Maintain electrolyte balance** Check electrolytes preoperatively Replace depleted electrolytes Administer blood that is less than 3 days old when giving more than 5 units	Potassium, calcium, sodium, and chloride will be within normal range; cardiac rate and rhythm will be within normal limits
High risk for anxiety Related to unfamiliar environment, concern for family/significant other, surgical procedure, planned anesthesia, belief that one will feel pain	**Promote coping strategies for anxiety** Orient patient to surroundings Make patient aware of the plan of care Keep patient, family, friends informed of patient status Comfort and support family/significant other	Physical and emotional factors increasing the patient's risk for surgery will be evaluated
High risk for injury and impaired tissue integrity Neuromuscular damage, related to improper positioning, extended length of surgery Burns, related to improper grounding of electrocautery equipment Nosocomial infection, related to leaving a foreign object in wound	**Protect patient from environmental hazards** Pad all bony prominences Position patient in a manner in which no pressure or abnormal stretching of nerves occurs Apply grounding pads securely; perform safety check on electrosurgical equipment Adhere to strict aseptic technique Prepare surgical site with appropriate antiseptic Remove road gravel, dirt from patient's back before positioning supine Place dry pads under patient after prepping skin	Patient will be free of neuromuscular damage Patient will be free of injury, as exhibited by correct needle, sponge, and instrument counts Patient will be free of infection
High risk for ineffective thermoregulation Related to a cool operating room environment, cool temperature of resuscitation fluids, surgical exposure	**Promote effective thermoregulation** Provide warm irrigation fluid Limit area of surgical exposure Have warming pad in place Adjust room temperature as needed Monitor patient core temperature	Patient will have normal temperature
High risk for pain Related to surgical incision, untreated injuries	**Promote comfort** Observe patient for signs indicating pain, and give appropriate medication	Patient will be reasonably comfortable and not overly sedated
High risk for fluid volume deficit Related to blood loss during surgery	**Maintain blood volume** Communicate and document estimated blood loss to surgical and anesthesia team Communicate and document estimated blood loss to postanesthesia care unit so that fluid replacement may be planned Monitor and document intake and urinary output	Patient will be hemodynamically stable

From Neff JA, Kidd PS: *Trauma nursing: the art and science*, St Louis, 1993, Mosby.

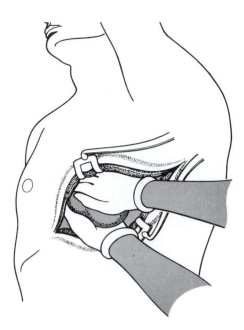

Fig. 21-7 Anterolateral thoracotomy allows internal cardiac massage (two hands are recommended). (From Neff JA: Perfusion: cardiac and vascular injuries. In Neff JA, Kidd PS: *Trauma nursing: the art and science,* St Louis, 1993, Mosby.)

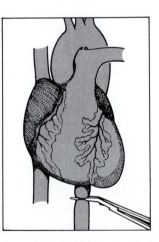

Fig. 21-8 Occlusion of the descending thoracic aorta in severely hypovolemic patients can improve blood flow to the coronary arteries and the brain. (From Neff JA: Perfusion: cardiac and vascular injuries. In Neff JA, Kidd PS: *Trauma nursing: the art and science,* St Louis, 1993, Mosby.)

enteric injuries. A median sternotomy and lateral thoracotomy may also be performed when the injury has been localized, but often it is difficult to determine the precise location of injuries, and the exposure is not as good as it is with the anterolateral approach (Mattox, 1993). Subxyphoid pericardiotomies are not recommended, because they limit exposure and can delay definitive repair (Box 21-2). Pericardiocentesis (insertion of a large-bore needle into the pericardium to drain blood) may provide emergency relief until surgery can be performed, but it should not delay opening of the chest and performance of a definitive repair.

In addition to release of the tamponade and control of the site of bleeding, internal cardiac massage (Fig. 21-7) may be necessary to decompress an arrested or fibrillating heart that has become distended and to perfuse distal organs until cardiac activity can be resumed. In markedly hypovolemic patients, cross-clamping the descending thoracic aorta (Fig. 21-8) may be done to enhance coronary and cerebral blood flow (Mattox, 1993). Vascular clamps should not be placed on ventricular walls; doing so could cause injury to the myocardium. Partial-occlusion clamps may be used on atrial tissue and on blood vessels with small, discrete injuries that can be repaired primarily.

Internal defibrillation paddles should be available on the surgical field. CPB is usually available on a standby basis, although it can be contraindicated in patients with head or other injuries where increased bleeding would result from systemic anticoagulation.

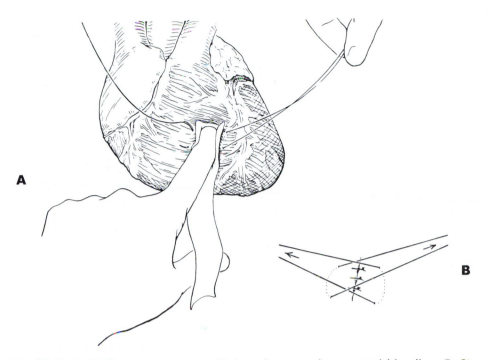

Fig. 21-9 **A,** Digital pressure is applied to the wound to control bleeding. **B,** Stay sutures are inserted (avoiding major coronary arteries) for traction and closure of the wound while the repair is performed. (From Waldhausen JA, Pierce WS: *Johnson's surgery of the chest*, ed 5, St Louis, 1985, Mosby.)

Nurses should be prepared to institute CPB quickly if necessary.

Operative procedure: suture of a heart wound

1. An anterolateral (or midsternal) incision is made.
2. The pericardium is opened, and blood clots are removed. Very brisk hemorrhage may be evident; autotransfusion suctions should be available to salvage and reinfuse as much blood as possible.
3. The wound(s) is located after a careful search. Occasionally a discrete wound can be covered with a finger (Fig. 21-9, *A*). If digital control is difficult to achieve, a urinary drainage catheter with a 5 cc inflatable balloon can be inserted through the wound; the balloon can then be inflated and gently pulled against the inside of the heart (the catheter lumen is occluded to prevent back bleeding).

   Lifting the hypovolemic heart may kink the vena cava, reducing venous return (preload). Ventricular fibrillation may occur, especially if the patient is hypothermic and acidotic, and has electrolyte imbalances (Mattox, 1993). Cardiac massage is performed, and underlying metabolic alterations are corrected. Defibrillation is attempted but may be unsuccessful in the presence of severely altered blood values.
4. Deep traction sutures are placed on either side of the wound, avoiding coronary arteries if possible. Crossing the sutures may close the wound sufficiently to permit removal of the finger and allow

suture repair under direct vision (Fig. 21-9, *B*). Polypropylene (4-0, 5-0) may be used with or without pledgets to bolster the suture line; pledgets may be required, especially if coexisting myocardial contusion has weakened the tissue. More extensive lacerations require multiple sutures (Waldhausen and Pierce, 1985).

   If a major coronary artery has been lacerated or ligated, bypass grafting (Chapter 12) with CPB may be necessary.
5. After hemostasis has been achieved, the traction sutures are removed. Chest tubes are inserted and the incision is closed.

Penetrating wounds to major arteries and veins

Stab and bullet wounds to the thoracic aorta and its major branches, or to veins within the chest, may cause rapid exsanguinating hemorrhage unless occlusive vascular clamps can be quickly placed across the proximal and distal segments of the injured vessel. This maneuver allows the surgeon to control the bleeding while the repair is being made. The incision depends on the location of the injury. Generally, a median sternotomy affords the best exposure to the pulmonary artery, the ascending aorta, and the proximal arch vessels. The incision can be angled at either side of the neck, if necessary, for access to vessels in that area. A thoracotomy may be indicated for subclavian injuries (Waldhausen and Pierce, 1985). Repair depends on the site and extent of the injury. Either primary suture repair or interposition of a tube graft to bridge the defect may be done (Cohn and Braunwald, 1992).

INADVERTENT HYPOTHERMIA

Prolonged exposure to cold temperatures or submersion in cold water can produce hypothermia (core temperatures below 32° C [90° F]). Hypothermia due to submersion can occur as a consequence of falling through the ice into water or being in a motor vehicle accident wherein the car veers into a body of cold water. Patients become apneic and pulseless, with fixed and dilated pupils.

Conventional warming techniques, such as heating blankets, radiant warmers, body cavity lavage, and airway rewarming, are usually not capable of increasing the body temperature by more than 1° C (34° F) per hour. Children are more likely to recover than adults. Institution of CPB has been an effective method in the absence of associated traumatic injuries that would preclude the use of systemic heparinization (Letsou and others, 1992). The patient may be placed on bypass with a portable system in the emergency department (see Chapter 11) or brought to the OR.

When there is a risk of bleeding from heparinization, an alternative method (devised by Gentilello and Rifley, 1991) is continuous arteriovenous rewarming. The system uses a rapid fluid warmer to increase the temperature of the endogenous blood volume 1° C approximately every 15 minutes.

Procedure for rewarming

The femoral artery and contralateral femoral vein are percutaneously cannulated with a standard renal arteriovenous hemofiltration catheter. Venous access can also be achieved by cannulating the ipsilateral femoral, internal jugular, or subclavian vein. The catheters are connected to a fluid warmer with an in-line filter to create a circulatory fistula through the heating mechanism. A blood pump, membrane oxygenator, or systemic heparinization is not required. The core temperature can be monitored with a pulmonary artery catheter and/or urinary bladder thermistor. After rewarming, the catheters are withdrawn, and digital pressure is applied for at least 20 minutes. Full neurologic recovery has been demonstrated with this technique (Gentilello and Rifley, 1991).

PULMONARY EMBOLUS

Pulmonary embolus is not a distinct disease but a complication of many medical and surgical disorders (Currie, 1990). Deep venous thrombosis (DVT) of the lower extremities is often a precursor to acute pulmonary thromboembolism in trauma patients as well as in patients who have been on prolonged bed rest or who have indwelling femoral intravenous catheters. In patients at risk for pulmonary embolus, prophylactic measures include insertion under fluoroscopy of a filter in the inferior vena cava (IVC) to trap emboli migrating from the IVC to the heart and thereby prevent their entry into the pulmonary circulation. The device may be especially useful in the patient with bleeding complications from anticoagulation therapy or a history of recurrent thromboembolism (Calligaro and others, 1991).

Studies by Shackford and colleagues (1990) have shown that high-risk factors in trauma patients related to venous thrombosis include stasis, local venous injury, hypercoagulability, and age greater than 45 years. Diagnosis relies on the clinical signs and symptoms of calf swelling, tenderness, warmth, and pedal edema. Doppler echocardiography and magnetic resonance imaging (MRI) have replaced venography for assessing pelvic and thigh DVT (Neff and Neff, 1993).

Acute pulmonary embolus (APE) occurs when a portion of thrombus in a systemic vein, right atrial appendage, or right ventricle dislodges and migrates to the pulmonary artery (PA) or one of its major branches. When approximately 60% or more of the pulmonary circulation is occluded, the right ventricle is unable to eject the blood returning from the systemic circulation. The obstruction causes acute right ventricular dilatation with right-sided congestive failure if the obstruction is unrelieved. Clinical signs of APE often include distended neck veins, engorgement of the liver, tachypnea, dyspnea, cough, and wheezing. Massive air emboli or fat emboli (associated with large bone fractures) can produce a similar clinical picture.

In addition to clinical signs and symptoms, the ECG, chest x-ray film, perfusion lung scanning, and pulmonary arteriography may be performed to determine the diagnosis. The ECG may show signs of right ventricular strain, anatomic rotation, axis shifts of the heart, acute myocardial infarction of the inferior portion of the heart, right bundle-branch block, and dysrhythmias such as sinus tachycardia and atrial flutter. Chest radiographs may show nonspecific changes, but the diaphragm is often elevated on the affected side. Pleural effusion, PA dilatation, and infiltrates may be apparent (Sabiston, 1991).

Perfusion scans using radioisotopes are performed to detect changes in the areas supplied by the occluded PA. With APE, defects appear in the scan. Normal perfusion scans exclude the possibility of massive APE. However, other conditions (e.g., pneumonia, emphysema) can also produce abnormal findings. The most accurate test for diagnosis of APE is right-sided heart catheterization with pulmonary arteriography. A positive study shows an intraluminal defect. A sharp reduction in flow may also be seen, although this needs to be distinguished from concomitant pulmonary or cardiac disease (Goldenberger, 1990).

Arterial blood gasses (ABGs) are used to monitor ventilation-perfusion defects. Arterial oxygen saturation is decreased as expected; compensatory hyperventilation produces a decreased level of carbon dioxide.

Initial treatment

Initial therapy for APE in trauma patients consists of oxygen administration, intravenous thrombolytic therapy (except in the presence of head injury), and pharmacologic treatment for shock. Monitoring is achieved with a central venous and/or pulmonary artery blood pressure catheter. If the patient does not respond to medical therapy and remains in critical condition (e.g., right-sided heart failure, significant pulmonary obstruction of the pulmonary vasculature), pulmonary embolectomy may be necessary. This is often the case with a massive "saddle" embolus, named for the characteristic shape of a clot that sits at the bifurcation of the main PA.

Perioperative considerations

Surgical mortality is high; in one series of 96 patients mortality was almost 38% (Meyer and others, 1991). Cardiac arrest and associated cardiopulmonary disease, as well as massive pulmonary hemorrhage, increase mortality.

Pulmonary embolectomy may be performed on one or both PA branches. Primarily unilateral involvement may be an indication for anterior thoracotomy on the affected side. In patients with bilateral emboli, or emboli within the main PA, median sternotomy and CPB are generally indicated (Sabiston, 1991). The risk of bleeding may be increased with systemic heparinization. Intrabronchial bleeding may occur, and in anticipation of this complication a double-lumen endotracheal tube is inserted so that the unaffected side may continue to be ventilated (Sabiston, 1991).

Operative procedure: pulmonary embolectomy with cardiopulmonary bypass

1. A median sternotomy is performed.
2. A venous cannula can be placed in either the right atrium or the right ventricular outflow tract; an arterial cannula is placed in the ascending aorta. CPB is instituted.

   In some cases the aorta is not clamped and the procedure is performed under normothermic conditions. In more complex cases aortic occlusion and cardioplegic arrest with hypothermia may be used. Occasionally, circulatory arrest is required.
3. The PA is dissected medially from the aorta.
4. An incision is made in the main PA, and the thrombus is removed.
5. If the thrombus is in the left or right PA, a second incision may be made, and the branches of the main embolus are removed. Peripheral emboli may be extracted with common bile duct forceps and standard suction tips (Meyer and others, 1991). When the thrombus has been removed, back bleeding of bright red blood will be seen (Sabiston, 1991).
6. The arteriotomies are closed; a pericardial or synthetic patch may be inserted to avoid constriction of the PA lumen during closure.

   Ligation or clipping of the IVC, or insertion of a vena caval filter may be performed in patients at risk for recurrent DVT or APE.
7. CPB is discontinued, chest tubes are inserted, and the incision is closed after hemostasis has been achieved.

Before heparin reversal with protamine, intrabronchial hemorrhage may occur; a balloon-tipped occlusion catheter can be inserted into the affected mainstem bronchus to tamponade the bleeding until coagulation and hemostasis can be achieved (Sabiston, 1991).

Postoperative complications include right ventricular failure in patients with pulmonary hypertension and pulmonary hemorrhage. A few patients may have recurrent pulmonary emboli. Anticoagulation and/or a vena caval filter may be inserted prophylactically in patients predisposed to DVT.

POSTOPERATIVE COMPLICATIONS OF CARDIAC SURGERY

In addition to APE, there are several postoperative complications of cardiac surgery, including hemorrhage with or without tamponade, low cardiac output syndrome, and lethal dysrhythmias that may require emergency management. When there is excessive bleeding from the chest tubes, correction of existing coagulopathies, volume replacement, and pharmacologic manipulation of cardiac output are first attempted. If the patient continues to deteriorate rapidly and becomes profoundly hypotensive or shows signs of tamponade, the chest may have to be reopened in the postoperative intensive care unit (ICU) (Fairman and Edmunds, 1981). If the patient has fibrillated, direct cardiac massage (see Fig. 21-7) can help to decompress the heart and perfuse peripheral organs. Internal defibrillation may be necessary.

When possible, mediastinal exploration is performed within the controlled environment of the OR. However, some patients are unable to tolerate transfer, and exploration in the ICU may be necessary. With some preplanning, these procedures can be performed in the ICU in a manner that is safe, effective, convenient, and less costly, without increasing morbidity and mortality (Kaiser and others, 1990). Important advantages of performing surgery in the ICU are that it saves time, reduces the possibility of further hemodynamic deterioration, and obviates the necessity of disconnecting the reattaching monitors and intravenous infusion lines (Fairman and Edmunds, 1981).

Procedural considerations

Having sterile instrumentation and supplies in the ICU is critical in order to avoid delays and enhance preparedness for such emergencies. Communication and coordination among hospital staff members in the OR and ICU are important for establishing protocols, developing instrument and supply inventories, and outlining roles and responsibilities during emergencies (Seifert and Speir, 1990). Perioperative and critical care nursing responsibilities should be outlined, but there must be flexibility built into any policy or protocol.

A number of questions can arise, and these should be discussed and clarified:

- Are perioperative nurses routinely expected to assist with ICU emergency sternotomy? If they are, how will they be notified?
- What are the critical care nurse's responsibilities? Monitoring? Documenting? Volume/medication infusion?
- What constraints exist in the number of personnel, availability of supplies and equipment, and knowledge of procedures?

A system to alert perioperative cardiac nurses when there is a need for sternal exploration in the ICU (or the OR) should be available at all times. Late-night emergencies may mean a delay in arrival of the perioperative nurses. In this case the critical care nurse may have to assist the surgeon temporarily in opening the chest. Perioperative nurses can provide inservices to critical care personnel about the indications for emergency sternotomy and the goal of exploration. Emphasis should be placed on the basic steps necessary for reopening the chest and the minimum requirements: a knife (or scissors), wire cutters, a sternal retractor, and suction.

The following items may be needed for ICU emergencies and are often found in the unit: privacy screens, sterile gowns and gloves, skin antiseptics, hats and masks, sterile suction tubing and tips, and internal defibrillator paddles. Internal defibrillator cords and paddles must be appropriate for the ICU defibrillator, which may be different from the one used in the OR. Cables from one unit may not be interchangeable with those of another unit; different models from the same manufacturer may not be interchangeable. Occasionally the defibrillator and the cords and cables from the OR may have to be brought to the ICU for internal defibrillation.

Other items that may have to be added to the ICU inventory (or brought to the unit) include a headlight and light source, suture material, and temporary pacing wires (Kern, 1990). Some units keep an electrosurgical unit (and dispersive pads), but more often a unit is brought from the OR (or an eye cautery is used), along with the surgeon's headlight and light source. Additional lighting is especially useful if it is difficult to achieve adequate illumination of the pericardial cavity.

When the chest must be opened, the chest instrument set can be placed on an overbed table and opened. The ICU nurses may be requested to assist the surgeon until the OR staff arrives. Responsibilities should be jointly delineated by nursing staff from the ICU and the OR, surgeons, and other personnel likely to be involved in resuscitative efforts.

Operative procedure: sternal exploration in the intensive care unit

Ideally, there are two perioperative nurses available: one to perform the duties of the sterile nurse and one to act as a circulator. If only one perioperative nurse is available, she or he may perform "sterile" duties and direct a critical care nurse in preparing the skin and providing sterile supplies. Personnel should wear head coverings and masks.

Procedure

1. The emergency sternotomy tray is placed on a table (or counter) and opened; sterile gowns and gloves are opened. The patient's chest dressings are removed.
2. A sterile drape is opened on another surface (if available), and required sterile supplies (e.g., sponges, suture) are placed on the drape. If another table or counter is unavailable, supplies may have to be opened onto the set of instruments.
3. While a nurse expeditiously prepares the patient's chest with antimicrobial solution (using a spray bottle is the fastest method), the sterile nurse and surgeon wash their hands and then gown and glove.
4. The sterile nurse and the surgeon drape the patient.
5. While draping is performed, the nurse gathers a knife or scissors to open the skin incision and passes sterile suction tubing off the field; this is connected to the wall suction outlet and turned to "high." Sterile internal paddles are prepared, and the cords are passed off to be connected to the defibrillator. (These may have to be done while the surgeon is opening the chest.)
6. The skin incision is opened with the knife and/or scissors. If staples have been used for chest closure, a staple remover is necessary. Any patient whose chest is closed with staples must have a staple remover accompany him or her to the ICU, and the staple remover must be placed where it can be made available immediately (e.g., taped to the wall near the patient).
7. After the skin is opened, the nurse hands the wire cutters and a wire needle holder (or heavy clamp such as a Kocher clamp) to the surgeon, who cuts and removes the wires.
8. A chest retractor is inserted, and a suction is handed to the surgeon.
9. The surgeon performs cardiac massage if the heart is asystolic. If the heart is fibrillating, internal defibrillation may be attempted first, and the heart is then massaged if cardiac rhythm is not restored. While performing these maneuvers, the surgeon assesses the heart and surrounding structures for areas of bleeding. The sterile nurse or surgical assistant can suction the field and also look for bleeding sites.
10. When cardiac rhythm is restored and the site of bleeding is determined, the repair is performed. This may be application of a vascular ligating clip

or use of a suture ligature, or a more complex repair may be required.

Sternal and retrosternal (e.g., from an internal mammary artery pedicle) bleeding can be repaired without the need for CPB. Leaking from coronary artery bypass grafts on the anterior surface of the heart may not require CPB, but suturing a moving heart is difficult. In such a situation the patient may require transport to the OR, where the repair can be performed under more controlled conditions.

Lacerations of the ventricle, posterior coronary artery bypass anastomotic leaks, and other injuries may necessitate the use of extracorporeal circulation to decompress the heart and perfuse the body. Induced cardiac arrest (fibrillation or cardioplegic arrest) may be required.

11. After the repair has been completed, blood clots within the chest tubes are removed, and the drainage tube is repositioned in the chest. The epicardial pacing wires may have been detached; these are reattached to the heart.

The surgical site is reassessed for hemostasis, and the sternum is rewired. Fascia, subcutaneous tissue, and skin are closed, and dressings are applied. (The patient may be transported to the OR for closure, but this is often unnecessary.)

Postoperative course

Standard postoperative monitoring and management are performed after completion of the ICU procedure. Special attention is focused on detecting the recurrence of problems that required ICU sternotomy and signs of infection. Contrary to expectation, there is a low incidence of infection after such procedures (Kaiser and others, 1990; McKowen and others, 1985.)

Complications associated with pacemaker wire removal

The risk of sudden hemorrhage is also present a few days after surgery when temporary pacemaker wires are discontinued. Removal of the pacing wires (commonly attached to the right atrial and ventricular epicardium during surgery) can produce bleeding secondary to laceration of the myocardium, nearby blood vessels, or an adjacent bypass graft (Johnson, Brown, and Alligood, 1993).

If chest tubes are still in place, a sudden increase in drainage will be evident (and tamponade is less likely to develop). However, pacing wire removal is often done after the mediastinal drainage tubes have been removed, and rapid tamponade can develop because blood remains confined to the pericardium. Pericardial tamponade can occur, often within 60 minutes after pacing wire removal, and demonstrate symptoms described earlier in the chapter. Pericardiocentesis may be attempted, but mediastinal exploration in the patient unit or in the OR may be necessary to repair the site of injury and release the tamponade.

REFERENCES

Beck CS: Acute and chronic compression of the heart, *Am Heart J* 14:515, 1937.

Buchman TG, Phillips J, Menker JB: Recognition, resuscitation and management of patients with penetrating cardiac injuries, *Surg Gynecol Obstet* 174:205, 1992.

Calligaro KD and others: Thromboembolic complications in patients with advanced cancer: anticoagulation versus Greenfield filter placement, *Ann Vasc Surg* 5:186, 1991.

Cohn PF, Braunwald E: Traumatic heart disease. In Braunwald E, editor: *Heart disease*, ed 4, Philadelphia, 1992, WB Saunders.

Crawford FA: Penetrating cardiac injuries. In Sabiston DC, editor: *Textbook of surgery*, ed 14, Philadelphia, 1991, WB Saunders.

Currie DL: Pulmonary embolism: diagnosis and management, *Crit Care Nurs Q* 13(2):41, 1990.

Fairman RM, Edmunds LH: Emergency thoracotomy in the surgical intensive care unit after open cardiac operation, *Ann Thorac Surg* 32(4):386, 1981.

Fisher MM: The luck paradox, *Crit Care Med* 18(7):783, 1990 (editorial).

Foss J, Feistritzer N: Perioperative care of the trauma patient. In Neff JA, Kidd PS: *Trauma nursing: the art and science*, St Louis, 1993, Mosby.

Gentilello LM, Rifley WJ: Continuous arteriovenous rewarming: report of a new technique to treat hypothermia, *J Trauma* 31:1151, 1991.

Goldenberger E: *Treatment of cardiac emergencies*, ed 5, St Louis, 1990, Mosby.

Hammond SG: Chest injuries in the trauma patient, *Nurs Clin North Am* 25(1):35, 1990.

Harkin DE: Foreign bodies in, and in relation to, the thoracic blood vessels and heart. I. Techniques for approaching and removing foreign bodies from the chambers of the heart, *Surg Gynecol Obstet* 83:117, 1946.

Hefti D: Chest trauma, *RN* 54(5):28, 1991.

Hood RM: Trauma to the chest. In Sabiston DC, Spencer FC: *Surgery of the chest*, ed 5, Philadelphia, 1990, WB Saunders.

Huggins B: Trauma physiology, *Nurs Clin North Am* 25(1):1, 1990.

Johnson LG, Brown OF, Alligood MR: Complications of epicardial pacing wire removal, *J Cardiovasc Nurs* 7(2):32, 1993.

Kaiser GC and others: Reoperation in the intensive care unit, *Ann Thorac Surg* 49:903, 1990.

Kern LS: Emergency exploratory sternotomy: the nurse's role, *AACN Clin Issues Crit Care Nurs* 1(1):148, 1990.

Kidd PS: Assessment of the trauma patient. In Neff JA, Kidd PS: *Trauma nursing: the art and science*, St Louis, 1993, Mosby.

Letsou GV and others: Is cardiopulmonary bypass effective for treatment of hypothermic arrest due to drowning or exposure? *Arch Surg* 127:525, 1992.

Markovchick V, Duffens KR: Cardiovascular trauma. In Rosen P and others, editors: *Emergency medicine: concepts and clinical practice*, vol 1, ed 3, St Louis, 1992, Mosby.

Mattox KL: Penetrating heart trauma. In Champion HR and others, editors: *Rob and Smith's operative surgery, trauma surgery*, part I, ed 4, London, 1993, Butterworths.

McKowen RL and others: Infectious complications and cost-effectiveness of open resuscitation in the surgical intensive care unit after cardiac surgery, *Ann Thorac Surg* 40:388, 1985.

McSwain NE: Kinematics of chest trauma. In Webb WR, Besson A, editors: *Thoracic surgery: surgical management of chest injuries*, St Louis, 1993, Mosby.

Meyer G and others: Pulmonary embolectomy: a 20-year experience at one center, *Ann Thorac Surg* 51:232, 1991.

Millham FH, Grindlinger GA: Survival determinants in patients undergoing emergency room thoracotomy for penetrating chest injury, *J Trauma* 34(3):332, 1993.

Moore EE: Trauma and burns, *Am Coll Surg Bull* 77(11):55, 1992.

Morgan T and others: Trauma center and the OR: a cooperative approach to caring for the massively injured, *AORN J* 44(3):416, 1986.

Neff JA, Neff MJ: Perfusion: cardiac and vascular injuries. In Neff JA, Kidd PS: *Trauma nursing: the art and science,* St Louis, 1993, Mosby.

O'Connel WD: The resuscitation OR: priorities for the perioperative trauma nurse, *Todays OR Nurse* 14(12):9, 1992.

Reeder JM: Family perception: a key to intervention, *AACN Clin Issues Crit Care Nurs* 2(2):188, 1991.

Rice DP, McKenzie EJ: *Cost of injury in the United States: a report to Congress,* San Francisco, 1989, Institute for Health and Aging, University of California; and Baltimore, 1989, Injury Prevention Center, Johns Hopkins University.

Sabiston DC: Pulmonary embolism. In Sabiston DC, editor: *Textbook of surgery,* ed 14, Philadelphia, 1991, WB Saunders.

Seifert PC, Speir AM: Left ventricular rupture: a collaborative approach to emergency management, *AORN J* 51(3):714, 1990.

Shackford SR and others: Venous thromboembolism in patients with major trauma, *Am J Surg* 159:365, 1990.

Smith A, Fitzpatrick E: Penetrating cardiac trauma: surgical and nursing management, *J Cardiovasc Nurs* 7(2):52, 1993.

Symbas PN, Justicz AG: Quantum leap forward in the management of cardiac trauma: the pioneering work of Dwight E. Harkin, *Ann Thorac Surg* 55:789, 1993.

Trauma Nursing Coalition: *Resource document for nursing care of the trauma patient,* Chicago, 1992, Emergency Nurses Association.

Turner JA: Cardiovascular trauma, *Nurs Clin North Am* 25(1):119, 1990.

Turney SZ and others: Traumatic rupture of the aorta: a five-year experience, *J Thorac Cardiovasc Surg* 72:727, 1976.

Unkle D: Traumatic injury to the thorax, *Todays OR Nurse* 10(11):12, 1988.

Waldhausen JA, Pierce WS: *Johnson's surgery of the chest,* ed 5, St Louis, 1985, Mosby.

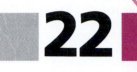

Miscellaneous Procedures

"It's great to be alive"—and to help others.

Motto of The Mended Hearts, Inc.*

CARDIAC TUMORS

Primary tumors originating in the heart and pericardium are rare and occur 10 to 40 times less frequently than metastatic neoplasms involving the heart (Chitwood, 1989; Smith, 1986). The most common cardiac tumor is the myxoma (Fig. 22-1); which was first resected under direct vision with cardiopulmonary bypass (CPB) by Crafoord (1955) in 1954.

To illustrate the rarity of cardiac tumors, in one series of over 52,500 patients undergoing surgery between 1961 and 1983, only 20 primary cardiac tumors (excluding myxomas) were found—an incidence of less than 1 in every 2500 cases. (Five of the 20 tumors were malignant.) In the same series, 51 benign myxomas were found (Reece and others, 1984). The types of cardiac tumors, benign and malignant (Box 22-1), occurring in the heart are typical of those that develop in any mass of striated muscle and connective tissue. Approximately 75% of cardiac tumors (mostly myxomas) are benign histologically, and the remainder (mostly sarcomas) are malignant (Lammers and Bloor, 1986; McAllister and Fenoglio, 1978). It has been observed that malignant tumors are more frequently found in the right side of the heart, whereas those in the left side tend to be benign (Rosai, 1989).

The etiology of most tumors is obscure, but immunosuppresion from drugs or disease, radiation, and chemotherapy are among the exogenous sources that have been implicated. Of significance to cardiac transplant recipients, long-term immunosuppression regimens have been associated with an increased incidence of malignant neoplasms (such as Kaposi's sarcoma). The incidence is 100 times greater in these patients as compared with the general population (Atkins, Bender, and Rippert, 1992; Washer and others, 1983).

Clinical Presentation

Many primary tumors are asymptomatic or have clinical features that mimic other cardiac conditions. Patients may have signs and symptoms of congestive heart failure: dyspnea, orthopnea, elevated venous pressure, and peripheral edema (Larrieu and others, 1982). Dysrhythmias may be present, but the site of origin may not correlate with the site of the lesion (Reece and others, 1984). Systemic and/or pulmonary embolism may occur as a result of fragments breaking off from the main tumor mass within the left or right side of the heart, respectively (McRae, 1987). Nonspecific findings are common and may include fever, cachexia (severe weight loss and muscle wasting), malaise, weakness, fatigue, arthralgias, and skin rash.

In patients with a left atrial myxoma, a heart murmur may be present if the tumor prolapses through the mitral valve. This murmur is often referred to as a tumor "plop" and may be audible early in the diastolic phase of the cardiac cycle when the tumor falls into the ventricle (Sellke and others, 1990). These (and other) tumors may cause symptoms of obstruction and/or insufficiency depending on the size and behavior of the myxoma.

Diagnostic Evaluation

Laboratory tests may show an elevated erythrocyte sedimentation rate and elevated serum gamma globulins. Deoxyribonucleic acid (DNA) analysis has been used to determine whether the lesion is a true neoplasm (Colucci and Braunwald, 1992.)

Chest radiography is often nonspecific, although a left atrial myxoma obstructing the mitral valve may produce a pattern similar to that of mitral stenosis. The electrocardiogram (ECG) may show atrial dysrhythmias and various degrees of heart block. Echocardiography has become the most useful noninvasive method of recognizing cardiac tumors; two-dimensional transthoracic and transesophageal echocardio-

*The Mended Hearts, Inc., 7320 Greenville Ave., Dallas, TX 75231.

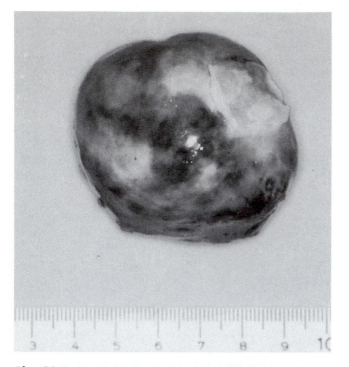

Fig. 22-1 Benign left atrial myxoma. The tumor is primarily composed of acid mucopolysaccharides and has a soft, smooth, glistening capsule. Myxomas may be small nodules or large masses that fill the atrium and are often attached by a stalk or pedicle to the atrial septum. Myxomas are often pale or, as shown, stained by bleeding into the tumor. (Courtesy Edward A. Lefrak, MD).

grams with color flow Doppler techniques can often provide precise information about the tumor(s). Radionuclide scanning, digital subtraction angiography with contrast, computed tomography (CT), and magnetic resonance imaging (MRI) are also valuable diagnostic tools (Kirklin and Barratt-Boyes, 1993).

If all four cardiac chambers cannot be visualized with the noninvasive methods listed above, cardiac catheterization and angiography may be necessary. Because of the danger of dislodging fragments from the tumor, catheterization, when necessary, is done with great caution. Coronary angiography may be indicated in older patients with suspected coronary artery disease.

Endomyocardial biopsy, first used to monitor the status of the transplanted heart, can be used to diagnose cardiac tumors. Direct histologic examination of biopsied tissue can confirm a diagnosis of cardiac malignancy (Flipse, Tazelaar, and Holmes, 1990).

Treatment

With improvements in diagnostic capabilities, cardiac tumors (especially benign tumors) can be detected early and successfully treated with surgery. Excision of an atrial myxoma (see later discussion) is the most common of the surgical procedures performed for

---

Box 22-1 Primary tumors of the heart*

Benign Tumors
Atrial myxoma
Lipoma
Papillary (valvular) fibroelastoma
Rhabdomyoma
Fibroma
Hemangioma
Teratoma
Atrioventricular nodal mesothelioma
Bronchogenic cyst

Malignant Tumors†
Angiosarcoma
Rhabdomyosarcoma
Mesothelioma
Fibrosarcoma
Malignant lymphoma
Osteosarcoma (arising in heart)

Modified from McAllister HA, Fenoglio JJ: Tumors of the cardiovascular system. In *Atlas of tumor pathology*, fasc 15, ser 2, Washington, DC, 1978, Armed Forces Institute of Pathology.
*Relative incidence; may involve the pericardium.
†Often involve both the heart and the pericardium.

---

cardiac tumors. Tumors located within the ventricle or the atrioventricular conduction system, or attached to the papillary muscles, chordae tendineae, and cardiac valves may also be excised.

Unfortunately, surgery for most malignant tumors is not as effective because of the large mass of cardiac tissue that is often involved, or because of the presence of metastases. Surgery may be performed to establish a diagnosis and to exclude the possibility of a benign tumor that can be cured. Palliation of hemodynamic derangements and/or physical symptoms can be achieved with aggressive therapy: partial resection of the tumor, chemotherapy, immunotherapy, and radiation therapy—alone or in combination (Colucci and Braunwald, 1992; Dein and others, 1987).

Nursing Considerations

Occasionally resection of tumors necessitates sacrificing a portion of normal tissue. When valve structures, for example, are involved, the perioperative nurse anticipates and prepares for the possibility of repair or replacement of the valve. Similarly, surgery in the area of conduction tissue may warrant having a permanent pacemaker lead available. Potential complications and possible treatment options should be discussed by the nurse and the surgeon.

Because the prognosis for primary malignant tumors of the heart and pericardium is often relatively poor, nursing interventions are aimed at maximizing the quality of life by helping the patient and family to cope with the fear of death, reduce emotional distress, retain some degree of control over one's life, and maintain as much physical, emotional, and physical comfort as possible.

An early case study by Motock (1966) focuses on a patient with sarcoma of the pericardium. Motock's conclusions in the study are as pertinent today as they were when she wrote them, and they reflect the importance of the nurse's behavior and attitude toward a patient (Box 22-2).

Atrial Myxoma

Atrial myxomas may appear at almost any age, but they occur predominantly in women. Most are benign, although malignant myxomas have been reported. Myxomas are usually located in the left atrium; they are solitary tumors that attach by a stalk or pedicle to the atrial septum, usually in the area of the fossa ovalis. Right atrial, ventricular, or mitral valve myxomas are less common (Colucci and Braunwald, 1992). Surgical removal is indicated soon after the diagnosis is made, because of the rapid deterioration, danger of embolization, and risk of sudden death in these patients.

Myxomas tend to be sporadic, but there may be a familial pattern. Patients with the familial type are more likely to have recurrence of the lesion after surgery; family members may also have myxomas. "Syndrome myxoma" is associated with the familial pattern; patients tend to be younger and may demonstrate extensive facial freckling. They may have noncardiac myxomas and endocrine neoplasms (Vidaillet and others, 1987).

Operative procedure: excision of a left atrial myxoma

Median sternotomy is the preferred incision, although right or left thoracotomy may be used for difficult reoperations (Sellke and others, 1990). To the basic chest set are added atrial retractors. Because complete removal of the tumor pedicle requires excison of the attached portion of the atrial septum, closure of the resulting atrial septal defect is necessary. This may be achieved by primary suture closure or, more commonly, with a patch of autologous pericardium or synthetic material.

Procedure
1. A median sternotomy is performed. If the surgeon plans to close the septum with pericardium, a piece is removed for later use. The tissue should be kept moist to retain its pliability.
2. CPB is instituted with bicaval cannulation for venous drainage. Caval tapes or clamps are used to divert all systemic venous return away from the right atrium and into the venous line. The aorta is cross-clamped. Minimal manipulation of the heart before cross-clamping lessens the risk of dislodging tumor fragments (Cleveland, Westaby, and Karp, 1983).
3. The left atrium is incised adjacent to the interatrial groove (a right atrial transseptal incision may be performed, depending on the location of the lesion and the surgeon's preference).
4. An atrial retractor is inserted, and the atrium is inspected. The tumor may bulge out of the atrium.
5. The tumor pedicle attached to the atrial septum is located. The pedicle and the full thickness of the atrial septum to which the pedicle is attached is excised. Occasionally, proximate conduction tracts must be sacrificed in order to achieve complete excision of the tumor (Edmunds, Norwood, and Low, 1990).
   The entire tumor and pedicle are removed.
6. The atria, atrioventricular valves, and ventricles are inspected. Remaining tumor fragments (and other particulate matter) are removed.
7. The septal patch is cut into the desired shape; closure of the interatrial septal defect with pericardium or a synthetic patch is performed with a running (3-0) polypropylene suture. Just before completion of the patch closure, the right atrium is irrigated or allowed to fill with blood to remove large amounts of air.
8. Patch closure is completed, and closure of the left atrial wall is started. Air is evacuated from the left atrium and openings of the pulmonary veins, the left ventricle, and the aortic root. Atrial closure is completed.

9. If the right atrial wall was incised, it is closed in a similar manner.
10. Temporary atrial and ventricular pacing wires are attached, and chest tubes are inserted for drainage.
11. The sternum and chest incision are closed.

Postoperative course

Temporary atrial dysrhythmias (due to the atriotomy and cardiac manipulation) are common postoperatively. If permanent heart block develops, a transvenous pacemaker system can be inserted (if a permanent epicardial lead was not inserted at operation). Antibiotic prophylaxis before invasive procedures is recommended in patients with synthetic patch material (Hupp, Shoaf, and Riggs, 1986).

Occasionally there is recurrence of an excised myxoma, usually within 1 to 5 years after surgery. This may be due to incomplete initial tumor excision or seeding of tumor cells during surgery, regrowth from the same cells of origin, or multifocal sites of origin unrecognized during the initial procedure (McRae, 1987). It is often related to the familial form of myxoma. Follow-up with annual echocardiograms for 5 years has been recommended (Cleveland, Westaby, and Karp, 1983). Family members of patients with the familial form should also be screened by echocardiography (Sellke and others, 1990).

PERICARDIAL DISEASE

The pericardium serves a number of purposes in order to enhance cardiac function. When disease affects either the sac itself or the fluid within it, the heart may be unable to function effectively.

The pericardial sac encloses the heart and consists of parietal and visceral layers between which is approximately 50 ml (although this can vary) of lubricating fluid. It is thought that the function of the pericardium is to stabilize the position of the heart within the chest, reduce friction between the surface of the heart and surrounding tissues, protect the heart against the spread of infection from adjacent structures, prevent cardiac overdilatation, and maintain the normal pressure-volume relationships of the cardiac chambers (Cox, 1992; Lorell and Braunwald, 1992).

Studies have demonstrated that pericardial fluid is an ultrafiltrate of plasma. When venous or lymphatic drainage of the heart is obstructed (as can occur with trauma or tumors), abnormal amounts of pericardial fluid can accumulate as a result of the altered balance of hydrostatic and osmotic forces. This leads to increased filtration of plasma across the visceral pericardium, producing pericardial effusion (Gibson and Segal, 1978). Production of excess pericardial fluid can also be stimulated by inflammation of the pericardium (Kirklin and Barratt-Boyes, 1993).

Pericarditis

There are numerous causes of pericarditis. The most common is idiopathic or viral pericarditis; other causes include bacterial infection, malignancy, trauma, irradiation, and inflammation secondary to drug reaction and autoimmune disease (Cox, 1992). Pericarditis may also occur after recent cardiac surgery ("postpericardiotomy syndrome"). "Dressler syndrome," another form of pericarditis, develops after acute myocardial infarction as a result of the body's immunologic response to damaged myocardium and pericardium; it is considered an autoimmune disorder.

Patients with acute pericarditis frequently complain of substernal chest pain that varies with respiration; it is usually relieved by sitting forward and is worsened by lying down. A **pericardial friction rub** and ECG abnormalities are often present. The rub is the hallmark of pericarditis and is caused by friction between either the inflamed or scarred visceral and parietal pericardium, or the parietal pericardium and the adjacent pleura. The sound of the rub is characterized as "scratchy" or "creaky."

The ECG goes through a series of changes that may resemble myocardial infarction. Sinus tachycardia is common. Other atrial dysrhythmias, conduction block, and ventricular tachycardias are not typical features of acute pericarditis. Laboratory studies may indicate inflammation, but the findings are nonspecific. The chest radiograph may show pericardial or pleural effusion, but it is less sensitive and accurate than the echocardiogram (Lorell and Braunwald, 1992).

If the underlying problem can be identified, specific therapy is instituted. Both nonsteroidal antiinflammatory agents and corticosteroids may be used to treat pain and inflammation. If pericardial effusion progresses, it can cause acute compression of the heart with tamponade (see Chapter 21). Pericardiocentesis with a large-bore needle (Fig. 22-2) or pericardial window may be performed to release the tamponade. Pericardiocentesis may also be performed diagnostically in cancer patients with chronic pericardial effusion to differentiate malignant effusion from postirradiation pericarditis (Shabetai, 1990).

Creation of a pericardial window

Pericardiotomy via an anterior thoracotomy or a subxiphoid approach can be used to drain the pericardium. With the release of the fluid, a dramatic improvement in systemic blood pressure can be expected. The pericardial drainage should be measured; culture tubes should also be available for bacteriologic and histologic evaluation. Elevating the head of the transport stretcher or the operating room bed may reduce some of the discomfort felt by the patient in the supine position prior to surgery.

Because there is a risk of sudden cardiac decompensation with positive-pressure ventilation and general anesthesia in these patients, it is recommended that patients be prepared and draped before anesthetic induction to minimize the time interval between ventilation and release of the tamponade. Initially, local anesthesia may be used to enhance the patient's hemodynamic status; once the patient has been stabilized, general anesthesia and ventilation may be initiated (Campbell and Larach, 1990).

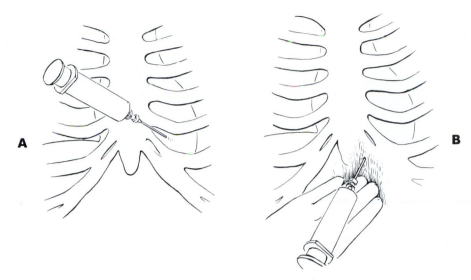

Fig. 22-2 Pericardiocentesis. Insertion through either **A** or **B** may be used. Advancement of the needle is halted when either intrapericardial blood appears or the motion of the heart is felt by the fingers. An ECG lead may be attached to the needle; a significant change in the ECG tracing alerts the surgeon that contact has been made with the myocardium. (From Waldhausen JA, Pierce WS: *Johnson's surgery of the chest*, ed 5, St Louis, 1985, Mosby.)

Operative procedure: creation of a pericardial window via an anterior thoracotomy

Thoracotomy instruments are used, and positioning equipment is assembled (usually a small roll under the left side is sufficient). The patient is placed in a semilateral position or supine with the left side slightly elevated. Internal defibrillator paddles should be available.

Procedure

1. An incision is made over the anterior left fifth rib; occasionally a segment of the rib is excised.
2. The pericardium and anterior surface of the heart are exposed by incising the posterior periosteum and parietal pleura.
3. As large a portion of pericardium as possible is removed from the right ventricle and left ventricle (anterior to the left phrenic nerve) with scissors and cautery to create a "window." The heart should be gently retracted to avoid injury during excision of the pericardium. Because a metal retractor may conduct electrical current and burn the heart, a sterile tongue blade has been recommended by some authors (Edmunds, Norwood, and Low, 1990.)

   Pericardial fluid and a portion of the excised pericardium are routinely sent for laboratory study.
4. Posterolateral and anterior chest tubes are brought out from the left pleural space through lower intercostal stab wounds (Kirklin and Barratt-Boyes, 1993), and the incision is closed.

Operative procedure: creation of a pericardial window via a subxiphoid approach

The patient is in the supine position; sternal instruments are used.

Procedure

1. A vertical midline incision, about 4 to 8 cm long, is made over the xiphoid process and upper abdomen.
2. The linea alba is divided. The xiphoid process is removed with bone cutters, or it is retracted upwardly with the distal sternum.
3. The diaphragm is dissected away from the undersurface of the sternum and xiphoid.
4. The pericardium is opened under direct vision.
5. Fluid is aspirated and measured, and cultures are taken.
6. As large a portion of pericardium as possible is excised to create the window; fluid and a specimen of tissue may be sent to the laboratory.
7. A small drain is inserted, and the incision is closed.

Constrictive Pericarditis

Constrictive pericarditis is produced when chronically inflamed, fibrotic (often calcified), noncompliant pericardium restricts diastolic ventricular filling. The etiology is often viral, although tuberculosis is once again becoming an important etiologic factor. Among patients with chronic renal disease, uremic pericardial disease is also seen.

Clinically the patient demonstrates signs and symptoms similar to those of congestive heart failure. The absence of a history of myocardial disease is important in the differential diagnosis. Dyspnea, fatigue, and weight gain are common complaints, and jugular venous distension, peripheral edema, hepatomegaly, or ascites may be evident. A striking abnormality of constrictive pericarditis, in contrast to the situation with cardiac tamponade (or in normal subjects), is the failure of intrathoracic pressure changes during respi-

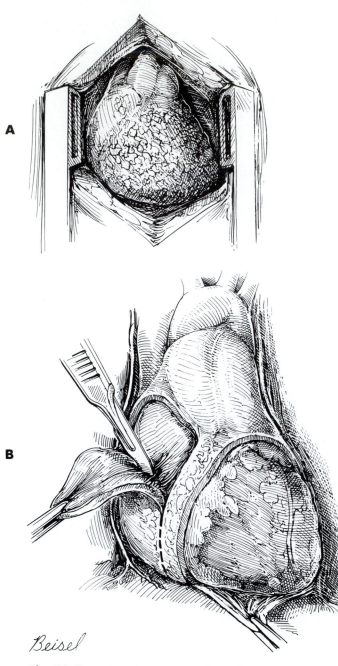

Fig. 22-3 Pericardiectomy. **A,** A median sternotomy exposes the fibrous pericardium. **B,** Dissection of the fibrous peel; the right and left phrenic nerves are protected during dissection. (From Waldhausen JA, Pierce WS: *Johnson's surgery of the chest,* ed 5, 1985, Mosby.)

ration to be transmitted to the pericardium and cardiac chambers. Thus with constrictive pericarditis, central venous pressure does not fall during inspiration, and venous return to the right atrium does not increase. In some patients systemic venous pressure may increase with respiration (e.g., **Kussmaul's sign**). Kussmaul's sign does not occur in acute cardiac tamponade (Lorell and Braunwald, 1992).

Radiographically the heart may be small; calcification of the pericardium may be seen. The ECG may show nonspecific ST-T wave changes, atrial dysrhythmias, and low QRS voltage. CT scanning may be used to distinguish between thickened pericardium and underlying myocardium; it is often more useful than echocardiography, which may not be able to make the distinction. Cardiac catherization (and endomyocardial biopsy) may be necessary to differentiate constrictive pericarditis from other cardiac disease, such as restrictive cardiomyopathy, and to assess the status of the coronary arteries (Cox, 1992).

Treatment

Because the disease is progressive and not reversible, the treatment of choice is pericardiectomy. Decortication of the visceral (epicardial) and parietal pericardium adhering to the cardiac chambers often produces dramatic improvement.

A median sternotomy provides excellent exposure and facilitates the repair of lacerations that may occur during removal of the fibrous layer (Waldhausen and Pierce, 1985). This incision also allows rapid institution of CPB if there is sudden cardiac decompensation; CPB should be available on a standby basis.

Basic sternotomy instruments are used; lung retractors are required. Ultrasonic debridement may be a useful adjunct when there is dense calcification (Johnson and others, 1989). Suture ligatures (4-0, 5-0 polypropylene, silk, or other material, depending on the surgeon's preference) and pledgets can be used to repair lacerations. Internal defibrillator paddles should be readily available, because manipulation of the heart may cause ventricular fibrillation.

Operative procedure: pericardiectomy (Waldhausen and Pierce, 1985)

1. A median sternotomy is performed to expose the heart and great vessels (Fig. 22-3, *A*). The pleurae are opened, and the lungs are displaced laterally. The phrenic nerves are identified and protected.
2. A knife or scissors are used to incise the pericardium. Multiple incisions may be made over different portions of the heart (Fig. 22-3, *B*).
3. Pericardial flaps are created and meticulously dissected. Inflation of the lungs is performed intermittently throughout the procedure.
4. Small lacerations of the myocardium can be repaired with pledgeted or nonpledgeted suture ligatures.
5. If pericardial and epicardial adhesions in the region of the right coronary artery pose too great a risk of laceration of the artery, a strip of scar tissue may be retained in the area of the right atrioventricular groove (Fig. 22-3, *B*).
6. Dissection is carried laterally over the left ventricle to beyond the left phrenic nerve, which is preserved as a pedicle.
7. The right atrium is freed to the right phrenic nerve, which is preserved as in step 6.

8. Drainage catheters are placed in the pericardium and each pleura, and the chest incision is closed.

Postoperative course

Postoperatively, low cardiac output syndrome may occur, especially in patients with more severe preoperative disability (e.g., functional class III or IV; marked elevation of right ventricular end-diastolic pressure). Preoperative functional status also influences long-term survival, and it is recommended that pericardial resection be performed early in the course of constrictive pericarditis. When performed early, patients can expect definite symptomatic improvement. However, some patients require weeks or months before relief is obtained and elevated venous filling pressures are reduced (Lorell and Braunwald, 1992).

REFERENCES

Atkins CR, Bender PS, Rippert L: Transplantation. In Dossey BM, Guzzetta CE, Kenner CV: *Critical care nursing: body—mind—spirit,* ed 3, Philadelphia, 1992, JB Lippincott.

Campbell DB, Larach DR: Management of cardiothoracic surgical emergencies. In Hensley FA, Martin DE, editors: *The practice of cardiac anesthesia,* Boston, 1990, Little, Brown.

Chitwood WR: Cardiac neoplasms, *Ann Thorac Surg* 48:451, 1989.

Cleveland DC, Westaby S, Karp RB: Treatment of intra-atrial cardiac tumors, *JAMA* 249(20):2799, 1983.

Colucci WS, Braunwald E: Primary tumors of the heart. In Braunwald E, editor: *Heart disease,* ed 4, Philadelphia, 1992, WB Saunders.

Cox GR: Pericardial and myocardial disease. In Rosen P, Barkin RM, Braen CR, editors: *Emergency medicine: concepts and clinical practice,* vol 2, ed 3, St Louis, 1992, Mosby.

Crafoord CL: Discussion of late results of mitral commissurotomy. In Lam CR, editor: *Proceedings: international symposium on cardiovascular surgery,* Philadelphia, 1955, WB Saunders.

Dein JR and others: Primary cardiac neoplasms: early and late results of surgical treatment in 42 patients, *J Thorac Cardiovasc Surg* 93(4):502, 1987.

Edmunds LH, Norwood WI, Low DW: *Atlas of cardiothoracic surgery,* Philadelphia, 1990, Lea & Febiger.

Flipse TR, Tazelaar HD, Holmes DR: Diagnosis of malignant cardiac disease by endomyocardial biopsy, *Mayo Clin Proc* 65:1415, 1990.

Gibson AT, Segal MB: A study of the composition of pericardial fluid, with special reference to the probable mechanisms of fluid formation, *Physiol* 277:367, 1978.

Hupp E, Shoaf B, Riggs TR: Cardiac myxomas: diagnosis, surgical excision, and nursing care, *AORN* 44(6):928, 1986.

Johnson RG and others: Ultrasonic debridement of calcified pericardium in constrictive pericarditis, *Ann Thorac Surg* 48:855, 1989.

Kirklin JW, Barratt-Boyes BG: *Cardiac surgery,* ed 2, New York, 1993, Churchill Livingstone.

Lammers RJ, Bloor CM: Tumors of the heart and pericardium, *Mod Concepts Cardiovasc Dis* 55(1):1, 1986.

Larrieu AJ and others: Primary cardiac tumors: experience with 25 cases, *J Thorac Cardiovasc Surg* 83(3):339, 1982.

Lorell BH, Braunwald E: Pericardial disease. In Braunwald E, editor: *Heart disease,* ed 4, Philadelphia, 1992, WB Saunders.

McAllister HA, Fenoglio JJ: Tumors of the cardiovascular system. In *Atlas of tumor pathology,* fasc 15, ser 2, Washington, DC, 1978, Armed Forces Institute of Pathology.

McRae ME: Care plan for the patient undergoing intracardiac myxoma excision, *Crit Care Nurse* 10(9):58, 1987.

Motock EC: A patient with sarcoma of the pericardium: a case study, *Nurs Clin North Am* 1(1):15, 1966.

Reece IJ and others: Cardiac tumors, *J Thorac Cardiovasc Surg* 88:439, 1984.

Rosai J: Cardiovascular system. In Rosai J: *Ackerman's surgical pathology,* ed 7, vol 2, St Louis, 1989, Mosby.

Sellke FW and others: Surgical treatment of cardiac myxomas: long-term results, *Ann Thorac Surg* 50:577, 1990.

Shabetai R: Pericardial disease. In Hurst JW, Schlant RC, editors: *The heart,* ed 7, New York, 1990, McGraw-Hill.

Smith C: Tumors of the heart, *Arch Pathol Lab Med* 110:1, 1986.

Vidaillet HJ and others: "Syndrome myxoma": a subset of patients with cardiac myxoma associated with pigmented skin lesions and peripheral and endocrine neoplasms, *Br Heart J* 57:247, 1987.

Waldhausen JA, Pierce WS: *Johnson's surgery of the chest,* ed 5, St Louis, 1985, Mosby.

Washer GF and others: Cause of death after transplantation, *JAMA* 250:49, 1983.

Index